CHRONIC DISEASE EPI
AND CONTR

American Public Health Association
800 I Street, NW
Washington, DC 20001-3710
www.apha.org

DISCLAIMER: Any discussion of medical or legal issues in this publication is being provided for informational purposes only. Nothing in this publication is intended to constitute medical or legal advice, and it should not be construed as such. This book is not intended to be and should not be used as a substitute for specific medical or legal advice, since medical and legal opinions may only be given in response to inquiries regarding specific factual situations. If medical or legal advice is desired by the reader of this book, a medical doctor or attorney should be consulted.

The use of trade names and commercial sources in this book does not imply endorsement by either the APHA or the editorial board of this volume.

While the publisher and author have used their best efforts in preparing this book, they make no representations with respect to the accuracy or completeness of the content.

Georges C. Benjamin, MD, FACP, FACEP (E) *Executive Director*
Norman A. Giesbrecht, PhD, *Chair, APHA Publications Board*
Carlos Castillo–Salgado, MD, JD, MPH, DrPH, *Publications Board Liaison*

Printed and bound in the United States of America
Interior Design and Typesetting: Manila Typesetting Company
Cover Design: Jennifer Strauss
Printing and Binding: United Book Press

Library of Congress Cataloging-in-Publication Data

Chronic disease epidemiology and control / [edited by] Patrick L. Remington,
Ross C. Brownson, Mark V. Wegner. — 3rd ed.
       p. ; cm.
   Includes bibliographical references.
   ISBN-13: 978-0-87553-192-2
   ISBN-10: 0-87553-192-X
   1. Chronic diseases—United States—Epidemiology. I. Remington, Patrick L. II. Brownson,
Ross C. III. Wegner, Mark V., 1972– IV. American Public Health Association.
   [DNLM: 1. Chronic Disease—epidemiology. 2. Chronic Disease—prevention & control.
   3. Epidemiologic Methods. WT 500 C556 2009]
   RA644.6.C475 2009
   614.4'273--dc22
                                                2009037680

ISBN 13: 978-0-87553-192-2
ISBN 10: 0-87553-192-X
5M/12/2009

TABLE OF CONTENTS

Foreword *with James S. Marks, MD, MPH and Janet L. Collins, PhD* v

Preface *with Patrick L. Remington, MD, MPH, Ross C. Brownson, PhD, and Mark V. Wegner, MD, MPH* vii

Contributors to Chronic Disease Epidemiology and Control ix

Section 1: Public Health Approaches

 1 Current Issues and Challenges in Chronic Disease Control
  with Matthew McKenna, MD, MPH and Janet Collins, PhD 1

 2 Methods in Chronic Disease Epidemiology
  with Patrick L. Remington, MD, MPH, Ross Brownson, PhD,
  and David Savitz, PhD.. 27

 3 Intervention Methods for Chronic Disease Control
  with Robert J. McDermott, PhD, Julie A. Baldwin, PhD,
  Carol A. Bryant, PhD, and Rita D. DeBate, PhD 59

 4 Chronic Disease Surveillance *with Mark V. Wegner, MD, MPH,*
  Angela Rohan, PhD, and Patrick L. Remington, MD, MPH........................... 95

Section 2: Selected Chronic Disease Risk Factors

 5 Tobacco Use *with Corinne G. Husten, MD, MPH* 117

 6 Diet and Nutrition *with Nasuh Malas, MD, MPH,*
  Kathleen M. Tharp, PhD, MPH, RD, and Susan B. Foerster, MPH, RD 159

 7 Physical Activity *with Barbara E. Ainsworth, PhD, MPH,*
  FACSM and Caroline A. Macera, PhD, FACSM.. 199

 8 Alcohol Use *with Mary C. Dufour, MD, MPH,*
  Rear Admiral, USPHS (retired).. 229

Section 3: Major Chronic Conditions

 9 Obesity and Overweight *with Deborah A. Galuska,*
  MPH and William H. Dietz, MD, MPH.. 269

 10 Diabetes *with Donald B. Bishop, PhD,*
  Patrick J. O'Connor, MD, MPH, and Jay Desai, MPH................................. 291

 11 High Blood Pressure *with Leonelo E. Bautista, MD, DrPH*.......................... 335

 12 High Blood Cholesterol *with Heather M. Johnson, MD and*
  Patrick E. McBride, MD, MPH.. 363

Section 4: Major Chronic Diseases

13   Cardiovascular Disease *with Craig J. Newschaffer, PhD, Longjian Liu, MD,*
     PhD, MSc, and Alan Sim, MS 383

14   Cancer *with Ross C. Brownson, PhD and Corinne Joshu, PhD, MPH, MA* 429

15   Chronic Respiratory Diseases *with Henry A. Anderson, MD*
     and Mark Werner, PhD 469

16   Mental Disorders *with Danny Wedding, PhD, MPH* 513

17   Neurological Disorders *with Edwin Trevathan, MD, MPH* 531

18   Arthritis and Other Musculoskeletal Diseases *with Rosemarie Hirsch, MD,*
     MPH and Marc C. Hochberg, MD, MPH 571

19   Chronic Liver Disease *with Adnan Said, MD, MS*
     and Jennifer Wells, MD 593

20   Kidney Disease *with Vishnu Moorthy, MD*
     and Jonathan B. Jaffery, MD, MS 623

Index 645

FOREWORD

Hardly a day goes by when there isn't something in the press or on the news about how the costs of medical care are affecting our ability to meet urgent health care needs, maintain a U.S. competitive advantage, or continue to underwrite the costs of Medicare or Medicaid. The fact that the nation's health care costs are driven by chronic diseases is becoming ever more apparent. Chronic diseases are common and costly, with new and expensive interventions and pharmaceuticals developed almost daily. Clearly, effective health policy will need to reduce the demand for chronic disease care to have any chance for success.

This book provides a crisp overview of current knowledge and best practices in the prevention and control of major chronic diseases and their risk factors. Chapter authors highlight many public health successes where evidence-based interventions have resulted in improved health and the reduction or elimination of disparities. Just as evident are the many opportunities where public health know-how goes underutilized due to limited resources or lack of political will.

Tackling chronic disease prevention requires a sophisticated analysis of the underlying causes and risk factors for illness. Such an analysis is provided throughout this volume. Chronic diseases generally do not arise from a lack of medical care, but rather from a complex array of personal and environmental forces. Lifestyle risks such as tobacco use and poor nutrition are defined in large part by how communities are designed—with sidewalks and markets or without . . . with safe places to play . . . where jobs are available and accessible by affordable public transportation . . . where schools ensure a high graduation rate and promote health. Simply put, societal policies and practices are fundamental causes of good or ill health.

It is increasingly clear that disparities in life expectancy between minority and majority, between rich and poor are heavily affected by differences in the incidence and severity of chronic disease. Efforts to eliminate disparities in health outcomes must have chronic disease prevention as a central focus. As part of that focus, communities must be empowered to establish supportive social and physical environments for individuals at greatest risk. Unfortunately, persons with the fewest financial and educational resources are often saddled with environments that are not conducive to good health.

This book, and its previous editions, tackles some of the most important and vexing public health problems of our time, including how to cope with the rising tide of chronic illness. Unfortunately, the aging of the population only adds to the managerial and fiscal crisis looming for our medical care system. The solution cannot be more of the same and the time for innovative solutions is now.

This text lays out the means for building a public health system for chronic disease prevention that is capable of reducing the growing pressures on an overwhelmed medical care system, while at the same time, delivering improved health outcomes. Both the public health system and the medical care system need to participate, as both perform vital functions the other cannot, or cannot perform as well. Unfortunately, the public health system is vastly underfinanced and underdeveloped to achieve its mission of optimal health for all through prevention.

Reducing disease, disparities, and cost, and improving quality of life will depend on having a robust and effective public health system that effectively addresses chronic disease. This simple fact places this volume and the issues it addresses right in the center of one of the highest priorities of our times.

James S. Marks, M.D., M.P.H.
Janet L. Collins, Ph.D.

PREFACE

Since the publication of the first edition of *Chronic Disease Epidemiology and Control* almost two decades ago, our understanding of the causes and consequences of chronic diseases has continued to progress. More importantly, researchers have continued to identify effective programs and policies to reduce the risk of chronic disease, or to control their consequences.

The 2002 report by the Institute of Medicine, *The Future of the Public's Health in the 21st Century*, points to the multiple determinants of disease with a call to action for nontraditional public health partners—such as health care, business, media, academia, and community groups—to engage in community health improvement efforts. Some health care systems are responding to this call with efforts to not only increase health care coverage and improve quality, but also develop incentives to reward population health improvement, rather than simply reward more and higher cost treatments.

In addition, information technology has continued to evolve, now able to provide an overwhelming amount of information on the web for those who are able to access and interpret it. Conflicting with the promise of better information for public health are concerns about patient privacy, confidentiality, and propriety rights to health information technology.

With this changing landscape, this third edition of *Chronic Disease Epidemiology and Control* has been updated to help students and practitioners keep abreast of advances in chronic disease prevention and control by providing up-to-date and practical information about the leading chronic diseases, conditions, and risk factors. This book is intended to support a broad range of chronic disease control activities, and it is designed to serve as a quick reference guide for students or practicing health professionals who need to locate critical background information and/or develop appropriate interventions.

This book is intended for several audiences. First, it can be useful to professionals involved in the practice and teaching of chronic disease epidemiology, prevention, and control at all levels. In state health agencies, the book can be helpful to staff involved in primary and secondary prevention of chronic diseases, including epidemiologists, physicians, nurses, health educators, and health promotion specialists. In local health agencies, administrators, physicians, nurses, health educators, and sanitarians should find it of value. In academic institutions, it can provide helpful background information on chronic diseases for students taking beginning and advanced public health courses. Although the book is intended primarily for a North American audience, there is literature drawn from all parts of the world, and we believe that much of the information covered will be applicable in any developed or developing country.

The authors of the various chapters in this book were selected for both their scientific expertise and their practical experience in carrying out chronic disease control programs at the community level. The new edition now includes 20 chapters and is organized into four major sections: (1) Public Health Approaches to Chronic Disease Control, (2) Selected Chronic Disease Risk Factors, (3) Major Chronic Disease Conditions, and (4) Major Chronic Diseases. In the new edition, we reflect feedback we have received informally from colleagues and have added four new chapters (i.e., obesity, mental illness, liver disease, and kidney disease).

Chapter 1 of this book provides a historical review of chronic disease control, a brief explanation of the current status of chronic disease control programs, and a discussion of the prospects and challenges for chronic disease control during the next decade and beyond. Chapters 2 and 3 briefly review the methods used in chronic disease epidemiology and chronic disease surveillance and provide a framework for the interpretation of the information in the following chapters. Chapter 4 provides an overview of chronic disease control intervention methods, providing a theoretical grounding for interventions that address the diseases and risk factors discussed in later chapters. It also summarizes some of the important features of successful interventions and provides practical examples.

In Section 2, Chapters 5–8 focus on "upstream" and potentially modifiable "risk factors" for chronic diseases. The chapters in this section examine the important areas of tobacco use, diet and nutrition, physical inactivity, and alcohol use. In Section 3, Chapters 9–12 focus on those "chronic disease conditions" that often result from high risk behaviors, and substantially increase the risk of chronic diseases. These conditions include obesity, diabetes, high blood pressure, and high blood cholesterol. In the final section of the book, Chapters 13–20 describe major "downstream" chronic diseases—cardiovascular disease, cancer, chronic lung diseases, mental disorders, chronic neurological disorders, arthritis and other musculoskeletal diseases, liver disease, and kidney disease.

A standard format has been used for all chapters that focus on specific risk factors and chronic diseases, to allow the reader quick and easy access to information. Each chapter begins with a brief introduction, reviewing the significance of the chronic condition and the underlying biological or physiological process of disease. The next section addresses descriptive epidemiology by examining high-risk groups (person), geographic variation (place), and secular trends (time). The third section describes the causes of the disease, condition, or risk factor under consideration. The final section discusses prevention and control measures. When available, specific examples of practical and effective public health interventions are reviewed as well as recommendations for future research and demonstration. A bibliography and list of resources are also included to facilitate access to additional information.

This book is not intended to provide a complete and final review of chronic disease epidemiology and control. Because the field is so broad, with overlapping issues, any division of the topic becomes somewhat arbitrary. There are literally thousands of different chronic diseases. We have chosen to focus on those that account for a large proportion of morbidity and mortality in the adult population and to emphasize risk factors that can be modified through public health interventions.

Future research will continue to expand our understanding of chronic disease epidemiology and control. Epidemiological studies will identify new risk factors and quantify their effects. Intervention studies underway will expand the array of interventions available for public health practitioners.

Chronic disease epidemiology and control is a rapidly expanding field. There is a clear and increasing need for public health professionals with knowledge and expertise in chronic disease control. We hope this book will become a useful resource for health professionals as they are called on to meet new challenges.

P.L.R., R.C.B., and M.W.

CONTRIBUTORS TO CHRONIC DISEASE EPIDEMIOLOGY AND CONTROL

Henry A. Anderson, MD
Wisconsin Division of Public Health
Department of Health Services
Madison, WI
Chapter 15: Chronic Respiratory Diseases

Barbara E. Ainsworth, PhD, MPH,
FACSM
College of Nursing & Health Innovation
Arizona State University
Tempe, AZ
Chapter 7: Physical Inactivity

Julie A. Baldwin, PhD
College of Public Health
University of South Florida
Tampa, FL
*Chapter 4: Intervention Methods for
Chronic Disease Control*

Leonelo E. Bautista, MD, MPH, DrPH
School of Medicine and Public Health
University of Wisconsin
Madison, WI
Chapter 11: High Blood Pressure

Donald B. Bishop, PhD
Minnesota Department of Health
St. Paul, MN
Chapter 10: Diabetes

Ross Brownson, PhD
Schools of Medicine and Social Work
Washington University in St. Louis
St. Louis, MO
*Chapter 2: Methods in Chronic Disease
Epidemiology*
Chapter 14: Cancer

Carol A. Bryant, PhD
College of Public Health
University of South Florida
Tampa, FL
*Chapter 4: Intervention Methods for
Chronic Disease Control*

Janet L. Collins, PhD
National Center for Chronic Disease
Prevention and Health Promotion
Centers for Disease Control and Prevention
Atlanta, GA
*Chapter 1: Current Issues and Challenges in
Chronic Disease Control*

Rita D. DeBate, PhD
College of Public Health
University of South Florida
Tampa, FL
*Chapter 4: Intervention Methods for
Chronic Disease Control*

Jay Desai, MPH
Center for Health Promotion
Minnesota Department of Health
St. Paul, MN
Chapter 10: Diabetes

William H. Dietz, MD, PhD
Division of Nutrition, Physical Activity,
and Obesity
Centers for Disease Control and Prevention
Atlanta, GA
Chapter 9: Obesity
Chapter 10: Diabetes

Mary C. Dufour, MD, MPH
The Madrillon Group Inc.
Bethesda, MD
Chapter 8: Alcohol Use

Susan B. Foerster, MPH, RD
Cancer Control Branch
California Department of Public Health
Sacramento, CA
Chapter 6: Diet and Nutrition

Deborah A. Galuska, MPH, PhD
Division of Nutrition, Physical Activity,
and Obesity
Centers for Disease Control and Prevention
Atlanta, GA
Chapter 9: Obesity

Rosemarie Hirsch, MD, MPH
National Center for Health Statistics,
Centers for Disease Control
and Prevention
Hyattsville, Maryland
*Chapter 18: Arthritis and Other
Musculoskeletal Diseases*

Marc C. Hochberg, M.D., M.P.H.
Division of Rheumatology
and Clinical Immunology
University of Maryland
School of Medicine
Baltimore, Maryland
*Chapter 18: Arthritis and Other
Musculoskeletal Diseases*

Corinne G. Husten, MD, MPH
Partnership for Prevention
Washington D.C.
Chapter 5: Tobacco Use

Jonathan B. Jaffery, MD, MS
School of Medicine and Public Health
University of Wisconsin
Madison, WI
Chapter 20: Kidney Disease

Heather M. Johnson, MD
School of Medicine and Public Health
University of Wisconsin
Madison, WI
Chapter 12: High Blood Cholesterol

Corinne Joshu, PhD, MPH, MA
Department of Epidemiology
Bloomberg School of Public Health
Johns Hopkins University
Baltimore, MD
Chapter 14: Cancer

Longjian Liu, MD, PhD, MSc
Department of Epidemiology and
Biostatistics
Drexel University School of Public Health
Philadelphia, PA
Chapter 13: Cardiovascular Disease

Caroline A. Macera, PhD, FACSM
Graduate School of Public Health
San Diego State University
San Diego, CA
Chapter 7: Physical Inactivity

Nasuh Malas, MD, MPH
School of Medicine and Public Health
University of Wisconsin
Madison, WI
Chapter 6: Diet and Nutrition

James Marks, MD, MPH
Robert Wood Johnson Foundation
Princeton, NJ
Foreword

Patrick E. McBride, MD, MPH
School of Medicine and Public Health
University of Wisconsin
Madison, WI
Chapter 12: High Blood Cholesterol

Robert J. McDermott, PhD
College of Public Health
University of South Florida
Tampa, FL
*Chapter 4: Intervention Methods for
Chronic Disease Control*

Matthew McKenna, MD, MPH
National Center for Chronic Disease
Prevention and Health Promotion
Centers for Disease Control and
Prevention
Atlanta, GA
*Chapter 1: Current Issues and Challenges in
Chronic Disease Control*

Vishnu Moorthy, MD
School of Medicine and Public Health
University of Wisconsin
Madison, WI
Chapter 20: Kidney Disease

Craig J. Newschaffer, PhD
Department of Epidemiology and
Biostatistics
Drexel University School of Public Health
Philadelphia, PA
Chapter 13: Cardiovascular Disease

Patrick J. O'Connor, MD, MPH
HealthPartners Research Foundation
Minneapolis, MN
Chapter 10: Diabetes

Patrick Remington, MD, MPH
School of Medicine and Public Health
University of Wisconsin
Madison, WI
*Chapter 2: Methods in Chronic Disease
Epidemiology*
Chapter 3: Chronic Disease Surveillance

Angela Rohan, PhD
Wisconsin Division of Public Health
Department of Health Services
Madison, WI
Chapter 3: Chronic Disease Surveillance

Adnan Said, MD, MS
School of Medicine and Public Health
University of Wisconsin
Madison, WI
Chapter 19: Chronic Liver Disease

David A. Savitz, PhD
Center of Excellence in Epidemiology,
Biostatistics, and Disease Prevention
Mount Sinai School of Medicine
New York, NY
*Chapter 2: Methods in Chronic Disease
Epidemiology*

Alan Sim, MS
Department of Epidemiology and
Biostatistics
Drexel University School of Public Health
Philadelphia, PA
Chapter 13: Cardiovascular Disease

Kathleen M. Tharp, PhD, MPH, RD
Cancer Control Branch
California Department of Public Health
Sacramento, CA
Chapter 6: Diet and Nutrition

Edwin Trevathan, MD, MPH
National Center on Birth Defects &
Developmental Disabilities
Centers for Disease Control and
Prevention
Atlanta, GA
Chapter 17: Chronic Neurological Disorders

Danny Wedding, PhD, MPH
Missouri Institute of Mental Health
University of Missouri-Columbia School
of Medicine
Saint Louis, MO
Chapter 16: Mental Disorders

Mark V. Wegner, MD, MPH
Wisconsin Division of Public Health
Department of Health Services
Madison, WI
Chapter 3: Chronic Disease Surveillance

Jennifer Wells, MD
School of Medicine and Public Health
University of Wisconsin
Madison, WI
Chapter 19: Chronic Liver Disease

Mark Werner, PhD
Wisconsin Division of Public Health
Department of Health Services
Madison, WI
Chapter 15: Chronic Respiratory Diseases

CHAPTER 1

CURRENT ISSUES AND CHALLENGES IN CHRONIC DISEASE CONTROL

Matthew McKenna, M.D., M.P.H. and Janet Collins, Ph.D.

Introduction

At the turn of the twenty-first century, and soon after the destruction of the World Trade Towers in New York City, the capacities of the public health institutions within the United States were precipitously stressed by a series of intentional biological attacks using *Bacillus anthracis* spores that resulted in the deaths of five Americans, and involved the treatment of tens of thousands of exposed individuals (Gerberding, Hughes, and Koplan 2002). The policy response to these events has been the investment of billions of dollars in public health planning, research, and infrastructure designed to protect citizens against similar terrorist uses of biologic, chemical, or radiologic agents (Cohen, Gould, and Sidel 2004). Paradoxically, the urgent, renewed investment and focus on infectious and environmental contaminants is occurring in the context of overall improvements in population level indicators for infectious and environmental diseases. These trends have been evident since the beginning of the twentieth century, and the improvements are largely attributable to the public health agencies and institutions currently undergoing renewed scrutiny for their ability to protect the American public against acute infectious and environmental threats—whether these threats are man-made (e.g., weaponized anthrax) or products of nature (e.g., pandemic influenza).

Infant mortality has fallen from 150 deaths per 1,000 live births in 1900 to 6.9 per 1,000 in 2005. Life expectancy from birth has risen from 47 years in 1900 to almost 78 years in 2005—an increase of slightly more than two days for every week that has passed since the beginning of the twentieth century (Kung, Xu, and Murphy 2007). However, despite the marked reductions in overall mortality, disparities remain among certain subpopulations in the United States—most notably people of low socioeconomic status, African Americans, and American Indians—and an epidemic of obesity that exacerbates these disparities has surged on the scene (Harper et al. 2007; Minkler et al. 2006; Murray et al. 2006; Ogden et al. 2006).

The heightened concern about the potential use of infectious agents as bioweapons has emerged when the reality is that the leading causes of death have changed dramatically since the initial establishment of public health as an essential societal institution in America. In 1900, the three leading causes of death were pneumonia and influenza; tuberculosis; and gastritis, enteritis, and colitis. These diseases accounted for nearly one-third of all deaths (Table 1.1). Today, heart disease, malignant neoplasms, and cerebrovascular

Disclaimer: The findings and conclusions in this report are those of the authors and do not necessarily represent the views of the Centers for Disease Control and Prevention.

Table 1.1. Death Rates and Percent of Total Deaths for the 10 Leading Causes of Death in the United States, 1900

Cause of Death	Death Rate per 100,000	Percent of Total Deaths
All causes	1719	100.0
Pneumonia and influenza	202	11.8
Tuberculosis	194	11.3
Gastritis, enteritis, colitis	143	8.3
Heart diseases	137	8.0
Symptoms, senility, ill-defined conditions	118	6.8
Vascular lesions affecting central nervous system	107	6.2
Chronic nephritis and renal sclerosis	81	4.7
Unintentional injuries	72	4.2
Malignant neoplasms	64	3.7
Diphtheria	40	2.3
All other causes		32.6

Note: Data compiled from National Office of Vital Statistics (U.S. Department of Health, Education, and Welfare 1954).

diseases (stroke) are the three leading causes of death, accounting for over half of all deaths (Table 1.2). These changes are known as the "epidemiologic transition" and they predictably occur in populations that move through stages of technologic and economic development (Omran 1971). With these changes in the leading causes of mortality, the primary emphasis of societal systems designed to address health concerns has generally shifted from microbiologic investigation of communicable diseases to a focus on the role of behavioral and environmental risk factors and methods for preventing disease, disability, and death in a population.

The landmark 1988 Institute of Medicine (IOM) report, entitled *The Future of Public Health*, described the mission of public health as assuring conditions in which people can be healthy (IOM 1988). The distinctive roles of public health agencies in this mission are to assess the health needs of the community, to develop comprehensive public health policies, and to assure that the services necessary to achieve this goal are being provided to the community. Subsequent to the publication of this report, comprehensive national

Table 1.2. Death Rates and Percent of Total Deaths for the 10 Leading Causes of Death in the United States, 2005

Cause of Death	Death Rate per 100,000	Percent of Total Deaths
All causes	826	100.0
Diseases of heart	219	26.5
Malignant neoplasms	189	22.8
Cerebrovascular diseases	48	5.9
Chronic obstructive pulmonary diseases	44	5.3
Accidents (unintentional injuries)	39	4.7
Diabetes mellitus	25	3.1
Alzheimer's disease	24	2.9
Influenza and pneumonia	21	2.6
Kidney disease	15	1.8
Septicemia	12	1.4
All other causes		22.0

Note: Data compiled from National Center for Health Statistics (NCHS 2007).

legislation for the United States to address health care reform was proposed, vigorously debated, and then abandoned in the early 1990s. Health care financing was then left to various market-oriented and state-level initiatives—principally in the form of managed care—that initially demonstrated some promise in slowing the growth in health care costs. However, by the beginning of the new century the uncontrolled growth in the cost of medical care in the United States resumed and now consumes greater than 15% of all goods and services purchased—by far the largest proportion of any economy in the developed world (Woolhandler and Himmelstein 2007; White 2007). Despite these expenditures, more than 40 million Americans were consistently left without financing for access to health care, health indicators such as life expectancy and infant mortality remained among the lowest in the developed world, and a systematic overview of health systems' performance around the world ranked the system in the United States as number 37 among 155 nations (WHO 2000).

In the context of the urgent threats of biological terrorism and a health care system expending huge sums on the urgent realities associated with providing medical services for chronic diseases, the IOM revisited the status and role of the American public health system in 2003. The new report, entitled *The Future of the Public's Health in the 21st*

Century, emphasized that in order to meet the responsibility of the core function of assuring the health of the public articulated in the first report, many parties would have to collaborate with governmental public health agencies because ". . . in a society as diverse and decentralized as that of the United States, achieving population health requires contributions from all levels of government, the private business sector, and the variety of institutions and organizations that shape opportunities, attitudes, behaviors, and resources affecting health" (IOM 2003).

The challenge to the public health practitioner is daunting, yet the opportunities are vast. There is growing evidence that enormous savings are being realized in health care expenditures among the older population in the United States covered by Medicare because of lower than expected levels of disability resulting from more favorable risk factor profiles achieved by members of this cohort when they were younger (Daviglus et al. 1998; Manton, Lamb, and Gu 2007). Much of this success can be attributed to concerted clinical and community efforts to prevent and control the impact of chronic diseases (Ford et al. 2007; Fries 2003). In fulfilling the general mission outlined by the IOM, public health practitioners must tackle an expanded role in developing and implementing effective community-based prevention programs and in mobilizing social support for the prevention and control of chronic diseases. The purpose of this book is to provide a detailed and comprehensive overview of the state of the evidence regarding the best methods for accomplishing these tasks in order to assist public health practitioners with this essential role in American society.

Definition of Chronic Disease

Chronic diseases have been referred to as chronic illnesses, noncommunicable diseases, and degenerative diseases. They are generally characterized by uncertain etiology, multiple risk factors, a long latency period, a prolonged course of illness, noncontagious origin, functional impairment or disability, and incurability. Though these characteristics help to delineate deficits in health generally regarded as "chronic," it is clear that many of these attributes are also found in infectious diseases such as tuberculosis, and human immunodeficiency virus (HIV) infection in the era of highly active anti-retroviral therapy (Kuller 1987; Barrett-Connor 1979). In addition, now that immunizations are included in the armamentarium of interventions designed to prevent cervical and hepatocellular cancer, and antibiotic regimens are available to treat peptic ulcer disease, some of the distinctions between infectious, acute, and chronic diseases must be considered provisional in the context of emerging scientific discoveries (O'Connor, Taylor, and Hughes 2006).

In more general terms, a chronic disease can be defined as a disease that has a prolonged temporal course, that does not resolve spontaneously, and for which a complete cure is rarely achieved. Although this definition of chronic disease encompasses a wide range of diverse disease processes, it provides a practical framework for their control.

The course of a chronic disease can be viewed as a continuum from the "upstream" social and environmental determinants, to behavioral risk factors, chronic conditions, chronic diseases, and finally, impairment, disability, and ultimately death (Figure 1.1). This book is organized along this continuum, with chapters addressing not only chronic diseases, but their associated chronic disease conditions and risk factors.

The causes of many chronic diseases remain obscure, but epidemiologists have identified risk factors for many of the most common chronic diseases (Table 1.3). The com-

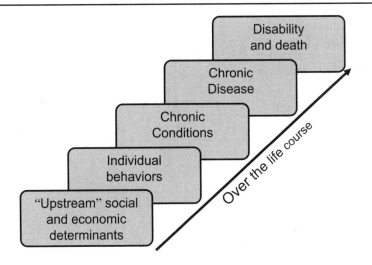

Figure 1.1. The Chronic Disease Continuum.

plexity of chronic disease control is also apparent. For example, control of a single risk factor, such as direct and secondhand exposure to cigarette smoke, can often reduce the risk of many chronic diseases. However, a single disease designation, such as cancer, may actually consist of hundreds of different diseases, some with shared—but many with separate—risk factors. Chronic conditions such as obesity or diabetes that result in substantial decrements in function and health-related quality of life are the result of multiple risk factors, such as poor diet and a sedentary lifestyle. And these conditions, in turn, serve as important and independent risk factors for related conditions such as cardiovascular disease (Alley and Chang 2007; Flegal et al. 2007). In addition to the many modifiable environmental and behavioral risk factors, many genetic and physiological factors increase the risk of chronic diseases (Khoury et al. 2005; Mackenbach 2006).

The extended time frame associated with the development and duration of chronic diseases implies, almost by definition, that rapid changes in disease trends are difficult to achieve. However, highly effective interventions that focus on later stages of the disease process can quickly translate into improved outcomes at the population level (Berkelman and Buehler 1990). A recent example of such an event was the rapid decrease in use by women of post-menopausal estrogens after the publication of a definitive clinical trial demonstrating that this therapy resulted in unexpectedly harmful cardiovascular outcomes (Berry and Ravdin 2007). This change was followed by an 11% drop in the incidence of breast cancer within four years among women older than age 50 years in the United States (Ravdin et al. 2007). The use of exogenous estrogen and progesterone is a known promoter of latent breast cancer (Collaborative Group on Hormonal Factors in Breast Cancer 1997). However, more frequently, health promotion efforts involve interventions that influence behavioral and lifestyle modifications to either avoid or delay the initiation of disease processes, or mitigate the disability associated with existing conditions. The length of time required to demonstrate the effect of risk factor modification at the individual and population level can take several years (Ford et al. 2007; Multiple Risk Factor Intervention Trial Research Group 1990). Therefore, the prevention and control of chronic diseases generally must be implemented with a persistent, long-term perspective.

Table 1.3. Interrelationships among Various Chronic Diseases and Modifiable Risk Factors, United States

	Cardiovascular Disease	Cancer	Chronic Lung Disease	Diabetes	Cirrhosis	Musculoskeletal Diseases	Neurologic Disorders
Tobacco use	+	+	+			+	+
Alcohol use	+	+			+	+	+
High cholesterol	+						
High blood pressure	+						+
Diet	+	+		+		+	?
Physical inactivity	+	+		+		+	+
Obesity	+	+	+	+		+	+
Stress	+	?					
Environmental tobacco smoke	+	+	+				?
Occupation	?	+	+		?	+	?
Pollution	+	+	+				+
Low socioeconomic status	+	+	+	+	+	+	+

Note: + = established risk factor; ? = possible risk factor.

Correspondingly, systems designed to measure the "downstream" outcomes are unlikely to detect changes in the development of chronic disease or changes in their impact on the quality of life within the first few years after the implementation of interventions.

Goals of Chronic Disease Prevention and Control

The goals of chronic disease prevention and control are to reduce the incidence of disease, delay the onset of disease and disability, alleviate the severity of disease, and improve the health-related quality and duration of the individual's life (Doll 1985). One traditional view of aging is that chronic disease prevalence and disability inevitably increase as life expectancy increases and the lethal outcomes of disease are controlled (Verbrugge 1984). Often termed the "failure of success," this perspective predicts exploding health care costs and dour plights for the growing population of elderly who are faced with longer lives, but lower quality existence during the extended years. An alternative hypothesis was offered by Fries. He and his colleagues suggested that the maximum life span has limits. Hence, the proportion of people who will live to very old ages (i.e., older than 85 years) will not substantially increase (Fries et al. 1993). Besides the assumption that the human life span is relatively fixed, the Fries model also assumes that the onset of chronic diseases and disabilities can be delayed or at least modified so that the effects of aging are compressed into a shorter time span before death. Therefore, chronic disease could occupy a smaller and less debilitated portion of a person's life span, and the need for medical care in later life could decrease.

These alternate hypotheses give rise to three models of the future chronic disease burden (Figure 1.2). In the first model (life extension), the average age at onset of chronic conditions remains unchanged, whereas mortality is delayed and chronic conditions occupy a greater proportion of extended life. The second model (shift to the right) predicts a delay in the onset of morbidity, and an extension of the life span. The third and final model (compression of morbidity) is consistent with Fries hypothesis that prevention and control of chronic diseases can have a more profound impact on the initiation of disability with relatively modest gains in life expectancy. Whichever model or combination of models proves most accurate, preventing disability from chronic diseases should be a prime goal of public health efforts. Chronic disease prevention and control should focus on morbidity as well as mortality; it should emphasize postponement of occurrence, and it should have the goal of improving the quality of life (Fries 2003).

A strategic objective for chronic disease control is to change the public's perception of chronic diseases and their complications from one of inevitability to one of preventability. A reduction in chronic disease burden may best be achieved by altering factors that place a person at higher risk for chronic diseases, such as tobacco use, lack of physical activity, and poor nutrition across the life span. Unfortunately, changing a person's fundamental and ingrained behaviors can be difficult. However, empirical information assessed as part of systematic, evidence-based reviews has demonstrated that successful implementation of effective interventions can result in timely reductions in the impact of chronic diseases (Zaza 2008). For example, smoking cessation is associated with a 40–60% decline in the risk of a myocardial infarction within just one year (Lightwood and Glantz 1997; McElduff et al. 1998).

An important dimension of chronic disease prevention is that behavioral change that promotes health and prevents chronic disease usually requires more than just providing

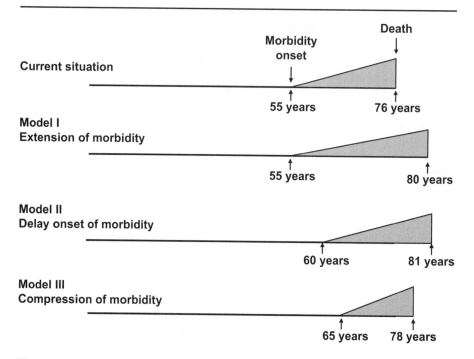

Figure 1.2. Present lifetime morbidity, portrayed as the shaded area, is contrasted with three possible future scenarios. Used with permission of the American College of Physicians, from Fries, J. F. Measuring and Monitoring Success in Compressing Morbidity. *Ann Intern Med* (2003):139:455–459. Permission conveyed through Copyright Clearance Center, Inc.

accurate information about the benefits of physical activity, good nutrition, or avoiding exposure to tobacco smoke. Environmental and structural interventions that result from societal and governmental policies are also necessary and powerful tools for assuring population health (Brownson, Haire-Joshu, and Luke 2006). Just as municipal water purification systems have been profoundly effective in diminishing the impact of waterborne infections and environmental diseases, societal investments and policies that facilitate clean air free from industrial pollutants as well as tobacco smoke, provide open spaces for safe, pleasant physical activity, and mandate the availability of accurate information about, as well as access to, nutritious food have been documented to result in behavioral change and biological outcomes that promote health and prevent chronic diseases (Brownson, Haire-Joshu, and Luke 2006). However, deleterious environmental influences are also promoting negative influences on health-related behaviors. Recreational and transportation activities that are increasingly automated and hence sedentary have combined with the surge in the availability of inexpensive, calorie-laden foods high in saturated fats and refined sugars to create an unprecedented epidemic of obesity in the United States—an epidemic that is also becoming increasingly evident on a global scale (Caballero 2007).

Definitions of Prevention and Control

The distinction between treatment of disease and promotion of health has been recognized since early times. In classical Greek mythology, Asklepios and his two daughters,

Panacea and Hygeia, were deities of medicine and health. Panacea represented the treatment of people who were ill, and Hygeia embodied living wisely and preserving health. Today, Panacea could represent the usual activities of the medical care system, and Hygeia could embody disease prevention and health promotion.

Accepting that chronic diseases are not an inevitable consequence of aging, but can be delayed in onset and ameliorated in impact, is the first step toward chronic disease control. Understanding the natural history of a disease provides the heuristic framework for the design of prevention methods. The course of a chronic disease can be viewed as a continuum from the disease-free state to asymptomatic biological change, clinical illness, impairment and disability, and ultimately death (Figure 1.1). Although this simple linear model illustrates the basic concept of chronic disease progression, the physical and social manifestations of chronic diseases result from the simultaneous and complex interaction of several risk factors and diseases at different stages on this continuum.

Prevention and control are interrelated, and the two terms are often used interchangeably. Prevention suggests that an intervention occurs before the onset of a disease or early in the course of a disease, whereas control efforts may occur later in the disease course and are often focused on reducing the sequelae of diseases, such as amputation, blindness, or renal failure in persons with diabetes. The precise boundary between prevention and control is not distinct, however.

A commonly used system classifies prevention efforts according to the target population and what stage of the disease continuum is influenced. Traditionally, only primary, secondary, and tertiary stages of prevention were identified. However, this taxonomy did not adequately distinguish between interventions that intervene on risk factors in otherwise healthy individuals, and promotion of environmental and behavioral interventions that prevent the onset of risk factors. In order to clarify this distinction, the Centers for Disease Control and Prevention (CDC) recently recommended the use of the classification schema for cardiovascular disease prevention that included health promotion, which

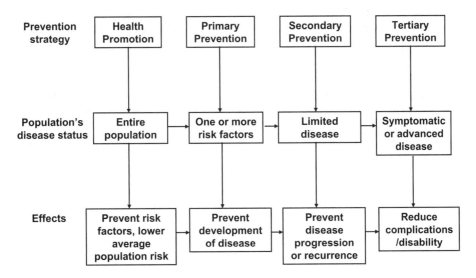

Figure 1.3. Classification schema for chronic disease prevention and control methods that include health promotion.

is sometimes called "primordial prevention" (Mensah et al. 2005). The target group for this type of prevention is the entire population with the goal to lower the overall average risk of ill health. When health promotion is added to the prevention continuum, as in Figure 1.3, primary prevention reduces disease incidence by identifying persons with risk factors and intervening more intensively in order to prevent the onset of disease; secondary prevention decreases the duration and severity of disease through early detection and treatment either before signs and symptoms occur, or by preventing recurrence of disease by intensively intervening on risk factors in those who have had symptomatic disease; and tertiary prevention reduces complications of existing disease.

Health promotion efforts are wide ranging and aim to maintain the health and well-being of the populace. Examples of health promotion include the environmental and societal policies delineated in the previous section of this chapter as well as occupational and informational campaigns that reinforce the immediate and long-term benefits of a healthy lifestyle (Brownson, Haire-Joshu, and Luke 2006).

Primary prevention is directed at identifying and intervening with high-risk people before they develop a particular chronic disease. These preventive interventions reduce the incidence of disease and, consequently, its sequelae. The antecedent causes or risk factors for a disease must be established for primary prevention to be feasible. Examples of primary prevention interventions include telephone counseling programs that support smoking cessation and hypertension control activities (Chobanian et al. 2003; Keller et al. 2007).

Secondary prevention is directed to people who are asymptomatic, but who have developed biologic changes resulting from the disease. Strategies for secondary prevention may be referred to as "disease control" because the goal is to reduce the consequences of the disease. Secondary prevention generally does not reduce the incidence of disease but instead detects the condition at an earlier, more treatable stage. Screening for cervical and breast cancers are examples of secondary prevention. Screening programs are recommended only under certain conditions: if the natural history of the disease permits early detection; if a screening test is available to accurately detect the disease at an early stage; if treatment at early stages can alter the consequences of the disease; and if the screening test is acceptable to the populations at highest risk for the disease (Morrison 1992).

Tertiary prevention is directed at preventing disability in people who have symptomatic disease. Strategies for tertiary prevention may be to prevent the progression of a disease and its complications or to provide rehabilitation. For example, eye examinations for people with diabetes can detect retinopathy early when this condition can be promptly treated, preventing progression to blindness. Although the public health system has less frequently focused on developing strategies for tertiary prevention, issues such as quality of life, the cost of long-term health care, and the aging population's demand for health care services make prevention of disabilities an emerging priority for chronic disease control (Fries et al. 1998).

Potential and Effectiveness

As stated previously, in the United States during 2005, heart disease, cancer, and cerebrovascular disease were the three most common causes listed on death certificates, accounting for over half of all deaths. Recently, several investigators have reported on reclassifications of all deaths in the United States and other developed countries according to the contributing risk factors rather than the attributed diseases (Ezzati et al. 2006; Mokdad et al.

2004). These analyses consistently estimated that smoking, poor diet and physical activity patterns, and alcohol use were the actual causes of about 40% of all deaths. Though there is not universal consensus within the public health community regarding the details of the assumptions and methods that underpin such an analysis, there is agreement that interventions aimed at changing the impact of these underlying factors on health status have the potential to prevent disability and death due to chronic diseases (Flegal et al. 2004; Schroeder 2007). Thus, the potential for prevention remains high. Public health agencies need to support programs in chronic disease prevention and health promotion and develop more effective strategies to help people adopt healthier lifestyles.

The urgent treatment of people with acute illness and injury will always remain a priority in health care. However, additional health care investments in health promotion are critical to maintain health and prevent chronic diseases. Growing evidence documents the cost-effectiveness of these interventions in controlling chronic disease. A recent, comprehensive economic assessment of clinical preventive services ranked health promotion interventions based on cost-effectiveness and the potential impact of each intervention to reduce the overall burden of ill health in the population (Maciosek et al. 2006). These two criteria were scored on a scale from one to five with interventions demonstrating the greatest results given higher scores. Two of the three services found to be cost saving (i.e., a score of five on cost-effectiveness) and having the greatest potential for population impact on burden involve prevention of chronic diseases. These are smoking cessation counseling and low-dose aspirin therapy to prevent myocardial infarctions in high-risk patients. In other studies dietary interventions to reduce levels of serum cholesterol have been shown to be at least as cost-effective as coronary artery bypass surgery (Tengs et al. 1995).

Unlike the extensive literature on the economic characteristics of clinical services, information from economic evaluations of community prevention and health promotion interventions is more limited (Schwappach, Boluarte, and Suhrcke 2007; Carande-Kulis et al. 2000). In general, such evaluations find that there are substantial gains in population health to be made through investments that are small in comparison to the expenditures devoted to clinical care. One of the challenges is that chronic disease prevention requires shifting the focus from episodic care for acute illnesses to emphasis on a continuum of services and activities across a variety of settings that often involve many societal institutions outside of the medical care community, such as professionals in the fields of education, transportation, law, economics, and mental health. Assessment of these efforts also requires long-term follow-up to determine the impact of the prevention efforts.

Priorities and Strategies

The current priorities and strategies for chronic disease control are the result of a complex relationship among government agencies, health provider organizations, and other medical provider groups and voluntary health organizations. Government health agencies fund and conduct health education and research, develop policies, establish standards, provide financing for medical care, deliver medical services to the poor, and monitor the health status of the population. Voluntary health agencies fund research, provide public and professional education, stimulate social and legislative changes, and create visibility for prevention and treatment through their large cadre of volunteers. The medical care sector delivers services, provides preventive medicine through primary care, and establishes professional guidelines that improve the quality of services.

In 1979, *Healthy People: The Surgeon General's Report on Health Promotion and Disease Prevention* set the direction for chronic disease control (USDHEW 1979). This report concluded that further improvements in health were most likely to be achieved through disease prevention and health promotion rather than through increased medical care services and health expenditures. After a review of age-specific risks for mortality, actions were recommended in five priority areas: smoking, high blood pressure, alcohol consumption, nutrition, and physical activity. Though completed almost 30 years ago, the conclusions from this report were recently substantiated for coronary artery heart disease in a study where simulation models were used to analyze the determinants of the 50% decline in mortality from this disease in the United States between 1980 and 2000. The authors in this study concluded that about half of the decline was attributable to reductions in risk factors for persons with and without coronary artery heart disease (Ford et al. 2007).

Standard guidelines for prevention and health promotion interventions have been established. The U.S. Preventive Services Task Force, which is supported by the Agency for Healthcare Research and Quality, first published the *Guide to Clinical Preventive Services* in 1989 (USDHHS 1989). The reviews in this compendium are now regularly updated and published on the Internet (USDHHS 2007).

A more recent authoritative compendium of recommendations organized and maintained by the CDC is known as the *Guide to Community Preventive Services*. This effort provides evidenced-based guidelines derived through systematic assessments of programs and policies to promote population health (Briss et al. 2000). First published in 2000, subsequent reviews and updates are also made available on a stand-alone website (CDC 2007).

Health Care Cost and Access

The control and prevention of chronic disease is inextricably linked with issues of the current and future cost of health care. The dimensions of the health care "cost crisis" in the United States were alluded to in earlier sections of this chapter. Chronic diseases consume over 80% of the two trillion dollars spent on health care in the United States (Anderson et al. 2004). These expenditures can be expected to grow substantially because of the inevitable increase in the number of elderly residents resulting from the aging of the "baby boom" generation (Garrett and Martini 2007). However, there is evidence that much of the recent growth in costs is attributable to increases in the frequency of treatment for various chronic diseases beyond that which can be explained by the average aging of the population (Thorpe 2006). These dynamics suggest that prevention and health promotion should be a major component of the policy and resource allocation deliberations devoted to damping this rise in costs (White 2007; Thorpe 2006). Yet, most proposed solutions for containing these expenditures focus on various financing mechanisms to optimize the quality of care, and diminish the provision of unnecessary and ineffective treatments (Hsiao 2007). These latter components of the health care debate are important, but clearly not sufficient to address the looming problems associated with the cost of medical care in the United States and other developed nations. Finally, the focus on financing has continued to drive incentives for private health care providers to avoid covering socioeconomically disadvantaged and high-risk populations. The result is that 40–45 million Americans remain uninsured, and many more are vulnerable to economic disaster because of unstable, work-related insurance coverage that can disappear with the onset of a disabling, high-cost condition (Woolhandler and Himmelstein 2007).

Activities to promote prevention of chronic disease (e.g., water fluoridation and installation of walking trails in public parks) have traditionally been funded through public revenues. Such activities deserve support from all health care organizations because they effectively prevent conditions that would be expensive to treat in the medical setting. In keeping with the recommendations of the most recent IOM report, *The Future of the Public's Health in the 21st Century*, public agencies need to explore the development of partnership arrangements between multiple private health care delivery organizations as well as governmental entities such as public health, education, and transportation departments in their area to coordinate community as well as clinical programs for preventing chronic disease in all the members of the community (IOM 2003). Initiatives and demonstration projects such as those funded through the CDC *Steps* and Racial and Ethnic Approaches to Community Health (REACH) programs foster this type of collaboration and provide the much needed evidence base to encourage wider dissemination of such efforts (CDC 1997; Giles and Liburd 2006). Such a community-based approach with a long-term perspective could benefit health care organizations because all citizens are potential clients.

Current Challenges in Chronic Disease Control

Information on Chronic Diseases

An epidemiologic surveillance system for monitoring trends in chronic diseases is an essential part of chronic disease control. The system is needed for three key reasons: (1) to identify groups of people who are at risk of developing chronic disease or who experience fewer benefits from interventions, (2) to measure the effect of program interventions, and (3) to identify newly emerging chronic diseases. Reliable and geographically specific data on the burden from many self-reported chronic diseases and risk factors are available for every state and nearly 200 communities in the United States through the CDC Behavioral Risk Factor Surveillance System (Chowdhury et al. 2007). This state-based, but federally coordinated system provides information on self-reported chronic disease and health-related quality of life measures that enrich the understanding between risk factors and nonfatal health outcomes. However, there are limited data available from administrative sources or surveys using biomedical diagnostic technology that can be used at the local or community level to monitor effectiveness of treatment and prevention for chronic diseases such as diabetes or hypertension (Frieden 2004). Also, data are clearly inadequate to assess the status of many socioeconomically disadvantaged groups (Isaacs and Schroeder 2004).

Although mortality data are a major source of information for measuring the impact of chronic diseases, measures of morbidity and quality of life are more relevant for estimating the total burden from chronic diseases. Since the last edition of this book, there have been improvements in some chronic disease surveillance systems. In particular, implementation of a national system of cancer registries provides useful epidemiologic information about the incidence, stage of disease at diagnosis, and survival of patients diagnosed with this disease in almost every community in this country. This data system is also large enough to enable precise and detailed analyses of population subgroups inequitably affected by cancer (Espey et al. 2007). More limited information on the clinical presentation of strokes has also been implemented within a coordinated system of registries (Labarthe et al. 2006). The goal of these stroke registries is to identify the determinants of quality care for this devastating condition.

Two approaches that attempt to combine monitoring data on the incidence of, and morbidity and mortality from, diseases use the number of years of life lost from premature death and the loss of health from disease and disability. These are the quality-adjusted life year (QALY), which is often used in cost-effectiveness analyses, and the disability-adjusted life-year (DALY) (IOM 1998). The DALY was initially presented in the *World Development Report*, which was issued by the World Bank in 1993, and has subsequently been regularly used by the World Health Organization (WHO) to assess distributions and determinants of population health and the performance of health systems across the world (WHO 2000). Both of these measures express disability as a proportion of healthy life years based on the severity and duration of nonfatal health conditions. A detailed analysis using the DALY in the United States found that 50% of the burden of disease arises from the disabilities associated with predominantly nonfatal conditions (e.g., arthritis) and that 75% of this disability burden results from chronic diseases (Michaud et al. 2006).

Traditionally, many health care priorities have been developed only on the basis of diseases that cause the most deaths. These results suggest that control of chronic diseases can be optimally pursued as a high priority only when there are better measures of the incidence and prevalence of a broader range of chronic diseases, their effects on independent living, their costs, and the effectiveness of control measures.

Research Dissemination, Translation, and Diffusion

Research has provided a strong scientific base for many public health interventions. Often, the most important research issue is not the efficacy of the prevention technology itself, but the effectiveness of the application of the intervention to the general population and the adaptation of the technology to population subgroups at highest risk. Research in this area reflects the need to increase the benefits that can be realized from prevention by bringing it into more widespread use in the community and in the health care system. Public health professionals should continue to move from developing the scientific base of prevention to implementing and evaluating public health programs for the control of chronic diseases. The barriers to moving a health promotion intervention from the point of demonstrated efficacy, to translation based on the particular characteristics of the target community, and ultimate diffusion and institutionalization as part of ongoing public health practice require ongoing evaluation and research. More attention to an applied research agenda that addresses these types of issues is definitely needed (Glasgow and Emmons 2007).

Reducing Disparities in Special Populations

Death and disability rates remain elevated among socioeconomically disadvantaged groups and some minority populations, particularly blacks and persons with low income and education levels (Minkler et al. 2006; Isaacs and Schroeder 2004). Woolf and colleagues have demonstrated that during the last decade of the twentieth century 886,202 lives could have been saved in the United States by eliminating the disparity in death rates between blacks and whites—far more than could have been averted by population level advances in health care achieved during the same decade (Woolf et al. 2008). Other investigators have noted that the gaps between the poorest and richest Americans are much greater than the disparities in mortality between the races at all levels of income or education (Isaacs and Schroeder 2004).

The association between poverty and higher rates of morbidity, disability, and mortality has been observed since the twelfth century. Possible explanations for these higher rates include not only the disproportionate burden of established risk factors associated with poverty, but also a constellation of conditions, such as inadequate or crowded housing, poor education, substandard medical care, and exposure to a hazardous environment including air pollution. In the United States, the additional legacy of racial discrimination further exacerbates the disparities in social status and health for minorities (Murray et al. 2006). In disadvantaged populations, increased susceptibility to diseases may also result from stressful life events, social and cultural changes, and behaviors that have been adopted to cope with stress. For example, several studies have shown that experiences of racial discrimination are associated with health outcomes such as elevated blood pressure and preterm births (Krieger and Sidney 1996; Mustillo et al. 2004).

Racial and ethnic health disparities frequently provide opportunities, some might say moral imperatives, to ensure that all persons experience the level of health achievable within the majority group. Unfortunately, some of the greatest disparities in public health arise in the area of chronic disease. To mitigate such disparities, community-based efforts such as the Racial and Ethnic Approaches to Community Health (REACH) program involve the populations most disparately impacted. This program is designed to be culturally sensitive and has demonstrated that disparities in risk factors and conditions can be eliminated (Giles and Liburd 2006).

Social and Health Policies

Individual behaviors affect a person's risk of developing chronic diseases. People need to assume responsibility for their health in order to enjoy the full fruits of healthy lifestyles, but it is important that supportive social norms and health policies facilitate healthy behaviors. Reinforcing messages from many sources must be available, and their implementation should address a broad range of health issues. Environmental and structural policies such as the elimination of smoking in public places, and regulations to require adequate food labeling as well as reduced fat, sodium, and sugar content in food can help in prevention efforts directed at a variety of diseases (Brownson, Haire-Joshu, and Luke 2006).

Communication of Health Risk

Mobilizing support for policies designed to prevent chronic disease and disability will require accurate communication of health risks and the benefits of healthy behaviors. The perceived threat from a health risk may be exaggerated when exposure to the risk is considered involuntary, as in environmental exposure to hazardous wastes; when effects of the risk are unknown or unfamiliar; or when exposure to the risk is associated with dramatic and immediate consequences, as in an airplane crash. Often, this tendency to exaggerate a risk is aided by intense media coverage of the event. Unfortunately, the reverse is true for voluntary or familiar exposures and those that have delayed or long-term consequences.

For example, the health risk associated with smoking is underestimated by society because (1) smoking tobacco is considered to be an individual's choice, (2) it has been an accepted social behavior, and (3) it leads to disease only after years of exposure.

Providing accurate information by itself is usually not sufficient, however, to change behaviors. Packaging messages using methods developed by product and media marketers is essential to attain the attention and emotional impact necessary to affect demonstrable change in behaviors and outcome. This approach, known as social marketing, is being more widely used by the public health community. Messages that contain new, persuasive information delivered through personal testimony and graphic representations have the greatest effect. However, the costs of using ever-increasingly complex media and communication venues often make this approach prohibitive and difficult to sustain for public agencies with limited budgets (Huhman et al. 2007).

Global Health and Chronic Diseases

The changes described in the opening of this chapter in the major sources of disease and death seen in the United States and other high-income countries during the 20th century are now being seen throughout the world at an accelerated rate. Conditions such as malaria, diarrhea and parasitic diseases, malnutrition, HIV, and tuberculosis continue to exact a tremendous toll on the health of persons living in low- and middle-income countries. However, as many of these nations continue to struggle with the conditions traditionally associated with international public health work, they are simultaneously experiencing the emergence of chronic disease epidemics. The World Health Organization (WHO) estimated that in 2005 chronic diseases – mainly cardiovascular disease, cancer, chronic respiratory diseases, and diabetes – caused 60% of all the deaths worldwide, and more than 80% of these deaths occurred in low-income and middle-income countries (Abegunde et al. 2007). It is not just the large population size in many of these countries that accounts for this disproportionate burden. For most, the age-standardized rates for chronic diseases exceed those observed in wealthier nations (Figure 1.4). This documents an enormous toll in premature mortality that will continue to increase unless there are major changes in health policy, training and resource allocation.

Just as the traditional public health infrastructure in the United States still devotes disproportionate resources to infectious diseases, the international donor community has predominately focused on communicable conditions (Dear et al. 2007). To raise awareness about the burden and preventability of the chronic disease epidemic in the developing world, in 2005 the WHO set a goal of reducing chronic disease death rates by an additional 2% per year over existing trends in order to avert 36 million deaths between 2005 and 2015 (Strong et al. 2005). The WHO estimated that this goal could be accomplished by addressing the major risk factors of tobacco use, physical inactivity, and the consumption of processed, calorie-dense foods in a coordinated fashion through known behavioral and pharmaceutical interventions (WHO 2005). In addition to developing policies and health systems priorities that address these health problems, there will also need to be a major restructuring of the training received by health care and public health workers. The current medical and public health workforce in developing countries is not only inadequate in terms of the quantity of professionals, but has also been primarily trained to address acute health problems. Effective care for older patients and populations requires ongoing attention to lifestyle behaviors as well as coordinated care for complex,

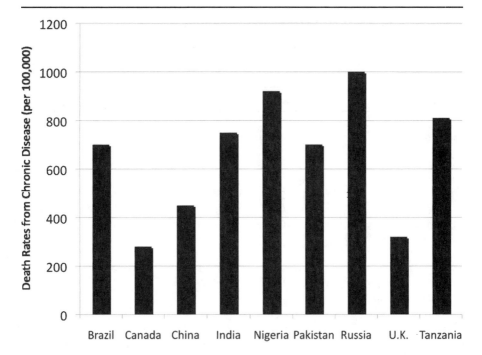

Figure 1.4. Age-standardized death rates from chronic disease (per 100,000) by country for ages 30–69 years. Reprinted from *The Lancet,* Vol. 366, Strong, K., C. Mathers, S. Leeder, and R. Beaglehole. Preventing Chronic Diseases: How Many Lives Can We Save? (2005):1578–1582, with permission from Elsevier.

chronic conditions that often require multiple providers and interventions across a variety of settings (Pruitt and Epping-Jordan 2005). The science, strategies, and public health approaches that are described in this book, while based on evidence from high-income nations, hold promise for applicability in the global context (Koplan et al. 2009).

In response to documented success in global chronic disease prevention and control, support appears to be growing. Major recent exemplary efforts include the Bloomberg Initiative to Reduce Tobacco, the Oxford Health Alliance, and the Global Alliance for Chronic Diseases (Frieden and Bloomberg 2007; Stevens, Siegel and Smith 2007; Anonymous 2009). These efforts have committed resources, and brought together major international donors, research institutions, and public health practitioners to address the major determinants of the worldwide chronic disease problem. This activity provides hope that further resources will be identified to realize the goals set by WHO.

Disability as a Consequence of Chronic Disease

Effective interventions need to be developed to reduce the prevalence of disability and to help people with disabilities to adapt and become self-sufficient. Disability is defined as a limiting health condition that interferes with the performance of socially defined activities and roles such as work (NCHS 2007).

Disability results from the complex interaction between the level of impairment or actual anatomically determined functional limitation and a person's expected roles and

Table 1.4. Distribution of Usual Activity Limitation and Limitation Due to Chronic Conditions, United States, 2006

Category	Individuals with Activity Limitation[a]		Individuals with Limitation Due to Chronic Condition[b]	
	Number, thousands	%	Number, thousands	%
All persons	35 776	12.1	34 776	11.7
Age group	5 458	7.4	5 323	7.2
Under 18 years	6 375	5.8	6 056	5.5
18–44 years	12 023	16.2	11 562	15.7
45–64 years	4 810	25.5	4 655	24.8
65–74 years	7 110	42.9	6 816	41.6
75 years and over				
Sex	16 857	12.1	16 267	11.7
Male	18 919	12.0	18 919	11.5
Female				
Family income	11 962	24.4	11 585	23.8
Under $20 000	6 121	15.3	5 980	15.0
$20 000–$34 999	4 449	11.5	4 338	11.3
$35 000–$54 999	2 295	8.5	2 188	8.2
$55 000–$74 999	3 749	7.5	3 627	7.3
$75 000 or more				

[a] Includes usual activities such as work, play, school, or other activities for health reasons.
[b] Subset of "limited" category; conditions lasting 3 months are classified as chronic; selected conditions such as arthritis, diabetes, cancer, heart disease, etc. are considered chronic regardless of duration.
Note: Data compiled from National Center for Health Statistics 2007.

tasks in the social environment. In the United States in 2006, more than 34 million people reported a limitation in activity due to a chronic condition (Table 1.4) (NCHS 2007). Limitations in activity are more common among older adults, women, and persons in low-income groups. As stated earlier in this chapter, with the aging of the population and the increase in the prevalence of disability with age, chronic disease control will become more important (Garrett and Martini 2007).

Workforce and Training Issues

Skills in epidemiology, public health management, communication, and community organization are considered increasingly essential for the public health practitioner. However, assessments of the workforce engaged in institutional public health routinely identify major deficiencies in the education, training, and experience of the practitioners in this workforce (Thacker 2005). In 2002, the IOM published a report, *Who Will Keep the Public Healthy? Educating Public Health Professionals for the 21st Century,* that targeted the training needs of the public health workforce in this century (Gebbie, Rosenstock, and Hernandez 2003). This report called for a greater need for funding and support for training and developing the public health workforce. Achieving this in the face of the added complexity of dealing with the issues involved in chronic disease prevention will be a massive challenge for the foreseeable future.

High-Risk and Population-Based Approaches

A general population-based approach to chronic disease prevention has several advantages. The common risk factors for chronic diseases are usually present in a large proportion of the population. Therefore, most of the cases of chronic disease arise from the large populations that possess intermediate- and low-risk profiles. The implication for prevention efforts is that small changes in risk in the total population will result in a greater overall disease reduction than will greater changes in a specified and limited high-risk group (Rose 1992). Further, a targeted high-risk approach requires the correct classification of people at high risk (Murray, Gakidou, and Frenk 1999). The efficiency of this approach depends on the cost of identifying the high-risk group and the ability to reach them with an effective intervention.

An intervention to reduce levels of excess body weight illustrates the differences between population-based and high-risk approaches. During the period 1999 through 2000, the prevalence of overweight (body mass index [BMI] ≥ 25) and obesity (BMI ≥ 30) among adults in the United States was 64.5% and 30.5%, respectively (Flegal et al. 2002). The objective in the population-based nutrition and physical activity program would be to reduce the overall distribution of body weight for all people. The population-based approach supports individuals' efforts to change their diets and increase their activity levels by increasing their knowledge and skills and by changing their environment. This effort is accomplished by providing nutrition information, labeling foods, developing healthier food products, pricing foods consistent with desired consumption patterns, creating a social context of positive reinforcement, encouraging changes in food preparation in restaurants and by food services, and supporting a physical environment that facilitates activity. In contrast, a high-risk approach attempts to reduce body weight only in those persons who have elevated body weight.

In practice, population-based and high-risk approaches are often combined. People in the population at large are encouraged to reduce their level of risk, and those in the high-risk population receive a more intensive intervention through public health efforts and/or the traditional medical care system. Often, the community milieu created by the population-based intervention will help those at high risk to initiate and maintain behavioral changes. Major challenges for chronic disease control specialists are to develop better tools for identifying those at high risk and to develop population-specific interventions that can be integrated into a comprehensive, population-based program. For directors of population-based programs, the challenge is to harness the energies and interests of the many community organizations whose policies can affect the health decisions of the community. Interventions must include consistent, reinforcing messages in both the health care setting and nontraditional settings, such as schools, community organizations, and work sites.

One important challenge when using either technique is to ensure that all individuals in the population targeted have equal access to the intervention. Otherwise, a well-intentioned public health campaign could have the undesirable effect of increasing disparities in health outcomes. For example, if the message delivered is not written at the proper literacy level, or if an intervention is established in such a way that an individual needs to have good access to the health care system to access it, those who are better educated or are already established in the health care system will preferentially benefit from the intervention, thus increasing disparities among disadvantaged populations.

Advances in Genomics

During the last decade, there have been unprecedented advances in the ability of medical science to assess genetic susceptibility to human diseases. The Human Genome Project, which has sequenced the entire human genome, will further accelerate the availability of numerous tests aimed at identifying specific genetic variants and their function (Collins and McKusick 2001). Many chronic diseases are the result of interactions between genetic and environmental risk factors (e.g., hypertension, atherosclerosis, and breast cancer). Genetic tests can identify people who may be susceptible to development of many of these conditions. In some classical genetic disorders, a single-point mutation can confer life-threatening consequences (e.g., sickle cell anemia or cystic fibrosis), but the interpretation of the newer tests is very complex and requires integration of information from multiple sources. Although many of these discoveries have the ultimate goal of facilitating prevention, early detection, accurate diagnosis, and effective treatment, there is limited knowledge about how most of the emerging information should be used in the context of current public health programs. Nevertheless, family health history is being increasingly used as a tool for identifying individuals with elevated risk as part of chronic disease prevention and control programs (Khoury and Mensah 2005).

In the near future, the public health impact of any particular genetic test will probably be limited compared with those of population-based health promotion programs. Current information suggests that the proportion of burden associated with any chronic disease attributable to a specific gene is limited (Kraft and Hunter 2009). However, the long-term potential for genomics technology is profound. The identification of increased susceptibility to chronic diseases through family history, genetic testing, and new biomarkers of disease classification and early detection has the potential to affect virtually everyone (provided access to these technologies is made universal) and can improve the efficiency of preventive interventions (Evans 2007). Additionally, the ability to track high-risk genetic patterns through families raises issues analogous to the classic public health activity of tracing contacts to persons with infectious diseases such as tuberculosis, infection with the human immunodeficiency virus, or sexually transmitted diseases. On the basis of their experience with these disease control programs, public health officials clearly have much to offer in the development of policies on issues such as determining when genetic tests are ready for widespread public health practice, the confidentiality of test results, assessing the impact of these technologies on population health outcomes and the potential for difficulties in obtaining employment and insurance for those with a high risk for developing conditions that are costly to treat (Evans 2007).

Integration of Chronic Disease Prevention Programs

In order to successfully address the prevention of the leading chronic diseases by intervening on the underlying risk factors, it is important to reemphasize that these diseases and determinants are often interrelated (Table 1.3). As just one example, persons with diabetes are more likely to die of heart disease than any other cause (Morrish et al. 2001). In general, persons at risk for diabetes, heart disease, and cancer tend to be from the same populations due to age, race, ethnicity, shared risk factors such as tobacco use, and other underlying social factors such as education or poverty. The implications of the enormous scope of the problem of preventing and controlling chronic disease and the overlap among the populations affected suggest the need for a more integrated and hence, potentially more efficient approach to public health practice. As a result, the field of chronic disease public health appears to be moving toward an integrated model as its way of doing business in the future.

How can improved integration be achieved? First, public health strategies need to focus as far upstream as possible by focusing on social determinants of health and the major shared risk factors of tobacco use, nutrition, physical activity, and overweight.

Second, interventions need to be coordinated within key settings to address multiple chronic diseases simultaneously. Settings where interventions can be most effectively implemented such as workplaces, schools, and communities are often unable to assimilate and maintain numerous unrelated or duplicative public health strategies. A workplace program focusing on cardiovascular health could be expanded or thoughtfully linked to programs to build an integrated chronic disease intervention. Such approaches could emulate the eight-component model for coordinated school health, which has long provided an exemplary framework for comprehensively orienting multiple functions of educational institutions (e.g., food service and physical education as well as health education and health services) toward promoting student health (Allensworth and Kolbe 1987).

Third, populations at greatest risk for one or more common chronic illnesses need to be identified, and the most effective approaches for reducing the incidence of chronic disease and its complications among these groups need to be launched in a coordinated fashion.

More practice-based evidence is needed to develop and test integrated interventions and to understand their effect on specific chronic diseases and on chronic disease as a whole. To be successful, it is anticipated that the integrated strategy will need to maintain highly specific interventions from categorical programs. Broad and diffuse interventions designed to "do it all" are unlikely to have much effect. Nevertheless, chronic disease public health will benefit from the hard work of examining how to improve its reach and effectiveness through better coordination and integration of prevention programs.

Future Directions

Appropriate responses to the stresses on the medical care and public health communities that will arise from an aging population will require continuing dynamism in the health care delivery system, and new strategies for preventing chronic diseases and disabilities in older adults and among the poor. These efforts can only be achieved through more aggressive and robust implementation of evidence-based, population-oriented, health promotion and chronic disease prevention interventions such as those identified by the *Guide to Community Preventive Services*, and engagement of a wide array of social institutions beyond the medical care community (Schroeder 2007; CDC 2007).

A better understanding of the psychological and social factors that affect behavior and of the relationship between behavior and chronic disease is necessary if the public health system is to fulfill its mission. The exploding cost of acute care medical services has prompted transformation in the structure of financing and the delivery of medical care with limited impact on the economic costs of these services. During this transition the number of persons without health care insurance coverage has remained stubbornly high. However, the cost-saving potential of chronic disease control and health promotion can only be realized if disease prevention is established as a major priority and access to medical and preventive health services is made widely available (Manton, Lamb, and Gu 2007; Fries 2003).

Current preventive strategies have targeted diseases and risk factors that cause the greatest mortality, and successful programs have resulted in increased life expectancy. Additional preventive strategies that incorporate considerations of patient satisfaction, and emerging technologies such as genetic testing, need to be developed to reduce disability and improve the quality of life associated with chronic diseases and aging. Measures of morbidity and quality of life such as QALYs and DALYs will serve as important outcomes for programs that address chronic disease control and the prevention of disabilities (Kindig 1997).

The existing level of knowledge about chronic diseases and their risk factors is sufficient to significantly reduce morbidity and mortality. This book outlines that knowledge and challenges the public and private health system to improve the prevention and management of chronic diseases in the United States.

References

Abegunde, D.O., C.D. Mathers, T. Adam, M. Ortegan, and K. Strong. The Burden and Costs of Chronic Disease in Low-Income and Middle Income Countries. *Lancet* (2007):370:1929–1938.

Allensworth, D.D., and L.J. Kolbe. The Comprehensive School Health Program: Exploring an Expanded Concept. *The Journal of School Health* (1987):57:409–412.

Alley, D.E., and V.W. Chang. The Changing Relationship of Obesity and Disability, 1988–2004. *JAMA* (2007):298:2020–2027.

Anderson, G., R. Herbert, T. Zeffiro, and N. Johnson. *Chronic Conditions: Making the Case for Ongoing Care.* Baltimore, MD: Johns Hopkins University (2004).

Anonymous. The Global Alliance for Chronic Diseases. *Lancet* (2009):373:2084.

Barrett-Connor, E. Infectious and Chronic Disease Epidemiology: Separate and Unequal? *Am J Epidemiol* (1979):109:245–249.

Berkelman, R.R.L., and J.J.W. Buehler. Public Health Surveillance of Non-Infectious Chronic Diseases: The Potential to Detect Rapid Changes in Disease Burden. *Int J Epidemiol* (1990):19:628–635.

Berry, D.A., and P.M. Ravdin. Breast Cancer Trends: A Marriage between Clinical Trial Evidence and Epidemiology. *J Natl Cancer Inst* (2007):99:1139–1141.

Briss, P.A., S. Zaza, M. Pappaioanou, J. Fielding, L. Wright-De Agüero, B.I. Truman, et al. Developing an Evidence-Based Guide to Community Preventive Services—Methods. The Task Force on Community Preventive Services. *Am J Prev Med* (2000):18(1 Suppl):35–43.

Brownson, R.C., D. Haire-Joshu, and D.A. Luke. Shaping the Context of Health: A Review of Environmental and Policy Approaches in the Prevention of Chronic Diseases. *Annual Rev Public Health* (2006):27:341–370.

Caballero, B. The Global Epidemic of Obesity: An Overview. *Epidemiol Rev* (2007):29:1–5.

Carande-Kulis, V.G., M.V. Maciosek, P.A. Briss, S.M. Teutsch, S. Zaza, B.I. Truman, et al. Methods for Systematic Reviews of Economic Evaluations for the Guide to Community Preventive Services. Task Force on Community Preventive Services. *Am J Prev Med* (2000):18(1 Suppl):75–91.

Centers for Disease Control and Prevention (CDC). *CDC's Steps Program.* 1997. Available at http://www.cdc.gov/steps/index.htm. Accessed December 3, 2007.

Centers for Disease Control and Prevention (CDC). *Guide to Community Preventive Services.* Atlanta, GA: National Center for Health Marketing, CDC, and the Community Guide Partners (2007).

Chobanian, A.V., G.L. Bakris, H.R. Black, W.C. Cushman, L.A. Green, J.L. Izzo, Jr., et al. The Seventh Report of the Joint National Committee on Prevention, Detection, Evaluation, and Treatment of High Blood Pressure: The JNC 7 Report. *JAMA* (2003):289:2560–2571.

Chowdhury, P.P., L. Balluz, W. Murphy, X.J. Wen, Y. Zhong, C. Okoro, et al. Surveillance of Certain Health Behaviors Among States and Selected Local Areas—United States, 2005. *MMWR*, CDC Surveillance Summaries (2007):56:1–160.

Cohen, H.W., R.M. Gould, and V.W. Sidel. The Pitfalls of Bioterrorism Preparedness: The Anthrax and Smallpox Experiences. *AJPH* (2004):94:1667–1671.

Collaborative Group on Hormonal Factors in Breast Cancer. Breast Cancer and Hormone Replacement Therapy: Collaborative Reanalysis of Data from 51 Epidemiological Studies of 52,705 Women with Breast Cancer and 108,411 Women without Breast Cancer. *Lancet* (1997):350:1047–1059.

Collins, F.S., and V.A. McKusick. Implications of the Human Genome Project for Medical Science. *JAMA* (2001):285:540–544.

Daviglus, M.L., K. Liu, P. Greenland, A.R. Dyer, D.B. Garside, L. Manheim, et al. Benefit of a Favorable Cardiovascular Risk-Factor Profile in Middle Age with Respect to Medicare Costs. *N Engl J Med* (1998):339:1122–1129.

Dear, A.S., P.A. Singer, D.L. Persad, S.K. Prammig, D.R. Matthews, R. Beaglehole, et al. Grand challenges in chronic non-communicable disease. *Nature* (2007):450:494–496.

Doll, R. *The Value of Preventive Medicine.* London: Pitman (1985).

Espey, D.K., X.C. Wu, J. Swan, et al. Annual Report to the Nation on the Status of Cancer, 1975–2004, Featuring Cancer in American Indians and Alaska Natives. *Cancer* (2007):110:2119–2152.

Evans, J.P. Health Care in the Age of Genetic Medicine. *JAMA* (2007):298:2670–2672.

Ezzati, M., S. Vander Hoorn, A.D. Lopez, G. Danaei, A. Rodgers, C.D. Mathers, et al. Comparative Quantification of Mortality and Burden of Disease Attributable to Selected Risk Factors. In: Lopez, A.D., C.D. Mathers, M. Ezzati, D.T. Jamison, and C.J.L. Murray, editors, *Global Burden of Disease and Risk Factors.* New York: Oxford University Press (2006).

Flegal, K.M., M.D. Carroll, C.L. Ogden, and C.L. Johnson. Prevalence and Trends in Obesity among U.S. Adults, 1999–2000. *JAMA* (2002):288:1723–1727.

Flegal, K.M., B.I. Graubard, D.F. Williamson, and M.H. Gail. Cause-Specific Excess Deaths Associated with Underweight, Overweight, and Obesity. *JAMA* (2007):298:2028–2037.

Flegal, K.M., D.F. Williamson, E.R. Pamuk, and H.M. Rosenberg. Estimating Deaths Attributable to Obesity in the United States. *AJPH* (2004):94:1486–1489.

Ford, E.S., U.A. Ajani, J.B. Croft, J.A. Critchley, D.R. Labarthe, T.E. Kottke, et al. Explaining the Decrease in U.S. Deaths from Coronary Disease, 1980–2000. *N Engl J Med* (2007):356:2388–2398.

Frieden, T.R. Asleep at the Switch: Local Public Health and Chronic Disease. *AJPH* (2004):94:2059–2061.

Frieden, T.R., and M.R. Bloomberg. How to Prevent 100 Million Deaths from Tobacco. *Lancet* (2007):369:1758–1761.

Fries, J.F. Measuring and Monitoring Success in Compressing Morbidity. *Ann Intern Med* (2003):139:455–459.

Fries, J.F., C.E. Koop, C.E. Beadle, P.P. Cooper, M.J. England, R.F. Greaves, et al. Reducing Health Care Costs by Reducing the Need and Demand for Medical Services. The Health Project Consortium. *N Engl J Med* (1993):329:321–325.

Fries, J.F., C.E. Koop, J. Sokolov, C.E. Beadle, and D. Wright. Beyond Health Promotion: Reducing Need and Demand for Medical Care. *Health Aff* (1998):17:70–84.

Garrett, N.N., and E.M. Martini. The Boomers are Coming: A Total Cost of Care Model of the Impact of Population Aging on the Cost of Chronic Conditions in the United States. *Dis Manag* (2007):10:51–60.

Gebbie, K., L. Rosenstock, and L.M. Hernandez, editors. *Who Will Keep the Public Healthy? Educating Public Health Professionals for the 21st Century.* Washington, D.C.: National Academies Press (2003).

Gerberding, J.L., J.M. Hughes, and J.P. Koplan. Bioterrorism Preparedness and Response: Clinicians and Public Health Agencies as Essential Partners. *JAMA* (2002):287:898–900.

Giles, W.H., and L. Liburd. Reflections on the Past, Reaching for the Future: REACH 2010—The First 7 Years. *Health Promot Pract* (2006):7(3 Suppl):179S–180.

Glasgow, R.E., and K.M. Emmons. How Can We Increase Translation of Research into Practice? Types of Evidence Needed. *Annu Rev Public Health* (2007):28:413–433.

Harper, S., J. Lynch, S. Burris, and G. Davey Smith. Trends in the Black-White Life Expectancy Gap in the United States, 1983–2003. *JAMA* (2007):297:1224–1232.

Hsiao, W.C. Why is a Systemic View of Health Financing Necessary? *Health Aff* (2007):26:950–961.

Huhman, M.E., L.D. Potter, J.C. Duke, D.R. Judkins, C.D. Heitzler, and F.L. Wong. Evaluation of a National Physical Activity Intervention for Children: VERB(TM) Campaign, 2002–2004. *Am J Prev Med* (2007):32:38–43.

Institute of Medicine (IOM). *The Future of Public Health.* Washington, D.C.: National Academy Press (1988).

Institute of Medicine (IOM). *Summarizing Population Health. Directions for the Development and Application of Population Metrics.* Washington, D.C.: National Academy Press (1998).

Institute of Medicine (IOM). *The Future of the Public's Health in the 21st Century.* Washington, D.C.: National Academy Press (2003).

Isaacs, S.L., and S.A. Schroeder. Class—The Ignored Determinant of the Nation's Health. *N Engl J Med* (2004):351:1137–1142.

Keller, P.A., L.A. Bailey, K.J. Koss, T.B. Baker, and M.C. Fiore. Organization, Financing, Promotion, and Cost of U.S. Quitlines, 2004. *Am J Prev Med* (2007):32:32–37.

Khoury, M.J., R. Davis, M. Gwinn, M.L. Lindegren, and P. Yoon. Do We Need Genomic Research for the Prevention of Common Diseases with Environmental Causes? *Am J Epidemiol* (2005):161:799–805.

Khoury, M.J., and G.A. Mensah. Genomics and the Prevention and Control of Common Chronic Diseases: Emerging Priorities for Public Health Action. *Prev Chronic Dis* (2005):2:A33.

Kindig, D. Purchasing Population Health: Paying for Results. Ann Arbor, MI: University of Michigan Press (1997).

Kraft, P., and D.J. Hunter. Genetic Risk Prediction—Are We There Yet?. *N Engl J Med* (2009):360:1701–1703.

Krieger, N., and S. Sidney. Racial Discrimination and Blood Pressure: The CARDIA Study of Young Black and White Adults. *AJPH* (1996):86:1370–1378.

Kuller, L.H. Relationship between Acute and Chronic Disease Epidemiology. *Yale J Biol Med* (1987):60:363–377.

Kung, H.C., D.L. Hoyert, J. Xu, and S.L. Murphy. *Deaths: Preliminary Data for 2005.* Atlanta, GA: National Center for Health Statistics, Centers for Disease Control and Prevention (2007).

Labarthe, D.R., A. Biggers, T. LaPier, and M.G. George. The Paul Coverdell National Acute Stroke Registry (PCNASR): A Public Health Initiative. *Am J Prev Med* (2006):31(6, Supplement 2): S192–S195.

Lightwood, J.M., and S.A. Glantz. Short-Term Economic and Health Benefits of Smoking Cessation: Myocardial Infarction and Stroke. *Circulation* (1997):96:1089–1096.

Maciosek, M.V., A.B. Coffield, N.M. Edwards, T.J. Flottemesch, M.J. Goodman, and L.I. Solberg. Priorities among Effective Clinical Preventive Services: Results of a Systematic Review and Analysis. *Am J Prev Med* (2006):31:52–61.

Mackenbach, J.P. The Origins of Human Disease: A Short Story on "Where Diseases Come From." *J Epidemiol Commun Health* (2006):60:81–86.

Manton, K.G., V.L. Lamb, and X. Gu. Medicare Cost Effects of Recent U.S. Disability Trends in the Elderly: Future Implications. *J Aging Health* (2007):19:359–381.

McElduff, P., A. Dobson, R. Beaglehole, and R. Jackson. Rapid Reduction in Coronary Risk for Those Who Quit Cigarette Smoking. *Aust N Z J Public Health* (1998):22:787–791.

Mensah, G.A., W.H. Dietz, V.B. Harris, R. Henson, D.R. Labarthe, F. Vinicor, et al. Prevention and Control of Coronary Heart Disease and Stroke—Nomenclature for Prevention Approaches in Public Health: A Statement for Public Health Practice from the Centers for Disease Control and Prevention. *Am J Prev Med* (2005):29(5 Suppl 1):152–157.

Michaud, C., M. McKenna, S. Begg, N. Tomijima, M. Majmudar, M. Bulzacchelli, et al. The Burden of Disease and Injury in the United States 1996. *Popul Health Metrics* (2006): 4:11.

Minkler, M., E. Fuller-Thomson, and J.M. Guralnik. Gradient of Disability across the Socioeconomic Spectrum in the United States. *N Engl J Med* (2006):355:695–703.

Mokdad, A.H., J.S. Marks, D.F. Stroup, and J.L. Gerberding. Actual Causes of Death in the United States, 2000. *JAMA* (2004):291:1238–1245.

Morrish, N.J., S.L. Wang, L.K. Stevens, J.H. Fuller, and H. Keen. Mortality and Causes of Death in the WHO Multinational Study of Vascular Disease in Diabetes. *Diabetologia* (2001):44 (Suppl 2):21.

Morrison, A. *Screening in Chronic Disease.* New York: Oxford University Press (1992).

Multiple Risk Factor Intervention Trial Research Group. Mortality Rates After 10.5 Years for Participants in the Multiple Risk Factor Intervention Trial. Findings Related to a priori Hypotheses of the Trial. The Multiple Risk Factor Intervention Trial Research Group. *JAMA* (1990):263(13):1795–1801.

Murray, C.J., E.E. Gakidou, and J. Frenk. Health Inequalities and Social Group Differences: What Should We Measure? *Bull WHO* (1999):77:537–543.

Murray, C.J.L., S.C. Kulkarni, C. Michaud, N. Tomijima, M.T. Bulzacchelli, T.J. Iandiorio, et al. Eight Americas: Investigating Mortality Disparities across Races, Counties, and Race-Counties in the United States. *PLoS Medicine* (2006):3:e260.

Mustillo, S., N. Krieger, E.P. Gunderson, S. Sidney, H. McCreath, C.I. Kiefe. Self-Reported Experiences of Racial Discrimination and Black-White Differences in Preterm and Low-Birthweight Deliveries: The CARDIA Study. *AJPH* (2004):94:2125–2131.

National Center for Health Statistics (NCHS). *Summary Health Statistics for the U.S. Population: National Health Interview Survey, 2006.* Hyattsville, MD: National Center for Health Statistics (2007).

O'Connor, S.M., C.E. Taylor, and J.M. Hughes. Emerging Infectious Determinants of Chronic Diseases. *Emerg Infect Dis* (2006):12:1051–1057.

Ogden, C.L., M.D. Carroll, L.R. Curtin, M.A. McDowell, C.J. Tabak, and K.M. Flegal. Prevalence of Overweight and Obesity in the United States, 1999–2004. *JAMA* (2006):295:1549–1555.

Omran, A.R. The Epidemiologic Transition: A Theory of the Epidemiology of Population Change. *Milbank Quarterly* (1971):49:509–538.

Pruitt, S.D., and J.E. Epping-Jordan. Preparing the 21st Century Global Healthcare Workforce. *BMJ* (2005):330:637–639.

Ravdin, P.M., K.A. Cronin, N. Howlader, C.D. Berg, R.T. Chlebowski, E.J. Feuer, et al. The Decrease in Breast-Cancer Incidence in 2003 in the United States. *N Engl J Med* (2007):356:1670–1674.

Rose, G. *The Strategy of Preventive Medicine.* New York: Oxford University Press (1992).

Schroeder, S.A. We Can Do Better—Improving the Health of the American People. *N Engl J Med* (2007):357:1221–1228.

Schwappach, D.L., T.A. Boluarte, and M. Suhrcke. The Economics of Primary Prevention of Cardiovascular Disease—A Systematic Review of Economic Evaluations. *Cost Eff Resour Alloc* (2007):5:5.

Stevens, D., K. Siegel, and R. Smith. Global Interest in Addressing Non-communicable Disease. *Lancet* (2007):370:1901–1902.

Strong, K., C. Mathers, S. Leeder, and R. Beaglehole. Preventing Chronic Diseases: How Many Lives Can We Save? *Lancet* (2005):366:1578–1582.

Tengs, T.O., M.E. Adams, J.S. Pliskin, D.G. Safran, J.E. Siegel, M.C. Weinstein, et al. Five-Hundred Life-Saving Interventions and Their Cost-Effectiveness. *Risk Anal* (1995):15:369–390.

Thacker, S.B. How Do We Ensure the Quality of the Public Health Workforce? *Prev Chronic Dis* (2005):2:A06.

Thorpe, K.E. Factors Accounting for the Rise in Health-Care Spending in the United States: The Role of Rising Disease Prevalence and Treatment Intensity. *Public Health* (2006):120:1002–1007.

U.S. Department of Health and Human Services (USDHHS). *Guide to Clinical Preventive Services: Report of the U.S. Preventive Services Task Force*. Washington, D.C.: U.S. Department of Health and Human Services (1989).

U.S. Department of Health and Human Services (USDHHS). U.S. Preventive Services Task Force. Agency for Healthcare Research and Quality. Rockville, Maryland: U.S. Department of Health and Human Services (2007).

U.S. Department of Health, Education, and Welfare (USDHEW). *Vital Statistics Special Reports, National Summaries, 1950*. Washington, D.C.: U.S. Department of Health, Education, and Welfare (1954).

U.S. Department of Health, Education, and Welfare (USDHEW). *Healthy People: The Surgeon General's Report on Health Promotion and Disease Prevention*. Washington, D.C.: U.S. Department of Health, Education, and Welfare (1979).

Verbrugge, L.L.M. Longer Life but Worsening Health? Trends in Health and Mortality of Middle-Aged and Older Persons. *Milbank Memorial Fund Quarterly*. Health and Society (1984):62:475–519.

White, C. Health Care Spending Growth: How Different is the United States from the Rest of the OECD? *Health Aff* (2007):26:154–161.

Woolf, S.H., R.E. Johnson, G.E. Fryer Jr., G. Rust, and D. Satcher. The Health Impact of Resolving Racial Disparities: An Analysis of U.S. Mortality Data. *AJPH* (2008):98(9 Suppl):S26–S28.

Woolhandler, S., and D.U. Himmelstein. Competition in a Publicly Funded Healthcare System. *BMJ* (2007):335:1126–1129.

World Health Organization (WHO). *The World Health Report 2000—Health Systems: Improving Performance*. Geneva: World Health Organization (2000).

World Health Organization (WHO). Preventing Chronic Diseases: A Vital Investment: WHO Global Report. Geneva: World Health Organization, 2005. Available at http://www.who.int/chp/chronic_disease_report/media/. Accessed August 9, 2009.

Zaza, S. Community Health Promotion and Disease Prevention. In: Wallace, R.B., editor, *Wallace/Maxcy-Rosenau-Last: Public Health and Preventive Medicine* (15th ed.). New York: McGraw-Hill (2008):1023–1028.

CHAPTER 2

METHODS IN CHRONIC DISEASE EPIDEMIOLOGY

Patrick L. Remington, M.D., M.P.H., Ross Brownson, Ph.D., and David Savitz, Ph.D.

Introduction

Purpose

As noted in Chapter 1, chronic diseases are distinguished from other health problems by their multiple and interrelated causes often rooted in early life and related to individual behavioral risk factors, such as smoking, physical inactivity, or poor diet. As public health advances have reduced the burden from infectious diseases, chronic diseases have become the leading causes of death and disability in the United States. In addition, many people are surviving with chronic diseases, since most are controlled through health care or lifestyle interventions, rather than being cured or rapidly fatal.

The field of epidemiology has been invaluable in understanding the causes of chronic diseases and designing interventions to prevent chronic diseases. Each of the chapters in this book, describing chronic diseases, conditions, and risk factors, is organized to address these two basic questions:

- What is the epidemiology of this problem? That is, what do we know about the burden of chronic diseases, their distribution in populations, and their causes? This question is addressed in this chapter.
- What can be done to control this problem in the population? That is, what are effective strategies to prevent, detect, and treat this problem in populations? This question is addressed in Chapter 3.

The purpose of this chapter is to provide a brief overview of the methods that can be used to answer this first question. This chapter summarizes the methods used to understand the epidemiology of chronic diseases, conditions, and risk factors. Breast cancer and tobacco use will be used to illustrate the various methods used in chronic disease epidemiology and control. The methods used to develop effective programs and monitor progress in populations are described in Chapters 3 and 4, respectively.

Definition of Epidemiology

Epidemiology is considered the "science of public health." The word comes from the Greek terms *epi* (upon), *demos* (people), and *logos* (study); thus, it is literally the study upon people. Traditionally, epidemiology was defined as the "study of the distribution and determinants of disease in populations." Over time, this definition broadened to include the study of other health states, such as injury, disability, risk factors, and health-related quality of life.

More than 30 years ago, William Foege coined the term "consequential epidemiology" to further broaden the definition of the term, to go from the study of disease to the use of epidemiology in disease control (Koplan and Thacker 2001). He stated that "the reason for collecting, analyzing, and disseminating information on a disease is to control that disease. Collection and analysis should not be allowed to consume resources if action does not follow" (Foege, Hogan, and Newton 1976).

The Centers for Disease Control and Prevention (CDC) currently defines epidemiology as "the study of the distribution and determinants of health-related states in specified populations, and the application of this study to control health problems." The key words include the following (CDC 2008; http://www.cdc.gov/excite/classroom/intro_epi.htm#defined):

- *Study*—Epidemiology is a quantitative discipline based on principles of statistics and research methods.
- *Distribution*—Epidemiologists study the "distribution" of health events within groups in a population, characterizing health events in terms of person, place, and time. This type of epidemiology is referred to as descriptive epidemiology.
- *Determinants*—Epidemiologists also search for "determinants" (i.e., causes or factors) that are associated with increased risk or probability of disease. This type of epidemiology, where we move from questions of "who," "what," "where," and "when" and start trying to answer "how" and "why," is referred to as "analytical epidemiology."
- *Health-related states*—Although infectious diseases were clearly the focus of much of the early epidemiological work, the field is no longer limited in this way. Epidemiology as it is practiced today is applied to the whole spectrum of health-related events, which includes chronic diseases, conditions, and risk factors.
- *Populations*—One of the most important distinguishing characteristics of epidemiology is that it deals with groups of people rather than with individual patients.
- *Control*—Finally, although epidemiology can be used simply as an analytical tool for studying diseases and their determinants, it can also play a more active role. Epidemiological data and methods steer public health decision-making and aids in developing and evaluating interventions to control and prevent health problems. This is the primary function of applied, field, or consequential epidemiology.

Brownson and Petitti (2006) define "applied epidemiology" according to the intended purpose. In their view, the field can be defined based on five core purposes: (1) the synthesis of the results of etiologic studies as input to practice-oriented policies; (2) the description of disease and risk factor patterns as information to set priorities; (3) the evaluation of public health programs, laws, and policies; (4) the measurement of the patterns and outcomes of health care; and (5) the communication of epidemiological findings effectively to health professionals and the public.

The Chronic Disease Continuum

For diseases of known infectious origin, such as AIDS, measles, and influenza, the presence of a single, known, necessary cause (e.g., the microorganism) helps to focus epidemiological research and intervention strategies. For injuries, the cause is often acute and leads to immediate health consequences, such as drinking and driving or a child drowning.

In contrast, the wide variety of chronic diseases lacks such unifying causal agents and often develops over the life course. Research has demonstrated that many chronic diseases have their origins early in the life course (Felitti et al. 1998). These early life experiences and exposures to social and economic factors increase the risk of unhealthy behaviors later in life. These unhealthy behaviors eventually lead to conditions such as hypertension, obesity, or high blood cholesterol. Finally, individuals with these conditions are at increased risk for developing chronic diseases, such as heart disease, cancer, or diabetes.

This model of a chronic disease continuum is shown in Figure 2.1 and has been used to organize this text, with three different parts for chronic diseases, chronic disease conditions, and chronic disease risk factors. The chronic disease continuum also requires special methods for chronic disease epidemiology and control. Because the causal process is prolonged and typically complex, many modest influences, rather than a single predominant cause, often affect the probability of developing disease. The prolonged duration of these diseases, which often includes a presymptomatic phase and subsequent development of chronic disease conditions, provides numerous overlapping opportunities for intervention. For most chronic diseases, the large number of modest risk factors and the diverse opportunities for intervention make their control difficult and typically require a multifaceted approach.

Because disease is the end result of a continuum, it is sometimes difficult to determine whether "disease" is even present at all. For example, the large increase in mammography

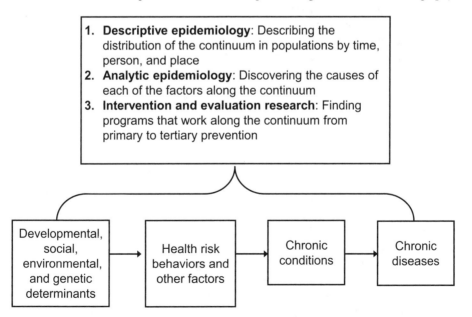

Figure 2.1. Methods used in chronic disease epidemiology and control, applied along the chronic disease continuum.

over the late 1980s and 1990s has led to a large increase in the incidence of a pathological lesion known as "ductal carcinoma in situ" (DCIS). Although DCIS is not invasive breast cancer, and although many women with DCIS will not develop invasive breast cancer, DCIS is often treated the same way as invasive cancer, that is, by surgical excision. Many women with DCIS consider themselves to have "breast cancer." Similarly, many men with "prostate cancer" actually have a pathological lesion that would never have progressed to clinical disease. In general, as our ability to detect earlier and earlier stages of the disease process improves, the point at which disease truly begins becomes increasingly unclear (Fryback et al. 2006).

Another important consideration for chronic disease is the meaning of "control" or what it is we are trying to prevent. Chronic disease often affects the quality of life long before it affects the duration of life, if it affects duration at all. People with diabetes, for example, do have higher mortality, but only many years after diagnosis. In the interim, however, they may experience blindness, kidney failure, painful feet ulcers, leg amputation, or premature heart disease, all as a direct result of having diabetes. For example, "controlling" diabetes implies not only decreasing mortality from this disease but also decreasing the detrimental effects on quality of life that occur rather than focusing solely on prolonging life. Both disease-specific and general measures of quality of life have been developed and validated (McDowell and Newell 1996), and these measures are being used increasingly to describe the course ("natural history") of disease as well as the effect of various methods of control.

There is a need to pay careful attention to methodological principles in many areas of the study and control of chronic disease. The need for clarity of terminology and thought is enhanced by the advancements that have been made and the expansion of options for tackling chronic disease through public health measures. In this chapter, we provide some basic terms and concepts common in epidemiological literature on the etiology (i.e., causes), consequences, and control of chronic diseases. We also describe how epidemiology has been used to understand the epidemiology (distribution and determinants) and control of chronic disease, along the chronic disease continuum shown in Figure 2.1.

Building on this continuum, each chapter in Parts 2–4 of this text has the following sections:

(1) Significance: The first section of each chapter provides an overview of the "significance" of the disease, condition, or risk factor in populations. This section measures the burden to public health by estimating the number of people affected, rates, and economic costs.

(2) Pathophysiology: The second section of each chapter describes the biology and pathophysiology of the disease, condition, or risk factor. This information is important to understand when interpreting epidemiological information or designing interventions.

(3) Descriptive epidemiology: The third section of each chapter provides an overview of the "distribution" of the disease, condition, or risk factor in populations. This section uses "descriptive epidemiology" to identify high-risk groups (person), geographic variation (place), and secular trends (time).

(4) Causes: The fourth section of each chapter provides an overview of the "causes" of the disease, condition, or risk factor in populations. This section used "analytic epidemiology" to identify those factors that increase the risk of an individual developing a chronic disease, condition, or risk factor. Special techniques, de-

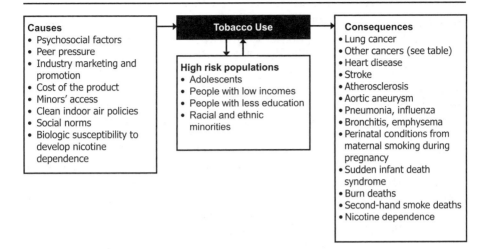

Figure 2.2. Tobacco use: causes, consequences, and high-risk groups.

scribed below, are used to go beyond finding associations to finding factors that are causally related to the outcome of interest.

(5) Interventions: The final section of each chapter provides an overview of the interventions that may be used to prevent or control the chronic disease, condition, or risk factor. These methods go beyond the use of epidemiology to determine the causes to finding programs that work, along the continuum from primary prevention to secondary and tertiary prevention. The final section of this chapter describes methods that can be used to move from descriptive and analytic epidemiological research to developing effective interventions. Intervention methods are described in detail in Chapter 3 of this text.

The epidemiology of each chronic disease, condition, or risk factor is summarized in a figure in each chapter, as shown in Figure 2.2. This figure shows the "upstream causes" on the left side, the "high-risk groups" in the middle, and the "downstream consequences" on the right side. The sections below will provide a brief overview of the methods used to measure the burden, describe high-risk groups and trends in the population, and identify modifiable risk factors.

Descriptive Epidemiology: Describing the Burden and Distribution in Populations

The first step in developing approaches to chronic disease control is to understand the nature and extent of the problem. The Institute of Medicine (1988), in its landmark report on the future of public health, stressed the importance of epidemiology in carrying out public health assessment—one of the core functions of public health. This report focused on the governmental role in public health and stated that every public health agency should regularly and systematically collect, analyze, interpret, and disseminate information on the health of the community, including statistics on health status, community health needs, and epidemiological and other studies of health problems.

The type of epidemiological studies used to support this assessment function varies, depending on the nature of the public health program. Descriptive epidemiology makes use of available data to examine the distribution of diseases in populations by time, person, or place. This type of information can be used to assess the burden of disease, identify high-risk groups, or monitor trends over time. The public and health policy makers frequently underestimate the health and economic burden from chronic diseases. Research has demonstrated that the public is more concerned about diseases and exposures that are unknown or out of one's individual control. For example, although tobacco use, poor nutrition, and physical inactivity account for nearly two thirds of preventable deaths in the United States (Mokdad et al. 2004), the public often perceives much greater risk from AIDS, homicide, and environmental pollution (Tinker and Vaughan 2002) (so-called involuntary risks).

In the first part of each chapter of this text, the authors describe the burden of the chronic disease, condition, or risk factor in the population and how it is distributed by "person, place, and time." For example, in Chapter 14, the following questions are addressed for breast cancer:

(1) *Significance: What are the "downstream consequences" of this problem?* This is addressed through measures of disease occurrence: incidence rate, cumulative incidence, and prevalence. Both incidence rate and cumulative incidence indicate the risk of newly acquiring the disease, whereas prevalence is the number of people who have the disease at a point in time. Mortality rates are often used when incidence rates are unavailable.

(2) *What populations have the highest risk?* This question is addressed by comparing the risk or incidence of disease among people within the population who have some characteristic (e.g., older age) with those who do not have the characteristic. To do this, we use measures of association—rate ratio—and difference measures.

(3) *Geographic distribution: How does the burden of disease in one area compare with that in other areas?* In calculating statistics that quantify the disease burden in one area versus other areas, consider the potential for distortion due to such factors as differing age, sex, and race in your population. To avoid distortion, you may need to divide measures of disease occurrence into categories to make them age-, sex-, or race-specific or standardize (adjust) them to make the populations comparable.

(4) *Time trends: What are the trends in the disease cancer over time?* Monitoring trends over time can provide insight on the etiology of chronic diseases (e.g., increases in lung cancer followed increases in smoking), burden (e.g., increasing rates of obesity), and control (e.g., declines in breast cancer mortality). The methods used to answer these questions are described in more detail below.

Measuring the Burden of Disease

Several measures are used to quantify the magnitude of disease occurrence, each one valid for a slightly different purpose. The number or actual count of persons affected by a chronic disease, condition, or risk factor is often used as the most fundamental measure of burden in the population. This measure is useful when assessing the need for health care or public health services as a direct measure of the burden on these systems. The actual burden of cancer is described in Chapter 14:

- Cancer is the leading cause of death among persons younger than 85 years old and the second leading cause of death overall in the United States.
- Cancer accounts for an estimated 1.4 million new cases and 560,000 deaths in 2007.
- Breast cancer is the most common cancer type among women in the United States and the second leading cause of cancer death.
- Breast cancer accounted for about 178,000 new cases and 40,000 deaths in 2007.
- Worldwide, breast cancer is the second most common cancer and the fifth among cancer deaths.
- Breast cancer rarely occurs in men, with only 2,000 new cases and 450 deaths in 2007.

The actual number of people with a chronic disease or the number of deaths is an easy way to communicate burden to the general public and to policy makers. However, the absolute number of people affected is almost entirely dependent on the size of the population under consideration. Therefore, other measures must be used when making comparisons across populations and over time.

Calculating Rates in Populations

Rates must be calculated in order to compare populations of various sizes and characteristics. The principal rates used in chronic disease epidemiology and control are incidence and prevalence. Measures such as rate ratios and rate difference are then used to compare these different measures of risk across populations.

Incidence (or incidence rate) refers to the number of new cases over a defined period divided by the "person-time experience of the population"—that is, the number of persons multiplied by the period over which they were monitored; this is often called "person-years." However, in practice, the incidence rate is typically used to describe the number of new cases that develops in a year in a specified population. For example, if 500 women develop breast cancer in a year in a population of 342,000 women, the incidence rate would be 146 cases of breast cancer per 100,000 population of women. For many chronic diseases, such as coronary heart disease and diabetes, mortality rates are calculated because incidence data are unavailable.

Cumulative incidence is defined as the probability or risk of developing a disease over a defined period. It ranges from 0 to 1 and indicates the probability that the disease will develop in a population that is monitored over a set period. For example, according to a 2006 report from the National Cancer Institute (Ries et al. 2006), a woman's lifetime risk of developing breast cancer is 0.127, or about 1 in 8. Thus, we can estimate that a girl born today has a 12.7% chance of eventually being diagnosed with breast cancer, although such estimates ignore any competing causes of mortality and are based on the somewhat unrealistic assumption that the present incidence rates will persist over time.

Prevalence also is measured as a proportion—that is, existing cases of disease divided by total population—but the occurrence of disease is measured at a point in time rather than over some interval. At the time of a disease survey, prevalence is defined as the number of existing cases divided by the population count. The prevalence of disease is influenced by the incidence (more new cases yield more existent cases) and persistence of the disease (rapid recovery or rapid death reduces the number of affected individuals at any point in time). For breast cancer, for example, the prevalence greatly exceeds the annual incidence because most women diagnosed with breast cancer survive for at least five years.

Because it is influenced by survival and recovery, prevalence is less valuable than incidence for identifying etiologic factors. For assessing public health needs, however, prevalence may be exactly the measure of interest. For example, women diagnosed with breast cancer are at a higher risk of a second breast cancer. Therefore, a prevalence estimate of the number of breast cancer survivors in a given area may be useful in targeting limited public health resources to women in high-risk groups.

Comparing Rates Across Populations

Many local, state, and federal health agencies now calculate incidence rates for various conditions. Likewise, mortality rates (which can be viewed as incidence rates of death) are also published, often for such geographic areas as counties or cities. Public health officials have a natural interest in comparing incidence or mortality rates from other areas with their own to determine which areas have a greater problem.

Once rates have been calculated for various populations or population subgroups, these rates can be compared using rate ratios or relative risks. For example, data from the Surveillance, Epidemiology, and End Results program of the National Cancer Institute provide breast cancer incidence rates for men and women. From 2001 to 2005, for example, the age adjusted incidence rate for women was 126.1 per 100,000 person-years (Ries et al. 2006). The comparable incidence rate for men was 1.2 cases per 100,000 person-years. Having determined the incidence rate in each of the two groups we wish to compare, our next challenge is to determine how that comparison should be summarized.

The ratio of the incidence rate in one group to that in another is referred to as a rate ratio. Likewise, the ratio of the cumulative incidence or risk in two groups is termed the "risk ratio" or "relative risk." Considering the incidence rate in men as the reference, we can calculate the rate ratio for women compared with men as 126.1/1.2 = 105. Thus, we can say that women have an incidence rate 105 times that of men: breast cancer is predominantly a disease of women, although it does occur infrequently in men.

One advantage of such ratio measures is the ease of intuitive understanding (i.e., disease occurrence is increased about 100-fold among the women). Also, this ratio is independent of the absolute incidence rates in the two groups and, therefore, is directly interpretable: there is a strong association between sex and breast cancer.

Other risk factors besides sex can be discussed in similar terms. For example, research has demonstrated that the risk of breast cancer increases, as the age of first birth increases. The five-year risk of breast cancer among women who have their first child before the age of 20 years is 0.7%, compared with a risk of 1.3% for women who have their first child after the age of 30 years (Table 2.1). In this instance, the relative risk for developing breast cancer in the next five years is 1.86 times (1.3/0.7 = 1.86).

An alternative to the ratio measure is the rate difference, calculated by subtracting the rates from one another. For example, the rate difference between women who have their first child after the age of 30 years, compared with women who have their first child before the age of 20 years, is calculated as follows: 1.3% − 0.7% = 0.6%, or 0.6 more cases

Table 2.1. Five-Year Breast Cancer Risk, Rate Ratios, Rate Differences for Women[a] Based on Age at First Pregnancy

Age at First Pregnancy (years)	Rate[b] (%)	Rate Ratio	Rate Difference (%)
<20	0.7	Reference group	Reference group
20–24	0.9	0.9/0.7 = 1.29	0.9 – 0.7 = 0.2
25–29	1.1	1.1/0.7 = 1.57	1.1 – 0.7 = 0.4
30+	1.3	1.3/0.7 = 1.86	1.3 – 0.7 = 0.6
None	1.1	1.1/0.7 = 1.57	1.1 – 0.7 = 0.4

[a]Based on women who are 50 years old with no family or personal history of breast cancer.
[b]Rate = percentage of those who will develop breast cancer in the next five years.
Source: http://www.cancer.gov/bcrisktool/Default.aspx.

per 100 women (or six cases per 1,000 women) over the next five years. This difference indicates how much, in absolute rather than relative terms, the risk differs depending on child-bearing histories. The advantage of this measure is that the actual amount by which the disease has increased in one group as opposed to another has public health importance beyond the ratio of the two rates.

A doubling or even tripling of rate of a disease (e.g., the incidence or mortality rate) may not indicate an important public health problem if the baseline rate is extremely low. That is, the increment in disease burden from doubling a very small number would be very small. The difference in incidence rates, however, provides direct information about the public health effects of a particular exposure. A large difference indicates an important problem, regardless of the size of the baseline rate.

The difference between rate ratios and rate differences is shown in Table 2.2. Comparing smokers with nonsmokers, the relative risk is much greater for developing lung cancer than for coronary heart disease. However, the rate difference for heart disease (the rate in smokers minus the rate in nonsmokers) is actually greater than the rate difference

Table 2.2. Smoking-Related Rate Ratio and Rate Difference Estimates for Coronary Heart Disease and Lung Cancer among Women

Disease	Mortality Rate		Ratio (*a*/*b*)	Difference (*a* – *b*)
	Smokers (*a*)	Nonsmokers (*b*)		
Lung cancer	131	11	11.9	120
Coronary heart disease	275	153	1.8	122

Note: Adapted from the second edition of this text.

for lung cancer because the baseline mortality rate of heart disease is so much greater than that for lung cancer. The public health impact due to increasing heart disease risk twofold is similar to the impact of increasing lung cancer risk tenfold. Both ratio and difference measures contribute to our understanding of the effect of an exposure on disease occurrence, and both measures should be examined when the data permit.

Finally, rates can be used to identify subgroups at need for program targeting. For example, identifying factors associated with compliance with cancer screening (CDC 2003, 2007) helps program planners and managers to select subpopulations at greater risk for negative outcomes. Also, identifying these associations simultaneously with that of health-related behaviors (Liang et al. 2006; Coughlin et al. 2007) and other screening practices provides managers with practical information on whom and how to offer joint interventions.

Controlling for Differences in Age When Comparing Populations

Perhaps the most important issue to consider when comparing rates across populations is the potential that the two populations differ in average age. The risk of most chronic diseases increases dramatically with increasing age. For example, a retirement community may have a higher rate of breast cancer because they have a greater proportion of older women. Thus, this higher rate might not be due to some risk factors (e.g., genetics, child-bearing practices). How then could we compare the rates in one area with those in another area, accounting for the differing ages, to determine whether some other factors are influencing the rate of breast cancer?

We have two options. First, age-specific rates can be calculated. That is, incidence rates may be given only for people in a specific age range. If the incidence rate of breast cancer for women aged 50 through 59 years is much greater in one area than in another, the difference could not have been caused by differences in age distributions between the two groups. A drawback with such calculations is that the problem of precision may be worsened: fewer cases are diagnosed (therefore, the numerator for the incidence rate is smaller) in a narrow age range than in the entire population. Such age-specific calculations typically require cases diagnosed over longer periods or from larger populations.

A second way to ease comparison of incidence rates is to adjust the rate to a standard population. This, in effect, combines many age-specific rates into a single age-adjusted rate. For example, the breast cancer incidence rate given in the previous example (110 cases per 100,000 women) is age-adjusted to the 1970 U.S. standard population. This means that statistical adjustments were made to the initial calculations to provide the rate that would be expected in the area's population if it had the same age distribution as did the U.S. population in 1970. Rates adjusted to the same standard population can be compared directly: they refer to rates calculated for populations with the same age structure.

Small Area Analyses

Once differences in the ages of populations have been taken into account (either by comparing age-specific rates or through age adjustment), the problem of precision must be addressed by considering the statistical precision of the incidence or mortality rate. When rates are calculated for small areas such as a county, the numerator of the rate will be small (for most counties). When a numerator is smaller than 20, rates are unstable. If only a few cases are detected a year early or a year late, the incidence rate calculated for a particular year may appear much higher or much lower than it is on average over a longer period.

For example, if the incidence rate for breast cancer is 110 new cases per 100,000 women, a county with 25,000 women would be expected to have about 27 new cases each year (27/25,000 = 110 cases per 100,000). If only four cases were diagnosed too late to be counted for a particular year, the rate would decrease to 23 cases that year (23/25,000 = 92 cases/100,000), yielding an incidence rate ratio of 92/110 or 0.84. If only six cases from the next year were diagnosed a bit early, the rate would appear to increase dramatically to 33 cases per year (33/25,000 = 132 cases/100,000 women), for an incidence rate ratio of 1.20 and an apparent 20% increase in breast cancer incidence.

Thus, rates calculated from cases diagnosed in a single year from an area with a small population are subject to a large amount of variation from year to year and are said to be imprecise. For this reason, one should calculate rates from cases diagnosed over several years to increase the number of cases in the numerator of the incidence rate, thereby increasing the precision of the calculated rate.

The use of these methods can be seen in the maps of breast mortality for white women and lung cancer mortality for white men for the United States (produced by the National Cancer Institute; see http://www3.cancer.gov/atlasplus/).

These maps compare the breast cancer mortality rates for white women and lung cancer mortality for white men for 1970–1994. First, notice that rates are presented by

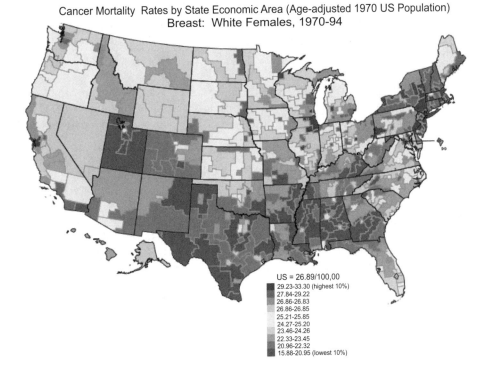

Cancer Mortality Rates by State Economic Area (Age-adjusted 1970 US Population)
Breast: White Females, 1970-94

US = 26.89/100,00
29.23-33.30 (highest 10%)
27.84-29.22
26.86-26.83
26.86-26.85
25.21-25.85
24.27-25.20
23.46-24.26
22.33-23.45
20.96-22.32
15.88-20.95 (lowest 10%)

Figure 2.3. Breast cancer mortality rates by state economic area, white women, United States, 1970–1994. Rates are age-adjusted to the 1970 U.S. population.

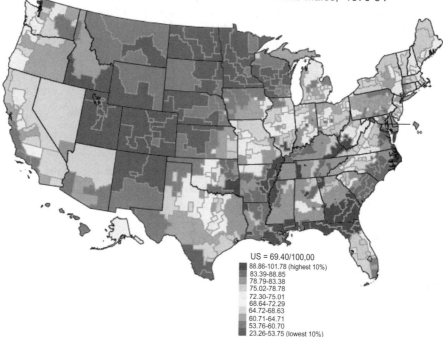

Cancer Mortality Rates by State Economic Area (Age-adjusted 1970 US Population)
Lung, Trachea, Bronchus, and Pleura: White Males, 1970-94

US = 69.40/100,00
88.86-101.78 (highest 10%)
83.39-88.85
78.79-83.38
75.02-78.78
72.30-75.01
68.64-72.29
64.72-68.63
60.71-64.71
53.76-60.70
23.26-53.75 (lowest 10%)

Figure 2.4. Lung cancer mortality rates by state economic areas, white men, United States, 1970–1994. Rates are age-adjusted to the 1970 U.S. population.

grouping counties into "state economic areas" and that many years of data were combined to produce more reliable rates. In addition, these rates are age-adjusted (to the 1970 U.S. population) to account for differences in the ages of the populations, not only among counties but also over time.

These maps provide insight into the epidemiology of breast and lung cancer. First, the mortality rates for breast cancer are higher in the northeastern United States. Research has shown that differences in cancer incidence and survival explain some, but not all, of these geographic differences (Goodwin et al. 1998). Considerable interest remains in the possibility that environmental exposures contribute to these differences (Reynolds et al. 2005). In contrast, the reasons for the higher rates of lung cancer mortality among white men are almost entirely due to higher rates of smoking among men living in the southeastern United States.

Analytic Epidemiology: Finding the Causes of Chronic Disease

The second major function for epidemiology in chronic disease prevention and control is to understand the "determinants" (i.e., causes) of chronic diseases—with a focus on those determinants that can be modified. In the second section of each of the chapters in this text, authors describe the modifiable factors for each of the major chronic diseases, conditions, and, when possible, chronic disease risk factors.

One of the most important and challenging roles for epidemiology is to differentiate between factors that are simply associated with chronic diseases and those factors that actually cause those chronic diseases. Criteria have been established to help epidemiologists determine which associations are truly causal and which are not. Experimental evidence provides the strongest evidence for a causal association, but it is most useful in examining the effects of drugs and clinical interventions, rather than the complex associations between environmental, social, or lifestyle factors and chronic diseases. Ultimately, subjective judgments must be made.

After finding modifiable risk factors for chronic diseases, epidemiology can be used to estimate the morbidity and mortality that might be prevented by interventions. Although interventions such as education and screening programs often seem valuable, many have little effect on the number of people with the disease. Therefore, we need to evaluate the effects of intervention programs and use those results to design new and better programs for controlling chronic diseases. Even when there are strong theoretical reasons to expect benefit, a determination is needed that the intervention reduces mortality or improves quality of life when applied in a real setting. Every intervention, even those that reduce the burden of disease, has a "downside," both through undesired consequences and by consuming resources. Calculating the proportion of a disease that is attributable to a particular risk factor may help to quantify the effect of its reduction or elimination (i.e., the population attributable risk).

Study Designs in Chronic Disease Epidemiology

Experimental Studies

Randomized controlled trials (RCTs) are considered the most scientifically rigorous type of epidemiological study. In an RCT, subjects are randomly assigned to either receive or not receive a preventive or therapeutic procedure, such as a clinical smoking cessation intervention or a new drug. The disease course or mortality patterns are then observed over time to assess the effectiveness of the preventive or therapeutic procedure.

The advantage of using a clinical trial, when possible, was best demonstrated by an RCT of the health effects of estrogen replacement therapy among women, called the Women's Health Initiative. This study was halted in 2002, when, contrary to its original hypothesis, the estrogen replacement therapy actually increased risk of breast cancer and heart disease (Writing Group for the Women's Health Initiative Investigators 2002). These results were definitive and conflicted with results that had been obtained from observational research decades before.

In practice, however, RCTs are either impossible or impractical when studying many interventions, especially those based outside of clinical settings and in the community. For example, it may be impractical to design a study to examine the effects of a community-wide educational intervention encouraging women to get a mammogram. In these situations, interventions can be tested in "quasi-experimental studies," in which a program (e.g., education program, screening program, new treatment regimen) is systematically offered to a population and the effect on health is measured. One key objective of such a study is to draw specific conclusions about the intervention. If the health of the population receiving the intervention improves, the investigators must demonstrate that a similar population that did not receive the intervention did not improve, at least to the same extent. This implies that to clearly interpret the results, such studies require comparison groups, which, unfortunately, are often lacking.

Comparison groups vary in their appropriateness for disease intervention studies. Least convincing are comparisons with national data or populations in other studies. Previous data on the same population are most appropriate if the disease can be shown to have been stable for a long period and if there are no other reasons for a change in disease incidence. The best control groups are those that can be shown to be similar to the intervention population and from which disease information is collected concurrently.

Despite certain limitations, quasi-experimental studies have shown that low-cost interventions can significantly improve the population's health. In one such study, low-cost community-based information campaigns were conducted in four low-income rural counties to encourage women to get routine breast and cervical cancer screening examinations. The rates of screening from baseline to follow-up were significantly higher among women living in these counties, compared with the trends among women living in four similar rural counties in Wisconsin (Eaker et al. 2001; Jaros, Eaker, and Remington 2001). The strengths and limitations of the different types of experimental studies are summarized in Table 2.3.

Observational Studies

RCTs or quasi-experimental interventions are either impossible or impractical when studying many of the causes of chronic diseases in the population. In some cases, it would be unethical or impossible to randomly assign the exposure (e.g., asbestos exposure, cigarette smoking, hypertension). In other cases, it is impractical to design a study to examine the effects of a randomly assigned exposure (e.g., effects of exercise during adolescence on the risk of postmenopausal breast cancer). In these instances, investigators must use observational methods. In observational studies, in contrast to RCTs (which are considered experimental studies), the risk factor or disease process is allowed to take its course without intervention from the researcher.

The observational study that is closest to an experiment is the prospective cohort design. In this approach, exposed and unexposed subjects are identified and then observed over time for the development of disease. Unlike a true experiment, however, the exposures are observed rather than randomly assigned. Exposures are implicitly "assigned" based on physician recommendations (e.g., x-ray use), genetic heritage (e.g., family history of breast cancer), or individual behavior (e.g., dietary fat intake). Having obtained measures of disease occurrence (incidence rates or cumulative incidence) for both exposed and unexposed groups, the influence of exposure can be quantified as either the ratio of exposed to unexposed (the relative risk) or the difference between exposed and unexposed (the rate difference), as discussed earlier.

The primary advantage of a true prospective study over other observational designs is the opportunity to actively and intensively measure the exposures of interest before the period of disease induction. For example, instead of having subjects recall dietary fat intake over many years, intake could be calculated more accurately if periodic direct measurements were made. For rare diseases and those with a prolonged period between exposure and the manifestation of adverse effects (typical of chronic diseases), however, true prospective studies must be extremely large and prolonged and, therefore, are very expensive.

Table 2.3. Summary of Strengths and Limitations of Various Study Designs

Study Type	Strengths	Limitations
Experimental studies		
Randomized clinical trial	-Controls for bias by random assignment	-High cost -Not practical for many exposures (e.g., lifestyle, environmental, social/economic) -Not practical for long latency periods
Randomized community trial	-Can examine population wide exposures -Multicomponent interventions may be more effective	-Very high cost -Often involves small number of study groups
Quasi-experimental studies	-Can be used to study real world program and policy interventions -Can use multiple comparison groups, repeated baseline measures to strengthen design	-Potential for bias in comparison groups -Lack of control of confounding factors
Observational studies		
Prospective cohort	-Opportunity to measure risk factors before disease occurs -Can study multiple disease outcomes -Can yield incidence rates as well as relative risk estimates	-Often expensive -Requires large number of subjects -Requires long follow-up period -Difficult to control for all factors related to exposure
Case-control	-Useful for rare diseases -Relatively inexpensive -Relatively quick results	-Possible bias in measuring risk factors after disease has occurred -Possible bias in selecting control group -Identified cases may not represent all cases

One way to overcome these problems is to study exposures that occurred in the past and to monitor disease either up to the present or into the future. The ability to conduct these historical (or retrospective) cohort studies depends on the availability of exposure records that can be linked to disease outcomes. For example, in a study of the effect of chest x-ray and the subsequent rate of breast cancer occurrence, Andrieu et al. (2006) were able to identify a roster of exposed and unexposed subjects from an earlier study of women with a gene that increases the risk of breast cancer (*BRCA1* and *BRCA2*) This study demonstrated that women who had had a chest x-ray were 1.5 times more likely to develop breast cancer compared with women who had not had a previous chest x-ray.

A case-control study is another type of observational study that can be used to investigate the causes of chronic diseases. Case-control studies study subjects on the basis of their health outcomes (e.g., disease); this design intentionally oversamples subjects who have developed the disease of interest. In case-control studies, researchers identify a sample of subjects with the disease, or case patients (often, all available case patients), and a sample of people without the disease, or control subjects, from the same population that yielded the case patients.

The historical exposures that may have influenced disease risk are ascertained for all subjects, and the frequency of exposure among case patients is compared with that among control subjects. Such studies cannot yield incidence rates or cumulative incidence because the population at risk is not comprehensively defined; the control subjects are typically a sample of that source population, but the sampling fraction is unknown. An estimate of the ratio of incidence rates or risks can be obtained, however, by calculating the ratio of the odds of exposure among cases (the number exposed divided by the number not exposed) to the odds of exposure among controls, referred to as the odds ratio. The odds ratio is intended to approximate the relative risk. No estimate of the risk difference can be obtained from a case-control study.

The obvious advantages of case-control studies are the relative speed with which they can be conducted, because the latent period is all in the past, and the small number of subjects who have to be enrolled. In contrast to a cohort study, in which many subjects who never develop the disease must be monitored, a case-control study includes only a small but adequate fraction of the nondiseased population. The principal weakness is the study's vulnerability to some forms of bias that arise from the fact that the disease has usually occurred before risk factor information was ascertained. The strengths and limitations of prospective and case-control studies are summarized in Table 2.3.

To evaluate the potential causes of breast cancer mortality, the National Cancer Institute has supported an ongoing case-control study of breast cancer among residents of Wisconsin, Massachusetts, and New Hampshire since 1988 (Eliassen et al. 2006). These studies compare the exposures (e.g., physical activity patterns during adolescence, childbearing history) of women diagnosed with breast cancer (i.e., cases) with the exposure histories of women of the same age, who have not had breast cancer (i.e., controls). These studies have led to the identification of potentially modifiable risk factors for breast cancer, including a long menstrual history (early menarche and late menopause), having no children or not having breastfed, previous chest irradiation, postmenopausal hormone therapy use, obesity (particularly postmenopausal), and moderate to heavy alcohol intake.

How Do We Measure Associations between Exposures and Outcomes?

Relative risk is the primary measure used to determine if there is an association between an exposure (e.g., cigarette smoking) and a health outcome (e.g., lung cancer). As described above, the ratio of the risk in two groups is termed the "relative risk." Associations can be assessed anywhere along the continuum shown in Figure 2.1. For example, the risk of lung cancer mortality among smokers is 131 deaths per 100,000 persons, compared with only 11 deaths per 100,000 persons—yielding a relative risk of 11.9.

Similarly, studies have shown that the risk of becoming a smoker is higher among children who view smoking in the movies, versus children who do not view smoking in the movies (Charlesworth and Glantz 2005). For example, if 34% of children who view smoking become smokers, compared with only 20% of students who do not view smoking in the movies, the relative risk of smoking would be 34%/20% = 1.7. If this association is causal, one could say that children who view smoking in the movies are 1.7 times more likely to become smokers, compared with students who do not view smoking in the movies.

How Do We Evaluate whether the Study Results Are Valid?

Despite the increasing sophistication of research studies, uncertainty continues to exist in our understanding of the causes and consequences of chronic diseases. As most chronic disease epidemiology studies use observational methods, it is possible that errors in measurement or in selection of study subjects lead to spurious results. For example, there may be uncertainty in epidemiological studies about a measure of association, such as relative risk. If we obtain an odds ratio or relative risk of 2.0, are we fully confident that becoming exposed will truly double the risk of disease or that removing exposure will cut the risk in half?

Considerable expertise is needed in order to address uncertainty in research and to determine the quality of a research study. Riegelman uses an organizing framework to evaluate whether results from a research study are valid (Riegelman 2005). Two of the most important factors to consider include "confounding" and "bias."

Confounding

One reason for uncertainty is the possibility for confounding, in which the influence of an exposure of interest is mixed with the effect of another. This arises when a risk factor for the disease of interest is also associated with the exposure of interest. For example, people who drink alcohol are also more likely to drink coffee. When a study is conducted to examine alcohol use and breast cancer, the possible confounding role of coffee and caffeine must be taken into consideration. The estimated effect of alcohol on breast cancer will be confounded by caffeine intake if (1) caffeine and alcohol use are correlated and (2) caffeine use independently influences the risk of breast cancer.

In an experiment or RCT, these potential confounders can be balanced among the study groups through the design of the study and the random manner in which the exposure is assigned. Conversely, in an observational study, potential confounders must be measured and adjusted statistically. The strategy involves creating groups that are similar with respect to the potential confounder and examining the impact of the exposure of interest within each of those groups. For example, we could measure caffeine consumption and create strata of nonconsumers, low caffeine consumers, and high caffeine consumers and assess the role of alcohol use on breast cancer within each of those strata. As long as the potential confounder can be measured, the adjustments will be effective; however, some potential confounders, such as psychological stress, health consciousness, or dietary intake, may be difficult to measure, or we simply may be unaware of the risk factors that should be considered for adjustment.

Selection and Information Bias

A different source error comes from bias regarding how the subjects enter in the study or information is collected from study subjects. A faulty sampling mechanism, caused by such problems as nonresponse or refusal to participate, could produce a sample that has a higher or lower disease risk. Note that the only kind of sampling distortion that matters is the selection that influences disease risk. Similarly, in a case-control study, the selected case patients should reflect the exposure distribution of all case patients of interest, and the selected control subjects should reflect exposure in the overall population that produced the cases. The potential for a poorly constituted control group is a major threat to the validity of case-control studies. For example, when we choose control subjects from a hospital, health problems that lead to their hospitalization may be associated with the exposure of interest. Similarly, when we choose control subjects by telephone screening, omitting households without telephones could introduce a bias.

Another category of bias that can occur in epidemiological studies is the result of errors in classification of exposure or disease; this is referred to as information bias. Although efforts should be made to minimize such bias, errors in classification of exposure are unavoidable. Past exposures such as dietary intake, alcohol use, or physical activity are impossible to measure perfectly, even if we know what aspect of such exposures was the most relevant to disease causation. In many instances, the errors in exposure classification can be assumed to be similar for those who do and do not develop disease. This situation, referred to as nondifferential misclassification of exposure, results in a predictable bias in which the measure of association (such as odds ratio or relative risk) will be biased toward the null value of no association (1.0 for ratio measures, 0 for difference measures). This means that virtually all reported associations between exposure and disease will be diluted to some degree or missed entirely.

When the patterns of misclassification are different for the study groups, this is referred to as differential misclassification. This can occur when exposure is classified differently for diseased and nondiseased subjects or when disease is classified differently for exposed and unexposed subjects. Now the distortion in the measure of association can be in either direction (exaggerated or understated), depending on the precise pattern of error. A particular worry in case-control studies is the possibility of recall bias, which is a particular type of differential misclassification. Recall bias exists when the recall of exposure information is different for case patients than for control subjects, presumably because the illness experience of the case patients has in some way altered their memory or reporting of past events. Intuitively, one might expect case patients to overreport exposures that did not occur in an effort to explain their illness. Also, studies suggest that case patients may report accurately (presumably because their memory search is more thorough), whereas control subjects tend to underreport past exposures. In either situation, the reported exposures of case patients are artificially greater than the reported exposures of control subjects, and the relative risk is falsely elevated.

Information bias was thought to be responsible for the apparent association between breast cancer and abortion. Case-control studies demonstrated that women with breast cancer were more likely to report having had an abortion in the past, compared with similar women who did not have breast cancer. In contrast, prospective studies comparing the future risk of breast cancer among women who had an abortion with women who had not had an abortion did not find an association. Researchers suspect that information bias in the case-control studies led to a spurious association—since women may underreport having had an abortion. This underreporting may be more common among controls, since women diagnosed with breast cancer may have provided a more accurate history (Rookus and van Leeuwen 1996).

How Do We Assess whether Associations between Potential Etiologic Factors and Disease Are Causal?

Any intervention program or public health action is based on the presumption that the associations found in epidemiological studies are causal rather than arising through bias or for some other spurious reason. Unfortunately, in most instances in observational epidemiology, such as the research showing an association between viewing smoking in the movies and becoming a smoker, there is no opportunity to absolutely prove that an association is causal. Nonetheless, some principles are helpful when one must make this judgment.

The Bradford Hill criteria (Hill 1965) are often cited as a checklist for causality in epidemiological studies. These criteria have value but only as general guidelines. Most of Hill's nine criteria relate to particular cases of refuting biases or drawing on nonepidemiological evidence.

(1) Strength of association: Stronger associations are less likely to be the result of some subtle confounding or bias, presuming that major distorting influences would be more readily recognized than small ones.

(2) Consistency of association: The association is observed across diverse populations and circumstances, making a particular bias unlikely to explain a series of such observations.

(3) Specificity of association: The exposure causes one rather than many diseases, and the disease is associated with one rather than many exposures, suggesting that the association is not the result of bias. This is the weakest of the criteria for chronic diseases and might as well be eliminated since we now know that many, perhaps most, exposures that influence one health outcome affect others (e.g., tobacco, radiation, diet) and that virtually all diseases have multiple causes.

(4) Temporality: The exposure must precede the disease. This is the only absolute criterion for causality.

(5) Biological gradient: A dose–response curve, in which the risk of disease increases with increasing exposure, indicates that an association probably is not the result of a confounder or other bias. This criterion is generally valid, but the absence of a perfect dose–response pattern does not negate the possibility of a causal explanation because true thresholds or ceilings of effects may exist. Conversely, the presence of a dose–response gradient may be the result of a strong confounder that closely tracks the exposure.

(6) Plausibility: Evidence from other disciplines suggests the agent is biologically capable of influencing the disease. This is a useful supportive evidence when it is available, but the lack of advancements in the other biological sciences should not be used to negate an epidemiological observation.

(7) Coherence: The evidence should not be contradictory to the known biology and natural history of the disease (similar to the plausibility criterion).

(8) Experimental evidence: When attainable, experimental evidence for causality—obtained by removing or randomly assigning exposure—is very strong because both known and unknown confounders are controlled when exposure is randomly allocated.

(9) Analogy: When other similar agents have been established as causes of disease, then the credibility of theories regarding a new disease operating in a similar manner is enhanced. This is the epidemiological counterpart to plausibility; however, the supportive evidence comes from other areas of epidemiology rather than from other disciplines.

In practice, the establishment of evidence for causality is largely through the elimination of noncausal explanations for an observed association. Consider, for example, the evidence that alcohol use may increase the risk of breast cancer. A series of further studies might confirm that this relationship is valid and not a result of confounding or other biases such as detection bias (in which disease is more thoroughly diagnosed among alcohol users) or nonresponse bias. By whittling away alternative explanations, the hypothesis that asserts alcohol use causes breast cancer becomes increasingly credible. It is the job of critics to propose and test noncausal explanations, so that when the association has withstood a series of such challenges, the case for causality is strengthened.

The danger of formalizing the process of declaring causality on the basis of a checklist or any other mechanistic process is that it can only lead to endless debates about the degree of certainty and can impede needed public health actions. Those who argue that causality must be established with absolute certainty before interventions can begin fail to appreciate that their two alternatives—action and inaction—each have risks and benefits. Decisions must therefore be based on evidence that exposure causes diseases and must take into account the costs of intervention, the potential for the intervention to produce adverse side effects, and the potential costs of failing to act.

For example, the tobacco companies have argued, until recently, that the association between smoking and disease is uncertain. In a technical sense, we will always have some degree of uncertainty, especially with no definitive data from large numbers of subjects randomly assigned to be smokers and nonsmokers. We have no doubt, however, that the evidence indicates a need to intervene because smoking has no clear health benefits and scientists have exhausted all reasonable noncausal explanations for the strong associations observed between smoking and a number of diseases. Nonetheless, to the extent that tobacco companies continue to argue that the evidence for causality is not definitive, they create enough controversy to distract some policy makers from supporting needed interventions. Establishing causality is an important goal for epidemiological research, but absolute proof is not needed to justify action.

How Much Morbidity and Mortality Might Be Prevented by Interventions?

In each chapter in this text, authors report the relative risk (discussed previously) and the "population attributable risk." The population attributable risk is particularly useful in evaluating the potential benefits of intervention. When presented with an array of potential causal factors for disease, we need to evaluate how much might be gained by reducing or eliminating each of the hazards. Relative risk estimates indicate how strongly exposure and disease are associated, but this measure does not indicate directly the benefits that could be gained through modifying the exposure.

Attributable Risk

The attributable risk is a measure of how much of the disease burden could be eliminated if the exposure were eliminated. The attributable risk represents the proportion of disease among exposed people that actually results from the exposure. This issue might arise in a court case in which an exposed individual claims that the agent to which he or she was exposed caused the disease. Note that we are presuming that the associations reflect causality for the purposes of estimation. The attributable risk among exposed individuals is calculated as follows:

$$\frac{\text{relative risk} - 1}{\text{relative risk}}$$

Thus, a relative risk of 2.0 (risk is doubled by exposure) yields an attributable proportion among exposed people of 0.5. This suggests a 50% chance that the disease resulted from the exposure in this study population.

Population Attributable Risk

Of still greater potential value is the incorporation of information on how common the exposure is. Although some exposures exert a powerful influence on individuals (i.e., a large relative risk), they are so rare that their public health impact is minimal. Conversely, some exposures have a modest impact but are so widespread that their elimination could have great benefit. To answer the question, "what proportion of disease in the total population is a result of the exposure?" the population attributable risk or etiologic fraction is used. The population attributable risk can be calculated in two ways. First, if the rate in the exposed and unexposed population is known, then the population attributable risk is

$$\frac{\text{rate (total population)} - \text{rate (unexposed)}}{\text{rate (total population)}}$$

The population attributable risk can also be calculated with information only about the relative risk (usually obtained from research studies) and exposure in the population (often obtained from surveys). It is calculated as follows:

$$\frac{P_e \, (\text{relative risk} - 1)}{1 + P_e \, (\text{relative risk} - 1)}$$

where P_e represents the proportion of the population that is exposed.

The population attributable risk is used most commonly to estimate the proportion of disease caused by a certain risk factor, such as the proportion of lung cancer due to smoking. Assuming that the relative risk of lung cancer due to cigarette smoking is 15 and that 30% of the population are smokers, the population attributable risk is 0.81, or 81%. This would suggest that 81% of the lung cancer burden in the population is caused by cigarette smoking and could be eliminated if the exposure were eliminated.

Population attributable risk could also be used to estimate the proportion of a risk factor due to various "upstream" determinants. As described above, research has shown the children exposed to smoking are at increased risk of become regular smokers (Charlesworth and Glantz 2005). Assuming that this is a causal relationship, about 35% of smoking among adolescents could be attributed to exposure to smoking in the movies. This is illustrated in Figure 2.5, a hypothetical example for 100 children, which shows the relationship among

- risk (e.g., 34% of children exposed to smoking in the movies become smokers, compared with 20% of children not exposed to smoking in the movies)
- relative risk (e.g., children exposed to smoking in the movies are 1.7 times more likely to become smokers)
- population attributable risk (e.g., 35% of smoking among adolescents is because of smoking in the movies)

Because of the effects of interactions between various risk factors, population attributable risk estimates for a given disease can sometimes add up to more than 100%. Although population attributable risk estimates provide a useful estimate of the public health burden, they may be unrealistic as absolute goals because only rarely can a risk factor be completely eliminated.

Interactions among exposures, also known as effect modification, in the causation of disease are of particular importance in fully understanding etiology. Effect modification occurs when the effect of one exposure on disease risk is modified by the presence of another exposure. In the purest form, which is rarely observed, each of two exposures

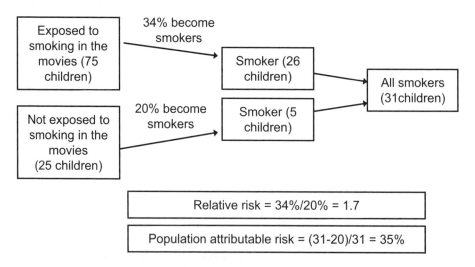

Figure 2.5. Risks of becoming a smoker among 100 children exposed/not exposed to smoking in the movies.

Table 2.4. Relative Risk Estimates for Lung Cancer Associated with Smoking and Asbestos Exposure among Insulation Workers

	Relative Risk Estimate	
Smoking Category	No Asbestos Exposure	Asbestos Exposure
Nonsmoker	1.0	5.2
Smoker	10.8	53.2

Saracci, R. The Interactions of Tobacco Smoking and Other Agents in Cancer Etiology. *Epidemiol Rev* (1987):9:175–193. Used by permission of Oxford University Press.

alone may have no effect on disease, but when the two are combined, a synergism occurs, causing an increase in disease. Conversely, two exposures that each can influence disease risk independently may be antagonistic, so that in combination they have a smaller effect on disease risk.

In epidemiological studies, interaction is measured as a combined effect of exposures that is larger than would be expected by simply adding the effects of the two separate exposures. Interaction is most easily detected by comparing the disease risk in groups with all combinations of exposure to the group exposed to neither agent. For example, cigarette smoking and asbestos exposure have been demonstrated to multiply the risk of lung cancer (Table 2.4). The risk of lung cancer among nonsmokers who are exposed to asbestos (relative risk = 5.2) is approximately half that of smokers who are not exposed to asbestos (relative risk = 10.8). However, a multiplicative effect is observed among smokers who are exposed to asbestos (relative risk = 53.2).

This measure of interaction has direct implications for developing intervention and prevention programs. If two factors interact, then the benefit of removing a given exposure will be greater if the other exposure is also present. For example, eliminating smoking has even more benefit for a group of workers exposed to asbestos than for individuals who are not exposed to asbestos.

Obviously, many factors enter into decisions about interventions, including certainty of causality, amenability to intervention, and social and political issues. However, in the traditional role of epidemiology as the basic science of public health, quantitative considerations of preventable disease can help us make a rational choice. How can we predict what benefits one or more of these interventions might yield in the community? This is where estimates of population attributable risk may be particularly useful. If one considers the earlier example of smoking and lung cancer, it is apparent that lung cancer incidence could be reduced by more than 80% if cigarette smoking were eliminated.

Additional Uses of Epidemiology in Chronic Disease Control

Although the use of epidemiology to describe the distribution and determinants of chronic diseases is necessary, it is not sufficient to prevent and control chronic diseases in populations. Developing evidence-based interventions require going beyond epidemiology to use other disciplines, such as behavioral and social sciences, environmental health sciences, health management, and policy analysis. This section briefly describes a set of questions and issues to be considered when interpreting data in chronic disease epidemiology. It also describes several analytic tools and processes of interest to practitioners (e.g., meta-analysis, expert panels).

Why Should Action Not Be Taken on the Basis of a Single Epidemiological Study?

As scientists and practitioners committed to improving the public's health, there is a natural tendency to scrutinize the epidemiological literature for new findings that would serve as the basis for prevention or intervention programs. In fact, application to public health practice is a principal motive for conducting such research. Adding to this inclination to intervene may be claims from investigators regarding the critical importance of their findings, media interpretation of the findings as the basis for immediate action, and even community support for responding to the striking new research findings with new or modified programs or elimination of existing programs. Appreciation of epidemiological methods applied to chronic disease prevention and control leads to the inevitable conclusion that a single epidemiological study is never sufficient for making such decisions. Well-designed and carefully conducted research adds evidence to assist in setting policy, but the stakes are so high in economic terms and public credibility that cautious interpretation of research findings that have not been replicated is required.

We have already discussed the validity of epidemiological research and criteria for causality, but a more direct consideration of why a single study is insufficient for action should be helpful. Breast cancer had rarely been considered a disease that might be affected by environmental pollutants, in contrast, for example, to lung or bladder cancer. However, a paper published in 1993 by Wolff et al. (1993) changed that perception. This study, which was well designed, carefully conducted, and certainly worthy of publication, reported that pesticide residues from dichlorodiphenyltrichloroethane (DDT) in the blood were positively associated with the risk of breast cancer, with relative risks on the order of 3.0. Media interest was high, and the notion that a common, life-threatening disease could be related in part to environmental agents was both terrifying and promising of the potential for intervention. Although these exposures had been accrued over a lifetime, if found to be related to breast cancer, interventions to reduce body burden would be worthy of consideration. For other reasons, largely based on adverse effects on wildlife, DDT was banned more than 20 years ago.

How could a study be "good epidemiology," published in a reputable journal, generate substantial media and public interest, and yet not be worthy of any action on the part of public health practitioners? First, despite the talents of the investigators and quality of the resulting study, its findings may simply be wrong or misleading. That is, for reasons discussed earlier, even within the population studied, there may well be no causal association between DDT residues and breast cancer. One critical concern is whether the measured levels of DDT residues were affected by early stages of breast cancer rather than the reverse. Also, potential confounding by lactation was examined but produced rather anomalous results, and the number of cases available for analysis was small.

Second, even if valid for the population under study, the generalizability of the findings has to be examined. Can results from women in the New York area be applied to other populations with different exposure histories, ethnic backgrounds, and risk factor profiles? Although we look for universal explanations for disease and occasionally find strong causal factors that account for most of the disease in most populations (e.g., smoking and lung cancer), these successes are rare. More often, there are a multitude of interacting factors that must be considered for extrapolating findings from one population to apply to another.

Finally, even if valid and generalizable, thus making a contribution to public health decision, what action should be taken for an agent that was banned long ago? At the margins, in evaluating costs and benefits, this research would (if valid) add to the evidence of health harm from exposure, but in this case, there is not a clear decision to be made. If we had two comparably effective pesticides, one of which was associated with health harm and one was not, such evidence might tip the balance. Public health decisions must integrate the full array of considerations regarding risks and benefits of different courses of action, as discussed below.

How Do We Assess a Series of Epidemiological Studies and Integrate the Evidence to Make Decisions?

Several important methods and tools are available to epidemiologists and practitioners to assist in determining when public health action is warranted. It is often necessary to use these because exposure-disease relationships in chronic disease epidemiology typically show relatively weak associations, in which the relative risk estimate is not too different from the null value of 1.0. Most accepted risk factors for breast cancer are associated with relative risks of less than 5.0, and often less than 3.0, considered by some to be weak (Wynder 1987). The closer a relative risk estimate comes to unity (i.e., 1.0), the more likely that it can be explained by methodological limitations such as confounding, misclassification, and other sources of bias. Yet, as noted earlier in the description of population attributable risk, even when a risk factor is weak, if highly prevalent in the population, the public health impact can be large. Therefore, we have great interest in determining when even relatively weak associations provide the basis for public health intervention, which can only come from a series of well-designed studies.

Although it is tempting to intervene rather than conduct yet more studies in the face of a serious health problem, in the long run, evaluation of all major interventions is essential. To conduct such an evaluation, investigators must study a comparison group and rule out other factors as the cause of any observed change. The diagnosis of breast cancer in a prominent local citizen, for example, could be the main cause of increased breast cancer screening, rather than a community education program. In programs that combine several interventions, investigators may be able to determine which intervention(s) actually produced the health benefits and whether the results of an evaluation are generalizable to a different population. The debate continues, for example, as to whether the results of studies of reduced serum cholesterol in men can be applied to women. Thus, determining whether a proposed intervention will actually bring about more good than harm can be difficult.

It is important to note that even ostensibly useful interventions may not have positive effects and that almost all programs may have unintended negative effects. An education program to increase breast cancer screening, for example, could have no effect on women who need screening, yet it could raise anxiety among younger women at low risk who do not need screening. The usefulness of a particular screening test is based on several characteristics, including its accuracy, reproducibility, sensitivity, and specificity.

This section provides an overview of three related methods that have proven useful in assimilating large bodies of evidence in chronic disease epidemiology. In turn, the summarized evidence can be useful in shaping public health interventions and policies. Because this consideration is necessarily brief, readers are referred to other sources for more detail.

Systematic Reviews and Meta-analysis

The volume of information published about chronic diseases and their risk factors in journals every day is far beyond what any person can remain current. In order to address this problem, researchers conduct "systematic reviews" to consolidate all the information from studies addressing a single clinical or public health question. Systematic reviews use explicit and comprehensive (systematic) methods to identify, select, and critically assess all relevant research on the issue under consideration. To avoid bias, all Cochrane reviews start as a published protocol stating in advance how the review will be carried out (searching for data, appraising and combining study data). Over the past two decades, systematic reviews have been increasingly using "meta-analysis" to provide a more quantitative approach for integrating the findings of individual studies (Petitti 2000). Petitti describes four steps in undertaking a meta-analysis.

(1) Identify relevant studies. Relevant studies must first be identified for inclusion in the meta-analysis. These can be identified through computerized sources such as MEDLINE, review articles, other journal articles, doctoral dissertations, and personal communications with other researchers.

(2) Inclusion/exclusion criteria. Explicit criteria distinguish a meta-analysis from a qualitative literature review. Criteria for inclusion should specify the study designs to be included; the years of publication or of data collection; the languages in which the articles are written (e.g., English only or English plus other specified languages); the minimum sample size and the extent of follow-up; the treatments and/or exposures; the manner in which the exposures, treatment, and outcomes were measured; and the completeness of information. Study quality should also be considered. As a minimum, studies whose quality falls below some specified rating criteria should be excluded. Rating scales may be developed to assess the quality of the included studies, although the basis for rating can be controversial and it may be preferable to consider the actual study attributes rather than a summary quality score.

(3) Data abstraction. In this step, important features of each study are abstracted such as design, number of participants, and key findings. The abstraction summary should produce findings that are reliable, valid, and free of bias. Blinding of abstractors and reabstraction of a sample of studies by multiple abstractors may be beneficial.

(4) Statistical analysis and exploration of heterogeneity. The data are combined to produce a summary estimate of the measure of association along with confidence intervals. Data are also examined to determine if the effect across studies was homogeneous and, if not, the reasons for heterogeneity.

Meta-analysis is most useful for combining the results of multiple, small, RCTs whose results are generally consistent yet imprecision is a problem in each individual trial. The method is less useful in situations where trials have found truly heterogeneous results through different methods or because the relationship of interest varies across populations. Partly for that reason, one must be careful not to be overwhelmed by the impressively large numbers that can be accrued in a meta-analysis. While the improved precision is a strength, one must also consider the validity of combining results across studies and whether the estimated size of the effect is large enough to warrant action.

Risk Assessment

Quantitative risk assessment is a widely used term for a systematic approach to characterizing the risks posed to individuals and populations by environmental pollutants and other potentially adverse exposures. Risk assessment has been described as a "bridge" between science and policy making. In the United States, its use is either explicitly or implicitly required by a number of federal statutes, and its application worldwide is increasing. There has been considerable debate over the U.S. risk assessment policies, and the most widely recognized difficulties in risk assessment are because of extrapolation-related uncertainties (i.e., extrapolating low-dose effects from higher exposure levels). Risk assessment has become an established process through which expert scientific input is provided to agencies that regulate environmental or occupational exposures.

Four key steps in risk assessment are hazard identification, risk characterization, exposure assessment, and risk estimation (U.S. EPA 2005). An important aspect of risk assessment is that it frequently results in classification schemes that take into account uncertainties about exposure-disease relationships. For example, the U.S. EPA has developed a five-tier scheme for classifying potential and proven cancer-causing agents, which includes the following: (1) group A, carcinogenic to humans; (2) group B, probably carcinogenic to humans; (3) group C, possibly carcinogenic to humans; (4) group D, not classifiable as to human carcinogenicity; and (5) group E, evidence of noncarcinogenicity for humans.

Expert Panels and Consensus Conferences

Most government agencies, in both executive and legislative branches, and voluntary health organizations, such as the American Cancer Society, use expert panels when examining epidemiological studies and their relevance to health policies and interventions (Brownson 2006). Ideally, the goal of expert panels is to provide peer review by scientific experts of the quality of the science and scientific interpretations that underlie public health recommendations, regulations, and policy decisions. If conducted well, peer review can provide an important set of checks and balances for the regulatory process. Optimally, the expert review process has the following common properties: experts are sought in epidemiology and related disciplines (e.g., clinical medicine, biomedical sciences, biostatistics, economics, ethics); panels typically consist of 8 to 15 members and meet in person to review scientific data (written guidance is provided to panel members); panel members should not have financial or professional conflicts of interest; draft findings from expert panels are frequently released for public review and comment before final recommendations. One of the successful outcomes of expert panels has been the production of guidelines for public health and medical care. A recent example is the publication of the second edition of the *Guide to Clinical Preventive Services* (AHRQ 2005). This document is a careful review of the scientific evidence for and against hundreds of preventive services (e.g., childhood immunizations, tobacco cessation counseling). Its production was overseen by a ten-member expert advisory committee. A related effort is presently underway to

Table 2.5. Key Concepts in Chronic Disease Epidemiology

Term	Definition
Incidence rate	$$\frac{\text{Number of new events in a specified period}}{\text{Number of persons exposed to risk during this period}}$$
Relative risk	$$\frac{\text{Risk of disease or death in the exposed population}}{\text{Risk of disease or death in the unexposed population}}$$
Population attributable risk	$$\frac{\text{Rate of a disease in a population that is associated with (attributed to) a certain risk factor}}{\text{Total rate of a disease in the population}}$$

develop a *Guide to Community Preventive Services* (available at www.thecommunityguide. org).

Consensus conferences are a related mechanism that is commonly used to review epidemiological evidence. The National Institutes of Health have used consensus conferences since 1977 to resolve controversial issues in medicine and public health. For example, a highly publicized consensus conference on breast cancer screening was held to determine whether mammography screening for women ages 40 to 49 years reduces breast cancer mortality.

There is one important difference between expert panels such as the U.S. Preventive Services Task Force and a consensus development panel, such as the one for breast cancer screening for women in their forties. Expert panels can take time to develop their recommendations, while the consensus development panel must make its decision within a 2.5-day conference, risking some sacrifice of careful judgment for speed.

Both expert panels and consensus development panels work best when they publish along with their recommendations the rationale for their recommendation and the process used to arrive at that rationale. In considering the recommendations of such panels, one should examine the extent to which they are evidence-based or instead rely on "expert" opinion. Evidence-based recommendations should be given much greater weight.

Conclusions

In this chapter, we have discussed the issues that help to determine whether associations are causal, the role of intervention research in disease control, and the uses of epidemiological evidence to make public health decisions. We have also outlined several types of epidemiological study designs and the biases that can complicate interpretation of results. We have discussed issues that help to determine whether associations are causal, as well as the role of intervention research in disease control. Such information serves as a foundation that will help readers address the more complex issues of chronic disease etiology and control. Some of the key epidemiological concepts that the reader will encounter in other chapters are summarized in Table 2.5.

The final section in each chapter of this book describes the evidence that exists for effective programs and policies. Epidemiological, behavioral, social science, and other research methods have been used to identify effective intervention strategies that can be implemented at the individual (Saha et al. 2001) and, more recently, community level (Truman et al. 2000). These methods are described in more detail in the following two chapters.

Suggested Reading

Brownson, R.C., and D.B. Petitti, editors. *Applied Epidemiology* (2nd ed.). New York: Oxford University Press (2006).

Cochran Collaboration and Library website. Available at: http://www.cochrane.org.

Friss, R.H., and T.A. Sellers. *Epidemiology for Public Health Practice.* Frederick, MD: Aspen (1996).

Gordis, L. *Epidemiology* (2nd ed.). Philadelphia: W.B. Saunders (2000).

Riegelman, R.K. *Studying a Study and Testing a Test: How to Read the Medical Evidence* (5th ed.). Philadelphia.

Szklo, M., and F.J. Nieto. *Epidemiology: Beyond the Basics.* Gaithersburg, MD: Aspen (2000).

References

Agency for Healthcare Research and Quality (AHRQ). *Guide to Clinical Preventive Services, 2005: Recommendations of the U.S. Preventive Services Task Force.* AHRQ Publication No. 05-0570. Rockville, MD: AHRQ (2005 June). Available at http://www.ahrq.gov/clinic/pocketgd05/. Accessed January 19, 2009.

Andrieu, N., D.F. Easton, J. Chang-Claude, et al. Effect of Chest X-Rays on the Risk of Breast Cancer among BRCA1/2 Mutation Carriers in the International BRCA1/2 Carrier Cohort Study. *J Clin Oncol* (2006):24(21):3361–3366.

Brownson, R.C. Epidemiology and Health Policy. In: Brownson, R.C., and D.B. Petitti, editors, *Applied Epidemiology: Theory to Practice* (2nd ed.). New York: Oxford University Press (2006):361–363.

Brownson, R.C., and D.B. Petitti, editors. *Applied Epidemiology* (2nd ed.). New York: Oxford University Press (2006).

Charlesworth, A., and S.A. Glantz. Smoking in the Movies Increases Adolescent Smoking: A Review. *Pediatrics* (2005):116(6):1516–1528.

Centers for Disease Control and Prevention (CDC). Colorectal Cancer Test Use among Persons Aged >50 Years—United States, 2001. *Morbid Mortal Weekly Rep.* (2003):52(10):193–196.

Centers for Disease Control and Prevention (CDC). Use of Mammograms among Women Aged >40 Years—United States, 2000–2005. *Morbid Mortal Weekly Rep.* (2007):56(3):49–51.

Centers for Disease Control and Prevention (CDC). *An Introduction to Epidemiology.* Available at http://www.cdc.gov/excite/classroom/intro_epi.htm#defined. Accessed August 1, 2008.

Coughlin, S.S., Z. Berkowitz, N.A. Hawkins, and F. Tangka. Breast and Colorectal Cancer Screening and Sources of Cancer Information among Older Women in the United States: Results from the 2003 Health Information National Trends Survey. *Prev Chronic Dis* (2007 Jul):4(3): A57. Erratum in: *Prev Chronic Dis* (2007 Oct):4(4):A114.

Eaker, E.D., L. Jaros, R.A. Vierkant, P. Lantz, and P.L. Remington. Women's Health Alliance Intervention Study: Increasing Community Breast and Cervical Cancer Screening. *J Public Health Manag Pract* (2001 Sep):7(5):20–30.

Eliassen, A.H., G.A. Colditz, B. Rosner, W.C. Willett, and S.E. Hankinson. Adult Weight Change and Risk of Postmenopausal Breast Cancer. *JAMA* (2006):296(2):193–201.

Felitti, V.J., R.F. Anda, D. Nordenberg, D.F. Williamson, A.M. Spitz, V. Edwards, et al. Relationship of Childhood Abuse and Household Dysfunction to Many of the Leading Causes of Death in Adults. The Adverse Childhood Experiences (ACE) Study. *Am J Prev Med* (1998 May):14(4):245–258.

Foege, W.H., R.C. Hogan, and L.H. Newton. Surveillance Projects for Selected Diseases. *Int J Epidemiol* (1976):5:29–37.

Fryback, D.G., N.K. Stout, M.A. Rosenberg, A. Trentham-Dietz, V. Kuruchittham, and P.L. Remington. Chapter 7: The Wisconsin Breast Cancer Epidemiology Simulation Model. *J Natl Cancer Inst Monogr* (2006):(36):37–47.

Goodwin, J.S., J.L. Freeman, D. Freeman, and A.B. Nattinger. Geographic Variations in Breast Cancer Mortality: Do Higher Rates Imply Higher Incidence or Poorer Survival? *Am J Public Health* (1998):88(3):458–460.

Hill, A.B. The Environment and Disease: Association or Causation? *Proc R Soc Med* (1965):58:295–300.

Institute of Medicine. *The Future of Public Health*. Washington, D.C.: National Academy Press (1988).

Jaros, L., E.D. Eaker, and P.L. Remington. Women's Health Alliance Intervention Study: Description of a Breast and Cervical Cancer Screening Program. *J Public Health Manag Pract* (2001):7(5):31–35.

Koplan, J.P., and S.B. Thacker. Fifty Years of Epidemiology at the Centers for Disease Control and Prevention: Significant and Consequential. *Am J Epidemiol* (2001 Dec 1):154(11):982–984.

Liang, S.Y., K.A. Phillips, M. Nagamine, U. Ladabaum, and J.S. Haas. Rates and Predictors of Colorectal Cancer Screening. *Prev Chronic Dis* (2006 Oct):3(4):A117.

McDowell, I., and C. Newell. *Measuring Health: A Guide to Rating Scales and Questionnaires*. New York: Oxford University Press (1996).

Mokdad, A.H., J.S. Marks, D.F. Stroup, and J.L. Gerberding. Actual Causes of Death in the United States, 2000. *JAMA* (2004):291:1238–1245.

Petitti, D.B. *Meta-Analysis, Decision Analysis, and Cost-Effectiveness Analysis: Methods for Quantitative Synthesis in Medicine* (2nd ed.). New York: Oxford University Press (2000).

Reynolds, P., S.E. Hurley, R.B. Gunier, S. Yerabati, T. Quach, and A. Hertz. Residential Proximity to Agricultural Pesticide Use and Incidence of Breast Cancer in California, 1988–1997. *Environ Health Perspect* (2005):113(8):993–1000.

Riegelman, R.K. *Studying a Study and Testing a Test: How to Read the Medical Evidence* (5th ed.). Philadelphia: Lippincott Williams & Wilkins (2005). Available at www.studyingastudy.com.

Ries, L.A.G., D. Harkins, M. Krapcho, et al. *SEER Cancer Statistics Review, 1975–2003*. Bethesda, MD: National Cancer Institute (2006).

Ries, L.A.G., D. Melbert, M. Krapcho, et al. *SEER Cancer Statistics Review, 1975–2005*. Bethesda, MD: National Cancer Institute (2008). Available at http://seer.cancer.gov/csr/1975_2005/ (based on November 2007 SEER data submission). Accessed July 19, 2009.

Rookus, M.A., and F.E. van Leeuwen. Induced Abortion and Risk for Breast Cancer: Reporting (Recall) Bias in a Dutch Case-Control Study. *J Natl Cancer Inst* (1996):88(23):1759–1764.

Saha, S., T.J. Hoerger, M.P. Pignone, S.M. Teutsch, M. Helfand, J.S. Mandelblatt, and Cost Work Group, Third US Preventive Services Task Force. The Art and Science of Incorporating Cost Effectiveness into Evidence-Based Recommendations for Clinical Preventive Services. *Am J Prev Med* (2001 Apr):20(3 Suppl):36–43.

Saracci, R. The Interactions of Tobacco Smoking and Other Agents in Cancer Etiology. *Epidemiol Rev* (1987):9:175–193.

Tinker, T., and E. Vaughan. Risk Communication. In: Nelson, D.E., R.C. Brownson, P.L. Remington, and C. Parvanta, editors, *Communicating Public Health Information Effectively: A Guide for Practitioners*. Washington, D.C.: American Public Health Association (2002):185–203.

Truman, B.I., C.K. Smith-Akin, A.R. Hinman, K.M. Gebbie, R. Brownson, L.F. Novick, et al. Developing the Guide to Community Preventive Services—Overview and Rationale. The Task Force on Community Preventive Services. *Am J Prev Med* (2000 Jan):18(1 Suppl):18–26.

U.S. Environmental Protection Agency (EPA). *Guidelines for Carcinogen Risk Assessment. Risk Assessment Forum.* PA/630/P-03/001F. Washington, D.C.: U.S. EPA (2005 March).

Wolff, M., P. Toniolo, E. Lee, M. Rivera, and N. Bubinn. Blood Levels of Organo Chlorine Residues and Risk of Breast Cancer. *J Natl Cancer Inst* (1993):85:648–652.

Writing Group for the Women's Health Initiative Investigators. Risks and Benefits of Estrogen Plus Progestin in Healthy Postmenopausal Women. Principal Results from the Women's Health Initiative Randomized Controlled Trial. *JAMA* (2002):288(3):321–333.

Wynder, E.L. Workshop on Guidelines to the Epidemiology of Weak Associations. Introduction. *Prev Med* (1987):16:139–141.

CHAPTER 3

INTERVENTION METHODS FOR CHRONIC DISEASE CONTROL

Robert J. McDermott, Ph.D., Julie A. Baldwin, Ph.D.,
Carol A. Bryant, Ph.D., and Rita D. DeBate, Ph.D.

Introduction

D espite the fact that the leading chronic diseases often have well-known risk factors, preventing them from occurring is an arduous task. This challenge stems from the fact that most chronic diseases have their origins in social, cultural, environmental, and behavioral factors, thereby making their causes (and potential interventions) both complex and multilevel. Social and cultural factors influencing the development, dissemination, and consequences of chronic diseases include, but are not limited to, social and economic status, race, education, income, and access to health care (McQueen 2007).

Interventions to prevent or control chronic diseases can address the individual level, the system level, or the community level, where both system- and individual-level strategies are organized to become multilevel or comprehensive programs. Moreover, interventions can address primary prevention (e.g., reducing the risk of disease through exercise, healthy eating, nonsmoking), secondary prevention (e.g., early detection through mammograms for women, prostate exams for men, blood pressure checks for all), or tertiary prevention (e.g., management of disease to minimize confounding complications through carefully monitored insulin intake for diabetes management, adherence to a prescribed diet, or moderate to vigorous exercise several days per week for patients who have had a heart attack).

Interventions seeking to alter a health risk profile may address behaviors at the individual level—such as poor diet, tobacco use, excessive alcohol consumption, physical inactivity, unsafe sexual activity, and so on. Health-promoting messages can be presented through print and electronic media, including Internet, or directly from people such as health care providers and health education prevention specialists, teachers, employers, members of the faith-based community, or a host of other individuals.

Other chronic disease interventions focus on system-level changes, including policy development or change, economic incentives, and specific actions within the health care system. Examples of these interventions include food product labeling of nutrition content, enactment of tobacco excise taxes to reduce purchases by new users, and insurance coverage for screening mammograms, among other actions.

Multilevel interventions seek to change many aspects of the environment that contribute to development of chronic diseases in people. These interventions include a combination of activities that prioritize change at the individual level as well as the system level.

Sometimes, comprehensive interventions also address root causes of some chronic diseases, such as poverty, low literacy, or limited education. In addition, they may attempt to garner social support for positive health behaviors. These interventions often involve health advocacy groups and empower coalitions comprised of individuals or whole communities to take action.

Multiple Determinants of Chronic Disease

To be effective, chronic disease prevention and control efforts must consider the multiple determinants of chronic disease, including lifestyle and health risk behaviors, the health care system, the physical environment, and social and economic factors. The influence of these determinants on chronic disease is described briefly below.

Behavioral Determinants

Many chronic diseases can be prevented, have their onset delayed, or have their symptoms significantly reduced through modest changes in individual behaviors. For example, the Centers for Disease Control and Prevention (CDC) estimates that by eliminating three risk behaviors—poor diet, physical inactivity, and smoking—80% of heart disease and stroke, 80% of type 2 diabetes, and 40% of cancers would be eliminated.

Americans have experienced significant increases in obesity during the past three decades. According to the CDC, 30% of U.S. adults 20 years and older—more than 60 million people—are obese. People with a Body Mass Index (BMI) greater than 30 have an increased risk of developing chronic diseases, including hypertension, hyperlipidemia (e.g., high total cholesterol or high levels of triglycerides), type 2 diabetes, coronary heart disease, stroke, gallbladder disease, osteoarthritis, sleep apnea and respiratory problems, and some cancers (endometrial, breast, and colon). Threats to health caused by obesity can be reduced through proper nutrition and physical activity.

Adults are not alone in experiencing obesity. Since the 1980s, the prevalence of obesity has more than doubled in preschool children between the ages of 2 and 5 years and in youth between 12 and 19 years. Moreover, it has more than tripled in children ages 6–11 years (Committee on Prevention of Obesity in Children and Youth 2005). Based on 2003–2004 data, 18.8% of children 6–11 years and 17.4% of youth 12–19 years were overweight (BMI ≥ 95th percentile for age and sex). In addition, 37.2% of children 6–11 years and 34.3% of youth 12–19 years were at risk for being overweight (BMI ≥ 85th percentile but <95th percentile for age and sex) (Ogden et al. 2006).

Many Americans are not following a healthy diet. The American Cancer Society reports that more than three-quarters (77%) of adults eat fewer than five servings of fruits and vegetables a day. Many Americans are also not active. CDC research indicates that the direct medical costs associated with physical inactivity totaled nearly $77 billion in 2000. Almost 25% of Americans participate in no physical activity. Smoking adversely affects nearly every organ in the body. Whereas smoking is causally linked to various types of cancers, smokers are also at risk of developing cardiovascular disease, respiratory illness, and other health problems. This relationship notwithstanding, one in five American adults is a current smoker.

Health Care Determinants

Medicare spending is expected to double by 2016 to $863 billion. U.S. health care spending is nearly $2 trillion a year and could double in the next decade (Henry J. Kaiser Family

Foundation 2007). The cost of treating chronic diseases contributes significantly to these increases. If the health care system reallocated funds to focus more on primary prevention, including broader reimbursement for prevention services, the overall cost of health care might be more manageable. With secondary prevention (e.g., screening for hypertension, hyperlipidemia, breast cancer, prostate cancer), asymptomatic problems can be detected early when they are more responsive to less invasive and less costly treatment and more likely to benefit from accompanying lifestyle changes. In addition, when people do get sick, more resources directed toward helping them manage their chronic diseases (tertiary prevention) will minimize hospitalizations and provider visits, thereby minimizing associated health care costs.

Although the health care system has the resources to provide preventive services, health care providers have few, if any, financial incentives to focus on prevention. Of the approximately 15,000 Medicare reimbursement codes, only a fraction of these are for preventive services (Shurney 2007). The U.S. health care system is designed around treating patients once they become chronically ill. Adding patient education billing codes would offer an incentive to health care providers to rely more on teaching patients about the benefits of physical activity, better nutrition, and other health promoting activities. Such education would be especially beneficial as part of primary and secondary prevention initiatives.

Environmental Determinants

Americans have witnessed many discussions during the past few years, in both scholarly literature and the popular press, about the obesity epidemic. One cause attributed to the rise in obesity is the role of the so-called built environment—those aspects of a person's surroundings that contribute favorably or unfavorably to his or her individual health initiatives. These elements broadly encompass not only one's local environment (e.g., inside the home and school), but also one's surroundings, such as neighborhoods, urban development, land use, transportation, industry, and agriculture. An environment that has accessible and safe sidewalks, nearby parks, and such entities as bike trails and community swimming pools will encourage people to engage in physical activity. Likewise, stairways at work that are aesthetically pleasing, signs reminding people to use the stairs, and such amenities as showers and facilities for changing clothes at work after exercising are pro-health surroundings. In contrast, an environment that lacks aesthetics and is dangerous (e.g., sidewalks in need of repair, no sidewalks, heavy vehicular traffic, poor lighting) will discourage people from being physically active. A person's home environment also has an important influence on activity level—a point that has become more evident with the presence of multiple-television households, desktop computers, and sophisticated video games—all of which contribute to sedentary behavior.

The built environment also influences what one chooses nutritionally. Menu choices in schools, restaurants, and work site cafeterias may offer healthy choices, but perhaps too often, less healthy alternatives. Neighborhoods lacking grocery stores or convenient farmers' markets may be devoid of fresh fruit and vegetable options, thereby forcing people to purchase what is cheap or available, regardless of its nutritional value. The many linkages between the built environment and obesity have resulted in diverse considerations for health promotion programming (Papas et al. 2007).

Social Determinants

According to Freudenberg (2007), "Health promotion provides a powerful tool for improving health in the twenty-first century, but researchers and practitioners have yet to achieve consensus on its scope. Globalization, urbanization, an aging population, and rising rates of chronic diseases are creating new health challenges throughout the world. How can health professionals respond to these changing circumstances? What are the relevant paradigms for promoting health today?"

For the past three decades, public health professionals have viewed individual behaviors (e.g., smoking, alcohol and other substance abuse, sexual activity, physical activity, nutrition) as contributing to most of the suboptimal health of Americans. Consequently, most interventions have been focused on change at the individual level. Although individual behaviors are clearly determinants of health status, focusing on the individual presents a limited and inefficient view of change on a population scale.

Population health is the science of variations in health status among segments within a society or culture. Population health scientists study the indicators of health behavior and health status as they relate to a social determinants' perspective. These indicators encompass social, economic, political, and environmental factors. Therefore, issues such as level of education, level of social or economic stressors, access to health care, transportation, housing, income inequality, or social inclusion or exclusion stemming from sex, race, or age are relevant matters. Policymakers and health professionals often blame persons at high risk for poor health on their own "lifestyles" or "choices" when, in fact, their available lifestyle choices are limited, and their behaviors are strongly influenced by their social, economic, cultural, or physical environment (CDC 2005). The many observed health disparities are largely a result of these social determinants.

If the United States is to achieve the goal of reducing the burden of chronic disease and eliminating health disparities, there will need to be a better understanding of the relationship between individual health behaviors and social context. Advertising, pricing, and retail practices of the food, alcohol, and tobacco industries that target particular population segments strongly influence health choices. In addition, the lack of public transportation may deter persons with less income and people on fixed incomes from meeting health care appointments. The high cost of insurance or the limits in insurance coverage may prohibit persons from taking advantage of secondary prevention screening technologies. More education correlates with better health and longevity, yet in many American cities, half of all youth who enter high school fail to graduate (Freudenberg 2007). Whereas improvement in school graduation rates could reduce disparities in health, especially among the most disadvantaged, public health agencies and law and policymakers rarely make the school dropout problem a priority for altering the status quo in health matters. Stronger alliances among public health authorities, policymakers, and educators may profoundly influence population health. The study of such mechanisms ought to be an academic priority for the first part of the twenty-first century.

Levels of Intervention: An Ecological Perspective

An ecological perspective takes into consideration the fact that health decisions are influenced by numerous factors (Figure 3.1). Therefore, this perspective addresses individual as well as social and environmental factors as the foci of chronic disease interventions.

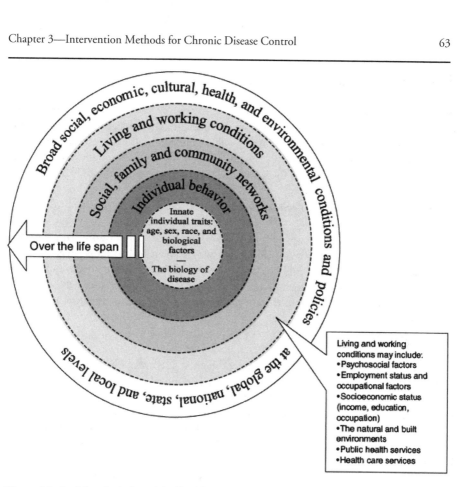

Figure 3.1. Social ecological model of health.

Whereas individual health behaviors are popular targets of interventions, they often result in a "victim blaming" culture that fails to take into account the influence of the social and physical environment that may also need to be modified. Using an ecological approach acknowledges the interaction of an individual and the environment and takes into account the following elements that influence health behavior:

- *Intrapersonal factors*—altering knowledge, attitudes, skills, and future behavioral intentions at the level of the individual person.
- *Interpersonal factors*—understanding and accessing the relationships that people have with other individuals in their social network such as friends, peers, and co-workers, family members, neighbors, and others from whom behavioral patterns and behavioral norms are acquired.
- *Organizational factors*—using organizations such as schools, faith-based groups, work sites, or health care facilities to direct, influence, or support health behavior change and help to define health behavior norms.
- *Community factors*—catalyzing interest within an area having geographic or political boundaries to leverage power structures to achieve a particular set of health objectives, perhaps to address the most serious health problems among persons

typically in the weakest position to advocate on their own behalf (e.g., the rural poor, members of underrepresented minorities, less educated, physically or mentally disabled).

- *Policy factors*—advocating for and organizing and analyzing policies and procedures, regulations, and laws that favorably influence the fight against chronic diseases.

These factors are examined further in this chapter.

Intrapersonal (Individual) Approaches to Chronic Disease Intervention

Intrapersonal models or theoretical frameworks draw on the assumption that people can be motivated to take individual action that changes their health knowledge, attitudes, skills, behavioral intentions, and eventual behavior. Although there are many such approaches, the potential usefulness of four popular theoretical approaches will be demonstrated here for their potential in chronic disease prevention and intervention.

Health Belief Model

The Health Belief Model (HBM) was one of the first attempts of behavioral scientists to use theory to study preventive health behaviors. The model was developed by a group of social psychologists at the U.S. Public Health Service in the 1950s to explain the failure of people to participate in programs designed to prevent or detect disease (Hochbaum 1958). According to the original model, the likelihood of someone taking a preventive action to avoid disease is enhanced if they perceive themselves to be susceptible to the disease, perceive the consequences of contracting the disease to be at least of moderate severity, recognize the benefits of choosing a preventive action, view the benefits as being superior to the costs and barriers of adopting the behavior, and receive cues to action, the cumulative internal or external messages that affect their readiness to take action. In the 1980s, another component was added to the HBM—self-efficacy, or one's beliefs that she or he can perform the activity of interest.

A simple illustration of the HBM in action can be seen in the following example of a 50-year-old woman deciding whether to seek a baseline mammogram, a health behavior in the category of secondary prevention. She may see herself as susceptible (e.g., past her 49th birthday, no previous baseline mammogram). She may see breast cancer as being severe (e.g., in the event of disease, possible mastectomy, physical disfigurement, loss of self-esteem, and even death). She may perceive the benefits of mammography (e.g., early detection of disease, and consequently, easier intervention, peace of mind that there is no disease) to outweigh any perceived costs or barriers (e.g., fear of disease, fear or embarrassment related to the examination). Her motivation may be inspired by cues to action (e.g., reminder postcard received in the mail, recommendation by a physician, message seen or heard through mass media, learning that an acquaintance just had a mammogram or recently received a breast cancer diagnosis). Finally, her likelihood of following through is enhanced if she possesses the confidence and ability (i.e., self-efficacy) to ask her physician about receiving a baseline mammogram, to know where to obtain one, to feel comfortable with calling for an appointment, and to know she can get herself to the facility. Whereas the HBM has been used largely to explain the failure of people to adopt preventive behaviors, the model can be useful for intervening at points along the way to develop targeted messages and other intervention strategies (i.e., changing perceptions of susceptibility and severity, assessing benefits and costs/barriers accurately, creating effective cues to action to which women will respond, and increasing women's confidence to follow through in receiving the procedure).

Transtheoretical Model and Stages of Change

The Transtheoretical Model, more commonly referred to as the Stages of Change Model, was developed by James O. Prochaska and Carlo C. DiClemente (1983) through their work on understanding how people quit smoking. The essence of the model is that not everyone is at an equivalent stage of readiness to change health behavior, and thus, interventions need to take on different characteristics to be responsive to these various stages.

The model is comprised of a series of stages, the exact number of which may vary. In the precontemplation stage, there is no intention to change behavior, perhaps not even any awareness that change is an alternative or something that can result in an improvement of health or lifestyle. In the contemplation stage, an individual may recognize that change is a possibility but is still thinking about making the change or adaptation and has not fully committed to doing so. In the preparation stage, people may gather information about the consequences of altering their lifestyle, affirming the need to change, and possibly, making a plan to do so at a specified time in the future—usually, in the next 30 days. At the action stage, the person actually implements the change, shifting the plan from one that is theoretical to one that is operational—a period that may last up to 6 months. If the action stage becomes routinized, one moves on into the maintenance stage—the consolidation of the behaviors initiated previously into one's typical lifestyle. At this point, people can go in one of two possible directions—enter the termination stage, where the former problem behavior is no longer perceived as being acceptable, or the relapse stage, where there is recidivism and a resumption of former, less healthy behavior.

With respect to planning and designing interventions, taking a person's stage of readiness to change into account can enhance the likelihood of moving them along the behavioral continuum, and ultimately improving success. For example, addressing the needs of a person who has a long history of physical inactivity and is contemplating change is quite different than intervening with someone who is in the preparation stage or who has moved back and forth between that stage and the action stage. Whereas the contemplative individual may require encouragement to evaluate the pros and cons of behavior change and identification of positive outcomes and expectations, the person who has already "tested the waters" instead may need to find social support, receive specific suggestions for overcoming obstacles to cementing the change, and seek satisfaction from small, incremental successes in the direction of the desired behavior. It is important to realize that this model is more circular or spiral in nature than linear. People may advance a stage but then fall back. Moreover, individuals may go through multiple cycles of contemplation, preparation, and action before reaching a terminal stage or exiting the system altogether. Understanding "where people are at" will assist intervention efforts.

Theory of Planned Behavior

The Theory of Planned Behavior (TPB) posits that individual behavior is driven by behavioral intentions (Ajzen 1985, 1991). Behavioral intentions are influenced by a person's collective attitudes about the behavior in question, the subjective norms with respect to carrying out the behavior, and the person's perception of the ease with which the behavior can be carried out (behavioral control). This theory has its roots in Fishbein's model of behavioral intentions (1967) and the theory of reasoned action (Ajzen and Fishbein 1973; Fishbein and Ajzen 1975).

With the TPB, one's attitude toward the behavior (e.g., daily exercise) is the sum of all the positive feelings (e.g., doing something good for one's health, feeling better about one's self, exercise is a popular activity) or negative feelings (e.g., exercise wears me out, exercise is inconvenient, exercise will make me sore) about performing the behavior. This sum comes from determining one's beliefs about the consequences arising from a behavior and an evaluation of the desirability of these consequences. A person's overall attitude is expressed as the sum of the individual consequences x desirability assessments for all expected consequences of the behavior.

The beliefs underlying a person's subjective norms are called normative beliefs. The subjective norm is defined as a person's perception of whether people important to him or her value the behavior and think the person should engage in it. The opinion of any significant other is weighted by the motivation that the person has to comply with the wishes of that significant other. The overall subjective norm is expressed as the sum of the individual perceptions x motivation assessments for all significant others who may influence the person considering the behavior.

Behavioral control is a person's perception of the difficulty of carrying out the behavior (e.g., skills, available time, sacrifice of other activities for this particular behavior). In the TPB, the control that people have over their behavior is a continuum of behaviors from ones that are easily carried out to ones requiring much time, effort, resources, and so on. The link between behavior and behavioral control in the TPB should be between behavior and actual behavioral control rather than perceived behavioral control. However, the difficulty of assessing actual behavioral control has resulted in behavioral scientists using perceived control as a proxy measure.

Health Locus of Control Model

Locus of control refers to a person's expectations about where control over events in life resides. In a health context, who or what is responsible for that which happens to one's health? Expectancy, which concerns future events, is an important part of the locus of control construct. Locus of control is grounded in expectancy value theory, that is, if a person values a particular outcome and believes that carrying out a particular behavior will result in that outcome, then they are more likely to pursue that behavior.

Rotter (1966) classified beliefs concerning who or what influences things along a continuum from completely internal control to completely external control. Whereas internal control is the expectancy that future events are largely under the control of the individual, external control refers to the belief that future events are outside of individual control—such as under the control of others or due entirely to fate or chance.

Since its introduction more than 40 years ago, the locus of control construct has seen many permutations and iterations through the work of behavioral scientists in numerous fields. However, health behavior researchers have used the locus of control idea extensively. Among the most widely used health-specific measure is the Multidimensional Health Locus of Control Scale (Wallston, Wallston, and DeVellis 1978).

In practice, people who believe that their health status is largely within their own control are more likely to embrace preventive, positive health behaviors. Persons perceiving their locus of control to be more external are less inclined to take on preventive actions, concluding that a higher power, fate, luck, or other influences beyond their control ultimately will determine their health outcomes. Public health workers attempting to influence health behavior choices may have better success with a target group that possesses more of an internal locus of control perspective. Conversely, changing policies or using a systems approach may be more effective for individuals who perceive an external locus of control.

Interpersonal Approaches to Chronic Disease Intervention

Models of interpersonal health behavior assume that the interpersonal environment is one of the most powerful sources of influence for health-related behavior and health status. "People's environments provide the means, model, reinforcements, resources, and sources of influence from which people gain information, skills, self-confidence, self-management competencies, coping behavior, and support" (Glanz, Rimer, and Lewis 2002, p. 265).

Social Cognitive Theory

Social cognitive theory (SCT) is one interpersonal-level theory that has been readily used in a number of chronic disease prevention and control studies. SCT addresses both the psychosocial dynamics influencing health behavior and methods for promoting behavioral change. Within SCT, human behavior is explained in terms of a triadic, dynamic, and reciprocal model in which behavior, personal factors (including cognitions), and environmental influences all interact (Bandura 1977). Critical factors include the individual's ability to monitor behavior, to anticipate the outcomes of behavior (including overcoming the obstacles in performing a given behavior), to self-determine or self-regulate behavior, and to reflect on and analyze experiences (Bandura 1977).

SCT emphasizes the importance of enhancing a person's behavioral capability (knowledge and skills) and self-confidence (self-efficacy) to engage in a particular health behavior. Self-efficacy, one of the most important constructs in this theory, has been demonstrated to predict the initiation of a new health behavior, the continuation of the target behavior, and the maintenance of complex health behaviors. The most powerful and consistent way of enhancing self-efficacy is through mastery of a task. Successful SCT interventions engage participants in small steps of an enacted behavior, with self-monitoring as well as feedback from others. Bandura (1977, 1986) also developed a number of other SCT constructs that are important to understand and intervene in health behavior. These constructs include reciprocal determinism, environments and situations, observational learning, behavioral capability, reinforcement, outcome expectations, outcome expectancies, self-control of performance, and managing emotional arousal. Case studies and examples of how these constructs might be translated into intervention strategies are described in detail by Glanz, Rimer, and Lewis (2002).

SCT has wide applicability for different audiences and has been successfully used in physical activity promotion interventions (e.g., Marcus et al. 1998) in health education campaigns for people with chronic medical conditions such as arthritis (Lorig et al. 1998), and in a number of cardiovascular disease prevention programs for children and adults

(Bandura 1986; Farquhar et al. 1990; Puska and Uutela 2000). SCT is appealing for health promotion programs because it addresses both the causal mechanisms of individual behavior and guides the design of intervention approaches. By recognizing the importance of the environment, people, and behavior, SCT provides a framework for designing, implementing, and evaluating comprehensive behavioral change programs.

Family-Based Interventions

Family-based interventions often draw upon the enhancement of existing network linkages and entail training network members in skills for providing support and in mobilizing groups to maintain their networks. For example, family members have been trained to provide support to individuals who are in programs to stop smoking (Cohen and Lichtenstein 1990). A media campaign entitled "Friends Can Be Good Medicine" focused on informing people about the influence of social support on health and encouraging them to connect with their friends and family by telephone or in person (Hersey et al. 1984).

Family interventions have also been used to prevent adolescent smoking and alcohol use. "Family Matters" was a family-directed program focused on prevention of substance abuse (smoking and alcohol use) among teens age 12–14 years. The program was guided by social influence theories, persuasion theories, SCT, communication theory, and social development theory (Bauman et al. 2001). The core assumption of the program was that families could become engaged to influence adolescent substance abuse through constructive family interactions and communication that strengthened family and adolescent norms against substance abuse.

Friends and Social Networks

Another type of social network intervention entails developing new social network linkages through mentor programs, buddy systems, and self-help groups. Groups such as Alcoholics Anonymous, Overeaters Anonymous, and Weight Watchers provide access to new social networks designed to provide cognitive, instrumental, and emotional support for lifestyle change (Coreil, Bryant, and Henderson 2001).

Peer groups are critically important for adolescent-focused interventions. Social network characteristics have been shown to influence risk behaviors among youth (Ellen et al. 2005; Ennet, Bailey, and Federman 1999; Friedman and Aral 2001; Valente, Gallaher, and Mouttapa 2004). For example, studies have found that strong familial relationships among American Indian populations are protective against substance abuse (Baldwin et al. in press; Beauvais and Oetting 1999; Sanchez-Way and Johnson 2000). Peer relationships, self-esteem, and the importance of spirituality and religion also protect against substance abuse (Fisher, Storck, and Baco 1999; Sanchez-Way and Johnson 2000). Oman et al. (2004) found that having peer role models, family communication, use of time for religion, good health practices, future aspirations, and making responsible choices are protective for alcohol and drug use. Positive orientation to school and academic achievement are also consistently protective factors against substance abuse (Fergus and Zimmerman 2005). Having these assets creates a greater likelihood for feelings of hope, aspirations, and resilience, all of which have been found to be important for youth. Resources external to youth found to be protective include family connectedness and parental involvement with school (Fergus and Zimmerman 2005).

Social Support and Social Networks

The powerful influence that social relationships have on health has elicited a great deal of interest among public health researchers and practitioners. An understanding of the impact of social relationships on health status, health behaviors, and health decisions has the potential to make important contributions to the design of effective interventions. One important function of social relationships is the provision of social support. Social support has been defined and measured in numerous ways. According to House (1981), social support is the functional aspects of relationships that can be defined as four broad types of supportive behaviors: (1) emotional support, (2) instrumental support, (3) informational support, and (4) appraisal support. Social networks, in comparison, are linkages between people; social networks may or may not be supportive (Heaney and Israel 2002). Characteristics that describe a network include the extent to which network members are homogeneous in terms of demographic characteristics such as age, race, and socioeconomic status; the extent to which network members live in close proximity to each other (geographic dispersion); and the extent to which network members know and interact with each other (density) (Heaney and Israel 2002).

Several typologies of social network and social support interventions have been suggested (Gottlieb 2000; Israel 1982; McLeroy, Gottlieb, and Heaney 2001). These interventions include strengthening existing social network linkages, developing new social network linkages, enhancing networks through the use of indigenous natural helpers, and building networks at the community level through participatory community capacity development and problem-solving processes.

Natural Helpers

Natural helpers are respected and trusted members of social networks to whom other network members turn for advice, support, and other types of aid (Israel 1985). In addition to providing direct support, natural helpers also link social network members to each other and to resources outside of the network. Natural helper interventions have been conducted in a number of different communities, including urban neighborhoods, rural counties, residential institutions for the elderly, migrant farmworker communities, and churches (Israel 1985). For example, the Black Churches Project (Eng and Hatch 1991) identified natural helpers within congregations of black churches in North Carolina and provided health education training to the identified helpers. Likewise, the North Carolina Breast Cancer Screening Program built on the lessons learned through the "Save Our Sisters" program (Eng 1993) and extended the use of lay health advisors (LHAs) to five poor rural counties in North Carolina (Earp et al. 2002). Another study that used LHAs focused on migrant farmworker women serving as "promotores" to address maternal and child health issues of families in the Midwest (Booker et al. 1997) and the East Coast (Watkins et al. 1994). Village health workers in Detroit also have undertaken activities in their neighborhoods to improve the health of women and children (Parker et al. 1998). DeBate et al. (2004) found improvements in health practices and community competence after using LHAs in Charlotte, North Carolina, to reduce cardiovascular disease and diabetes among African Americans. In summary, the use of LHAs has emerged as an effective strategy in disease prevention programs.

Examples of Interpersonal-Level Interventions

As noted earlier, SCT has been used in a number of chronic disease prevention programs. For example, SCT was used to determine why fourth- and fifth-grade children were not eating sufficient servings of fruit, juice, and vegetables (Baranowski, Perry, and Parcel 2002). The research team creatively used SCT to design an intervention (called Gimme 5!—Fruit and Vegetables for Fun and Health) to increase availability and accessibility of these foods. Skills training activities, including role-playing, were taught to children to encourage them to ask their parents to purchase their favorite fruit, juice, or vegetable at the grocery store; to have their favorite fruit, juice, or vegetable available for meals and snacks; and to select restaurants that offer a variety of these healthy foods. Self-regulation skills were promoted by having students monitor their consumption, set goals for eating more, problem-solve when goals were not met, and reward oneself when goals were achieved. The intervention also effectively targeted home availability, accessibility, and consumption of fruits, juices, and vegetables.

Organizational-Level Venues for Intervention

Health Care System and Clinical Services

The health care system is an effective setting for providing screening and follow-up services that help to control chronic diseases. Historically, the health care setting has been used for blood pressure monitoring, diabetes control, cardiovascular health assessment, cancer screening, and various other secondary prevention measures. However, the health care setting is an ideal, although often underutilized, venue for patient education, including primary prevention. Research has firmly established that physician advice given in the health care setting provides a powerful and motivational message for cardiovascular disease risk reduction (CDC 1999), weight loss, dietary change, and physical activity improvement among adolescents (Kant and Miner 2007), tobacco control (Lancaster and Stead 2004), and alcohol consumption (Grossberg, Brown, and Fleming 2004).

An intervention that has shown effectiveness without being especially burdensome on health care providers or patients is known as the "brief intervention." Brief interventions usually last for 5–60 minutes and consist of counseling and education. Sometimes, there are multiple sessions, perhaps initiated by a primary care provider, and then transitioned to a health education specialist to carry on the intervention. However, a brief intervention can be as limited as 30 seconds and consist of just one "teachable moment" session conducted by an alert and opportunistic health care provider. The content, duration, and number of sessions may depend on the provider, the patient's receptivity and readiness to change, the setting, and previous patient–provider rapport.

There are a number of circumstances that lend themselves to brief interventions such as the ones listed in Table 3.1. However, a creative and alert health care provider will be able to note many other opportunities to intervene.

The brief intervention can be leveraged at any point in the health promotion–disease prevention–treatment continuum depending on the patient's readiness to change. For best results, the brief intervention is applied as early in the sequence as possible to prevent disease through structured advice. Brady (1995) points out some characteristics of brief interventions that make them adaptable in a number of situations:

- The interaction is private
- The process often involves the patient giving a personal account in his or her own words
- The process includes the provider sharing knowledge and talking about options, thereby offering the patient choices
- The health professional's role is nonjudgmental and nonconfrontational
- The patient's decision whether or not to change is his or hers to make

Schools

Schools are excellent venues for primary and secondary prevention. Philosophically, schools ought to convey health education along with the many other essential subjects that comprise modern education. Youth attend school for 12 or more years and are a captive audience for educators and health professionals to convey prevention messages and for health care providers to conduct selective health screenings. Moreover, establishing healthy habits in youth can help prevent many chronic health problems later in life that are attributable to unhealthy eating, sedentary lifestyle, sexual risk-taking, and other health-related issues. In addition to teaching health education, schools can offer services that promote health and monitor key health indicators in children and youth (e.g., height, weight, blood pressure). A coordinated or comprehensive school health program (Figure 3.2) offers an eight-component model illustrating a multitude of health promoting opportunities within the school setting for youth as well as adults (Allensworth and Kolbe 1987). Many public health care providers are interested in working with school systems, thus offering an opportunity for an effective partnership.

Prevention research focused on children and youth has yielded a number of evidence-based interventions that have applicability in school health education curricula. Several initiatives have emanated from the CDC's Prevention Research Centers, a network of 33 academic institutions that partner with public health agencies and community members

Table 3.1. Examples of Brief Interventions for Health Promotion

- When taking a blood pressure reading, sharing information about the causes and problems of high blood pressure, talking about exercise and proper diet as ways to reduce blood pressure

- Encouraging a patient at risk of developing diabetes to talk about the foods they eat, offering nutrition advice, talking about practical ways to shop for food and prepare healthy meals

- When treating an infant or child with a respiratory infection, talking to the mother who smokes to find out if she knows about passive smoking, recommending ways of reducing the child's exposure to smoking, and asking if she is thinking about quitting

- Finding out from a patient who drinks alcohol if they are drinking in a harmful way, and if they are, addressing the need to adjust their drinking to a healthier level, perhaps conveying factual information about the health effects of alcohol

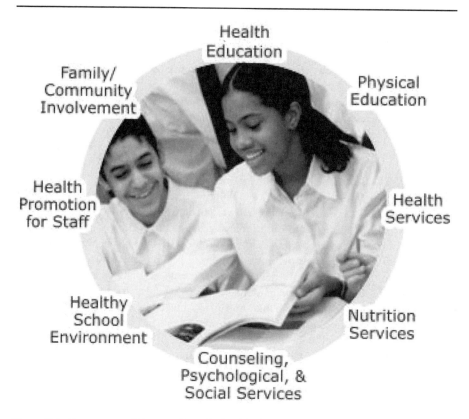

Figure 3.2. Components of the coordinated school health program (from CDC 2007b).

to conduct applied research in disease prevention and control (CDC 2007a). Three programs especially worth noting include one aimed at smoking cessation among adolescents (Not-On-Tobacco [N-O-T]) and two targeting physical activity and healthy eating for elementary and middle school children (Coordinated Approach to Child Health [CATCH] and Planet Health) (Franks et al. 2007). Shared features of these three programs include (1) identification of staff and resources that facilitate program implementation and dissemination; (2) stakeholder involvement (e.g., teachers, students, other school personnel, parents, nonprofit organizations, professional organizations) during all phases of program development and dissemination; (3) planning for dissemination of programs; and (4) rigorous evaluation (Franks et al. 2007).

Work Sites

The workplace is an excellent venue for health promotion interventions as a large proportion of the U.S. population typically spends half or more of its waking hours at work (Partnership for Prevention 2001). The 2000 census indicates that 130 million U.S. residents (65%) 16 years and older were employed by public or private employers (Clark et al. 2007). The number of work sites that have some form of work site health promotion program has grown from approximately 5% in the 1980s (O'Donnell and Harris 1994) to 95% of work sites with 50 or more employees in 1999 (Association for Worksite Health Promotion 1999). Work site health promotion programs offer benefits for both the employee as well as the employer by reducing the burden of employee health issues, moderating medical costs, reducing absenteeism, increasing productivity, and increasing employee morale (O'Donnell and Harris 1994). Research suggests that well-designed and implemented work site wellness programs can improve employee productivity, lower chronic disease health risks, and may have the potential for producing a positive return on the organization's investment (Goetzel et al. 2004).

Organizational leaders are becoming more aware of the economic burden of chronic disease conditions that impact employee absence, on the job productivity ("presenteeism"), disability program use, workers compensation use, turnover, and medical care costs (Goetzel et al. 2003, 2004). Employees with multiple risk factors for chronic disease (e.g., smoking, poor dietary habits, sedentary behaviors) are more likely to contribute to the health care expenditures via health care usage, absenteeism, disability, and overall loss of productivity (Partnership for Prevention 2001). Between 21% and 58% of medical claims are associated with modifiable health risk factors such as poor nutrition, lack of exercise, excess stress, and other lifestyle factors (Wellness Councils of America 2007).

A cost analysis of conditions affecting U.S. businesses revealed that physical and mental health expenditures averaged $3,703 (1999 U.S. dollars) per eligible employee (Goetzel et al. 2003). With regard to physical health conditions, employers paid an average of $2,505 per employee for medical care, $703 for absenteeism, and $316 for short-term disability use, resulting in a total of $3,524 in health and productivity expenditures (71% in medical care, 20% absenteeism, 9% short-term disability use) (Goetzel et al. 2003). Among physical health expenditures, 53% were because of chronic maintenance of angina pectoris, essential hypertension, and diabetes mellitus. Expenditures due to mental health conditions included $94 for medical care (53%), $61 for absenteeism (34%), and $24 for short-term disability (13%), for a total of $179 in health and productivity expenditures (Goetzel et al. 2003).

In addition to the aforementioned physical and mental health conditions, employee obesity is also related to increased health care costs and a barrier to providing affordable employee health insurance (Finkelstein, Fiebelkorn, and Wang 2005). In an analysis of overweight and obesity-attributable absenteeism and health care costs in 2005, the estimated cost of obesity in a workplace of 1,000 employees per year was $285,000 (Finkelstein, Fiebelkorn, and Wang 2005).

The aggregated medical, absence, short-term disability, and average loss of productivity costs per employee per year were highest for the following chronic disease conditions: hypertension ($368), heart disease ($368), depression/mental illness ($348), arthritis ($327), migraine headaches ($214), any cancer ($144), respiratory disorders ($134), and asthma ($100) (Goetzel et al. 2004). Interestingly, approximately 61% of the total costs associated with these chronic health conditions were because of on-the-job productivity losses (Goetzel et al. 2004).

Numerous benefits that can be garnered through workplace interventions to prevent and control chronic diseases, include the following:

- *Improved employee productivity.* Employees with multiple health risk factors have been found to be less productive than employees with fewer risk factors (Partnership for Prevention 2001).

- *Reduced absenteeism.* In an analysis of the effects of work site wellness programs and employee absenteeism, it was determined that there was an average savings of $5.00 for every dollar spent on employee wellness.
- *Reduced employee health risks.* For a cost of $32 per employee, the Coors Brewing Company "Lifecheck" program reduced employee risk for cardiovascular disease by decreasing high blood pressure, high cholesterol, and weight among its employees (Aldana 1998).
- *Reduced health care costs.* An analysis of eight work site wellness programs determined a reduction of health care expenses averaging $3.35 for every dollar spent on employee health promotion (Partnership for Prevention 2001).
- *Improved corporate image.* Work site wellness programs offer further gains to employers by demonstrating social responsibility in addition to promoting the health of employees and their families in addition to retirees (Partnership for Prevention 2001).

What are the barriers and reinforcing factors related to work site–based prevention programs? Analysis of the 2004 HealthStyles Survey revealed that the most preferred work site health promotion services are fitness centers, on-site exercise classes, weight loss programs, and policies related to paid time to exercise at work and healthy vending and/or cafeteria choices (Kruger et al. 2007). The greatest barrier to employee participation in work site wellness programs was time, more specifically, no time during the workday or after work hours (Kruger et al. 2007).

Faith-Based Organizations

Faith-based organizations have a long history of supporting health promotion programs in areas such as general health education, screening for and management of high blood pressure and diabetes, weight loss and smoking cessation, cancer prevention and control, geriatric care, nutritional guidance, and mental health care (DeHaven et al. 2004). DeHaven et al. (2004) examined the literature on health programs in faith-based organizations to determine the effectiveness of these programs and found that faith-based health programs can significantly increase knowledge of the disease, improve screening behavior and readiness to change, and reduce the risk associated with disease and disease symptoms.

Community-Level Interventions

"Community" has been defined in numerous ways. A community may refer to a group bounded geographically (a neighborhood, city, or other place) or one that shares special social ties (Stephens 2007). In either case, a shared identity and interdependency are extremely important. Not all neighborhoods or social groups are a community: rather, the group's members must share a sense of belonging, common symbols, norms and values, conditions and constraints, and mutual influence (Campbell and Jovchelovitch 2000). This section looks first at the physical aspects of community as a place, then examines the social features of community as an identity, and finally, how each influences chronic disease incidence and prevalence.

Intervention strategies should be selected based on the needs and priorities of the specific population so as to identify appropriate interventions that are compatible with the population's knowledge, attitudes, perceptions, and sociocultural and economic circumstances (Bartholomew et al. 2006). Many researchers also have stressed that chronic disease prevention and control programs will be more effective if the population of interest is actively involved in prioritizing, developing, and implementing all intervention activities (Bracht and Gleason 1990; Rothman 1970). A full partnership between public health professionals and local community members can lead to empowerment of individuals and groups and result in more effective management of health issues and economic, social, and political forces in the community (Minkler and Wallerstein 2003). Participation also facilitates community ownership of the intervention, which may provide better access to community leaders, and ultimately, lead to changes in community norms. Community members can play an important role in tailoring the intervention to fit the norms and values of the community and ensure that the proposed interventions are culturally sensitive and relevant. Communication messages that do not meet the needs of the specific population will likely not be well-received by the audience. Understanding the specific population is also essential for identifying appropriate communication channels.

Active Involvement of the Priority Population as Partners

With the increasing emphasis on partnership approaches to improving community health, community-based participatory research (CBPR) is rapidly becoming a more common approach in chronic disease prevention and control. CBPR is defined as "a collaborative process that equitably involves all partners in the research process and recognizes the unique strengths that each brings" (Minkler 2004, p. 686). The Institute of Medicine has identified CBPR as one of eight new areas in which all schools of public health should be offering training (Gebbie, Rosenstock, and Hernandez 2003). As outlined by Israel et al. (2005), the fundamental principles of CBPR are that (1) it is participatory, (2) it engages community members and researchers in a collaborative process to which each contributes equally, (3) it is a co-learning process, (4) it involves local capacity building and systems development, (5) it is an empowering process through which participants can gain increased control, and (6) it results in a balance between research and action.

Wallerstein and Duran (2003) explain that in CBPR, the relationship between researchers and communities requires trust and mutual commitment over time. "These relationships are subject to overall power relations in society, the history of research in the community, the immediate issues facing the community, and the origins of this particular research and the ability to negotiate relationships between the CBPR researchers and the community representatives" (Wallerstein and Duran 2003, p. 38). Thus, time is needed to develop both trust and the infrastructure to support it. Encouraging active participation in CBPR activities also requires the use of methods and approaches that help community members feel at ease and elicit local input. These methods may include nominal group processes, collaborative mapping of community indicators, risks, and assets, and support for bringing community viewpoints to the table (Wallerstein et al. 2005). Several CBPR assessment instruments have been developed to help provide guidance for CBPR projects (Brown and Vega 2003; Green et al. 2003).

Community Coalitions

Community coalitions offer promise for building capacity and competence among organizations and, ultimately, for increasing empowerment in the communities that coalitions serve (Chavis 2001; Kegler et al. 1998). Community coalitions are often initiated to assist communities in mobilizing resources and coordinating activities that improve the public's health. Coalitions may contribute to all phases of program delivery, from planning to implementation to evaluation to maintenance (Valente, Chou, and Pentz 2007). Depending on a given situation, a coalition can operate at different steps in a "continuum of decision making," ranging from an advisory role to full control over resources (Wandersman and Florin 2000).

The theoretical basis for the development and maintenance of community coalitions is derived from many fields, including community development, citizen participation, political science, interorganizational relations, and group process (Butterfoss and Kegler 2002). The increasing use of coalitions as a health promotion strategy parallels the growth of large-scale community-level health promotion and chronic disease prevention efforts over the past two decades, such as the National Heart, Lung, and Blood Institute's demonstration projects (Mittelmark 1999). These projects, which include the Stanford Three Community and Five City Projects and the Minnesota and Pawtucket Heart Health Programs, utilized community advisory boards to plan and implement cardiovascular disease prevention efforts (Carlaw et al. 1984; Farquhar et al. 1990; Lefebvre et al. 1987; Mittelmark et al. 1986; Shea and Basch 1990). Additionally, the CDC supported formation of community coalitions in the Planned Approach to Community Health (PATCH), which was widely adopted by state and local health departments in the late 1980s and early 1990s (Green and Kreuter 1992).

Media Advocacy

This section focuses on media advocacy, "the strategic use of mass media in combination with community organizing to advance healthy public policies" (Wallack 2000). Media advocacy differs from other uses of mass media in its attempt to shift power back to communities so they can change policies that affect their lives (i.e., addressing the power gap) rather than promote messages about the need for individual behavior change (Wallack 1997). By learning to use media to address system-level factors, communities are empowered to participate in the political process.

Like other forms of advocacy, a variety of tasks are used to create a shift in public opinion and bring about policy change: agenda setting, framing, and working with groups to reach opinion leaders to change public policies and address social inequities. Agenda setting refers to activities that shine the "spotlight on a particular issue and hold it there" (Wallack et al. 1993, p. 61). Media coverage is used to bring the policy issue to the public's attention and onto the official public agenda. News coverage is of special importance in this process because it can lend credibility to an issue. Media advocates also use paid advertising and other forms of media coverage to shape the nature of the debate.

How an issue is framed is of critical importance. Framing uses symbols, metaphors, and stories to define an issue, to suggest who is responsible for the problem, and to propose solutions. Media advocates try to frame public health issues in ways that direct attention to environmental- or system-level factors responsible for the problem, and suggest policy solutions rather than hold individual "victims" responsible for it.

Mass media also are used to place pressure on decision-makers (Wallack et al. 1993). As with media coverage designed to garner public support, media advocates frame policy positions to make them attractive to policymakers and use a variety of techniques to keep their issue in the news (e.g., by framing an event as a milestone, a breakthrough, or a controversial topic). Because policy battles often wage for years, media advocates must identify new opportunities to reintroduce an issue and keep it in the media spotlight over long periods of time (Wallack 2000).

Media advocacy in public health dates back to the 1980s when it was used by public health groups working to control tobacco and alcohol abuse. Tobacco control advocates, for instance, have used media advocacy to stop the distribution of Uptown cigarettes in Philadelphia and defuse a national public relations event organized by Phillip Morris. Since then, media advocacy has been applied to a number of public health topics, including gun control, suicide prevention, lead poisoning, and others (Wallack 2000). The major advantage of using media advocacy to address these issues is "escaping a traditional, limited focus on disease conditions and instead promote a greater understanding of the conditions that will support and improve the public's health" (Wallack 1997, p. 350).

Health Policy and Legal Interventions

The important role of policy in contributing to both individual and population health cannot be denied. Policies, regulations, and laws can have far-reaching consequences. The enactment of laws and enforcement of regulations are two mechanisms for promoting justice and ensuring that people's health rights are protected. A *policy* has been defined by some as "a course of action adopted and pursued by a government, party, statesman, or other individual or organization" (Subcommittee on Health and Environment of the Committee on Interstate Commerce 1976, p. 124).

Three broad domains of health policy and law include the areas of health care, public health, and bioethics (Teitelbaum and Wilensky 2007). Health care policy can be examined in terms of access to care, quality of care, and financing of care. The primary focus of public health policy concerns how, where, and under what circumstances government and law intervene in the name of protecting the public's health, safety, and general welfare. Finally, bioethics concerns itself with ethical issues about medical practice and biomedical research.

Health policy and law can also be examined in terms of the stakeholders whose lives or functions are impacted by particular regulatory measures. Where chronic disease issues are concerned, key stakeholder groups are likely to include patients and their families, health care providers, managed care organizations and insurance companies, pharmaceutical companies, medical supply companies, employers large and small, the research community, any of the organizational or community groups identified previously in this chapter, and more.

Health policies address a wide spectrum of issues, so how does one go about examining a proposed policy in a systematic fashion? Although formats may differ from situation to situation, almost all policy analyses contain the following elements (Teitelbaum and Wilensky 2007):

- A problem statement that defines the scope of the problem under analysis
- A background statement that provides as much factual information and data as possible for policymakers to understand the scope of the problem
- A description of the context or "landscape" that identifies primary stakeholders and the postures they may adopt and how they are likely to be affected by the proposed policy

- A statement that presents and analyzes the possible impact of all reasonable options
- A recommendation that offers the best case scenario or best option

Of these five elements, perhaps the most important one concerns the criteria for analyzing or weighing options. These criteria include such measures as cost and cost-benefit; feasibility within the political landscape and administrative obstacles, legality, fairness, timeliness; and the probability that the population of interest will actually benefit from the option (Teitelbaum and Wilensky 2007).

Several online resources exist to assist health policy advocates (Partners in Policymaking, 2007). An abbreviated listing of these includes the following:

- Centers for Medicare and Medicaid Services
  Comprehensive information on Medicare, Medicaid, and SCHIP, including coverage, laws, regulations, and extensive resource section.
  http://cms.hhs.gov
- Data Resource Center for Child and Adolescent Health
  Research tool for collecting demographic and other health-related data about this population and making state-by-state comparisons.
  http://www.childhealthdata.org
- Healthy People 2010
  Health care information and publications that challenge individuals, communities, and professionals to take specific steps to ensure good health is enjoyed by everyone.
  http://www.healthypeople.gov
- National Health Law Program (NHeLP)
  Provides extensive information on health care law affecting low-income people. The site is updated daily with health law news, legislative analysis, and health law Internet links.
  http://www.healthlaw.org
- Online Health Services
  Directory of disabilities-related websites
  http://www.onlinehealthresources.com/Disabilities/

Multilevel Approaches to Chronic Disease Control

Comprehensive interventions for controlling chronic diseases require primary, secondary, and tertiary prevention approaches. Moreover, these strategies must be directed at the individual, interpersonal, organizational, community, and policy levels. A relevant example is tobacco—as noted earlier (McGinnis and Foege 1993; Mokdad et al. 2004) the leading actual cause of death among Americans. Because of tobacco's important negative health consequences, a multilevel or comprehensive intervention to control tobacco must involve primary prevention education programs for youth in school settings, education programs for physicians, dentists, and other health care providers to inspire patient education in care settings through brief interventions and other mechanisms, free or low-cost cessation programs for smokers before the onset of disease (secondary prevention), health insurance cost reductions for nonsmokers as an economic incentive to eliminate tobacco use, tobacco excise taxes to bring an economic disincentive to continue use and raise revenue to finance care for affected individuals (tertiary prevention), rigorous enforcement of age restriction for purchase of cigarettes and careful monitoring of cigarette vending machines at the point of purchase, partnering with national and local voluntary organizations (e.g., American Heart Association, American Lung Association, American Cancer Society) for advocacy of anti-tobacco programs and policies, clean indoor air legislation, and restriction of smoking in public places. Whereas each one of these initiatives may have a modest influence on smoking and tobacco consumption, none is as singularly effective as a comprehensive program. Arguably, multilevel anti-tobacco programs have changed the cultural norm in the United States in the nearly five decades since the Surgeon General's first report on smoking and health and are beginning to do so in other countries that have had a history of high tobacco consumption. Today, comparable multicomponent approaches are likely to be necessary to combat obesity and the chronic disease conditions it spawns (e.g., diabetes), as well as for hypertension, the leading cause of stroke, coronary artery disease, heart attacks, and heart and kidney failure (Hajjar and Kotchen 2003).

Examples of Community-Level Health Planning Approaches

Various planning frameworks are used in chronic disease prevention and control. These frameworks can provide intervention planners with guidance in identifying and setting priorities, anticipating obstacles, and resolving them with the goal of improving the health and quality of life among selected populations (Green and Kreuter 2005). Although various intervention planning frameworks exist, most are comprised of similar principles. Breckon, Harvey, and Lancaster (1998) have described seven basic principles crucial to public health intervention program planning:

(1) *Plan the process.* Planning, implementing, and evaluating chronic disease interventions takes time and resources. Time spent at the beginning of the process dedicated to identifying key stakeholders, developing a mission and vision, gathering necessary data, and planning objectives and timelines will increase the likelihood that valuable resources are considered, needs are met, and a schedule for assessment, planning, implementation, and evaluation is prepared and followed.

(2) *Plan with people.* It is critical that the community be involved in the planning and evaluation process. Involving community members will increase the likelihood that needs are met, trust is established, and a sense of ownership and pride is created.

(3) *Plan with data.* Data regarding real and perceived needs of the community must drive the planning process. Data can be quantitative or qualitative in nature. Examples of data necessary for program planning include those pertaining to demographics, social indicators, perceived needs of the community, epidemiological indicators, behavioral risk factors and related knowledge, attitudes, beliefs, and skills necessary for behavior change. In addition, data regarding existing programs will decrease duplication of efforts in addition to providing valuable information on successful approaches.

(4) *Plan for institutionalization*. Due to the nature of chronic diseases, programs should be planned for ongoing implementation and evaluation. As such, coalitions should engage in long-range planning.

(5) *Plan for priorities*. Based upon the data representing real and perceived needs of the selected population, in addition to available resources, interventions should address identified and agreed upon priorities.

(6) *Plan for measurable short- and long-term outcomes*. Goals and measurable objectives must be developed. Establishing measurable objectives will facilitate the evaluation plan, and guide the coalition regarding changes in the direction and process of the intervention.

(7) *Plan for evaluation*. Evaluation should be built into the stages of program design and implementation. For example, evaluations of the planning process should include systems for documentation and assessment of community input, identification of priorities, and so on. In addition, as the program is being planned and implementation processes and procedures are being developed, evaluation plans, designs, and tools should be developed.

Planning models provide frameworks for putting the previously described principles into practice. Whereas numerous public health intervention planning models exist, the following ones illustrate popular or emerging strategies: PRECEDE-PROCEED, PATCH, Mobilizing Action through Planning and Partnerships (MAPP), Intervention Mapping, and Community-Based Prevention Marketing (CBPM).

PRECEDE-PROCEED Framework

The PRECEDE-PROCEED framework reflects an ecological and educational approach to intervention planning that respects both the real and perceived needs of the community of interest while following a systems approach to improving health and quality of life (Green and Kreuter 2005). The PRECEDE-PROCEED framework is comprised of two main components, each having a series of phases. The first component is referred to as PRECEDE (Predisposing, Reinforcing, and Enabling Constructs in Educational/Ecological Diagnosis and Evaluation) and is comprised of four phases:

Phase 1: Social assessment and situational analysis. During this phase, an assessment of the real and perceived needs of the community of interest. Data include both social indicators and subjective problems and priorities reflective of the community of interest.

Phase 2: Epidemiological assessment. During the epidemiological assessment, specification and prioritization of the health issue in addition to the etiologic genetic, behavioral, and environmental risk factors.

Phase 3: Educational and ecological assessment. Once the health issue and etiologic factors have been prioritized and selected, the educational and ecological assessment explores and prioritizes the predisposing, enabling, and reinforcing factors that influence the selected behavioral and environmental risk factors.

Phase 4: Administrative and policy assessment and intervention alignment. During this phase, the planner identifies the program components, interventions, and policy, organizational, and administrative resources needed to affect changes determined in Phases 1–3.

The second component referred to as PROCEED (Policy, Regulatory, and Organizational Constructs in Educational and Environmental Development) is comprised of the following phases:

Phase 5: Implementation. During this phase, organizational readiness and capacity is assessed before program implementation.
Phase 6: Process evaluation.
Phase 7: Impact evaluation.
Phase 8: Outcome evaluation. Phases 6–8 pertain to intervention evaluation. During these phases, the planning team determines the evaluation plan and design taking into account program processes (Phase 6), short-term impacts (Phase 7), and longer-term outcomes (Phase 8).

Planned Approach to Community Health

PATCH was developed by the CDC in partnership with community groups and state and local health departments (CDC 2007). Organized within the context of the PRECEDE model, the PATCH planning model provides a framework for increasing community capacity to plan, implement, and evaluate comprehensive community-based public health programs (CDC 2007). The PATCH model (Figure 3.3) contains five critical elements ensuring the program planning success:

Phase 1: Mobilizing the community
Phase 2: Collecting and organizing data
Phase 3: Choosing health priorities
Phase 4: Developing a comprehensive intervention plan
Phase 5: Evaluating PATCH

Mobilizing Action through Planning and Partnerships

MAPP is a planning framework developed in 2000 by the National Association of County and City Health Officials in cooperation with the Public Health Practice Program Office, CDC (2007). The guiding principles in the MAPP planning model include systems thinking, dialogue, shared vision, data, partnerships and collaboration, strategic thinking, and celebration for success. The MAPP planning model consists of four core assessments that drive the planning process (Figure 3.4). The main purposes of these four assessments are to provide insight concerning gaps between community wants and current circumstances, to provide information for identifying strategic issues, and to provide information for developing goals and strategies. These assessments include:

(1) *Community themes and strengths.* This assessment provides the planning team with an understanding of the perceived strengths and needs of the selected community.

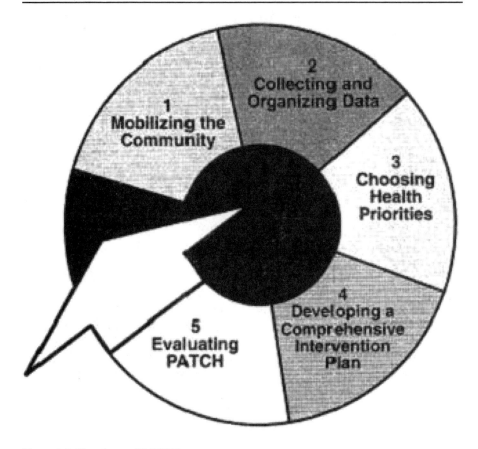

Figure 3.3. Five phases of PATCH.

(2) *Local public health system.* Assessment of the local public health system is comprised of a capacity assessment in addition to an overview of how essential services are being provided to the community.

(3) *Community health status.* Similar to the previously described planning models, the community health status assessment provides the planning team with the community health and quality of life status for determining health priorities.

(4) *Forces of change.* The forces of change assessment provides the planning team with information on legislation, technology, and other issues that may affect the priority health issue, the community functioning, and/or the operations of the public health system.

Intervention Mapping

Developed by Bartholomew and colleagues (2001), intervention mapping is a systematic and cumulative process for developing, implementing, and sustaining public health interventions. The steps and procedures within the intervention mapping framework facilitate

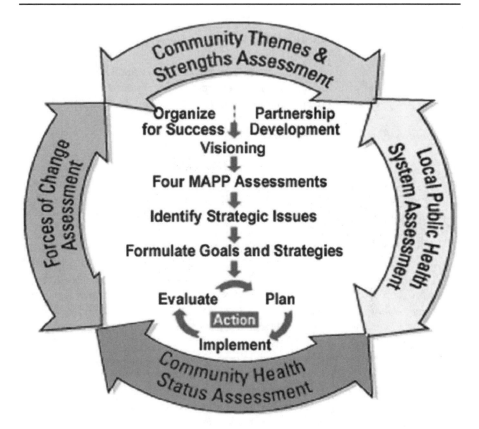

Figure 3.4. Mobilizing for Action through Planning and Partnerships planning model (from National Association of County and City Health Officials and Public Health Practice Program Office, CDC 2007).

the development of theory-based interventions based on the literature and population-specific data. Intervention mapping is a tool, then, that can serve as a blueprint for the design, implementation, and evaluation of an intervention once the planners have identified the health issue, behavioral and environmental risk factors, and associated determinates. The five core steps in the intervention mapping framework include:

(1) *Development of proximal program objectives based on the determinants of behavior and environmental conditions.* The first step in the intervention mapping process entails determining desired changes at each level of the ecological model and writing learning and change objectives.

(2) *Selection of theory-based intervention methods and strategies for change.* At this stage, intervention methods and strategies that relate to each of the proximal program objectives are developed.

(3) *Development of program components and processes.* Once intervention methods and strategies are developed, the processes and procedures of program implementation and program materials are developed and pilot tested.

(4) *Anticipation of program implementation, adoption, and sustainability.* At this stage a detailed plan based upon theory and evidence for accomplishing program adoption and implementation is developed.

(5) *Anticipation of process, impact, and outcome evaluation.* Similar to the previously described planning models, the final step in intervention mapping consists of the development of an evaluation plan, design, and procedures.

Community-Based Prevention Marketing

CBPM is a community-directed, social change planning framework that employs marketing techniques to design, implement, and evaluate health promotion and disease prevention programs (Bryant et al. 2007). CBPM draws from community organization principles and practices and marketing concepts and methods to create a synergistic behavior change planning framework.

From community organizing, CBPM borrows the principles of community participation, community capacity building and empowerment, and participatory research (Minkler and Wallerstein 1997). Community members select the issue to address and direct program planning, implementation, and evaluation activities. Academic-based researchers collaborate with local partners who represent the community, working together to analyze community problems, set goals, conduct research, design, implement, and evaluate interventions aimed at achieving their goals.

CBPM's primary objective is to build the community's capacity (Norton et al. 2002) to apply marketing principles, to set goals, and solve problems. Academic-based researchers provide training and technical assistance as community members analyze problems and design effective change strategies. During the process, local leaders are developed who can direct problem-solving activities and guide prevention activities.

CBPM uses participatory research in formative, pretesting, and evaluation research. Community partners provide academic researchers with a new perspective on local problems and present new research questions to explore. Academicians teach community members to develop research objectives, collect data, and interpret results. Community board members work with academic researchers to identify modifiable risks and prioritize health promoting behaviors.

The social marketing component refers to the application of commercial marketing concepts and techniques to promote voluntary behavior change (Grier and Bryant 2005). Social marketing provides the conceptual framework that guides strategy development—the use of formative research to gain input from the people the intervention plans to reach, analytical techniques for segmenting market audiences, and the use of program monitoring to identify ineffective activities that require modification and effective activities worthy of sustaining.

The steps of CBPM include:

- *Mobilizing the community.* The first step is devoted to building a community structure to guide the CBPM process. A local agency serves as a coordinating and fiduciary agency, working with academic researchers to define community boundaries and organize a community coalition or board.
- *Developing a community profile.* A community profile using local and national data is created to help the community assess its assets and needs.

- *Selecting the target behavior and audiences.* A community coalition identifies and prioritizes problems and selects the target issue(s) and audience(s) for the program.
- *Conducting formative research.* Following Israel et al.'s (2005) principles of CBPR, academicians work with community members to collect and interpret marketing data.
- *Developing strategy.* A marketing plan organized around the 4 P's (product, price, place, and promotion) and an implementation plan with timeline and organizational assignments are created to guide project development.
- *Developing the program.* Program materials are created and pretested. The community coalition mobilizes resources needed for program activities and creates the institutional foundation for sustaining the program.
- *Implementing the program.* A local program leader works closely with the community coalition to coordinate program launch and implementation.
- *Tracking and evaluation.* Academic and community researchers monitor program activities and assess program impact. Results are used to make program enhancements and identify new problems that require further attention.

Conclusions

Chronic diseases financially burden the American health care system and reduce the overall quality of life for as many as 90 million U.S. citizens. Intervention science for the prevention of chronic diseases has increased in precision during the past decade, making it possible for many of these disease threats to be prevented, delayed, or have their overall impact lessened. Today, there is excellent surveillance of diseases and an improved understanding of the interrelationships involving individual, social, environmental, and political factors. Moreover, there are sophisticated models, theories, and frameworks for intervening at the individual, interpersonal, organizational, community, and policy levels. The most promising of these interventions are multilevel ones that simultaneously address the complex disease causes. More case studies and applications of interventions are necessary to test the adaptability of previous findings in diverse settings. However, the evidence base gained to date through an abundance of demonstration projects can now be manifested and enlarged in scale to translate and disseminate these findings to broader audiences and address the major chronic disease issues facing Americans in the twenty-first century. Overall, the campaign against chronic disease threats appears to be entering a new and more optimistic era.

References

Ajzen, I. From Intentions to Actions: A Theory of Planned Behavior. In: Kuhl, J., and J. Beckmann, editors, *Springer Series in Social Psychology.* Berlin: Springer (1985):11–39.

Ajzen, I. The Theory of Planned Behavior. *Organ Behav Hum Decis Process* (1991):50(2):179–211.

Ajzen, I., and M. Fishbein. Attitudinal and Normative Variables as Predictors of Specific Behavior. *J Pers Soc Psychol* (1973):27(1):41–57.

Aldana, S. Financial Impact of Worksite Health Promotion and Methodological Quality of the Evidence. The Art of Health Promotion. Supplement. *Am J Health Promot* (1998):2(1):1–8.

Allensworth, D., and L.J. Kolbe. The Comprehensive School Health Program. *J Sch Health* (1987):57(10):409–412.

Association for Worksite Health Promotion. *1999 National Worksite Health Promotion Survey.* Northbrook, IL: Association for Worksite Health Promotion (1999).

Baldwin, J.A., B.G. Brown, H.A. Wayment, and R.A. Nez. Culture and Context: Buffering the Relationship between Stressful Life Events and Risky Behaviors in American Indian Youth. *Subst Use Misuse* (in press).

Bandura, A. *Social Learning Theory.* Englewood Cliffs, NJ: Prentice Hall (1977).

Bandura, A. *Social Foundations of Thought and Action.* Englewood Cliffs, NJ: Prentice Hall (1986).

Baranowski, T., C.L. Perry, and G.S. Parcel. How Individuals, Environments, and Health Behavior Interact: Social Cognitive Theory. In: Glanz, K., B.K., Rimer, and F.M. Lewis, editors, *Health Behavior and Health Education: Theory, Research, and Practice* (3rd ed.). San Francisco, CA: Jossey-Bass (2002):165–184.

Bartholomew, L.K., G.S. Parcel, G. Kok, and N.H. Gottlieb. *Intervention Mapping: Designing Theory and Evidence-Based Health Promotion Programs.* Mountain View, CA: Mayfield Publishing (2001).

Bartholomew, L. K., G.S. Parcel, G. Kok, and N.H. Gottlieb. *Planning Health Promotion Programs: An Intervention Mapping Approach* (2nd ed.). San Francisco, CA: Jossey-Bass (2006).

Bauman, K.E., V.A. Foshee, S.T. Ennett, K. Hicks, and M. Pemberton. Family Matters: A Family-Directed Program Designed to Prevent Adolescent Tobacco and Alcohol Use. *Health Promot Pract* (2001):2:81–96.

Beauvais, F., and E.R. Oetting. Drug Use, Resilience, and the Myth of the Golden Child. In: Glantz, M.D., and J.L. Johnson, editors, *Resilience and Development: Positive Life Adaptations.* New York: Kluwer Academic Publishers (1999):101–108.

Blackburn, H., R.V. Luepker, F.G. Kline, et al. The Minnesota Heart Health Program: A Research and Demonstration Project in Cardiovascular Disease Prevention. In: Matarazzo, J.D., S. M. Weiss, J.A. Herd, N.E. Miller, and S.M. Weiss, editors, *Behavioral Health: A Handbook of Health Enhancement and Disease Prevention.* New York: Wiley InterScience (1984):1171–1178.

Booker, V.K., J.G. Robinson, B.J. Kay, L.G. Nafera, and G. Steward. Changes in Empowerment: Effects of Participation in a Lay Health Promotion Program. *Health Educ Behav* (1997):4:452–464.

Bracht, N., and J. Gleason. Strategies and Structures for Citizen Partnerships. In: Bracht, N., editor, *Health Promotion at the Community Level.* Newbury Park, CA: Sage Publications (1990):109–124.

Brady, M. *Broadening the Base of Interventions for Aboriginal People with Alcohol Problems.* Technical Report No. 29. Sydney: National Drug and Alcohol Research Centre, University of NSW (1995).

Breckon, D.J., J.R. Harvey, and R.B. Lancaster. *Community Health Education: Setting Roles, and Skills for the 21st Century* (4th ed.). Gaithersburg, MD: Aspen Publishers (1998).

Britt, M., and C. Sharda. *The Business Interest in a Community's Health.* Washington, D.C.: Washington Business Group on Health (2000):30.

Brown, L., and W.A. Vega. A Protocol for Community-Based Research. In: Minkler, M., and N. Wallerstein, editors, *Community-Based Participatory Research in Health.* San Francisco, CA: Jossey-Bass (1996):407–409.

Bryant, C.A., K. McCormack Brown, R.J. McDermott, M.S. Forthofer, E.C. Bumpus, S. Calkins, and L.B. Zapata. Community-Based Prevention Marketing: A Framework for Facilitating Health Behavior Change. *Health Promot Pract* (2007):8:154–163.

Butterfoss, F.D., R.M. Goodman, and A. Wandersman. Community Coalitions for Prevention and Health Promotion: Factors Predicting Satisfaction, Participation, and Planning. *Health Educ Q* (1996):23:65–79.

Butterfoss, F.D., and M.C. Kegler. Toward a Comprehensive Understanding of Community Coalitions: Moving from Practice to Theory. In: DiClemente, R.J., R.A. Crosby, and M.C. Kegler, editors, *Emerging Theories in Health Promotion Practice and Research: Strategies for Improving Public Health*. San Francisco, CA: Jossey-Bass (2002):157–193.

Campbell, C., and S. Jovchelovitch. Health, Community, and Development: Towards a Social Psychology of Participation. *J Community Appl Soc Psychol* (2000):10:255–270.

Carlaw, R., M. Mittelmark, N. Bracht, and R. Luepker. Organization for a Community Cardiovascular Health Program: Experiences from the Minnesota Heart Health Program. *Health Educ Q* (1984):11:243–252.

Centers for Disease Control and Prevention (CDC). Physician Advice and Individual Behaviors about Cardiovascular Disease Risk Reduction—Seven States and Puerto Rico, 1997. *MMWR* (1999):48(4):74–77.

Centers for Disease Control and Prevention (CDC). *Social Determinants of Health* (2005). Available at www.cdc.gov/sdoh. Accessed September 4, 2007.

Centers for Disease Control and Prevention (CDC). *Prevention Research Centers* (2007a). Available at http://www.cdc.gov/prc. Accessed September 8, 2007.

Centers for Disease Control and Prevention (CDC). *Healthy Youth! Coordinated School Health Program* (2007b). Available at http://www.cdc.gov/HealthYouth/CSHP/. Accessed September 8, 2007.

Centers for Disease Control and Prevention (CDC). *Healthy Youth! YRBSS—Youth Risk Behavior Surveillance System* (2007c). Available at: http://www.cdc.gov/HealthyYouth/yrbs/index.htm. Accessed September 9, 2007.

Chavis, D.M. The Paradoxes and Promise of Community Coalitions. *Am J Community Psychol* (2001):29(2):309–320.

Chronic Disease Prevention. 2005. Atlanta, GA: U.S. Department of Health and Human Services, Centers for Disease Control and Prevention, National Center for Chronic Disease Prevention and Health Promotion [cited June 19, 2005]. Available at: http://www.cdc.gov/nccdphp/.

Clark, S., J. Iceland, T. Palumbo, K. Pose, and M. Weismantl. *Comparing Employment, Income, and Poverty: Census 2000 and the Current Population Survey* (2007).

Cohen, S., and E. Lichtenstein. Partner Behaviors that Support Quitting Smoking. *J Consult Clin Psychol* (1990):58:304–309.

Committee on Prevention of Obesity in Children and Youth. Executive Summary. In: Koplan, J.P., C.T. Liverman, and V.I. Kraak, editors, *Preventing Childhood Obesity: Health in the Balance*. Washington, D.C.: Institute of Medicine of the National Academies (2005):1–19.

Coreil, J., C.A. Bryant, and J.N. Henderson. *Social and Behavioral Foundations of Public Health*. Thousand Oaks, CA: Sage Publications (2001).

DeBate, R., M. Plescia, D. Joyner, and L. Spann. A Qualitative Assessment of Charlotte Reach: An Ecological Perspective for Decreasing CVD and Diabetes among African Americans. *Ethn Dis* (2004):14(3 Suppl 1):S1-77–S1-82.

DeHaven, M.J., I.B. Hunter, L. Wilder, J.W. Walton, and J. Berry. Health Programs in Faith-Based Organizations: Are They Effective? *Aust J Polit Hist* (2004):94(6):1030–1036.

Earp, J.A., E. Eng, M.S. O'Malley, et al. Increasing Use of Mammography among Older Rural African American Women: Initial Results from a Controlled Trial. *Aust J Polit Hist* (2002):92(4):646–654.

Elder, J.P., S.A. McGraw, and D.A. Abrams. Organizational and Community Approaches to Community-Wide Prevention of Heart Disease: The First Two Years of the Pawtucket Heart Health Program. *Prev Med* (1986):15:107–115.

Ellen, J., B. Brown, S. Chung, et al. Impact of Sexual Networks on Risk for Gonorrhea and Chlamydia among Low-Income Urban African American Adolescents. *J Pediatr* (2005):146:518–522.

Eng, E. The Save Our Sisters Project: A Social Network Strategy for Reaching Rural Black Women. *Cancer* (1993):72:1071–1077.

Eng, E., and J.W. Hatch. Networking between Agencies and Black Churches: The Lay Health Advisor Model. *Prev Hum Serv* (1991):10:123–146.

Ennett, S., S. Bailey, and E. Federman. Social Network Characteristics Associated with Risky Behaviors among Runaway and Homeless Youth. *J Health Soc Behav* (1999):40(1):63–78.

Farquhar, J., S. Fortmann, J. Flora, et al. Effects of Community-Wide Education on Cardiovascular Disease Risk Factors: The Five-City Project. *JAMA* (1990):264:359–365.

Fergus, S., and M. Zimmerman. Adolescent Resilience: A Framework for Understanding Healthy Development in the Face of Risk. *Annu Rev Public Health* (2005):26:399–419.

Finkelstein, E., I. Fiebelkorn, and G. Wang. The Costs of Obesity among Full-Time Employees. *Am J Health Promot* (2005):20(1):45–51.

Fishbein, M. Attitude and the Prediction of Behavior. In: Fishbein, M., editor, *Readings in Attitude Theory and Measurement.* New York: Wiley (1967):477–492.

Fishbein, M., and I. Ajzen. *Belief, Attitude, Intention, and Behavior: An Introduction to Theory and Research.* Reading, MA; Don Mills, Ontario: Addison-Wesley (1975).

Fisher, P., M. Storck, and J. Baco. In the Eye of the Beholder: Risk and Protective Factors in Rural American Indian and Caucasian Adolescents. *Am J Orthopsychiatry* (1999):69:294–304.

Flynn, B. Healthy Cities: A Model of Community Change. *Fam Community Health* (1992):15(1): 13–23.

Franks, A.L., S.H. Kelder, G.A. Dino, et al. School-Based Programs: Lessons Learned from CATCH, Planet Health, and Not-On-Tobacco. *Prev Chronic Dis* (2007). Available at: http://www.cdc. gov/pcd/issues/2007/apr/06_0105.htm. Accessed September 3, 2007.

French, S.A., M. Story, and R.W. Jeffery. Environmental Influences on Eating and Physical Activity. *Annu Rev Public Health* (2001):(22):309–325.

Freudenberg, N. From Lifestyle to Social Determinants: New Directions for Community Health Promotion Research and Practice. *Prev Chronic Dis* (2007). Available at: http://www.cdc.gov/ pcd/issues/2007/jul/06_0194.htm. Accessed September 9, 2007.

Friedman, S., and S. Aral. Social Networks, Risk Potential Networks, Health, and Disease. *J Urban Health* (2001):78(3):411–418.

Gebbie, K., L. Rosenstock, and L.M. Hernandez, editors. *Who Will Keep the Public Healthy? Educating Public Health Professionals for the 21st Century.* Institute of Medicine of the National Academies. Washington, D.C.: National Academies Press (2003).

Giles, W.H., P. Tucker, L. Brown, et al. Racial and Ethnic Approaches to Community Health (REACH 2010): An Overview. *Ethn Dis* (2004):14(3):S1-5–S1-8.

Glanz, K., B.K. Rimer, and F.M. Lewis, editors. *Health Behavior and Health Education: Theory, Research, and Practice* (3rd ed.). San Francisco, CA: Jossey-Bass (2002).

Goetzel, R., K. Hawkins, R. Ozminkowski, and S. Wang. The Health and Productivity Cost Burden of the "Top 10" Physical and Mental Health Conditions Affecting Six Large U.S. Employers in 1999. *J Occup Environ Med* (2003):45(1):5–14.

Goetzel, R., S. Long, R. Ozminkowski, et al. Health, Absence, Disability, and Presenteeism Cost Estimates of Certain Physical and Mental Health Conditions Affecting U.S. Employers. *J Occup Environ Med* (2004):46(4):398–412.

Goodman, R.M., et al. Identifying and Defining the Dimensions of Community Capacity to Provide a Basis for Measurement. *Health Educ Behav* (1999):25(3):258–278.

Gottlieb, B.H. Selecting and Planning Support Interventions. In: Cohen, S., L.G. Underwood, and B.H. Gottlieb, editors, *Social Support Measurement and Intervention.* New York: Oxford University Press (2000).

Green, L.W., A. George, M. Daniel, et al. Guidelines for Participatory Research in Health Promotion. In: Minkler, M., and N. Wallerstein, editors, *Community-Based Participatory Research in Health.* San Francisco, CA: Jossey-Bass (2003):419–428.

Green, L.W., and M.W. Kreuter. CDC's Planned Approach to Community Health as an Application of PRECEDE and an Inspiration for PROCEED. *J Health Educ* (1992):23:140–147.

Green, L.W., and M.W. Kreuter. *Health Program Planning: An Educational and Ecological Approach.* New York: McGraw-Hill (2005).

Grier, S., and C.A. Bryant. Social Marketing in Public Health. *Annu Rev Public Health* (2005):26:319–339.

Grossberg, P.M., D.D. Brown, and M.F. Fleming. Brief Physician Advice for High-Risk Drinking among Young Adults. *Ann Fam Med* (2004):2:474–480.

Hajjar, I., and T.A. Kotchen. Trends in Prevalence, Awareness, Treatment, and Control of Hypertension in the United States, 1988–2000. *JAMA* (2003):290:199–206.

Hardy, G.E., Jr. The Burden of Chronic Disease: The Future is Prevention. *Prev Chronic Dis* (2004). Available at: http://www.cdc.gov/pcd/issues/2004/apr/04_0006.htm. Accessed September 3, 2007.

Hatch, H.W., and K. Lovelace. Involving the Southern Rural Church and Students of the Health Professions in Health Education. *Public Health Rep* (1980):95:23–25.

Hawe, P., and A. Sheill. Social Capital and Health Promotion: A Review. *Soc Sci Med* (2000):51: 871–885.

Heaney, C.A., and B.A. Israel. Social Networks and Social Support. In: Glanz, K., B.K. Rimer, and F.M. Lewis, editors, *Health Behavior and Health Education: Theory, Research, and Practice* (3rd ed.). San Francisco, CA: Jossey-Bass (2002).

Henry J. Kaiser Family Foundation. *Medicare: The Basics* (2007). Available at: http://www.kff.org/medicare/7615.cfm. Accessed September 9, 2007.

Hersey, J.C., L.S. Klibanoff, D.J. Lam, and R.L. Taylor. Promoting Social Support: The Impact of California's "Friends Can Be Good Medicine" Campaign. *Health Educ Q* (1984):11:293–311.

Hochbaum, G.M. *Public Participation in Medical Screening Programs: A Socio-Psychological Study.* Washington, D.C.: U.S. Government Printing Office (1958). *Public Health Service Publication No. 572.*

House, J.S. *Work Stress and Social Support.* Reading, MA: Addison-Wesley (1981).

Hovell, M.F., D.R. Wahlgren, and C.A. Gehrman. The Behavioral Ecological Model: Integrating Public Health and Behavioral Science. In: DiClemente, R. J., R.A. Crosby, and M.C. Kegler, editors, *Emerging Theories in Health Promotion Practice and Research: Strategies for Improving Public Health.* San Francisco, CA: Jossey-Bass (2002):347–385.

Hoyert, D.L., M.P. Heron, S.L. Murphy, and H. Kung. *Deaths: Final Data for 2003.* National Vital Statistics Reports, vol. 54, no. 13. Hyattsville, MD: National Center for Health Statistics (2006).

Israel, B.A. Social Networks and Health Status: Linking Theory, Research, and Practice. *Patient Couns Health Educ* (1982):4(2):65–79.

Israel, B.A. Social Networks and Social Support: Implications for Natural Helper and Community Level Interventions. *Health Educ Q* (1985):12:65–80.

Israel, B.A., B. Checkoway, A. Schulz, and M. Zimmerman. Health Education and Community Empowerment: Conceptualizing and Measuring Perceptions of Individual, Organizational, and Community Control. *Health Educ Q* (1994):21:149–170.

Israel, B.A., A.J. Schulz, E.A. Parker, et al. Critical Issues in Developing and Following Community-Based Participatory Research Principles. In: Minkler, M., and N. Wallerstein, editors, *Community-Based Participatory Research for Health.* San Francisco, CA: Jossey Bass (2005):53–79.

Kant, A.K., and P. Miner. Physician Advice About Being Overweight: Association with Self-Reported Weight Loss, Dietary, and Physical Activity Behaviors of U.S. Adolescents in the National Health and Nutrition Examination Survey, 1999–2002. *Pediatrics* (2007):119(1):e142–e146. (doi:10.1542/peds.2006-1116). Available at http://pediatrics.aappublications.org/cgi/content/abstract/119/1/e142. Accessed September 7, 2007.

Kawachi, I., B.P. Kennedy, and R. Glass. Social Capital and Self-Rated Health: A Contextual Analysis. *Aust J Polit Hist* (1999):89:1187–1193.

Kawachi, I., B.P. Kennedy, K. Lochner, and D. Prothrow-Stith. Social Capital, Income Inequality, and Mortality. *Aust J Polit Hist* (1997):87:1491–1497.

Kawachi, I., B.P. Kennedy, and R.G. Wilkinson. Crime: Social Disorganization and Relative Deprivation. *Soc Sci Med* (1999):48:719–731.

Kegler, M., A. Steckler, K. McLeroy, and S.H. Malek. Factors that Contribute to Effective Community Health Promotion Coalitions: A Study of 10 Project ASSIST Coalitions in North Carolina, *Health Educ Res* (1998):13:225–238.

Kennedy, B.P., I. Kawachi, D. Prothrow-Stith, K. Lochner, and V. Gupta. Social Capital, Income Inequality, and Firearm Violent Crime. *Soc Sci Med* (1998):47:7–17.

Kreuter, M.W., and N. Lezin. Social Capital Theory: Implications for Community-Based Health Promotion. In: DiClemente, R.J., R.A. Crosby, and M.C. Kegler, editors, *Emerging Theories in Health Promotion Practice and Research: Strategies for Improving Public Health*. San Francisco, CA: Jossey-Bass (2002):228–254.

Kreuter, M.W., N. Lezin, and L. Young. Evaluating Community-Based Collaborative Mechanisms: Implications for Practitioners. *Health Promot Pract* (2000):1:49–63.

Kruger, J., M. Yore, D. Bauer, and H. Kohl. Selected Barriers and Incentives for Worksite Health Promotion Services and Policies. *Am J Health Promot* (2007):21(5):439–447.

Lancaster, T., and L.F. Stead. Physician Advice for Smoking Cessation. *Cochrane Database Syst Rev* (2004):(4):CD000165. doi:10.1002/14651858.CD000165.pub2. Avaliable at: http://www.cochrane.org/reviews/en/ab000165.html. Accessed September 7, 2007.

Lasater, T., B.L. Wells, R.A. Carleton, and J.P. Elder. The Role of Churches in Disease Prevention Studies. *Public Health Rep* (1986):101:125–131.

Lefebvre, R., T. Lasater, R. Carleton, and G. Peterson. Theory and Delivery of Health Programming in the Community: The Pawtucket Heart Health Program. *Prev Med* (1987):16:80–95.

Levine, J.S. The Role of the Black Church in Community Medicine. *J Natl Med Assoc* (1984):76:477–483.

Lewin, L. Action Research and Minority Populations. *J Soc Issues*, (1946):2:34–46.

Linares, C., J. Díaz, A. Tobías, et al. Impact of Urban Air Pollutants and Noise Levels Over Daily Hospital Admissions in Children in Madrid: A Time Series Analysis. *Int Arch Occup Environ Health* (2006):79(2):143–152.

Lorig, K., V.M. Gonzalez, D.D. Laurent, L. Morgan, and B.A. Laris. Arthritis Self-Management Program Variations: Three Studies. *Arthritis Care Res* (1998):11:448–454.

Marcus, B.H., N. Owen, L.H. Forshyth, N.A. Cavill, and F. Fridinger. Physical Activity Interventions Using Mass Media, Print Media, and Information Technology. *Am J Prev Med* (1998):15:363–378.

McAlister, A., P. Puska, J.T. Salonen, J. Tuomilehto, and K. Koskela. Theory and Action for Health Promotion: Illustrations from the North Karelia Project. *Aust J Polit Hist* (1982):72:43–50.

McGinnis, J.M., and W.H. Foege. Actual Causes of Death in the United States. *JAMA* (1993):270:2207–2212.

McLeroy, K.R., N.H. Gottlieb, and C.A. Heaney. Social Health. In: O'Donnell, M.P., and J. S. Harris, editors, *Health Promotion in the Workplace* (3rd ed.). Albany, NY: Delmar (2001).

McQueen, D.V. Continuing Efforts in Global Chronic Disease Prevention. *Prev Chronic Dis* (2007). Available at http://www.cdc.gov/pcd/issues/2007/apr/07_0024.htm. Accessed September 3, 2007.

Milstein, B., T. Chapel, S.F. Wetterhall, and D.A. Cotton. Building Capacity for Program Evaluation at the Centers for Disease Control and Prevention. *New Dir Eval* (2002):93:27–46.

Minkler, M. Ethical Challenges for the "Outside" Researcher in Community-Based Participatory Research. *Health Educ Behav* (2004):31(6):684–697.

Minkler, M., and N. Wallerstein. Improving Health through Community Organization and Community Building: A Health Education Perspective. In: Minkler, M., editor, *Community Orga-*

nizing and Community Building for Health. Piscataway, New Jersey: Rutgers University Press (1997):30–52.

Minkler, M., and N. Wallerstein. Improving Health through Community Organization and Community Building. In: Glanz, K., B.K. Rimer, and F.M. Lewis, editors, *Health Behavior and Health Education: Theory, Research, and Practice* (3rd ed.). San Francisco, CA: Jossey-Bass (2002):279–311.

Minkler, M., and N. Wallerstein, editors. *Community-Based Participatory Research for Health.* San Francisco, CA: Jossey-Bass (2003).

Mittelmark, M.B. The Psychology of Social Influence and Healthy Public Policy. *Prev Med* (1999):29(6 Pt 2):S24–S29.

Mittelmark, M., R. Luepker, D. Jacobs, et al. Community-Wide Prevention of Cardiovascular Disease: Education Strategies of the Minnesota Heart Health Program. *Prev Med* (1986):15:1–17.

Mokdad, A.H., J.S. Marks, D.F. Stroup, and J.L. Gerberding. Actual Causes of Death in the United States—2000. *JAMA* (2004):291:1238–1245.

Mumane, J., R. Ozminkowski, and R. Gptze. Cost-Benefit Analysis of the Citibank, N.A. Health Management Program. In: *Art and Science of Health Promotion 1998 Conference of the American Journal of Health Promotion. Phoenix, AZ* (1998).

National Association of County and City Health Officials and Public Health Practice Program Office, Centers for Disease Control and Prevention (CDC). *Mobilizing for Action through Planning and Partnerships* (2007).

Norris, T. *The Healthy Communities Handbook.* Denver, CO: The National Civic League (1993).

Norton, B.L., K.R. McLeroy, J.N. Burdine, et al. Community Capacity: Concept, Theory, and Methods. In: DiClemente, R.J., R.A. Crosby, and M.C. Kegler, editors, *Emerging Theories in Health Promotion Practice and Research: Strategies for Improving Public Health.* San Francisco, CA: Jossey-Bass (2002):194–227.

O'Donnell, M.P., and J.S. Harris. *Health Promotion in the Workplace* (2nd ed.). Albany, NY: Delmar Publishers (1994).

Ogden, C.L., M.D. Carroll, L.R. Curtin, et al. Prevalence of Overweight and Obesity in the United States, 1999–2004. *JAMA* (2006):295:1549–1555.

Oman, R., S. Vesel, C. Aspay, et al. The Potential Protective Effect of Youth Assets on Adolescent Alcohol and Drug Use. *Aust J Polit Hist* (2004):94(8):1425–1430.

Papas, M.A., A.J. Alberg, R. Ewing, et al. The Built Environment and Obesity. *Epidemiol Rev* (2007). Advance access published online on May 28, 2007 (doi:10.1093/epirev/mxm009).

Parker, E.A., B.A. Israel, A.J. Schulz, and R. Hollis. East Side Detroit Village Health Worker Partnership: Community-Based Lay Health Adviser Intervention in an Urban Area. *Health Educ Behav* (1998):25:24–45.

Partners in Policymaking. (2007). Available at: http://www.partnersinpolicymaking.com/resources.html#top. Accessed September 9, 2007.

Partnership for Prevention. *Healthy Workforce 2010: An Essential Health Promotion Sourcebook for Employers, Large and Small.* U.S. Department of Health and Human Services, Office of Disease Prevention and Health Promotion (2001):1–63.

Portes, A. Social Capital: Its Origins and Applications in Modern Sociology. *Annu Rev Sociol* (1998):24:1–24.

Prochaska, J.O., and C.C. DiClemente. Stages and Processes of Self-Change of Smoking: Toward an Integrative Model of Change. *J Consult Clin Psychol* (1983):51(3):390–395.

Puska, P., and A. Uutela. Community Intervention in Cardiovascular Health Promotion: North Karelia, 1972–1999. In: Schneiderman, N., M.A. Speers, J.M. Silva, H. Tomes, and J.H. Gentry, editors, *Integrating Behavioral and Social Sciences with Public Health.* Arlington, VA: American Psychological Association (2000):73–96.

Putnam, R.D. The Prosperous Community: Social Capital and Public Life. *Am Prospect* (1993):13:35–42.

Rothman, J. Three Models of Community Organization Practice. In: Cox, F.M., J.L. Erlich, J. Rothman, and J.E. Tropman, editors, *Strategies of Community Organization*. Itasca, IL: Peacock Press (1970).

Rotter, J.B. Generalized Expectancies for Internal versus External Control of Reinforcement. *Psychol Monogr* (1966):80:(1):1–28.

Sallis, J.F., M.F. Hovell, C.R. Hofstetter, et al. Distance between Homes and Exercise Facilities Related to Frequency of Exercise among San Diego Residents. *Public Health Rep* (1990):105:179–185.

Sampson, R.J., S.W. Raudensbush, and F. Earls. Neighborhoods and Violent Crime: A Multilevel Study of Collective Efficacy. *Science* (1997):277:918–924.

Sanchez-Way, R., and S. Johnson. Cultural Practices in American Indian Prevention Programs. *Juvenile Justice* (2000):7(2):20–30.

Shea, S., and C.E. Basch. A Review of the Five Major Community-Based Cardiovascular Prevention Programs. Part I: Rationale, Design, and Theoretical Framework. *Am J Health Promot* (1990):4:203–213.

Shurney, D. *Prevention Works* (2007). Available at: http://seattlepi.nwsource.com/opinion/314862_prevent09.html. Accessed September 3, 2007.

Stephens, C. Community as Practice: Social Representations of Community and Their Implications for Health Promotion. *J Community Appl Soc Psychol* (2007):17:103–114.

Stokols, A.J., and R.L. Ballingham. The Social Ecology of Health Promotion: Implications for Research and Practice. *Am J Health Promot* (1996):19(4):247–251.

Subcommittee on Health and Environment of the Committee on Interstate Commerce, U.S. House of Representatives. *A Discursive Dictionary of Health Care*. Washington, D.C.: U.S. Government Printing Office (1976).

Syme, S.L. Social Determinants of Health: The Community as an Empowered Partner. *Prev Chronic Dis* (2004):1(1):1–5.

Teitelbaum, J.B., and S.E. Wilensky. *Essentials of Health Policy and Law*. Sudbury, MA: Jones and Bartlett Publishers (2007).

U.S. Department of Health and Human Services (USDHHS). *Strategies to Control Tobacco Use in the United States: A Blueprint for Public Health Action in the 1990s. Smoking and Tobacco Control Monographs 1*. Bethesda, MD: National Cancer Institute (1991). NIH Publication 92-3316.

U.S. Department of Health and Human Services (USDHHS). *Healthy People 2010: Understanding and Improving Health*. Washington, D.C.: U.S. Government Printing Office (2000).

U.S. Department of Health and Human Services (USDHHS). *Planned Approach to Community Health: Guide for the Local Coordinator*. Atlanta, GA: U.S. Department of Health and Human Services, Centers for Disease Control and Prevention, National Center for Chronic Disease Prevention and Health Promotion (2007).

Valente, T., C.P. Chou, and M.A. Pentz. Community Coalitions as a System: Effects of a Network Change on Adoption of Evidence-Based Substance Abuse Prevention. *Aust J Polit Hist* (2007):97(5):880–885.

Valente, T., P. Gallaher, and M. Mouttapa. Using Social Networks to Understand and Prevent Substance Use: A Transdisciplinary Perspective. *Subst Use Misuse* (2004):39(10–12):1685–1712.

Veale, B.M. Meeting the Challenge of Chronic Illness in General Practice. *Med J Aust* (2003):179:247–249.

Wallack, L. Media Advocacy. In Minkler, M., editor, *Community Organizing and Community Building for Health*. Piscataway, New Jersey: Rutgers University Press (1997):339–352.

Wallack, L. The Role of Mass Media in Creating Social Capital: A New Direction for Public Health. In: Smedly, B.D., and S.L. Syme, editors, *Promoting Health: Intervention Strategies from Social and Behavioral Research*. Washington, D.C.: National Academy Press (2000): 337–365.

Wallack, L., L. Dorfman, D. Jernigan, and M. Themba. *Media Advocacy and Public Health: Power for Prevention*. Thousand Oaks, CA: Sage Publications (1993).

Wallerstein, N., and B. Duran. The Conceptual, Historical, and Practice Roots of Community-Based Participatory Research and Related Participatory Traditions. In: Minkler, M., and N. Wallerstein, editors, *Community-Based Participatory Research for Health*. San Francisco, CA: Jossey-Bass (2003):27–52.

Wallerstein, N., B. Duran, M. Minkler, and K. Foley. Developing and Maintaining Partnerships with Communities. In: Israel, B., E. Eng, A. Schulz, and E. Parker, editors, *Methods in Community-Based Participatory Research for Health*. San Francisco, CA: Jossey-Bass (2005):31–51.

Wallston, K.A., B.S. Wallston, and R. DeVellis. Development of the Multidimensional Health Locus of Control (MHLC) Scales. *Health Educ Monogr* (1978):6:160–170.

Wandersman, A., and P. Florin. Citizen Participation and Community Organization. In: Rappaport, J., and E. Seidman, editors, *Handbook of Community Psychology*. New York: Academic/Plenum (2000):247–272.

Watkins, E.L., C. Harlan, E. Eng, et al. Assessing the Effectiveness of Lay Health Advisers with Migrant Farmworkers. *Fam Community Health* (1994):16:72–87.

Wellness Councils of America. A WELCOA Expert Interview with Larry Chapman, Principal and Co-founder, Summex from WebMD (2007), pp. 1–7.

CHAPTER 4

CHRONIC DISEASE SURVEILLANCE

Mark V. Wegner, M.D., M.P.H., Angela M. Rohan, Ph.D.,
and Patrick L. Remington, M.D., M.P.H.

Introduction

Public health surveillance is the ongoing, systematic collection, analysis, interpretation, and dissemination of data regarding a health-related event for use in public health action to reduce morbidity and mortality and to improve health (CDC 2001). The final link in the surveillance chain is the application of surveillance findings to disease prevention and health promotion programs (Figure 4.1). A public health surveillance "system" includes a functional capacity for data collection, analysis, and dissemination linked to public health programs (Thacker and Berkelman 1988).

Public health surveillance evolved during the twentieth century as the health burden from chronic diseases increased. In the early 1900s, surveillance described the practice of monitoring people who had been in contact with patients with certain infectious diseases, such as plague, smallpox, or typhus (Table 4.1). In the 1950s, practitioners began using surveillance to describe the practice of monitoring populations for the occurrence of specific infectious diseases, such as polio, measles, or tetanus (Langmuir 1963). By the 1970s, surveillance techniques were being applied to a broader array of diseases, including cancer, childhood lead poisoning, and congenital malformations (Thacker and Berkelman 1988).

After the events of September 11, 2001, surveillance again became strongly associated with infectious diseases, as bioterrorism preparedness and surveillance became national priorities, prompting more widespread use of syndromic surveillance methods and monitoring programs such as BioSense (Henning 2004; Loonsk 2004). However, at the same time, understanding of the complex causes of chronic diseases has continued to grow, and surveillance systems have also evolved to include monitoring trends in behavioral, occupational, and environmental risk factors, as well as other health conditions, such as disabilities. In addition, there has been a growing awareness of the impact the built environment has on our physical and mental health (Jackson 2003). Therefore, several interesting new surveillance methodologies have been developed that aim to monitor the health of individuals in the context of the communities in which they live, involving a complex interaction of health determinants, health outcomes, physical measurements, biological samples, policies, and the built environment (Survey of the Health of Wisconsin 2009).

This chapter describes the three basic elements of a chronic disease surveillance system: (1) data sources, (2) analysis and interpretation, and (3) dissemination to public health programs and other important constituents. The chapter concludes by

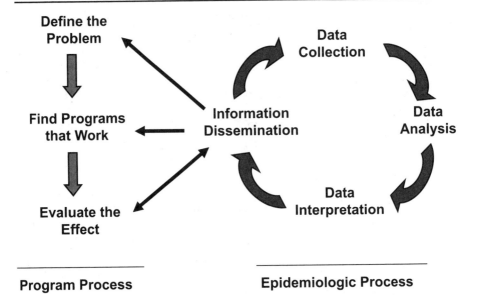

Program Process   **Epidemiologic Process**

Figure 4.1. Conceptual model for public health surveillance (epidemiologic process) and its link to the program planning process.

emphasizing the importance of linking these data to chronic disease prevention and control efforts.

Data Sources

Seven types of information systems exist in the United States that routinely provide data for surveillance (Stroup, Zack, and Wharton 1994). These data systems include notifiable diseases, vital statistics, sentinel surveillance, registries, health surveys, administrative data collection systems, and the U.S. census (Table 4.2). Chronic disease surveillance may use data from one or more of these systems. For example, surveillance of the health effects of tobacco use relies on data from vital statistics, cancer registries, telephone surveys about tobacco use, and administrative records of tobacco sales tax.

Notifiable Disease Systems

The Council of State and Territorial Epidemiologists, an organization consisting of public health epidemiologists working in states, territories, and local agencies in the United States, recommends modifications to the list of notifiable diseases annually, with input from the Centers for Disease Control and Prevention (CDC). This list of reportable diseases and illnesses (numbering 64 in 2009) includes primarily infectious diseases, such as measles, salmonella, and human immunodeficiency virus infection (CDC 2009a). Some noncommunicable diseases, such as lead poisoning, have historically been included. Using reports from clinicians and laboratories, public health agen-

Table 4.1. Trends in the Application of Surveillance to Public Health, 1900 to Present

Period	Application	Examples
1900s	Individual contacts of infected patients	Surveillance of individuals who came in contact with a case of smallpox is conducted
1950s	Communicable diseases	Cases of polio are reported to the public health agency as part of a communicable disease control program
1970s	Selected chronic diseases	Cancer registries are established as part of the Surveillance, Epidemiology, and End Results program
1990s	Behavioral, occupational, and environmental risk factors	Trends in the prevalence of cigarette smoking, determined through telephone surveys, are used to plan tobacco control programs
2000s	Bioterrorism and preparedness	Syndromic surveillance for early detection of outbreaks
	The built environment	Surveillance programs looking at both health status and the communities in which individuals live

cies follow up on people with high blood lead levels and provide appropriate control measures.

In 1996, the Council of State and Territorial Epidemiologists voted to include the prevalence of cigarette-smoking as an indicator for nationwide surveillance. This was the first time that a behavior, rather than a disease or illness, had been considered for national surveillance. The goals of this addition included monitoring the trends in tobacco use, guiding intervention resources, and evaluating public health interventions. Furthermore, a survey—the state-based Behavioral Risk Factor Surveillance System—was identified as the source of data for trends in smoking.

A uniform set of indicators for chronic disease surveillance has also been constructed by the CDC, the Council of State and Territorial Epidemiologists, and the Association of State and Territorial Chronic Disease Program Directors (CDC 2004a). The 2004 revision of this list includes 92 indicators covering cancer, cardiovascular disease, diabetes, alcohol, nutrition, tobacco, oral health, physical activity, renal disease, asthma, osteoporosis, immunizations, and overarching conditions such as poverty and health insurance. The Chronic Disease Indicators website provides access to state-level data and definitions of all indicators.

Vital Statistics

Information collected at the time of birth and death constitute one of the cornerstones of surveillance in the United States (Stroup, Zack, and Wharton 1994). Mortality records

Table 4.2. Selected Chronic Disease Data Sources and Surveillance Systems

Data System	Example	Strengths	Limitations
Notifiable diseases[a,b,c]	State-based lead poisoning reporting systems	• Data are available at the local level • Usually coupled with a public health response (e.g., lead paint removal) • Detailed information can be collected to aid in designing control programs • Laboratory-based systems are inexpensive and effective	• Requires participation by community-based clinicians • Clinician-based systems have low reporting rates • Active reporting systems are time-consuming and expensive
Vital statistics[a,b,c]	Death certificates	• Data are widely available at the local, state, and national levels • Population-based • Can monitor trends in age-adjusted disease rates • Can target areas with increased mortality rates	• Cause of death information may be inaccurate (e.g., lack of autopsy information) • Little to no information about risk factors
Sentinel Surveillance[b,c]	Sentinel Event Notification System for Occupational Risks	• Low-cost system to monitor selected diseases • Usually coupled with a public health response (e.g., asbestos removal following report of mesothelioma) • Provides information on risk factors and disease severity	• Requires motivated reporting providers • May not be representative
Disease registries[b,c]	Cancer registries	• Data are increasingly available throughout the United States • Includes accurate tissue-based diagnoses • Provides stage-of-diagnosis data when available	• Systems are expensive • Data are affected by patient out-migration from one geographic unit to another • Risk factor information is seldom available

Table 4.2. (*continued*)

Data System	Example	Strengths	Limitations
Health Surveys[b,c]	Behavioral risk factor surveillance telephone surveys	• Monitors trends in risk factor prevalence • Can be used for program design and evaluation	• Information is based on self-reports • May be too expensive to conduct at the local level • May not be representative due to nonresponse (e.g., telephone surveys)
Administrative data collection systems[b,c]	Hospital discharge systems	• Reflects regional differences on disease hospitalization rates • Can capture cost information • Data are readily available • One of few sources of morbidity data	• Often lacks personal identifiers • Rates may be affected by changing patterns of diagnosis based on reimbursement mechanisms • Difficult to separate initial from recurrent hospitalizations
U.S. Census[a,b,c]	Poverty rates by county	• Required to calculate rates • Important predictors of health status • Available to all communities and readily available online	• Historically collected infrequently (every 10 years) • May undercount certain populations (e.g., the poor, homeless persons)

[a] Data are available from most local public health agencies.
[b] Data are available from most state departments of health.
[c] Data are available from many U.S. Federal health agencies (e.g., CDC, National Cancer Institute, Health Care Financing Administration, etc).

are the records most often used for chronic disease surveillance and constitute the oldest data systems used for disease surveillance. In 1850, the Federal Government began publishing U.S. mortality statistics based on the decennial census of that year (Thacker and Berkelman 1988). By the early part of the century, the death registration system had become an integral part of efforts to control tuberculosis, typhoid fever, and diphtheria. It was viewed as the foundation of all public health work (Chapin 1916). Chronic diseases, such as heart disease, cancer, and stroke, account for many of the leading causes of death in the United States (Hsiang-Ching et al. 2008), indicating the importance of chronic disease mortality data for surveillance.

In the United States, mortality data are collected through the vital registration system. After a person dies, a physician or coroner completes the death certificate. He or she lists the immediate cause of death (e.g., pneumonia), the sequence of events that led to the death (e.g., lung cancer), and other contributing causes (e.g., tobacco use). The disease or condition that triggered the chain of events that eventually caused the death is considered to be the "underlying cause of death" (Kirscher and Anderson 1987; CDC 2003). In the example cited above, lung cancer would be listed as the underlying cause, and tobacco use and pneumonia would be listed as contributing causes.

One important limitation of using mortality data for surveillance is that death certificates are occasionally incomplete. The physician or coroner who is completing the certificate may not know the complete clinical history of the deceased person or may not take the time to properly complete the certificate. In addition, some conditions, such as diabetes, are often underreported as underlying or contributing causes (CDC 1991a, 1991b; Andresen et al. 1993; Cheng et al. 2008). Finally, even though death certificates provide a space to list contributing factors and a question asking specifically whether tobacco use contributed to the death, some physicians may be reluctant to list this information as a contributing cause of death.

In most states, mortality data are readily accessible for chronic disease surveillance. State-specific data are collected and maintained by vital statistics departments in a standard format. The CDC has developed guidelines for the use of mortality data for chronic disease surveillance (Office of Surveillance and Analysis 1992). In addition, these mortality data are easily accessible online (CDC 2009b). Birth certificate data can be used to identify the presence of some chronic conditions during pregnancy, such as hypertension, diabetes, and cardiac disease; however, hospital discharge or other data sources may perform better than vital statistics for identifying some chronic diseases in pregnancy (Devlin, Desai, and Walaszek 2008).

Sentinel Surveillance

The term *sentinel surveillance* encompasses a wide range of activities that focus on key health indicators in the population. A sentinel event could be a particular symptom or constellation of symptoms, preventable disease, disability, or untimely death whose occurrence serves as a warning that prevention may need to be improved, or steps need to be taken to prevent a widespread outbreak. This type of surveillance lends itself well to communicable disease issues, such as monitoring the spread of influenza-like illness (CDC 2009c), and has also been proposed as a method for early identification of symptom patterns that may be indicative of a naturally occurring outbreak or a bioterrorist attack. However, the effectiveness of this approach remains to be proven (Moran and Talan 2007; Stoto, Schonlau, and Mariano 2004).

When applied to chronic diseases, sentinel surveillance most often focuses on occupational-related health conditions. The National Institute for Occupational Safety and Health has developed the Sentinel Event Notification System for Occupational Risks, which depends on sentinel providers to report detailed information about people diagnosed with diseases such as silicosis, lead poisoning, or carpal tunnel syndrome (Baker 1989).

Chronic Disease Registries

Chronic disease registries are essential for monitoring trends in diseases. Collection of chronic disease information for surveillance is often mandated under state law, and the chronic disease registry is usually the entity charged with fulfilling that mandate. Detailed information about each disease can be collected, such as patient demographics, stage at diagnosis, or types of treatment provided. Given the scope and complexity of the data collection and processing, these registries require considerable financial resources to implement and maintain.

Cancer registries are the most common type of disease registry used for chronic disease surveillance. Hospitals, pathology laboratories, physician offices, and clinics collect data on patients after they have been diagnosed with or treated for cancer. Those data are then reported to a cancer registry. These data include demographic information, tumor information (primary site, histology, diagnostic confirmation, stage of disease at diagnosis, distant metastases at time of diagnosis, date of diagnosis, patient's residence at diagnosis, behavior, and grade), and treatment information (date and type of cancer–directed first course treatment).

The type of cancer registry varies according to the population on which data are collected, the standards followed for collection, and the extent of follow-up performed. Hospital-based registries collect information on patients diagnosed or treated at that facility; they are often able to collect follow-up information on their patients from time of diagnosis to death. In contrast, population-based registries collect information on all people residing in a specific geographic area, such as a county, region, or state. These registries are more appropriate for epidemiological analysis and research covering a particular population group because the data collected can be tailored to the defined population at risk; thus, cancer incidence rates can be calculated over time and among geographic regions, and for a variety of patient demographic groups. However, patient migration out of the area covered by a population-based registry for care can often limit the accuracy of these systems, necessitating follow-up work to improve completeness of the data (Walsh et al. 2006). Many population-based registries do not have sufficient funds to conduct such follow-up. Hospital-based registries have the ability, more often, to conduct patient follow-up, making it possible to calculate survival statistics.

Population-based cancer registries were established to identify regional differences in cancer incidence rates and to better understand the reasons for these differences (Austin 1983). The first population-based cancer registry was established in Connecticut in 1936. The Surveillance, Epidemiology, and End Results program of the National Cancer Institute, established in 1972, is composed of individual population-based registries in 18 separate geographic areas, covering approximately 26% of the U.S. population. This program provides data on national trends in both cancer incidence and mortality and is used by researchers to conduct epidemiologic studies of cancer (NCI 2009).

In October 1992, Congress established the National Program of Cancer Registries by enacting The Cancer Registries Amendment Act (Cancer Registries Amendment Act

1992). As a result of this law, the CDC provides annual financial support to state and territorial health departments and some universities to establish and improve population-based cancer registries. As of the writing of this text, 45 states, the District of Columbia, Puerto Rico, and the United States Pacific Island Jurisdictions receive CDC support for cancer registries, representing 96% of the United States population.

Health Surveys

Health surveys may be used to collect information about self-reported behaviors and health practices in the general population. In the United States, surveys such as the National Health Interview Survey are important sources of information for monitoring trends in the prevalence of health conditions and risk factors in the general population. These surveys, conducted annually since 1957, provide information on self-reported chronic conditions, health behaviors, and use of health services.

To obtain comparable information at the state or local level, CDC has developed an ongoing telephone surveillance system called the Behavioral Risk Factor Surveillance System. These data are collected using standardized methods and questionnaires, thus permitting comparison of the prevalence of behavioral risk factors, such as smoking and alcohol use, between states, over time, and for various sociodemographic groups.

Data are collected monthly, with more than 350,000 adults interviewed each year by random-digit dial telephone sampling. Each interview takes about 15–20 minutes to complete and addresses a variety of conditions and risk factors, including cardiovascular disease, asthma, cancer, tobacco use, alcohol consumption, exercise, diet, and the use of preventive health services. States may choose to include topical modules relevant to their local health issues in addition to core questions used by all states. These data are usually entered directly into a computer and are summarized annually by CDC and state health departments. Data quality concerns include validity and reliability of the questions, sample bias, reporting accuracy, and changing trends in telephone surveys, such as decreasing landline coverage (Jackson et al. 1992; Kempf and Remington 2007).

The CDC also supports the Youth Risk Behavior Surveillance System (CDC 2004b). Anonymous surveys are administered to a representative sample of 9th to 12th grade students in many states, territories, and cities across the United States. This surveillance system monitors six categories of priority chronic disease risk behaviors, including tobacco use, alcohol and other drug use, sexual behaviors, unhealthy dietary behaviors, and physical inactivity. Health and education officials are using these data to improve national, state, and local policies and programs designed to reduce risks associated with the leading causes of mortality and morbidity.

Some health surveys go beyond self-reported risk factors and conditions to include additional information collected through physical examinations and biologic samples. The National Health and Nutrition Examination Survey (NHANES) was created in the late 1950s to monitor the health status of the U.S. population. NHANES data collection has focused on different population age groups over time, but today it operates continuously and includes all ages.

Mobile examination centers are used to conduct interviews and physical examinations, collecting information on prevalence of chronic conditions, risk factors, body measurements, and blood samples. Because of the extensive amount of data collected on each individual, NHANES is most valuable for providing national information. One of the first state- and local-level adaptations of this approach was started in Wisconsin in 2008 (Survey of the Health of Wisconsin 2009).

In an effort to compensate for the fact that Hispanics were not traditionally included in NHANES in sufficient numbers to estimate the health of this rising segment of the U.S. population, the Hispanic Health and Nutrition Examination Survey was conducted from 1982 to 1984. This survey was a national probability sample that included approximately 16,000 individuals aged 6 months to 74 years and the information collected can be used as a reference database for current and future environmental health studies involving Hispanic populations.

Administrative Data Collection Systems

Many data on chronic diseases are collected as part of routine administration. Hospital discharge data are the most widely available of these types of data. In particular, hospital discharge data may be used to characterize hospitalization patterns and reasons for hospitalization for chronic diseases (CDC, 1988). Information is collected from the medical abstracts and billing records of each patient discharged from the hospital. Patient diagnoses and procedures are coded according to the *International Classification of Diseases, Ninth Revision, Clinical Modification* (ICD-9-CM 1980). It is anticipated that the next revision, ICD-10-CM, will replace ICD-9-CM as the standard in 2013 (CDC 2009d).

Unfortunately, the usefulness of administrative databases is limited by incomplete records, unreliable or invalid coding, and missing important clinical variables. Measurement errors associated with hospital discharge data arise chiefly in the coding process, which requires coders to know clinical diagnoses and the organization of the ICD coding scheme. Thus, misclassification may occur either unintentionally if providers lack understanding of diagnostic coding and grouping, or if providers code with an eye toward maximizing reimbursement via particular diagnosis-related groups (National Opinion Research Center 2005). Also, although diagnoses are often listed on the face sheet of the medical record, the principal diagnoses may not be cited accurately when the hospital discharge form is completed.

Another limitation is inherent in the fact that these data only capture events that occur in a hospital. Thus, the growing number of procedures that historically required hospitalization, but that now can be performed in outpatient settings, would not be captured. Additionally, information on injuries may be missed by this system if the injury is either serious enough that the patient dies before being admitted to a hospital, or not serious enough to warrant a hospital stay (Schoenman et al. 2007).

The principles of surveillance can also be applied by state and national agencies to monitor the quality of health care (Chassin et al. 1996). For example, consumers and purchasers of health care use HEDIS® (Healthcare Effectiveness Data and Information Set) data to assess the performance of managed health care plans (Iglehart 1996). HEDIS® is developed and maintained by the National Committee for Quality Assurance, and addresses eight performance domains, including effectiveness of care, access/availability of care, satisfaction with the experience of care, cost of care, health plan stability, informed health care choices, use of services, and health plan descriptive information. HEDIS® is one of the most widely used sets of health care performance measures in the United States.

Because a large percentage of the population is enrolled in managed care and because HEDIS® addresses many different topics and health conditions, the use of HEDIS® data has led to innovative uses of these data to improve public health. For example, the Wisconsin

Collaborative Diabetes Quality Improvement Project (the Collaborative), initiated in 1999 by the Wisconsin Department of Health Services, Diabetes Prevention and Control Program, has been able to achieve an extraordinary level of cooperation from diverse, competitive health maintenance organizations (HMOs) to improve diabetes care in Wisconsin (Siomos et al. 2005). The HMOs participating in the Collaborative use select HEDIS® measures to evaluate ongoing implementation of the *Wisconsin Diabetes Mellitus Essential Care Guidelines* (Wisconsin Department of Health Services 2008), as a means to ultimately improve the quality of diabetes care in Wisconsin. Yearly collection and analysis of HMOs HEDIS® data allows the Wisconsin Collaborative to implement specific targeted interventions. For example, the Collaborative implemented an eye care initiative in 2001 and in 2006 to increase the percentage of persons with diabetes who receive an annual dilated eye examination. The HMO quality improvement workgroup has met quarterly since its inception, and in 2006 Wisconsin was recognized as the top performing state in the nation for three of the seven Comprehensive Diabetes Care measures.

Census Data

Every 10 years, the U.S. government conducts a census of the entire U.S. population. In addition to counting the population, the census collects detailed information on individual and household characteristics, such as age, race, education, and income. These census data are essential for calculating rates in populations, in order to compare disease burden and trends among regions or over time.

Despite efforts to enumerate the entire population, however, the census misses some people in its count. In 2000, the census missed an estimated 3 million people, who were disproportionately from minority racial and ethnic groups and concentrated in a small number of geographic areas. The potential for errors in the census must be taken into account when examining rates in these special populations.

In an effort to improve the timeliness of population information, the U.S. Census has instituted the American Community Survey (ACS). The ACS uses monthly samples, combining data over multiple years when necessary, to create small area data on topics such as educational attainment, income, ancestry, and housing. This information was previously collected in the "long form" of the decennial census. More timely small area population estimates are especially important for population groups whose numbers are changing rapidly and for areas that may experience large, sustained population changes due to natural disasters, economic changes, or other causes.

In conclusion, chronic disease surveillance can be conducted using a wide variety of existing data sources. When using these data, public health practitioners must understand the advantages and limitations inherent in each system. Despite these limitations, a comprehensive surveillance system—using a wide variety of chronic disease data—can serve as a resource to improve the health of the entire population (Roos et al. 1993).

Data Analyses and Interpretation

Chronic disease surveillance systems must have the capacity to analyze data. Data analysis and interpretation require knowledge about chronic diseases and the relationship among risk factors, conditions, morbidity, and death. In addition, interpretation of analyses must include a thorough understanding of the data systems and statistical techniques used in all analyses. Because of the large number of cases involved, analysis at one time required the use of mainframe computers; however, today large data sets can be easily accommodated on personal computers, and powerful laptops have made data entry, surveillance, and analysis highly portable. Data are also frequently available in an online or electronic format. Internet-based query systems provide quick access to national (http://wonder.cdc. gov/), state (http://dhs.wisconsin.gov/wish/), and local (http://www.nyc.gov/html/doh/ html/vs/vs-epiquery.shtml) data. The CDC's Public Health Information Network initiative is aimed at improving electronic public health data capacity and exchange.

Chronic disease surveillance uses descriptive epidemiology and examines the distribution of diseases in the population by person, place, and time. Brief descriptions of these important analyses follow.

Person Analyses

Descriptive studies begin by examining how the distribution of a disease or condition varies in the population according to personal characteristics, such as age, race, or gender. For example, breast cancer morality rates in the United States by age and race are shown in the following table (Table 4.3). Breast cancer mortality rates increase with increasing age, from fewer than 1 death per hundred thousand women under the age of 35, to 185 deaths per hundred thousand women 85 years of age and older. In addition, blacks have a higher mortality rate compared with whites and persons of other races (Native Americans and Asian/Pacific Islanders). Recognizing and understanding the reasons for these differences is necessary for designing effective breast cancer prevention and control programs.

Table 4.3. Breast Cancer Mortality Rates, per 100, 000, in the United States, 2001–2005, by Race and Age

Age (year)	White	Black	Other	All Races
<35	0.5	1.1	0.4	0.6
35–44	10.7	20.9	7.1	11.9
45–54	28.3	49.4	20.0	30.5
55–64	54.4	79.4	32.7	56.1
65–74	82.9	99.8	38.7	82.7
75–84	124.0	136.2	50.5	122.8
85+	186.0	207.1	71.2	185.1
All ages[a]	26.7	36.0	13.7	27.3

[a] Age adjusted to the 2000 U.S. female population. Data obtained from CDC Wide-ranging ONline Data for Epidemiologic Research.

Place Analyses

A second type of analysis involves comparing the occurrence of a disease, condition, or risk factor between one geographic region and another. Typically, the rate in a city or county is compared with rates for the rest of the state or the nation. This information may be used to target a specific intervention in a region (Brownson et al. 1992). Figure 4.2 shows the differences in breast cancer mortality between states in the United States.

Regional analyses must account for differences in age structure between and among regions by using age-standardized rates. In addition, regional differences in disease rates may result from differences in diagnostic practices and/or disease definitions. Finally, these analyses are often limited because of the small number of cases typically occurring in small regions, such as cities, villages, or towns. See Chapter 2 for a more detailed discussion of the challenges created by working with small numbers of cases, and how to handle these types of analyses.

A specialized form of regional analysis involves the analysis of diseases that appear to "cluster" in a geographic area, such as a cluster of cancer cases that occur in a neighborhood. The investigation of these disease clusters poses a continuing challenge to state and local public health officials. Most often, these disease clusters are reported by members of the public or by clinicians who are looking for explanations for the apparent increase in the incidence of a disease. For example, in response to a request from a legislator, the Wisconsin Division of Health analyzed breast cancer rates among women living in neighborhoods north of Milwaukee. This analysis found higher-than-expected rates of breast cancer incidence and deaths in this community, opening the possibility that certain conditions within the community itself may put the residents at increased risk for developing breast cancer (Remington and Park 1997) (Table 4.4).

Public health agencies have developed systematic protocols to aid in the investigation of these apparent disease clusters (Fiore, Hanrahan, and Anderson 1990; Devier et

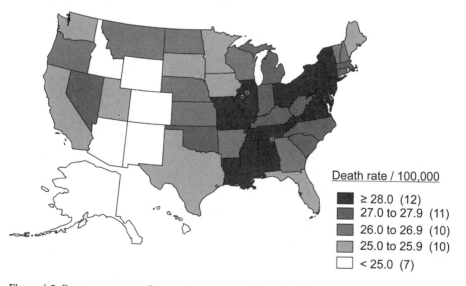

Figure 4.2. Breast cancer mortality rates by state, age-adjusted to the 2000 U.S. female population, 2001–2005.

Table 4.4. Breast Cancer Mortality and Incidence in Milwaukee's North Shore Communities, 1989–1994

	Observed Number	Expected Number	Difference	p Value
Cases	394	336	+58	0.01
Early stage	282	213	+69	<0.001
Late stage	94	104	−10	Not significant
Deaths	108	87	+21	<0.05

Remington, P. L., and S. Park. Breast Cancer Incidence and Mortality in Milwaukee's North Shore Communities. *Wis Med J* (1997):96(3):46–47.

al. 1990). These procedures involve defining the population at risk, ascertaining all cases, estimating rate ratios (i.e., observed versus expected), and assessing exposure and biologic plausibility. Using this approach, few investigations identify specific environmental exposures responsible for the disease cluster. A major difficulty in studying such clusters involves the small number of disease cases available for analysis. In fact, Rothman states that, with very few exceptions, there is little scientific or public health purpose in investigating individual disease clusters at all (Rothman 1990).

Time Analyses

Finally, and perhaps most importantly, chronic disease surveillance systems must monitor the trends in chronic disease rates over time. The epidemic curve has traditionally been used to detect outbreaks, to better characterize transmission patterns, and to determine appropriate intervention strategies. Similarly, trends in variables such as per capita cigarette sales can be used to monitor the effectiveness of interventions following the implementation of a statewide tobacco control program (Bandi, Remington, and Moberg 2006).

Temporal trend analyses must consider changes in the age structure of the population over time, usually by using age standardization with a standard reference population. In addition, changes in diagnostic practices and disease definitions may cause apparent trends in disease incidence over time. Both temporal trend and regional analyses may be conducted for specific subgroups of the population. For example, as mammography began to be widely implemented in the mid to late 1980s, and improvements in treatment were achieved in the 1990s, a significant gap developed in breast cancer mortality between white women and black women in the United States (Figure 4.3). Although more recently the rates of breast cancer appear to be declining among both white women and black women in the United States, the rate decline for black women began later and has been less pronounced than the decline for white women, and a large disparity gap continues to exist. These findings have important implications in the development of programs to ensure all demographic groups have equal access to advances in public health knowledge.

Age-adjusted rate/100,000

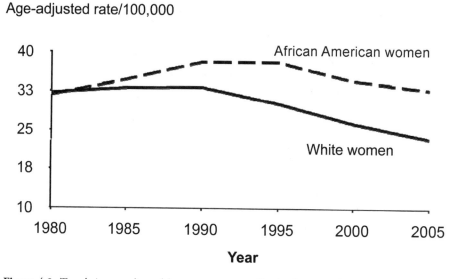

Figure 4.3. Trends in age-adjusted breast cancer mortality in the United States by race, 1980–2005.

Data Dissemination

The final step in chronic disease surveillance is to disseminate the information that has been collected. The increasing amount of surveillance data described above provides a wealth of information to public health agencies. However, too often these agencies simply analyze the data and report the results in agency reports or occasionally in state or national publications. These reports are often long and contain technical jargon. In addition, the information is seldom linked to program priorities, and the reports are seldom used to promote public health practice or as a vehicle for setting priorities for action.

In the past, communicable disease surveillance systems typically produced surveillance reports and distributed them to health care providers. Today's chronic disease programs address a broader constituency, including policymakers, voluntary health organizations, professional organizations, and the general public. Thus, the information must be communicated through several channels using different strategies to assure that it reaches the appropriate target groups.

Epidemiologists working in public health agencies are frequently asked to disseminate the results of a surveillance report, often by publishing the information in a health department report. To increase application of surveillance findings to disease prevention and health promotion programs, a basic framework for communicating surveillance information can be used (Remington 1998; Goodman and Remington 1993) (Table 4.5).

Once the analysis has been completed, this framework has five additional steps:

Establish the Message

This is perhaps the most important step in disseminating health and surveillance information. Like businesses, public health agencies have a product (i.e., information) that they need to sell (i.e., communicate). An epidemiologist must convince the audience that it is

Table 4.5. Steps in Communicating Public Health Surveillance Information

Step	Question	Action
1	What do the data show?	Conduct the analysis
2	What should be said?	Establish the message
3	What is the communication objective?	Set an objective
4	To whom should the message be directed?	Define the audience
5	What communications medium should be used?	Select the channel
6	Was the communication objective achieved?	Evaluate the impact

Remington, P. L. Communicating Epidemiologic Information. In: Brownson, R. C., and D. B. Petitti, editors, *Applied Epidemiology: Theory to Practice*. New York, NY: Oxford University Press (1998) pp. 323–348. Used by permission of Oxford University Press, Inc.

worth their time to read, understand, and act on the information. An important adage in marketing the message is "less is more."

Many reports produced by public health agencies are long, technical, and full of information. These reports might be mailed to the media, policymakers, or health care providers who, in turn, rarely take the time to read through the report to find the important information. To capture their attention, the main point of the report must be obvious and simple to understand. For example, the main message of the report describing the trends in breast cancer in the United States would be that these trends are different for black and white women, and a significant gap exists in mortality for these two groups.

Set an Objective

Why is the information being reported? Public health agencies often report information without any specific goal, but simply "because it is there." Other times, the purpose is to educate the general public about a health issue. This is a worthwhile, but challenging, goal given the complexity of the message and the inability to shape the message for the intended audience.

Occasionally, surveillance findings point to a needed public health action. For example, the finding of an increasing breast cancer mortality gap between black women and white women emphasizes the need for effective breast cancer screening initiatives that can be universally accessed and that do not preferentially benefit one segment of the population. Therefore, the intent of releasing this information might be to support a public health initiative, such as the National Breast and Cervical Cancer Early Detection Program.

Define the Audience

Once the objective for communicating the information has been established, one can define the appropriate target audience. Local health departments and health care providers have been the long-standing audience of communicable disease surveillance information, since these professionals were responsible for implementing disease control strategies. In addition, physicians were the source of these reports, and reporting back to them showed the usefulness of the system and helped maintain their continued reporting.

The audience for public health surveillance information is much broader today and includes policymakers, voluntary health organizations, professional organizations, and the general public. A report that breast cancer death rates are increasing among minorities, or low income women, or women who are uninsured or underinsured in a state could be communicated to the general public, or to women specifically. This would increase awareness of the importance of mammography and early detection. It might also be targeted to policymakers, such as legislators considering developing a breast cancer detection program focused on reducing breast cancer deaths among minorities or low income and uninsured women. Finally, the report could be given to an advocacy organization, such as a statewide minority health council, to use in their efforts to advocate for minority health.

Select the Channel

A "channel" can be considered the medium through which messages must travel to reach the intended audience. Examples of channels include professional journals, direct mail, television, radio, newspapers, blogs, and other Internet sources. Public health agencies traditionally report surveillance information in newsletters or statistical bulletins. These reports are routinely mailed to local public health agencies, physicians, health care institutions, the media, and other interested individuals in the community or the state. A press release is occasionally used to increase the media interest in the story.

Careful selection of a proper communication channel increases the likelihood that the information will reach the target audience. This requires a thorough understanding, based on market research, of how those individuals obtain their information. For example, children and teachers might best be reached through the school system newsletter. Policymakers might be reached through a direct mailing to their offices or via a constituent organization. Doctors might be reached through a state medical society journal. For most target groups, it is also helpful in disseminating a message through an effective presence on the internet, as Internet access has become nearly universal and is often the first source individuals turn to for information.

As an example of a targeted dissemination of information, the Wisconsin Comprehensive Cancer Control Program developed the Surveillance Brief, a document that highlights current research in cancer control at the University of Wisconsin in a format easily digestible by policymakers, clinicians, and public health leaders—groups whose time is often at a premium. The Surveillance Brief format consists of about two pages of text and one page of figures with an abstract containing critical information included on page one. Each Surveillance Brief includes a section describing program and policy implications related to the research highlighted. Historically, paper copies of the Surveillance Briefs had been mailed to a list of subscribers, but with the rapid adoption of internet usage as described above, starting in 2009 an all-electronic format will be used, with e-mail notifications to subscribers when the latest Surveillance Brief is available on the Wisconsin Comprehensive Cancer Control Program's website (http://wicancer.org/publications.html).

Creative presentation of information can also increase the media coverage of a health issue. For example, in support of a comprehensive smoking ban in Wisconsin, it was pointed out that in Wisconsin in a given year, the number of people who die from second hand smoke exposure (a harm viewed by many as an insignificant risk not requiring government intervention) and the number of people who die in motor vehicle accidents (a cause of death well recognized as a significant public health issue requiring government regulation) is approximately the same at about 800 individuals per year.

Evaluate the Impact

The final step in a communication plan is to evaluate how widely the information was disseminated and whether the information led to the intended outcome. The dissemination can be measured by determining the number of reports distributed, the readership of a journal, coverage in the media, or the number of hits on a particular website. Web searches can be an effective means of finding all articles on a particular topic in a defined geographic area. These articles can be reviewed by the program staff to assess the geographic distribution and extent of the media coverage. In addition, the content can be reviewed to assess both the accuracy and appropriateness of the messages as they were picked up by the media.

The above methods can provide early indicators of success of public health campaigns. However, one major drawback of evaluating interventions aimed at reducing chronic disease is that as a consequence of the slow progression from risk factors to physiologic changes to symptoms to eventual disease development, demonstrating definitive proof of disease reduction may take decades, while the typical political cycle is only every 2–6 years. Thus, if the political winds shift, potentially effective programs may be cut before they have had a chance to demonstrate their impact. In addition, evaluations of societal change and impact on disease are often expensive, time consuming, and difficult to interpret.

Conclusion

Data collection, analysis, and dissemination are vital components of a chronic disease surveillance system. The final link in surveillance is the application of the data to prevention and control (Thacker and Berkelman 1988). Unfortunately, the long latency period of most chronic diseases often results in a perceived lack of urgency in developing and implementing control measures. For example, at the onset of a potential influenza pandemic or an outbreak of an illness new to the world or a particular region of the world such as severe acute respiratory syndrome or monkeypox, media attention is intense and considerable amounts of resources are deployed within hours, days, and weeks to implement control measures and contain disease spread. In contrast, it has been 45 years since the First Surgeon General's Report on Smoking and Health was released, definitively linking smoking to cancer and other serious chronic diseases. However, about half of the states in the United States still lack comprehensive smoke-free laws. In those states where legislation has passed, it has come only after heavy sustained effort and occasionally compromises on issues where the strong weight of the evidence rests on the side of public health. This demonstrates that building up a definitive library of evidence and scientific data in support of a public health issue does not in and of itself constitute a "public health surveillance system" unless these data are disseminated in such a way that they can impact public health policies aimed at controlling chronic disease.

With the recent emergence of chronic disease program integration as a priority, chronic disease surveillance will play an even bigger role at state departments of health.

An integrated approach will require innovative new methods for tracking and reporting chronic diseases, with specific emphasis on how chronic disease risk factors and certain chronic diseases themselves are interrelated. As links among chronic diseases and risk factors are more clearly demonstrated to policymakers, there is significant potential to reframe the health care reform debate from a focus on access to a focus on prevention, and in the process increase the amount of state and Federal resources allocated to addressing the important chronic disease issues that exist in our society.

Resources

Information on the availability of routinely collected chronic disease surveillance data is available
    from a variety of Federal agencies and other sources:
Agency for Health Care Research and Quality (http://www.ahrq.gov/)
Behavioral Risk Factor Surveillance System (http://www.cdc.gov/BRFSS/)
Centers for Disease Control and Prevention (CDC), including the National Center for Health
    Statistics, the National Center for Chronic Disease Prevention and Health Promotion, and
    the Epidemiology Program Office (http://www.cdc.gov)
CDC WONDER (http://wonder.cdc.gov/)
Centers for Medicare and Medicaid Services (CMS) (http://www.cms.hhs.gov/)
Chronic Disease Indicators—CDC (http://apps.nccd.cdc.gov/cdi/)
National Institute of Health (NIH), including the National Cancer Institute (NCI), the Nation-
    al Heart, Lung, and Blood Institute (NHLBI), and the National Institute on Drug Abuse
    (NIDA) (http://www.nih.gov)
National Institute for Occupational Safety and Health (NIOSH)/SENSOR (http://www.cdc.gov/
    niosh/topics/surveillance/ords/default.html)
National Notifiable Diseases Surveillance System (http://www.cdc.gov/ncphi/disss/nndss/nndsshis.
    htm)
U.S. Census Bureau (http://www.census.gov/)
Youth Risk Behavior Surveillance System (http://www.cdc.gov/HealthyYouth/yrbs/index.htm)
Additional surveillance information and data can be obtained from state health departments and
    many local public health agencies.

Suggested Reading

Centers for Disease Control. Indicators for Chronic Disease Surveillance. *MMWR Recomm Rep*
    (2004):53(RR11):1–6.
Centers for Disease Control. Surveillance for Certain Health Behaviors among States and Selected
    Local Areas—Behavioral Risk Factor Surveillance System, United States (2004). Indicators for
    Chronic Disease Surveillance. *MMWR Surveill Summ* (2006):55(SS07):1–124.
Choi, B.C.K., D.V. McQueen, P. Puska, et al. Enhancing Global Capacity in the Surveillance,
    Prevention, and Control of Chronic Diseases: Seven Themes to Consider and Build upon.
    J Epidemiol Community Health (2008):62:391–397.
Lee, L.M., S.M. Teutsch, M.E. St. Louis, and S.B. Thacker, editors. *Principles and Practice of Public
    Health Surveillance*, 3rd ed. New York, NY: Oxford University Press (in press).
Pelletier, A.R., P.Z. Siegel, M.S. Baptiste, and C. Maylahn. Revisions to Chronic Disease Surveil-
    lance Indicators, United States, 2004. *Prev Chronic Dis* (2005):2(3):1–5.
Remington, P.L., E. Simoes, R.C. Brownson, and P.Z. Siegel. The Role of Epidemiology in
    Chronic Disease Prevention and Health Promotion Programs. *J Public Health Manag Pract*
    (2003):9(4):58–265.

References

Andresen, E.M., J.A.H. Lee, R.D. Pecoraro, T.D. Koepsell, A.P. Hallstrom, and D.S. Siscovick. Underreporting of Diabetes on Death Certificates, King County, Washington. *Am J Public Health* (1993):83:1020–1024.

Austin, D.F. Cancer Registries: A Tool in Epidemiology. *Rev Cancer Epidemiol* (1983):2:118–140.

Baker, E.L. Sentinel Event Notification System for Occupational Risks (SENSOR): The Concept. *Am J Public Health* (1989):79(Suppl):18–20.

Bandi, P., P.L. Remington, and D.P. Moberg. Progress in Reducing Cigarette Consumption: The Wisconsin Tobacco Control Program, 2001–2003. *Wis Med J* (2006):105:45–49.

Berkelman, R.L., and J.W. Buehler. Public Health Surveillance of Noninfectious Chronic Disease: The Potential to Detect Rapid Changes in Disease Burden. *Int J Epidemiol* (1990):19:628–635.

Boss, L.P., and L. Suarez. Uses of Data to Plan Cancer Prevention and Control Programs. *Public Health Rep* (1990):105:354–360.

Brownson, R.C., C.A. Smith, N.E. Jorge, et al. The Role of Data-Driven Planning and Coalition Development in Preventing Cardiovascular Disease. *Public Health Rep* (1992):107:32–37.

Cancer Registries Amendment Act. Public Law 102-515. 106 Stat. 3372 Oct. 24, 1992. Available at http://www.cdc.gov/cancer/npcr/npcrpdfs/publaw.pdf. Accessed June 19, 2009.

Centers for Disease Control and Prevention (CDC). Lower Extremity Amputations among Persons with Diabetes–Washington; 1988. *MMWR* (1991a):40:737–739.

Centers for Disease Control and Prevention (CDC). Sensitivity of Death Certificate Data for Monitoring Diabetes Mortality—Diabetic Eye Disease Follow-up Study, 1985–1990. *MMWR* (1991b):40:739–741.

Centers for Disease Control and Prevention (CDC). Updated Guidelines for Evaluating Public Health Surveillance Systems: Recommendations from the Guidelines Working Group. *MMWR* (2001a):50(No. RR-13).

Centers for Disease Control and Prevention (CDC). *Physicians' Handbook on Medical Certification of Death* (2003b). DHHS Publication No. (PHS) 2003-1108.

Centers for Disease Control and Prevention (CDC). Indicators for Chronic Disease Surveillance. *MMWR* (2004a):53(No. RR-11).

Centers for Disease Control and Prevention (CDC). Methodology of the Youth Risk Behavior Surveillance System. *MMWR* (2004b):53(No. RR-12).

Centers for Disease Control and Prevention (CDC). Nationally Notifiable Infectious Diseases: United States 2009. Available at http://www.cdc.gov/ncphi/disss/nndss/phs/infdis2009.htm. Accessed June 25, 2009a.

Centers for Disease Control and Prevention (CDC). Wide-ranging ONline Data for Epidemiologic Research (WONDER). Available at http://wonder.cdc.gov. Accessed May 15, 2009b.

Centers for Disease Control and Prevention (CDC). Overview of Influenza Surveillance in the United States. Available at http://www.cdc.gov/flu/weekly/pdf/flu-surveillance-overview.pdf. Accessed May 15, 2009c.

Centers for Disease Control and Prevention (CDC). National Center for Health Statistics. About the International Classification of Diseases, Tenth Revision, Clinical Modification (ICD-10-CM). Available at http://www.cdc.gov/nchs/about/otheract/icd9/abticd10.htm. Accessed June 19, 2009d.

Chapin, C.V. State Health Organization. *JAMA* (1916):66:699–703.

Chassin, M.R., E.L. Hannan, and B.A. DeBuono. Benefits and Hazards of Reporting Medical Outcomes Publicly. *New Engl J Med* (1996):334:394–398.

Cheng, W.S., D.L. Wingard, D. Kritz-Silverstein, and E. Barrett-Connor. Sensitivity and Specificity of Death Certificates for Diabetes. *Diabetes Care* (2008):31:279–284.

Devier, J.R., R.C. Brownson, J.R. Bagby, G.M. Carlson, and J.R. Crellin. A Public Health Response to Cancer Clusters in Missouri. *Am J Epidemiol* (1990):132(Suppl 1):S23–S31.

Devlin, H.M., J. Desai, and A. Walaszek. Reviewing Performance of Birth Certificate and Hospital Discharge Data to Identify Births Complicated by Maternal Diabetes. *Matern Child Health J* (2008 Sep 3). [Epub ahead of print]

Fiore, B.J., L.P. Hanrahan, and H.A. Anderson. State Health Department Response to Disease Cluster Reports: A Protocol for Investigation. *Am J Epidemiol* (1990):132(Suppl 1):S14–S22.

Goodman, R., and P.L. Remington. Disseminating Surveillance Information. In: Teutsch, S.M., and R.E. Churchill, editors, *Principles and Practice of Public Health Surveillance.* New York, NY: Oxford Univ. Press (1993).

Hsiang-Ching, K., D.L. Hoyert, J. Xu, and S.L. Murphy. *Deaths: Final Data for 2005. National Vital Statistics Reports*; Vol. 56 No. 10. Hyattsville, MD: National Center for Vital Statistics (2008).

Henning, K.J. Overview of Syndromic Surveillance: What is Syndromic Surveillance? *MMWR* (2004):53(Suppl):5–11.

Iglehart, J.K. The National Committee for Quality Assurance. *N Engl Med J* (1996):335:995–999.

International Classification of Diseases, 9th Revision, Clinical Modification (2nd ed.). Washington, D.C.: U.S. Department of Health and Human Services (1980). DHHS publication PHS 80-1260.

Kempf, A.M., and P.L. Remington. New Challenges for Telephone Survey Research in the Twenty-First Century. *Annu Rev Public Health* (2007):28:113–126.

Kirscher, T., and R.E. Anderson. Cause of Death: Proper Completion of the Death Certificate. *JAMA* (1987):258:349–352.

Jackson, C., D.E. Jatulis, and S.P. Fortmann. The Behavioral Risk Factor Survey and the Stanford Five-City Project Survey: A Comparison of Cardiovascular Risk Behavior Estimates. *Am J Public Health* (1992):82:412–416.

Jackson, R.J. The Impact of the Built Environment on Health: An Emerging Field. *Am J Public Health* (2003):93:1382–1383.

Langmuir, A.D. The Surveillance of Communicable Diseases of National Importance. *N Engl J Med* (1963):288:182–192.

Loonsk, J.W. BioSense—A National Initiative for Early Detection and Quantification of Public Health Emergencies. *MMWR* (2004):53(Suppl):53–55.

Moran, G.J., and D.A. Talan. Commentary. *Ann Emerg Med* (2007):50:54.

National Cancer Institute. Surveillance Epidemiology and End Results (SEER). Available at http://seer.cancer.gov/about/. Accessed May 15, 2009.

National Opinion Research Center. *The Value of Hospital Discharge Databases.* Bethesda, MD: NORC (2005).

Office of Surveillance and Analysis. *Using Chronic Disease Data: A Handbook for Public Health Practitioners.* Atlanta, GA: National Center for Chronic Disease Prevention and Health Promotion, Centers for Disease Control (1992).

Remington, P.L. Communicating Epidemiologic Information. In: Brownson, R.C., and D.B. Petitti, editors, *Applied Epidemiology: Theory to Practice.* New York, NY: Oxford Univ. Press (1998) pp. 323–348.

Remington, P.L., and S. Park. Breast Cancer Incidence and Mortality in Milwaukee's North Shore Communities. *Wis Med J* (1997):96(3):46–47.

Roos, L.L., C.A. Mustard, J.P. Nicol, et al. Registries and Administrative Data: Organization and Accuracy. *Med Care* (1993):31(3)201–212.

Rothman, K.J. A Sobering Start for the Cluster Buster's Conference. *Am J Epidemiol* (1990):132(Suppl 1):S6–S13.

Schoenman, J., J. Sutton, A. Elixhauser, and D. Love. Understanding and Enhancing the Value of Hospital Discharge Data. *Med Care Res Rev* (2007):64:449–468.

Siomos, E.E., R.S. Newsom, J. Camponeschi, and P.L. Remington. A Statewide Collaboration to Monitor Diabetes Quality Improvement among Wisconsin Health Plans. *Am J Manag Care* (2005):11(5):332–336.

Stoto, M.A., M. Schonlau, and L.T. Mariano. Syndromic Surveillance: Is It Worth the Effort? *Chance* (2004):17(1):19–24.

Stroup, N.E., M.M. Zack, and M. Wharton. Sources of Routinely Collected Data for Surveillance. In: Teutsch, S.M., and R.E. Churchill, editors, *Principles and Practice of Public Health Surveillance.* New York, NY: Oxford Univ. Press (1994).

Survey of the Health of Wisconsin (SHOW) home page. Available at http://www.show.wisc.edu/. Accessed May 15, 2009.

Thacker, S.B., and R.L. Berkelman. Public Health Surveillance in the United States. *Epidemiol Rev* (1988):10:164–190.

Walsh, M.C., L. Stephenson, J. Strickland, and A. Trentham-Dietz. *Enhancing the Completeness of the Wisconsin Cancer Reporting System—The Border County Pilot Project. Surveillance Brief.* University of Wisconsin Comprehensive Cancer Center (2006):2–3.

Wisconsin Department of Health Services, Diabetes Prevention and Control Program. Wisconsin Diabetes Mellitus Essential Care Guidelines 2008. Available at http://dhs.wisconsin.gov/health/diabetes/guidelines.htm. Accessed May 15, 2009.

CHAPTER 5

TOBACCO USE
(ICD-10 F17)

Corinne G. Husten, M.D., M.P.H.

Introduction

Tobacco use and dependence is a chronic disease and a leading cause of cancer, heart disease, and chronic lung disease (Fiore et al. 2008). In 1988, the Surgeon General concluded that nicotine met the primary criteria for drug dependency and that cigarettes and other forms of tobacco (including smokeless tobacco [SLT]) are addicting (USDHHS 1988). In 1996, the Council of State and Territorial Epidemiologists added prevalence of cigarette smoking to the list of conditions designated as reportable by states to the Centers for Disease Control and Prevention (CDC 1996a). Decades of research have elucidated the causes, consequences, and groups at high risk for tobacco use (see Figure 5.1). This chapter summarizes this information, as well as effective interventions to reduce tobacco use in children and adults and eliminate exposure to secondhand smoke (SHS).

Significance

The Surgeon General (USDHHS 2004) has concluded that smoking harms nearly every organ of the body causing a myriad of diseases, including

- Cardiovascular diseases, including coronary heart disease (CHD), atherosclerosis, abdominal aortic aneurysm, and cerebrovascular disease
- A variety of cancers, including lip, mouth, pharynx, esophagus, stomach, pancreas, larynx, trachea, lung, cervix, kidney, bladder, and acute myeloid leukemia
- Respiratory problems, including chronic obstructive pulmonary disease (COPD), pneumonia, reduced lung function in infants, impaired lung growth during childhood and adolescence, lung function decline in adolescents and young adults, respiratory symptoms in children and adolescents, asthma-related symptoms in childhood and adolescence, premature onset and accelerated age-related decline in lung function among adults, major respiratory symptoms in adults (coughing, phlegm, wheezing, shortness of breath), and poor asthma control
- Reproductive disorders, including reduced fertility, fetal death, stillbirth, low birthweight, and pregnancy complications
- Other diseases, such as sudden infant death syndrome (SIDS), cataracts, adverse surgical outcomes related to wound healing and respiratory complications, low

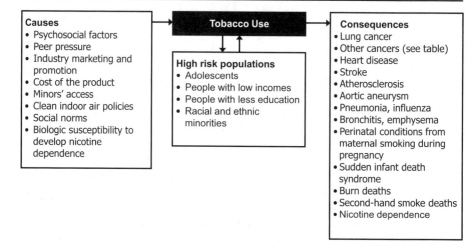

Figure 5.1. Tobacco use: causes, consequences, and high-risk groups.

bone density in postmenopausal women, hip fractures, and peptic ulcer disease in persons who are *Helicobacter pylori*–positive.

The Surgeon General (USDHHS 2006a) has also concluded that SHS (a mixture of sidestream smoke given off by a smoldering cigarette and the mainstream exhaled by the smoker) causes lung cancer, CHD, odor annoyance, and nasal irritation in adults and reduced birthweight, reduced lung function, lower respiratory infections (pneumonia, bronchitis), middle-ear disease (acute and recurrent otitis media and chronic middle-ear effusion), respiratory symptoms (cough, phlegm, wheeze, breathlessness), more severe asthma, and SIDS in children.

Use of SLT (defined as any finely cut, ground, powdered, or leaf tobacco that is intended to be placed in the oral cavity) causes cancer. The evidence is strongest for oral and pancreatic cancer (IARC 2005; USDHHS 2004), but increased risk for cancer of the stomach and esophagus has been reported (Chao et al. 2002). Some studies have shown a higher risk of hypertension, CHD, stroke, diabetes, hypercholesterolemia, lower high-density lipoprotein levels, and higher triglyceride levels with smokeless use (Bolinder, Ahlborg, and Lindell 1992; Gupta, Gurm, and Bartholomew 2004; Henley et al. 2005; USDHHS 1989). Adverse pregnancy outcomes have also been reported (England et al. 2003). SLT use causes periodontal disease, gingival recession, and oral leukoplakia (USDHHS 1986, 1994); changes in the hard and soft tissues of the mouth, discoloration of teeth, and decreased ability to taste and smell have also been reported (NIH 1988). SLT use may lead to subsequent cigarette use (Tomar 2003).

Cigar smoking causes oral, esophageal, laryngeal, and lung cancer (NCI 1998) and may increase the risk of pancreatic, bladder, and colon cancer (IARC 2004; Shapiro, Jacobs, and Thun 2000). Regular cigar smokers who inhale, particularly those who smoke several cigars a day, are at increased risk for COPD and CHD (Baker et al. 2000; Jacobs, Thun, and Apicella 1999). However, even those who do not inhale are at a higher risk of disease than those who never use tobacco. Cigar smoke contains a substantial proportion of its nicotine as un-ionized nicotine, which is easily absorbed through the oral mucosa.

Thus, cigar smokers do not need to inhale to ingest significant quantities of nicotine (NCI 1998), and cigars can deliver nicotine concentrations comparable with or higher than those from cigarettes and SLT.

Pipe smoking causes lip cancer (USDHHS 2004) and is also associated with COPD, oropharyngeal, laryngeal, esophageal, and lung cancer (Henley et al. 2004; IARC 2004; Lange et al. 1992). Some studies have suggested an increased risk of colorectal, pancreatic, and bladder cancer, and CHD (Henley et al. 2004; IARC 2004; Nyboe et al. 1991). It has been estimated that pipe smoking kills 1,100 Americans each year (Nelson et al. 1996).

Cigarette smoking causes more than 400,000 deaths each year (CDC 2008) (18% of all deaths in the United States) (Hoyert et al. 2006) and more than 5.1 million years of potential life lost (excluding SHS or burn deaths) each year (CDC 2008). The relative risks for death due to diseases caused by smoking and smoking-attributable mortality are shown in Table 5.1.

Smoking-attributable health care expenditures are estimated at $96 billion, and smoking-attributable productivity losses from premature deaths are estimated to be $97 billion per year (CDC 2007). These productivity costs are underestimates since they do not include lost productivity due to illness, disability, absenteeism, or reduced worker productivity. Health and productivity costs from SHS are estimated to be an additional $10 billion per year (Behan, Eriksen, and Lin 2005). One study assessed the cost burden to the smoker, his/her family (these costs are generally excluded from cost estimates), and to the society and found that these costs over 60 years were $220,000 for a male smoker and $106,000 for a female smoker, or $40 per pack of cigarettes (Sloan et al. 2004).

Smoking by employees is costly to employers. Smoking increases absenteeism, health and life insurance costs and claims, workers' compensation payments and occupational health awards, accidents, property damage and fires (and related insurance costs), cleaning and maintenance costs, and illness and discomfort among nonsmokers exposed to SHS (CDC 1996b). Male smokers are absent four days more each year than male nonsmokers (female smokers miss two additional days) (Warner et al. 1996). Among former smokers, absenteeism decreases with years of cessation (Halpern et al. 2001). One study reported that former smokers are 4.5% more productive than current smokers (Weis 1981).

Tobacco use may also increase poverty. A recent study estimated that, even after adjusting for a variety of demographic factors, each adult year of smoking was associated with a 4% reduction in net worth. The author concluded that smokers appear to pay for tobacco expenditures out of income that nonsmokers put into savings (Zagorsky 2004).

Pathophysiology

Cardiovascular Disease

Cigarette smoking is a major independent risk factor for CHD. Smoking-induced CHD results from at least five interrelated processes: atherosclerosis, thrombosis, coronary artery spasm, cardiac arrhythmia, and reduced oxygen-carrying capacity of the blood, although the exact components of cigarette smoke that cause each of these changes are not known (IARC 2005).

Data from animal and human studies suggest that nicotine causes endothelial damage (IARC 2005), increases in endothelial permeability to fibrinogen (Allen et al. 1988), and reductions in endothelium-dependent vasodilatation (Celermajer et al. 1993). Smoking

Table 5.1. Relative Risks[a] (RR) for Smoking-Attributable Mortality and Average Annual Number of Smoking-Attributable Mortalities (SAM[b]) among Current and Former Smokers, by Sex and Disease, United States, 2000–2004

	Men			Women			Total
	RR		SAM	RR		SAM	SAM
	Current Smoker	Former Smoker		Current Smoker	Former Smoker		
Cancers							
Lip, oral cavity, pharynx	10.9	3.4	3,749	5.1	2.3	1,144	4,893
Esophagus	6.8	4.5	6,961	7.8	2.8	1,631	8,592
Stomach	2.0	1.5	1,900	1.4	1.3	584	2,484
Pancreas	2.3	1.2	3,147	2.3	1.6	3,536	6,683
Larynx	14.6	6.3	2,446	13.0	5.2	563	3,009
Trachea, lung, bronchus	23.3	8.7	78,680	12.7	4.5	46,842	125,522
Cervix uteri	NA	NA	NA	1.6	1.1	447	447
Urinary bladder	3.3	2.1	3,907	2.2	1.9	1,076	3,903
Kidney or other part of urinary tract	2.7	1.7	2,827	1.3	1.1	216	4,123
Acute myeloid leukemia	1.9	1.3	855	1.1	1.4	337	1,192
Total			104,472			56,376	160,848
Cardiovascular diseases							
Ischemic heart disease							
Persons aged 35–64 years	2.8	1.6		3.1	1.3		
			50,884			29,121	79,965
Persons aged ≥65 years	1.5	1.2		1.6	1.2		
Other heart diseases	1.8	1.2	12,944	1.5	1.1	8,060	21,004

	Men			Women			Total
	RR		SAM	RR		SAM	SAM
	Current Smoker	Former Smoker		Current Smoker	Former Smoker		
Cerebrovascular disease							
Persons aged 35–64 years	3.3	1.0	7,896	4.0	1.3	8,026	15,922
Persons aged ≥65 years	1.6	1.0		1.5	1.0		
Atherosclerosis	2.4	1.3	1,282	1.8	1.0	611	1,893
Aortic aneurysm	6.2	3.1	5,628	7.1	2.1	2,791	8,419
Other arterial disease	2.1	1.0	505	2.2	1.1	749	1,254
Total			79,139			49,358	128,497
Respiratory diseases							
Pneumonia, influenza	1.8	1.4	6,042	2.2	1.1	4,381	10,423
Bronchitis, emphysema	17.1	15.6	7,536	12.0	11.8	6,391	13,927
Chronic airway obstruction	10.6	6.8	40,217	13.1	6.8	38,771	78,988
Total			53,795			49,543	103,338
Perinatal conditions from maternal smoking during pregnancy							
Short gestation/low birthweight	1.8		219	1.8		174	393
Respiratory distress syndrome	1.8		18	1.8		13	31
Other respiratory (newborn)	1.8		35	1.8		25	60
SIDS	1.5		173	1.5		119	292
Total			445			331	776

(continued on next page)

Table 5.1. (*continued*)

	Men			Women			Total
	RR		SAM	RR		SAM	SAM
	Current Smoker	Former Smoker		Current Smoker	Former Smoker		
Burn deaths			416			320	736
SHS deaths							
Lung cancer			2,131			1,269	3,400
Ischemic heart disease			29,256			16,744	46,000
Total			31,388			18,012	49,400
Total smoking-attributable mortality			269,655			173,940	443,595

[a]Relative to people who have never smoked.
[b]SAM is the estimated number of annual U.S. deaths due to smoking.
Source: CDC (2008b, 2008c).

also appears to stimulate smooth muscle cell proliferation and increase the adherence of platelets to arterial endothelium (IARC 2005). Smoking may also increase thrombus formation (Fusegawa et al. 1999). Current ideas about the pathogenesis of atherosclerosis increasingly emphasize a central role for inflammation (IARC 2005), and smoking induces a systemic inflammatory response (Friedman et al. 1973; Kuller et al. 1996). Additionally, a substantial body of evidence has demonstrated an association between smoking and adverse lipid profiles (IARC 2005; USDHHS 1990). Cigarette smoking also increases myocardial oxygen demand by increasing peripheral resistance, blood pressure, and heart rate (Benowitz and Gourlay 1997). In addition, the capacity of the blood to deliver oxygen is reduced by increased carboxyhemoglobin, greater viscosity, and higher coronary vascular resistance due to vasoconstrictor effects on the coronary arteries. Smoking has also been shown to lower the threshold for ventricular fibrillation (USDHHS 1990).

SHS increases the risk of cardiovascular disease among nonsmokers by causing prothrombotic effects and endothelial cell dysfunctions. Some studies have also found adverse effects on lipid profiles, reduced oxygen-carrying capacity, oxidative damage, and altered cardiac autonomic function. Studies have demonstrated these effects after even brief exposure to SHS (10–30 minutes), with effect sizes comparable with active smoking. Exposure to SHS causes atherosclerosis in animal models (USDHHS 2006a).

Cancer

Mainstream tobacco smoke (MS) contains nearly 5,000 chemicals (Repace 1993) and more than 60 known carcinogens (IARC 2004). Chemical analysis of the smoke from pipes, cigars, and cigarettes shows that carcinogens are found at comparable levels in the smoke of all these tobacco products. Carcinogens in tobacco smoke and SLT have been found in body fluids (saliva, urine, blood) and in multiple organ systems (IARC 2005). Specific carcinogens found in tobacco and tobacco smoke have been linked with specific tobacco-related cancers. For example, tobacco-specific nitrosamines and polyaromatic hydrocarbons cause lung cancer, benzo[a]pyrene causes squamous cell carcinoma of the esophagus (Kuratsune, Kohchi, and Horie 1965), and N-nitrosodimethylamine causes kidney tumors in animals (Shiao, Rice, and Anderson 1998). Pancreatic cancer can be produced in animals with the tobacco-specific nitrosamine NNK; aromatic amines may also play a role (IARC 2005). NNK has also been found in the cervical mucus (Prokopczyk et al. 1997), and smokers' cervical mucus is mutagenic (Holly et al. 1986). Similarly, the urine of smokers is more mutagenic than the urine of nonsmokers (Yamasaki and Ames 1977). Benzene, polonium-210, and lead-210 are known to cause myeloid leukemia; cigarette smoke is the major source of benzene exposure in the United States (Wallace 1996).

Less direct mechanisms of cancer causation are also implicated. For example, smoking may increase the infectivity or add to the pathogenicity of H. pylori, a known cause of stomach cancer. Smoking may also lower the plasma and serum concentrations of certain micronutrients that may protect against H. pylori infections or gastric cancer (IARC 2005).

Levels of tobacco-specific nitrosamines and other carcinogens in SLT are often at levels hundreds of times higher than what foods and beverages may legally contain. Tobacco-specific nitrosamines (NNN and NNK) are the most abundant, but not the only strong carcinogens in SLT. SLT also contains polonium-210, polynuclear aromatic hydrocarbons, uranium-235, nickel, and formaldehyde (IARC 1985; USDHHS 1992).

More than 50 carcinogens have been identified in SHS, and SHS is classified as a Group A (known human) carcinogen (USDHHS 2006a). SHS is qualitatively similar in composition to MS smoke, but many carcinogens found in MS appear in greater concentration in SHS. These carcinogens are absorbed by humans at measurable doses. For example, exposure to SHS causes a significant increase in urinary levels of NNK metabolites. The mechanisms by which SHS causes lung cancer are thought to be similar to those observed in smokers. The lower relative risk is due to the lower carcinogenic dose (USDHHS 2006a).

Chronic Lung and Other Respiratory Diseases

Smoking causes biologic processes (e.g., oxidant stress, inflammation, degradation of structural proteins) that result in airway and alveolar injury. If sustained, such injury results in COPD (IARC 2005; USDHHS 1984). The airflow obstruction leads to hypoxemia, which is further exacerbated by the inhaled carbon monoxide from cigarette smoke (USDHHS 1984). Abnormal lung function can occur as early as two years after smoking initiation (Beck, Doyle, and Schachter 1981). Smokers exhibit a more rapid, dose-related decline in pulmonary function with age than do nonsmokers (USDHHS 1984). Smoking decreases tracheal mucus velocity, increases mucus secretion, causes chronic airway inflammation and exaggerated airway responsiveness, increases epithelial permeability, and damages parenchymal cells (USDHHS 1990).

There are multiple mechanisms by which SHS causes injury to the respiratory tract. Increased airway wall thickness has been reported in infants exposed to maternal smoking, and SHS increases bronchial hyperreactivity in children and adults. Altered immune responses may also play a role in SHS-induced asthma exacerbation and enhanced susceptibility to respiratory infections (USDHHS 2006a).

Nicotine Dependence

In alkaline media, the nicotine molecule is un-ionized and readily absorbed. Thus, inhaled smoke is easily absorbed from the lung, and SLT's alkaline pH facilitates absorption from the mouth. Nicotine distributes rapidly to the brain whether administered orally or by inhalation. For example, when tobacco smoke is inhaled, nicotine is absorbed into the arterial bloodstream and reaches the brain within 10 seconds. Nicotine then crosses the blood-brain barrier and binds to specific receptors in the brain, resulting in the release of neurotransmitters and other chemicals, including acetylcholine, serotonin, dopamine, gamma aminobutyric acid, endogenous opioid peptides, pituitary hormones, and catecholamines (USDHHS 1988).

Nicotine is a psychoactive drug with stimulant and depressive effects. Nicotine's effects depend on the dose, rates of administration and elimination, and tolerance level of the person. Smokers dose themselves throughout the day, maintaining blood levels sufficient for them to avoid withdrawal symptoms. SLT users also maintain sustained levels of blood nicotine. Absorption is slower than with cigarettes, but more prolonged (USDHHS 1988).

Abstinence regularly produces a withdrawal syndrome that is attenuated by re-administration of nicotine. Among nicotine-dependent tobacco users, withdrawal symptoms (craving for nicotine; irritability, frustration, or anger; anxiety; difficulty concentrating; restlessness; decreased heart rate; increased appetite; and weight gain) begin within 24 hours of cessation and peak within a few days. Acute symptoms may persist for 10 days or more, but cravings for tobacco can persist for years. There is also a behavioral component to nicotine dependence. For regular smokers in particular, smoking has become so intertwined with activities of daily living, resulting in multiple "cues" each day that can trigger cravings and relapse (USDHHS 1988).

Descriptive Epidemiology

High-Risk Groups

In 2007, 43 million Americans were current smokers (ever smoked 100 cigarettes and smoked everyday or some days at the time of the survey). Smoking prevalence was higher for men (22%) than for women (17%) (Table 5.2). By age, prevalence was highest among those 18–44 years of age (23%). Smoking prevalence was 10% among Asians, 13% among Hispanics, 20% among African Americans, 21% among whites, and 36% among American Indians and Alaska Natives. Formal educational attainment is strongly associated with smoking prevalence and cessation rates. In 2007, smoking prevalence was highest among people with 9–11 years of education (33%) and lowest for persons with 16 or more years of education (<10%) (CDC 2008a), but this relationship is not linear. Persons with 0–8

Table 5.2. Percentage of Persons Aged 18 Years and Older Who Were Current Cigarette Smokers,[a] by Sex and Selected Characteristics: National Health Interview Survey, United States, 2007

Characteristics	Men (n=10,173)	Women (n=12,817)	Total (N=22,990)
Race/ethnicity[b]			
White, non-Hispanic	23.1 (21.6–24.6)	19.8 (18.7–20.9)	21.4 (20.4–22.4)
African American, non-Hispanic	24.8 (22.0–27.6)	15.8 (13.7–17.9)	19.8 (18.2–21.4)
Hispanic	18.0 (15.5–20.5)	8.3 (6.7–9.9)	13.3 (11.7–14.9)
American Indian/Alaska Native, non-Hispanic[c]	36.7 (19.0–54.5)	36.0 (20.2–51.8)	36.4 (22.9–49.9)
Asian, non-Hispanic[d]	15.9 (12.8–19.0)	4.0 (2.4–5.6)	9.6 (8.0–11.2)
Education[e]			
0–12 years (no diploma)	29.5 (26.9–32.1)	20.2 (18.0–22.4)	24.8 (23.1–26.5)
<8 years	20.4 (17.0–23.8)	10.0 (7.7–12.3)	15.4 (13.2–17.6)
9–11 years	36.9 (32.4–41.4)	30.0 (26.1–33.9)	33.3 (30.4–36.2)
12 years (no diploma)	33.1 (25.2–41.4)	14.8 (10.3–19.3)	22.7 (18.1–27.3)
GED diploma[f]	49.6 (42.0–57.2)	38.9 (31.8–46.0)	44.0 (39.0–49.0)
High school graduate	27.4 (24.9–29.9)	20.4 (18.3–22.5)	23.7 (22.0–25.4)
Associate degree	21.2 (18.1–24.3)	18.9 (16.4–21.4)	19.9 (17.8–22.0)
Some college	22.5 (20.2–24.8)	19.5 (18.0–21.0)	20.9 (19.5–22.3)
Undergraduate degree	13.4 (10.7–16.1)	9.4 (8.0–10.8)	11.4 (9.9–12.9)
Graduate degree	6.4 (4.7–8.1)	6.0 (4.5–7.5)	6.2 (5.1–7.3)
Age group (years)			
18–24	25.4 (22.1–28.7)	19.1 (16.2–22.0)	22.2 (19.9–24.5)
25–44	26.0 (24.1–27.9)	19.6 (18.1–21.1)	22.8 (21.5–24.1)
45–64	22.6 (20.8–24.4)	19.5 (18.0–21.0)	21.0 (19.7–22.3)
>65	9.3 (7.8–10.8)	7.6 (6.3–8.9)	8.3 (7.3–9.3)

(continued on next page)

Table 5.2. (*continued*)

Characteristics	Men (*n*=10,173)	Women (*n*=12,817)	Total (*N*=22,990)
Poverty status[g]			
At or above	22.8 (21.4–24.2)	17.8 (16.6–19.0)	20.3 (19.3–21.3)
Below	32.4 (28.3–36.5)	26.3 (23.3–29.3)	28.8 (26.2–31.4)
Unknown	17.6 (15.1–20.1)	13.4 (11.2–15.6)	15.2 (13.6–16.8)
Total	22.3 (21.1–23.5)	17.4 (16.5–18.3)	19.8 (19.0–20.6)

Values are % (95% Confidence Interval)
[a]Persons who reported smoking at least 100 cigarettes during their lifetimes and who, at the time of interview, reported smoking everyday or some days. Excludes 403 respondents whose smoking status was unknown.
[b]Excludes 317 respondents of unknown race or multiple racial categories.
[c]Wide variances in estimates reflect small sample sizes.
[d]Does not include native Hawaiians or other Pacific Islanders.
[e]Among persons 25 years and older. Excludes 1,770 persons whose educational level was unknown.
[f]General educational development.
[g]Based on family income reported by respondents and 2005 poverty thresholds published by the U.S. Census Bureau.
Source: CDC (2008a).

years of education have smoking prevalence and cessation rates similar to that found among people with 12 years of education, whereas persons with 9–11 years of education are the most likely to be ever, current, or heavy smokers, and the least likely to have quit smoking. Above 11 years of education, the likelihood of smoking decreases with each successive year of education (Zhu et al. 1996). In 2007, smoking prevalence was higher for persons living below the poverty level (29%) than for those living at or above that level (20%) (CDC 2008a). Despite these differences in smoking prevalence, however, the demographics of smokers still largely reflect the demographics of the U.S. population (white, 12 or more years of education, and half living at greater than 2.5 times the poverty level (CDC, unpublished data).

In 2005, the percentage of ever smokers who had quit was 51% for men and 50% for women and 53% for whites, 45% for Hispanics, 44% for Asians, 39% for African Americans, and 38% for American Indians and Alaska Natives (Malarcher et al. in press). African Americans are more likely than whites to try to quit smoking but are less likely to succeed, even after adjustment for demographic differences (USDHHS 1998). The percentage of ever smokers who have quit was lowest among the group with 9–11 years of education (44%) and highest among persons with 16 or more years of education (70%) (Malarcher et al. in press).

It is estimated that each year 4,000 young people smoke their first cigarette (USDHHS 2006b). Tobacco use generally begins in early adolescence and more than

80% of first use occurs before age 18 years. Little initiation occurs after age 24 years and essentially none after age 30 years (USDHHS 1994). In 2008, 20% of eighth graders, 32% of 10th graders, and 45% of 12th graders had tried cigarette smoking and 7%, 12%, and 20%, respectively, were current smokers (had smoked in the past 30 days). Among high school seniors, prevalence was somewhat higher for boys (22%) than girls (19%), and higher for whites (25%) than Hispanics (15%) or African Americans (10%) (Johnston et al. 2008). In 2008, 10% of eighth grade students, 12% of 10th grade students, and 16% of 12th grade students had tried SLT; current (past 30 days) use was 4% among eighth grade students, 5% among 10th grade students, and 6% among 12th grade students. SLT use among 12th grade students was much higher for boys (12%) than for girls (1%) and higher for whites (9%) than for Hispanics or African Americans (2%) (Johnston et al. 2008). In 2006, the prevalence of current cigar use was 4% for middle school students and 12% for high school students; use was higher for high school boys (17%) than girls (7%). In 2006, current use of any tobacco product was 26% for high school students and 10% for middle school students (CDC in press).

Geographic Distribution

In 2007, smoking prevalence varied more than twofold by state, ranging from 12% in Utah to 28% in Kentucky (CDC 2009b). In 2003, SLT use among adult men ranged from 1% in New Jersey to 13% in Wyoming (Current Population Survey 2003, unpublished data). These variations in use are reflected in state-specific smoking-attributable mortality rates. Annual smoking-attributable mortality ranges from 488 deaths in Alaska to 36,684 deaths in California; the SAM rate (number of smoking-attributable deaths per 100,000 population) varies from 138 in Utah to 371 in Kentucky (CDC 2009b). Youth smoking prevalence data are not available for all states, but in 2007, prevalence among high school students ranged from 8% in Utah to 28% in West Virginia; SLT use ranged from 4% in Maryland to 15% in West Virginia and Wyoming (36 states reporting) (CDC 2009b).

Time Trends

Annual per capita consumption of cigarettes reached a peak of 4,345 in 1963. Except for an increase from 1971 through 1973, consumption has steadily declined since then (Figure 5.2). Per capita cigarette consumption was 1,654 in 2006, the lowest level since 1935. Overall, the numbers of cigarettes sold in the United States declined from 640 billion in 1981 to 371 billion in 2006. Total consumption of cigars decreased from 8.1 billion in 1970 to 2.1 billion in 1993, but then increased to 5.3 billion in 2006. Per capita consumption of chewing tobacco among men 18 years and older decreased from 0.63 lb (285.76 g) in 1996 to 0.22 lb (99.79 g) in 2006 (Capehart 2004, 2007).

From 1965 to the late 1980s, adult smoking prevalence in the United States decreased an average of 0.5% per year (from 42% in 1965 to 26% in 1990); in the early 1990s, prevalence was flat, but then prevalence decreased from 25% in 1997 to 21% in 2004. Prevalence then remained flat from 2004 to 2006, declining to 20% in 2007 (Figure 5.3) (Malarcher et al. in press; CDC 2009c). If current patterns continue, the United States will not meet the *Healthy People 2010* (HP 2010) objective of a smoking prevalence of 12% (USDHHS 2000a).

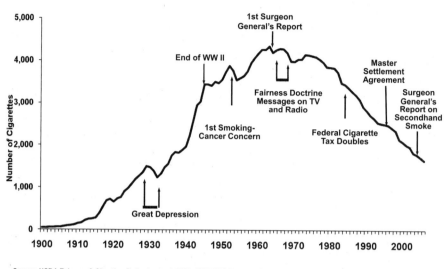

Source: USDA Tobacco & Situation Outlook report, 2006; 1986-2006 Surgeon General's Reports

Figure 5.2. Adult per capita cigarette consumption and major smoking-and-health events: United States, 1900–2006.

Although men historically had much higher smoking rates than women, the gap narrowed over time as more women started smoking. However, declines since 1985 are occurring at a comparable rate for women and men (Malarcher et al. in press). Smoking prevalence has declined faster for African Americans than for whites, so that prevalence among African American men (formerly higher than for white men) is now comparable with that among white men and the prevalence in African American women (formerly comparable with white women) is now lower than in white women. Smoking prevalence has declined fastest for persons with 16 or more years of education and slowest for persons with 9–11 years of education. The proportion of smokers who are heavy smokers (25 or more cigarettes per day) has been halved (from 25% in 1965 to 12% in 2005) (Malarcher et al. in press).

In 2002, for the first time, there were more former smokers than current smokers. Although historically, the percent of ever smokers who have quit was higher for men than for women (since men started quitting in larger numbers while uptake among women was still increasing), the sex gap has now closed. The increase in the percent of ever smokers who have quit was fastest for persons with 16 or more years of education and least for those with 9–11 years of education (Malarcher et al. in press).

The prevalence of current smoking (smoking within the past 30 days) among high school seniors decreased from 39% in 1976 to 29% in 1981, was then relatively stable until 1992, increased to 36% by 1997, and then decreased to 20% in 2008 (Figure 5.4). Similarly, prevalence among 10th graders increased from 21% in 1991 to 30% in 1996 and then decreased to 12% in 2008. The prevalence of smoking among eighth graders increased from 14% in 1991 to 21% in 1996 and then decreased to 7% in 2008. Similar patterns were seen for daily smoking. A larger decline in current smoking prevalence occurred

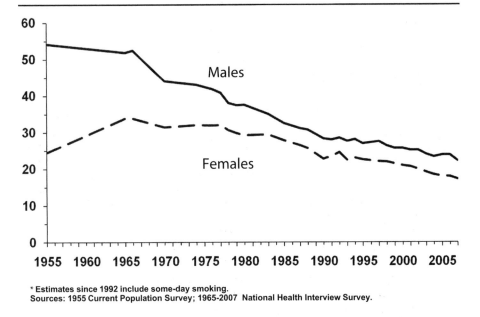

* Estimates since 1992 include some-day smoking.
Sources: 1955 Current Population Survey; 1965-2007 National Health Interview Survey.

Figure 5.3. Prevalence of cigarette smoking* among adults: United States, 1955–2007.

among African American high school seniors from 1977 to 1992 (37% to 9%) than among white high school students (38% to 32%). Smoking prevalence among African American high school students increased to 15% in 1998 but then decreased to 10% in 2008. Among high school seniors, smoking prevalence was higher for girls than for boys until 1990; since 1991, it has been somewhat higher for boys than girls (Johnston et al. 2008).

The decline in smoking prevalence among middle and high school students stalled from 2002 to 2005 but then declined in 2007. Although the decline from the early 1990s through 1997 suggested that the HP 2010 objective for high school students (a prevalence of 16%) would be met, the recent slowing of progress has raised concerns that this may no longer be true (CDC 2006, 2009b; USDHHS 2000a).

Birth certificate data suggest a continued decline in smoking prevalence among pregnant women (from 20% in 1989 to 11% in 2005). Prevalence is higher among adolescent mothers than older mothers (Malarcher et al. in press; Martin et al. 2007). However, birth certificate data appear to underreport smoking prevalence during pregnancy. Survey data from 2005 suggested that the prevalence was closer to 17% (USDHHS 2006b). Smoking among women of reproductive age (18–44 years) was 21% in 2006 (NHIS 2006, unpublished data).

Causes

Modifiable Risk Factors

No single factor causes a young person to begin using tobacco. In addition to sociodemographic factors, other important factors associated with tobacco use include the price of tobacco products, tobacco advertising and promotion, portrayal of tobacco in the popular

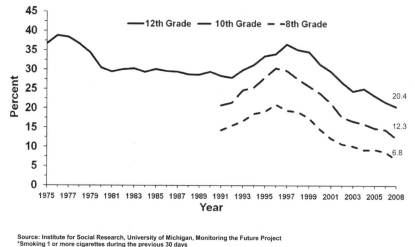

Source: Institute for Social Research, University of Michigan, Monitoring the Future Project
*Smoking 1 or more cigarettes during the previous 30 days

Figure 5.4. Trends in current cigarette smoking* by grade in school: United States, 1975–2008.

culture, countermarketing efforts, youth access to tobacco products, public attitudes and social norms around tobacco use, SHS policies, parental and peer influences, pharmacological effects of nicotine, and mental health issues (Figure 5.1). An emerging area of research interest is in biologic susceptibility to develop nicotine dependence. One study estimated that additive genetic effects account for 56% of the variance in risk to initiate smoking (Lerman and Berrettini 2003).

Societal and Individual Factors Increasing Tobacco Use among Youth

Societal factors that increase tobacco use among youth include tobacco industry advertising and promotion, exposure to tobacco images in movies and popular media, the perception that some tobacco products are "safe" or "safer," easy access to tobacco products, inadequate understanding of the health risks and risk of addiction, social norms promoting tobacco use, and parental and peer smoking.

Tobacco industry advertising and promotion

Youth are exposed to cigarette messages through a variety of media and promotional activities (e.g., sponsorship of events and entertainment, point-of-sale displays, distribution of specialty items). Tobacco companies maintain that their advertising and promotion are not intended to appeal to teen or preteen children. However, in 1997, the Liggett Group acknowledged that the tobacco industry marketed to youth under 18 years of age (Attorneys General Statement Agreement 1997).

Cigarette advertising uses images to portray the attractiveness and function of smoking (independence, maturity, slimness, glamour, self-confidence, adventure-seeking, and youthful activities). Such advertisements capitalize on the disparity between youth's ideal and actual self-image and imply that smoking may close that gap. The promotion of televised and live popular sporting and entertainment events also heavily exposes youth to tobacco advertising (Siegel 2001; USDHHS 1994, 2001).

In 2000, the tobacco industry spent nearly $60 million on advertising in youth-oriented magazines, and advertisements for the three most popular youth brands of cigarettes reached 80% of young people an average of 17 times (King and Siegel 2001). One study reported that nearly half of the U.S. Smokeless Tobacco Company's advertising budget was in youth-oriented magazines (Massachusetts Department of Health 2002). Tobacco industry discounting strategies (coupons, two-for-one offers) reduce the price of tobacco products and lower prices correlate with increased use by adolescents and young adults. Younger smokers are more likely than older smokers to use price discounts (Pierce et al. 2005; White et al. 2006).

Studies show an association among advertising expenditures and youth brand preference, tobacco marketing exposure and initiation, and favorable beliefs toward smoking in response to marketing exposure (Pechman and Ratneshawr 1994; Pierce et al. 1998; Pierce, Lee, and Gilpin 1994; Pollay et al. 1996; USDHHS 1994). The Surgeon General, the Institute of Medicine (IOM), the U.S. Food and Drug Administration (FDA), and the U.K. Scientific Committee on Tobacco and Health have all concluded that tobacco marketing influences young people to smoke (FDA 1996; Lynch and Bonnie 1994; Scientific Committee on Tobacco and Health 1998; USDHHS 1994, 2001). Teens appear to be three times more sensitive to cigarette advertising than adults (Pollay et al. 1996). One study reported that teens were more likely to be influenced to smoke by tobacco advertising than by peer pressure (Evans et al. 1995).

Smoking in the movies has emerged as a tobacco control issue. Several studies have reported that exposure to smoking in the movies increases youth initiation, particularly among adolescents with nonsmoking parents (Dalton et al. 2003; Distefan, Pierce, and Gilpin 2004). Smoking in the United States has declined since the 1950s, and smoking in the movies likewise decreased from 1950 to 1980–1982; however, it rebounded to 1950 levels in 2002 (10.9 incidents per hour) (Glantz, Kacirk, and McCulloch 2004). Other studies have shown that smoking is frequent even in G- or PG-rated movies (Polansky and Glantz 2005). A recent study estimated that from 1998 to 2002, U.S. adolescents ages 10–14 years were exposed to 13.9 billion gross smoking impressions (an average of 665 per adolescent) (Sargent, Tanski, and Gibson 2007).

The purported "prevention" media campaigns of the tobacco industry have been shown to actually increase youth smoking. For example, those exposed to the Philip Morris' "Think Don't Smoke" campaign were more likely to be open to the possibility of smoking (Farrelly et al. 2002). Youth exposed to tobacco industry parent-targeted advertisements (such as the Philip Morris "Talk to Your Kids" campaign) had lower perceived harm of smoking, stronger approval of smoking, stronger intentions to smoke in the future, and greater likelihood of having smoked in the past 30 days (Wakefield et al. 2006). Another study showed that tobacco company "prevention" ads engendered more favorable attitudes toward tobacco companies among adolescents (Henriksen et al. 2006).

Perception that Some Tobacco Products Are "Safe" or "Safer"

Products that are viewed as potentially "safer" can influence youth behavior. For example, youth who smoke low-tar cigarettes reported that they thought these products were safer, less addictive, and easier to quit than regular cigarettes (Kropp and Halpern-Felsher 2004). The belief that they are not harming themselves and can easily quit when they want to do so could lead to greater youth smoking.

Access

Commercial outlets are a readily available source of tobacco for minors. Numerous studies involving purchase attempts by minors confirm that, despite state and local laws banning such sales, youth can easily buy tobacco over the counter and from vending machines (Marshall et al. 2006; USDHHS 1994, 2000b). Ready access to cigarettes makes it easier for youth to progress from experimentation to regular smoking.

Inadequate Understanding of Health Risks and Risk of Dependence

Youth do not fully understand the risks of tobacco use. A 1999 survey of youth ages 14–22 years reported that 40% of smokers and 25% of nonsmokers underestimated or did not know the likelihood of smoking-related deaths; more than 40% did not know or underestimated the number of years of life lost to smoking. Young people assume that they will stop before harmful effects occur and do not believe that they personally are at risk from tobacco use (Romer and Jamieson 2001). Youth also underestimate the risks of becoming addicted to nicotine and do not expect to continue to smoke (USDHHS 1994). It may be only after the first failed quit attempt that youth realize they are nicotine-dependent and that quitting will not be easy.

Social Norms

Youth smoking behavior is influenced by societal norms, local community norms, parental and family behavior, and peer behavior. Social norms change over time. Smoking has gone from a common, accepted behavior to a less frequent and increasingly restricted one. However, community norms, such as living in a tobacco-producing state, clearly influence both youth and adult prevalence (CDC 2009c). Countermarketing campaigns help change social norms. There is also some evidence that smoke-free laws challenge the perception of smoking as a normal adult behavior (Siegel et al. 2005).

   Parental smoking increases the likelihood of children smoking by modeling the behavior and providing easy access to tobacco. Having several close friends who smoke is also associated with smoking among adolescents (USDHHS 1994), although the direction of the relationship is unclear (e.g., whether nonsmokers start smoking as a result of their friends smoking or whether adolescents who smoke start to associate with other smokers).

   Similarly, for SLT use, perceived approval of use by parents and peers; easy access to the product; use of cigarettes, alcohol, marijuana, or other drugs; engaging in other risky behaviors; living with someone else who uses SLT; and having peers who use SLT increases the risk of its use by young people (USDHHS 1994). Lower price also increases SLT use (Ohsfeldt, Boyle, and Capilouto 1997).

Individual Psychosocial Factors

Individual risk factors for tobacco use include weaker attachment to parents and family, strong attachment to peer and friends, perception that smoking is more common than is actually true, risk-taking and rebelliousness, weaker commitment to school and religion, the belief that smoking can control weight and moods, and having a positive image of smokers (USDHHS 2001).

Societal and Individual Factors Promoting Continued Tobacco Use among Adults

Societal factors that influence continued tobacco use include nicotine dependence, the perception that some tobacco products are "safer," tobacco industry advertising and promotion, inadequate understanding of the health risks, social norms around tobacco use, and lower prices for tobacco products. There is increasing interest in the role of genetics in treatment response (Lee et al. 2007).

Nicotine Dependence

Nicotine is a psychoactive drug. Once the smoker becomes nicotine-dependent, this dependence becomes a very strong factor for continued tobacco use (USDHHS 1988).

Perception that Some Tobacco Products Are "Safer"

Tobacco product changes that infer a reduced risk are appealing to smokers. For example, since their introduction to the U.S. market, the so-called low-tar, low-nicotine cigarettes have rapidly increased their market share. Low-tar cigarettes were specifically marketed to such smokers with such tags as "All the fuss about smoking got me thinking I'd either quit or smoke True. I smoke True" (Pollay Tobacco Ad Collection 2007), and evidence suggests that the persons most likely to initially use low-tar cigarettes were those most concerned about smoking and most interested in quitting. Product changes that imply a "safer" way to continue to consume tobacco may provide a rationalization for smokers to postpone quitting.

Tobacco Industry Advertising

Pro-tobacco advertising is thought to maintain adult smoking by (1) creating attitudes and images that reinforce the desirability of smoking and that remind smokers of enjoyable occasions associated with smoking, (2) reducing smokers' motivation to quit through attractive imagery and implicit alleviation of fears about the health consequences of smoking, and (3) reminding former smokers of the reasons and situations in which they smoked to encourage them to relapse (USDHHS 1989). Although the classic Marlboro ads target men, tobacco industry marketing efforts have also targeted women and minorities. The uptake of smoking among women beginning in 1967 was associated with the marketing of cigarette brands specific for women (Pierce, Lee, and Gilpin 1994).

Incomplete Understanding of Health Risks

Adults are not fully aware of the health hazards of tobacco use. For example, women's magazines, a source of medical information for many women, often downplay the hazards of smoking. A survey of 15 popular women's magazines in 2001–2002 found only 55 antismoking articles, compared with 726 on nutrition, 347 on fitness, and 268 on mental health. Only six articles focused on lung cancer, the leading cancer killer of women, and two of these articles did not address the importance of not smoking to prevent lung cancer. At the same time, there were 176 pro-smoking mentions (including photographs or illustrations) (Maroney et al. 2001).

Lower Price

Lower prices increase tobacco consumption. Young adults, adults with lower educational attainment or lower socioeconomic status, African Americans, and Hispanics are more sensitive to price increases (CDC 1998; USDHHS 2000b). These populations are also more likely to use coupons and other discounts to reduce the price (White et al. 2006).

Individual Factors Influencing Tobacco Use among Adults

Individual factors influencing tobacco use among adults include lower educational attainment and lower socioeconomic status. These may be accompanied by lower understanding of the health hazards of smoking and less supportive home and work environments for quitting (Sorensen et al. 2002). Smokers also vary in their confidence in being able to successfully quit.

Population-Attributable Risk

Although there are many studies estimating the population-attributable risk of smoking and various disease outcomes, few studies have estimated the relative influence of various modifiable risk factors on population risk of tobacco use. A California study suggested that one-third of all cigarette experimentation among youth could be attributed to tobacco promotional activities (Pierce et al. 1998). Two recent studies have estimated the attributable risk of adolescent smoking from exposure to smoking in the movies. One study estimated that 38% of initiation is attributable to such exposure (Sargent et al. 2005), and the other estimated that 52% of smoking initiation among adolescents with nonsmoking parents could be attributed to exposure to smoking in movies (Dalton et al. 2003; McDonald et al. 2003).

Prevention and Control

Prevention

The primary interventions to prevent tobacco use initiation are raising the prices of tobacco products, sustained media campaigns, community interventions to reduce minors' access to tobacco products, and smoke-free policies. Comprehensive school-based interventions are effective if implemented in conjunction with these other interventions. The primary intervention to prevent exposure to SHS is the implementation of comprehensive smoke-free policies.

Price

There is a robust body of evidence on the effectiveness of price increases on reducing youth initiation (USDHHS 1994). Price increases are also one of the most effective interventions to increase cessation. The Surgeon General, a National Cancer Institute (NCI) consensus panel, and the Community Preventive Services Task Force (CPSTF) all recommend price increases as a primary strategy to reduce youth and adult tobacco use (NCI 1993; USDHHS 2000b; Zaza, Briss, and Harris 2005). Youth are more sensitive to price increases than adults (NCI 1993; USDHHS 1994), probably because of lower discretionary incomes. It is estimated that a 10% increase in price would decrease total cigarette consumption among youth by 7%, reduce youth prevalence by 3.7%, decrease initiation by 3.8%, and decrease the amount smoked by adolescents who continued to smoke (NCI 1993; Zaza, Briss, and Harris 2005). For adults, a 10% increase in price decreases overall consumption 4% and increases cessation 1.5%. Other tobacco products also respond to price interventions (e.g., SLT use by adolescent boys) (USDHHS 2000b), but prices need to be kept aligned among various tobacco products or use merely shifts to less expensive forms of tobacco (Delnevo et al. 2004; USDHHS 2000b).

Countermarketing Campaigns

Media campaigns, when combined with other interventions, are an effective strategy to reduce youth initiation and prevalence (NCI 2008; USDHHS 1994, 2000b). The CPSTF reported that sustained (greater than two years) media countermarketing campaigns reduced youth tobacco prevalence by a median eight percentage points (74%) (Zaza, Briss, and Harris 2005). Youth-focused campaigns have been developed and evaluated in several states and nationally. It was estimated that 20% of the decline in youth smoking prevalence in the late 1990s was a result of the American Legacy Foundation's "truth" media campaign (Farrelly et al. 2005). However, these campaigns need to be sustained. In Minnesota, when a youth-focused media campaign was ended, youth susceptibility to initiate smoking increased from 43% to 53% within six months (CDC 2004a).

Countermarketing campaigns change social norms about tobacco use, increase awareness of the health hazards of smoking and exposure to SHS, educate about tobacco industry actions, provide motivations for people to quit, inform tobacco users about resources available to help them quit, and support policy efforts such as tobacco excise tax increases. The CPSTF recommends sustained countermarketing campaigns in conjunction with other interventions (such as tax increases, community education programs, cessation counseling or self-help materials, or other mass media efforts) as an effective strategy to increase cessation, estimating that such campaigns increase cessation by a median of two percentage points, reduce tobacco consumption by a median 13%, and reduce adult prevalence by a median of three percentage points (Zaza, Briss, and Harris 2005).

To be effective, warning labels need to stand out, have a visual impact, and be content-specific (not give just general information). There is some evidence that warning labels can impact smoking behavior. In South Africa, tobacco consumption decreased 15% over three years after new warning labels were introduced. Stronger warning labels in Australia appear to have had a larger effect on quitting behavior than the old labels, and half of Canadian smokers said that warning labels had contributed to their desire to quit or to cut back on their consumption (Kenkel and Chen 2000).

Advertising Bans

Evidence for the effectiveness of advertising bans is mixed. The apparent lack of effect in some studies may be due, in part, to these bans being frequently circumvented. For example, after the broadcast ban went into effect in the United States, tobacco advertising shifted to other media—newspapers, magazines, outdoor signs, transit, and point of sale (FTC 2007a). Studies suggest that partial bans are not effective, but that complete bans can decrease consumption (Saffer and Chaloupka 1999).

Minors' Access Restrictions

The CPSTF concluded that minors' access interventions are effective, but only in conjunction with other community interventions (Zaza, Briss, and Harris 2005).

Continued enforcement is critical in order to increase retailer compliance (Lynch and Bonnie 1994; USDHHS 1994). A Massachusetts evaluation reported that communities with a dramatic reduction in tobacco control funding saw an average increase of 74% in illegal sales to minors; communities that completely lost their programs had even larger increases (Tobacco Free Mass 2005).

School-Based Tobacco Prevention Programs

School-based tobacco prevention programs are effective when combined with concurrent, complementary community interventions (USDHHS 1994). Current recommendations on quality school-based prevention programs emphasize policy interventions, such as tobacco-free campuses and curricula that help children understand and effectively cope with social influences associated with smoking, highlight the immediate negative social consequences and inoculate youth against the effects of pressure to use tobacco (CDC 1994). Most prevention programs focus on students in grades six to eight. However, program effects decay without additional educational interventions, media campaigns, or supportive community programs, and comprehensive approaches are necessary for long-term success (USDHHS 1994).

Eliminating Exposure to SHS

In 2006, the Surgeon General concluded that eliminating smoking in indoor spaces fully protects nonsmokers, but that separating smokers from nonsmokers, cleaning the air, and ventilating buildings cannot eliminate exposure to SHS (USDHHS 2006a). Similarly, the CPSTF found that smoking bans reduced SHS exposure more than smoking restrictions (Zaza, Briss, and Harris 2005). The health impacts of statewide smoke-free laws have also been studied. Two studies showed dramatic declines in respirable particle and carcinogenic particulate polycyclic aromatic hydrocarbon levels after smoking bans were implemented (CDC 2004b; Repace 2004). Other studies have shown improvements in respiratory symptoms, sensory irritation, and lung function in hospitality workers after implementation of smoke-free laws (Eisner, Smith, and Blanc 1998; Farrelly et al. 2005). Several studies have reported decreased cardiovascular events (MIs) after smoke-free policies have been implemented (Cesaroni et al. 2008; Juster et al. 2007).

Concerns are often raised about possible adverse economic consequences of smoke-free policies on the hospitality industry. A review of studies that used objective outcomes (e.g., revenues, employment, restaurant sale price) generally showed a positive impact (Scollo et al. 2003), and the Surgeon General concluded that smoke-free policies do not have an adverse economic impact on the hospitality industry (USDHHS 2006a).

In addition to protecting nonsmokers from exposure to SHS, smoke-free policies reduce cigarette consumption and smoking initiation and increase cessation (Siegel et al. 2005; Zaza, Briss, and Harris 2005). Smoke-free venues such as schools and school campuses, public places, and restaurants help create nonsmoking social norms and reduce the "modeling" of smoking behavior by adult role models (CDC 1994). Smoke-free home rules help smokers who are trying to quit to maintain abstinence (Borland et al. 2006).

Screening

One of the most important screening strategies for health care professionals is to ask about a patient's tobacco use. Such information should be ascertained on every visit and documented in the medical record (Fiore et al. 2008). Routine screening for tobacco use is critical for ensuring that all tobacco users receive effective treatment every time they are seen by a health care professional.

Biochemical measures are available to assess whether a person is a smoker or is exposed to SHS. For example, cotinine (the major metabolite of nicotine) can be measured in blood, urine, and saliva (USDHHS 2006a). These measures are generally used in research or surveillance studies but are not recommended for use as part of routine clinical care of tobacco users. One potential exception is assessing pregnant women's tobacco use, since pregnant women often underreport their tobacco use to their clinician (Fiore et al. 2008).

Treatment

Interventions proven to increase cessation include increasing the price of tobacco products, sustained media campaigns, and smoke-free policies (discussed above) and reducing the out-of-pocket costs of treatment, telephone cessation quitlines, and health care system changes that ensure that all tobacco users are screened and treated every time they are seen by a health professional. There is also a robust evidence base about the specific clinical interventions that increase cessation rates.

Reducing Out-of-Pocket Costs of Treatment

Although 70% of smokers want to quit (CDC 2005) and more than 40% try to quit each year (CDC 2009c), most do not use available effective treatments (Cokkinides et al. 2005). Reducing the barriers to obtaining treatment is critical to increasing the number of smokers who successfully quit. The CPSTF and Public Health Service (PHS) Clinical Practice Guideline both recommend reducing the out-of-pocket costs for effective treatment interventions through comprehensive insurance coverage because such coverage increases use of treatment and the number of successful quitters (Fiore et al. 2008). The

CPSTF estimated the median increase in cessation with coverage was eight percentage points (Zaza, Briss, and Harris 2005).

Telephone Cessation Quitlines

Telephone cessation quitlines increase quitting success (Stead, Perera, and Lancaster 2006) and are recommended by the PHS guideline and by the CPSTF (Fiore et al. 2008; Zaza, Briss, and Harris 2005). Telephone quitlines provide practical advice to smokers interested in quitting about how to deal with withdrawal symptoms and the challenges of quitting. The quitlines increase access to treatment because they are free; generally available days, evenings, and weekends; do not require transportation or childcare arrangements; and provide individually tailored help. Some quitlines also provide free nicotine replacement therapy (CDC 2004c).

Individual Cessation Interventions

The 2008 PHS Clinical Practice Guideline reported the following findings: brief clinician advice to quit is effective (30% increase in cessation rates); more intensive counseling is even more effective (doubles the cessation rate). Counseling can be delivered as individual, group, or telephone counseling. FDA-approved medications increase cessation by twofold to threefold (Fiore et al. 2008). These findings are consistent with other published recommendations (USPSTF 2005).

Cessation counseling/coaching provides practical advice about quitting and provides social support to the tobacco user as they try to quit. Using counseling and medication together or combining medications results in higher cessation rates (Fiore et al. 2008). A major problem, however, is that few tobacco users use these effective treatments (Cokkinides et al. 2005), and there is also evidence that tobacco users use fewer doses of the medications and use medication for a shorter period than recommended, which may contribute to lower success rates (Fiore et al. 2008).

Since 70% of smokers see a physician and 53% see a dentist each year (Tomar, Husten, and Manley 1996), clinicians have frequent opportunities for treating tobacco users. The PHS Clinical Practice Guideline concluded that effective tobacco use treatments should be offered to every patient who uses tobacco, recommending a brief intervention (three minutes) called the "Five A's" (Fiore et al. 2008):

- Ask every patient at every visit if he or she uses tobacco and document the patient's status in the medical chart (e.g., as a vital sign)
- Advise all tobacco users to quit
- Assess patients' interest in quitting
- Assist smokers in quitting by helping them set a quit date; recommending and/or prescribing FDA-approved medications unless contraindicated; providing or referring patients to more intensive individual, group, or telephone counseling
- Arrange for follow-up (by telephone or by scheduling a return appointment) to assess progress and encourage relapsed smokers to try again

Patients not yet willing to quit smoking should receive a motivational intervention to promote later quit attempts. These recommendations assume that office systems will be developed to ensure the routine assessment of tobacco use and appropriate treatment (Fiore et al. 2008).

Unfortunately, studies have been mixed for youth cessation interventions (McDonald et al. 2003), although counseling interventions have some evidence of effectiveness (Fiore et al. 2008). Current recommendations are to provide opportunistic advice to quit and offer help to youth interested in quitting. Intensive efforts to recruit adolescents into treatment are not currently recommended, since this effort is difficult and expensive, and attrition is high (Backinger et al. 2003).

Tobacco-use treatment for adults is extremely cost-effective, more so than other commonly covered preventive interventions, such as mammography, treatment for mild-to-moderate hypertension, and treatment for hypercholesterolemia (Cromwell et al. 1997; Cummings, Rubin, and Oster 1989; Fiore et al. 2008). An analysis of recommended clinical preventive services that ranked the services based upon disease impact, treatment effectiveness, and cost-effectiveness concluded that treatment of tobacco use among adults ranked first (along with childhood immunizations and aspirin therapy to prevent cardiovascular events in high-risk adults). Tobacco-use treatment also had the lowest delivery rate among the top-ranked preventive services (Maciosek et al. 2006). One study found that the cost of a moderately priced cessation program (brief clinical interventions, free telephone counseling, and free nicotine replacement therapy) paid for itself within four years due to lower hospital costs among successful quitters compared with continuing smokers (Wagner et al. 1995). Provision of preventive services is also associated with increased patient satisfaction (Schauffler and Rodriguez 1994).

Examples of Evidence-Based Interventions

Comprehensive Tobacco Prevention and Control Programs

Although such analyses must be interpreted cautiously, it is estimated that because of interventions to reduce tobacco use since 1964, 1.6 million Americans gained an average of 21 years of additional life expectancy between 1964 and 1992, and an estimated 4.1 million additional Americans will reap the benefit from 1993 to 2015 (Office of Disease Prevention and Health Promotion 1994).

California had the first robustly funded tobacco prevention and control program, paid for with part of a 1989 cigarette excise tax increase. Evaluation of the program revealed that per capita consumption of cigarettes and smoking prevalence declined faster in California than the rest of the country. Additionally, the increase in youth smoking in the early 1990s was smaller in California than in the rest of the country (USDHHS 2000b). California now has the lowest per capita consumption in the United States (California Department of Health Services 2005), and has seen improved health outcomes. Lung cancer incidence has declined three times more rapidly in California than the rest of the country, and six tobacco-related cancers now have a lower incidence rate in California than in the rest of the United States (lung/bronchus, esophagus, larynx, bladder, kidney, and pancreas) (California Department of Health Services 2006). Faster reductions in cardiovascular disease than in the rest of the country have also been reported. It is estimated that the program was associated with 33,000 fewer heart disease deaths from 1989 to 1997 than would have been expected (Fichtenberg and Glantz 2000). California has reported that for every dollar spent on the program, statewide health care costs are reduced by more then $3.60 (California Department of Health Services 2000).

Massachusetts, the second state to implement a broad tobacco prevention and control program, experienced a greater decline in per capita cigarette consumption and smoking prevalence than the rest of the country (excluding California), and, like California, the increase in youth smoking prevalence in the early 1990s was less than in the rest of the country (USDHHS 2000b). Massachusetts reported that its program paid for itself through declines in smoking among pregnant women (Connolly 2005). Arizona and Oregon also reported positive findings after implementing their programs (USDHHS 2000b). Florida had a focused effort on youth ("truth" media campaign, youth community activities including youth advocacy groups, school programs, minors' access enforcement, and youth involvement in the design and implementation of the program). The state documented dramatic declines in current and ever smoking and large increases in the proportion of "committed never smokers" among middle and high school students (Florida Department of Health 2002).

Evidence from well-funded comprehensive state programs (particularly California and Massachusetts) and from controlled studies were analyzed and developed into CDC's "Best Practices" guideline. The annual cost to implement comprehensive state tobacco control programs is estimated to range from $9 to $18 per capita (CDC 2007). Subsequent to the infusion of billions of dollars to states from the Master Settlement Agreement (MSA), increases in state funding for tobacco control occurred, though generally not at CDC-recommended levels. Research has demonstrated that comprehensive tobacco prevention and control programs decrease consumption (Farrelly, Pechacek, and Chaloupka 2003), decrease youth prevalence (Tauras et al. 2005), decrease adult prevalence (Farrelley, Pechacek, et al. 2008), reduce disease burden, and are cost-effective (Connolly 2005). One study noted that larger, more established programs may be more efficient and concluded that if states had begun investing at the CDC-recommended minimum funding levels in 1994, the aggregate sales decline would have doubled by 2000 (Farrelly, Pechacek, and Chaloupka 2003). A second national analysis reported that had states spent the CDC-recommended minimum levels, youth smoking prevalence would have been between 3% and 14% lower than the observed rate (Tauras et al. 2005).

Evidence-based recommendations have outlined the specific interventions that comprise a comprehensive program. Effective interventions to decrease initiation include raising the price of tobacco products, media campaigns combined with other interventions (such as price increases or community interventions) and community mobilization around minors' access when combined with other interventions (Zaza, Briss, and Harris 2005). Effective interventions to reduce exposure to SHS include smoking bans or restrictions. Effective interventions to increase cessation include raising the price of tobacco products, sustained media campaigns (in conjunction with other interventions), telephone quitlines, reduced out-of-pocket costs of treatment (i.e., insurance coverage), and workplace smoke-free policies. Provider reminders alone or in combination with provider training also increase quitting (Zaza, Briss, and Harris 2005).

It is important that tobacco control efforts encompass all tobacco products, not just cigarettes. Components of a comprehensive approach include (CDC 2007):

- State and community interventions (policy interventions, coalition building, and community interventions with high-risk populations)

- Media interventions (youth and adult-focused campaigns, quitline marketing, and campaigns focused on SHS), restrictions on tobacco industry marketing, and stronger warning labels
- Cessation interventions (quitline services, comprehensive insurance coverage in both public and private sectors, working with health care systems to improve screening and treatment of tobacco use)
- Surveillance and evaluation (e.g., tobacco use, attributable disease and economic costs, program impact)
- Administration and management (accountability, monitor grants, and contracts)

Tobacco Excise Taxes

Increasing tobacco prices for all tobacco products is the single most effective intervention to prevent tobacco use and increase cessation. As of June 2009, the Federal cigarette tax was $1.01 per pack (increased from $0.39 in April 2009) and state excise taxes ranged from $0.07 cents per pack in South Carolina to $3.46 in Rhode Island, with an average state tax of $1.25 per pack (CTFK 2009a). In 2009, the Federal tax on SLT was $0.113 per can (CTFK 2009b). As of December 2008, 49 states and the District of Columbia taxed SLT (CDC 2009b). The effect of price attenuates over time (and with inflation), so regular increases are needed. Additionally, parity of taxation across tobacco products reduces switching to cheaper products. Tobacco industry discounting strategies (coupons, two-for-one offers) reduce the impact of tax increases. From 2002 to 2004, despite significant tax increases, the real price of cigarettes increased only 4% (U.S. Department of Labor 2007). There is evidence that the tobacco industry uses discounting strategies more heavily in states with more robust tobacco control programs (Loomis, Farrelly, and Mann 2006). Other tobacco control strategies that impact price include restrictions on free samples of tobacco products, restrictions on coupons or discounting, prohibiting the sale of single cigarettes ("loosies"), efforts to combat smuggling, and restrictions on Internet or mail-order sales.

Countermarketing Campaigns and Restrictions on Tobacco Industry Marketing

Tobacco industry spending on advertising nearly tripled from 1997 to 2001 (to $15.2 billion), with the proportion used for coupons and discounts increasing from 27% to 87%. Expenditures decreased slightly to $13.1 billion in 2005 (FTC 1997, 2007a). SLT companies spent $251 million on advertising in 2005; price discounts and free samples accounted for 60% of the advertising budget (FTC 2007b).

Other tobacco company promotional money goes toward supporting cultural and sporting events and minority organizations. The resulting financial dependence may buy silence or active opposition to tobacco control proposals. In 1994, arts organizations in New York that had been recipients of tobacco philanthropy spoke out against an ordinance to ban smoking in public places (Quindlen 1994). The inverse correlation between the percentage of a magazine's health articles that discuss smoking and cigarette advertising revenue as a percentage of the magazine's total advertising revenue suggests that tobacco money also affects editorial decisions (USDHHS 2001). Studies have also shown a correlation between tobacco industry donations to politicians and lack of support for tobacco prevention and control legislation (Givel and Glantz 2001).

Efforts have been made to reduce advertising that targets children. The Federal Trade Commission (FTC) filed suit against R. J. Reynolds in 1997, alleging that the Joe Camel symbol enticed children to smoke. Later that year, the company announced that they were discontinuing Joe Camel in the United States (Ono and Ingersoll 1997). In 2004, R. J. Reynolds settled a lawsuit with 13 states over their "Kool Mixx" marketing campaign, which the states alleged targeted urban minority youth in violation of the MSA (Maryland Attorney General 2007). In 2006, R.J. Reynolds settled a lawsuit with 38 states over their candy-, fruit-, and alcohol-flavored cigarettes and agreed to restrictions on the marketing of flavored cigarettes (Office of the New York State Attorney General 2007).

The 1997 MSA imposed some restrictions on cigarette marketing in the United States. There could no longer be (1) brand name sponsorship of concerts, team sporting events, or events with a significant youth audience; (2) sponsorship of events in which paid participants were underage; (3) tobacco brand names in stadiums and arenas; (4) cartoon characters in tobacco advertising, packaging, and promotions; (5) payments to promote tobacco products in entertainment settings, such as movies; (6) sale of merchandise with brand name tobacco logos; and (7) transit and outdoor advertising (including billboards) (USDHHS 2000b). The Federal Public Health Cigarette Smoking Act of 1969 preempts most state advertising restrictions (The Public Health Cigarette Smoking Act of 1969), and 18 states preempt localities from restricting the marketing of tobacco products (CDC 2009b).

Prohibiting retail products that have tobacco images or brands, eliminating images of tobacco use in television and the movies seen by children, restricting advertising in magazines and other print media with high youth readership, eliminating tobacco company sponsorship of school, cultural, or sporting events (and banning tobacco logos at such events), and eliminating candy cigarettes or shredded bubble gum that is packaged to look like SLT are other ways to reduce youth exposure to pro-tobacco messages. Stronger warning labels can increase consumer understanding of the health risks. Separating major league baseball and SLT use will also provide better role models for youth (USDHHS 1992).

Sustained countermarketing campaigns are important in order to counteract the promotion of tobacco products. Effective campaigns for youth include hard-hitting, "edgy" campaigns such as Florida's, and later Legacy's, "truth" campaign (Murphy-Hoefer, Hyland, and Higbee 2008). Effective campaigns for adults often tell the stories of real people who had been harmed by tobacco use. Media has also been shown to be very effective in driving calls to quitlines. In fact, limited quitline resources often require states to carefully titrate media buys to control call volume, so that demand does not overwhelm their ability to provide services (CDC 2004c).

Smoke-Free Policies

Although the purpose of smoke-free policies is to reduce SHS exposure, these policies also reduce consumption, increase quitting, decrease relapse, and reduce initiation (USDHHS 2006a, 2000b; Zaza, Briss, and Harris 2005). Smoke-free policies have been implemented in Federal facilities (U.S. Departments of Health and Human Services and Defense), by Federal law (in indoor facilities that are regularly or routinely used to provide services to children) (USDHHS 2006a), in transportation venues (airplanes, trains), and in the private sector (hospitals, some hotel chains, private workplaces) (Americans for Nonsmokers' Rights 2005).

As of December 2009, 16 states had comprehensive indoor smoke-free policies that included all workplaces, restaurants, and bars, and six more had statewide smoke-free policies that included workplaces and restaurants, but not bars (CDC 2009b). As of April 2009, 3,010 localities had passed some form of clean indoor air law, including 340 municipalities with a local law in effect that required workplaces, restaurants, and bars be 100% smoke-free (American Nonsmokers' Rights Foundation 2009). However, as of December 2008, 14 states had legislation that preempted localities from enacting laws to restrict smoking in public places that were more stringent than state laws (CDC 2009b). In addition to reducing the number and degree of protection afforded by local regulations, preemption prevents the public education that occurs as a result of the debate and community organization around the issue.

Despite substantial progress, 125 million Americans are still exposed to SHS. Homes and workplaces are the primary locations for adult exposure, and homes, schools, and public places are important sources for children (USDHHS 2006a). A study examining cotinine levels in a nationally representative survey reported that 12% of nonsmoking adults living in counties with extensive smoke-free laws were exposed to SHS, compared with 35% in counties with limited coverage and 46% in counties with no law (Pickett et al. 2006).

Improving Public and Private Insurance Coverage of Tobacco-Use Treatment

Although slowly improving, insurance coverage for tobacco-use treatment is poor in both public and private sectors. Medicare first included cessation counseling as a covered benefit in 2005, and with the prescription drug benefit, FDA-approved prescription medications are now also covered (Centers for Medicare and Medicaid Services 2007). In 2007, only one state (Oregon) offered comprehensive coverage of tobacco-use treatment to all Medicaid recipients, and eight states provided no Medicaid coverage for counseling or FDA-approved medications (CDC 2009a). Private coverage of tobacco dependence treatments is also limited. A survey of work sites having at least 10 employees and providing health insurance reported that only 4% offered coverage of screening, counseling, and medications (including over-the-counter medications) (Partnership for Prevention 2007). An analysis of state requirements for insurance coverage for tobacco-use treatment for state employees in 2009 found that only five states provided tobacco-use treatment coverage consistent with the PHS guideline for all state employees and seven states provided no cessation coverage (ALA 2009).

Minors' Access Restrictions

In 1992, Congress enacted the Synar amendment, requiring every state to have a law prohibiting tobacco sales to minors under age 18 years, to enforce the law, to conduct annual statewide inspections of tobacco outlets to assess the rate of illegal tobacco sales to minors, and to develop a strategy and time frame to reduce the statewide illegal sales rate to 20% or less (SAMHSA 2008). States not meeting the requirement are at risk to lose substance abuse and mental health grant funding. In 2007, all states and the District of Columbia met the overall goal of a 20% violation rate (USDHHS 2008), and the average retailer violation rate decreased from 40% in 1997 to 10.5% in 2007. However, as of the fourth quarter of 2008, 22 states had laws that included preemptive minors' access language preventing stronger local legislation (CDC 2009b).

The MSA also contained the following youth access restrictions: restricted free samples except where no underage persons were present, prohibited gifts to youth in exchange for buying tobacco products, prohibited gifts through the mail without proof of age, and prohibited sale or distribution of packs smaller than 20 for three years (USDHHS 2000b). Studies show that Internet sales provide easy access to cigarettes by minors because many Internet vendors don't have a valid age verification process (Ribisi, Williams, and Kim 2003). By the end of 2005, 29 states had passed laws prohibiting delivery of tobacco to individual consumers and/or restricting Internet sales in some way (ALA 2007).

As commercial sales to minors decrease, "social" sources (other adolescents, parents, and older friends) may become more important. Thus, a comprehensive approach is needed so that individuals, as well as retailers, do not provide tobacco to minors (USDHHS 2000b).

Telephone Cessation Quitlines

In 1992, California became the first state to have a quitline. Other states followed, although funding has been erratic, with some states losing and then regaining financial support. In 2004, the Federal Government developed a national network of quitlines. This network has a single portal number, 1-800-QUIT NOW, that routes callers to their state's quitline. As part of the initiative, CDC provided funding to states without these services (USDHHS 2007b) and as of August 2006, all states offered quitline services. Some quitlines offer free nicotine replacement therapy with the counseling service (North American Quitline Consortium 2009). However, for most states, funding is not robust enough to allow widespread promotion and the provision of counseling and medication to all tobacco users interested in quitting. It has been estimated that up to 15% of smokers would use a quitline service, but current quitlines have the capacity to only serve 1%–3% of smokers (Fiore et al. 2004).

Product Changes

The IOM concluded that an unsuccessful "harm reduction" strategy could lead to long-lasting and broadly distributed adverse consequences, suggesting that these interventions may need to be held to a higher standard of proof. The fact that it could take decades to be certain about the effects of potential reduced-exposure products was noted as a reason for particular caution. The IOM also recommended that any such strategy should occur only under comprehensive regulation of tobacco products and be implemented within a comprehensive tobacco control effort that emphasizes abstinence, prevention, and treatment (IOM 2001).

Current Status of Comprehensive Programs

Sustaining funding for state tobacco control programs has been a continued challenge. For example, all four of the initial tobacco control programs have sustained cuts. By 2004, the Massachusetts program had been virtually eliminated (a 92% cut) and the California, Arizona, and Oregon programs severely reduced (45%, 37%, and 69%, respectively) (CTFK 2006). Florida's campaign was cut 99%, eliminating the effective "truth" marketing campaign (Schroeder 2004).

In 1998, the MSA provided $246 billion over 25 years to the states to compensate them for Medicaid and Medicare costs for treating smokers (CTFK 2006). Although it was expected that states would fund comprehensive tobacco control programs with the proceeds, in most cases, the funds have been used for other purposes, particularly as states experienced budget deficits in the first few years of the twenty-first century. In 2009, no states were funding their programs at the CDC-recommended levels and 42 states were funding at less than half the recommended levels. National funding to the American Legacy Foundation through the MSA is decreasing, and other foundations have also decreased their investment in tobacco prevention and control. Total funding for to-bacco control programs dropped 27% between 2002 and 2005 and then increased 33% by 2009. However, funding was still below the maximum level of funding (achieved in 2002) (CTFK 2009c).

Areas of Future Research and Demonstration

Continued research on the effect of various public health actions on reducing tobacco use is important in adapting interventions to maintain and increase effectiveness. Key issues include the following:

- Research on promising public health interventions
- Evaluations of state tobacco prevention and control programs to inform best prac-tices
- Monitoring tobacco industry practices and developing interventions to counteract these practices
- Understanding the recent slowing of the decline in youth and adult prevalence
- Assessing tobacco use and developing effective interventions for reducing tobacco use in disparate populations
- Research to understand the population health impacts of product changes
- Improved tobacco-use treatment interventions
- Demonstration project to determine the most effective and cost-effective inter-ventions internationally, particularly in low- and middle-income countries

The reduction in tobacco use in the United States is considered a public health tri-umph (Eriksen et al. 2007). However, too many Americans are still dying from this totally preventable cause of disease and death, and mortality worldwide is projected to increase dramatically over the next 25 years (Gajalakshmi et al. 2000). With the implementation of the Framework Convention on Tobacco Control (WHO 2003), there is likely to be accelerated global action on tobacco prevention and control. The United States can learn from the successes of other countries, but many countries, particularly low- and middle-income countries, will need expertise and financial help from the developed world in order to effectively deal with the emerging epidemic of tobacco use.

A research agenda that adapts to the changing tobacco control landscape to continually identify the important emerging research needs, leads to improved tobacco control inter-ventions, and determines ways to quickly translate relevant research findings into action are critical. Careful evaluations of specific program interventions, timely evaluation of new and innovative strategies, and "macro"-level analyses of the impact of comprehensive programs on tobacco use, health outcomes, and health care and productivity costs are essential.

Economic incentives are one of the most effective strategies to reduce cigarette consumption, prevent initiation, and increase cessation (USDHHS 2000b; Zaza, Briss, and Harris 2005). The tobacco industry's dramatic increase in spending on coupons and two-for-one offers has effectively reduced the impact of recent state tobacco tax increases (U.S. Department of Labor 2007); effective strategies are needed to counteract this strategy. Health and public health professionals can support initiatives to raise tobacco taxes.

Nonsmoking is already an accepted norm in many socially defined groups in the United States, and continuing to change the social norms to reduce the acceptability of tobacco use offers great promise (California Department of Health Services 2006). Sustained media campaigns are a critical element for social norm change (Goldman and Glantz 1998). Smoke-free policies also change social norms and increase cessation rates (Zaza, Briss, and Harris 2005). Public health agencies and preventive medicine practitioners should support the enactment of comprehensive smoke-free laws and their enforcement in order to reduce exposure to SHS and to encourage quitting. However, tobacco industry promotion of SLT "for when you can't smoke" could negate the impact of smoke-free policies on increasing cessation.

Since 70% of current smokers want to quit smoking (CDC 2005) and nearly 40% attempt cessation each year (CDC 2009c), both public and private health organizations need to be prepared to assist them. Health care professionals should routinely assess tobacco use and advise users to quit. The PHS Clinical Practice Guideline recommends that treatment be fully covered under both public and private insurance and that use of medication and telephone quitlines should be strongly encouraged (Fiore et al. 2008). Promotion of the quitline is essential to increase call volume, but states currently carefully titrate their promotion of the quitline to ensure that demand does not overwhelm their capacity to provide services (CDC 2004c). Full implementation of comprehensive tobacco control programs would allow expansion of state quitline capacity to widely promote and deliver counseling services to all smokers interested in quitting (USDHHS 2000b).

Prevention programs have demonstrated the ability to delay smoking initiation. However, these programs are most effective when they are reinforced by policy interventions such as higher tobacco taxes, interventions to reduce adult tobacco use, media counter-marketing campaigns, and supportive community programs (USDHHS 1994, 2000b) that make smoking appear unattractive, socially unpopular, and sexually unappealing. Communication should also stress that tobacco is an addictive drug.

Three national studies have shown that comprehensive tobacco prevention and control programs reduce cigarette consumption overall and smoking prevalence among youth and adults, over and above the effect of any tax increase that funded the program or occurred concurrently (Farrelly, Pechacek, and Chaloupka 2003; Pechacek, Farrelley, et al. 2008; Tauras, Chaloupka, Farrelley 2005). To meet the HP 2010 goal of an adult smoking prevalence of 12% and a youth smoking prevalence of 16%, substantially increased funding for comprehensive tobacco control programs that use proven policy, countermarketing, and community interventions will be required (Committee on Reducing Tobacco Use 2007).

The decrease in cigarette consumption has been termed one of the greatest public health achievements of the twentieth century, but it is only half achieved (Eriksen et al. 2007). The challenge of the twenty-first century is to accelerate progress so that the morbidity, mortality, and disability caused by tobacco use no longer occur in the United States or internationally. Full implementation of proven interventions would accelerate the reduction in tobacco use among youth and adults; prevent disease, disability, and death for millions of Americans; increase productivity; and save health care costs. Reducing tobacco use is a shared responsibility of Federal, state, and local governments; the public health community; the health care system; the private sector; and individual communities. If each sector did its part, one could expect faster progress in reducing tobacco use. However, the power and money of the tobacco industry has influenced the political and public institutions responsible for implementing effective interventions and prevented full implementation of proven strategies. Additionally, tobacco industry responses to consumer health concerns have included the filter cigarette, reductions in machine-produced average tar and nicotine content, and, more recently, new cigarette and smokeless delivery systems (IOM 2001). However, because these innovations were perceived as "safer," it appears that smokers concerned about health issues switched to such products rather than quit tobacco use entirely and derived little or no health benefit. Rather than looking to product innovations as the "solution" to the tobacco epidemic, what is needed is a concerted public health effort to implement proven strategies to reduce tobacco use. As the Surgeon General said in 2000, "The issue is not that we don't know what to do, but the failure to implement what we know works" (USDHHS 2000b). A concerted effort is needed, analogous to the efforts to eliminate the morbidity and mortality from polio or smallpox. The leading preventable cause of death in Western societies (and soon, the world) deserves no less.

Resources

American Cancer Society, 250 Williams Street, NW, Atlanta, GA 30303-1002, tel.: 1-800-ACS-2345, www.cancer.org

American Heart Association, National Center, 7272 Greenville Avenue, Dallas, TX 75231, tel.: 1-800-AHA-USA-1 (1-800-242-8721), www.americanheart.org

American Lung Association, 61 Broadway, 6th Floor, New York, NY 10006, tel.: (212) 315-8700, http://www.lungusa.org

Americans for Nonsmokers Rights, 530 San Pablo Avenue, Suite J, Berkeley, CA 94702, tel.: (510) 841-3032, www.no-smoke.org

American Legacy Foundation, 1724 Massachusetts Avenue, NW, Washington, DC 20036, tel.: (202) 454-5555, info@americanlegacy.org

Campaign for Tobacco Free Kids, 1400 Eye Street, Suite 1200, Washington, DC 20005, tel.: (202) 296-5469, www.tobaccofreekids.org

National Cancer Institute, Cancer Information Service, 6116 Executive Boulevard, Room 3036A, Rockville, MD 20852, tel.: 1-800-4-CANCER

National Cancer Institute, Tobacco Control Research Branch, Behavioral Research Program, Division of Cancer Control and Population Sciences, National Cancer Institute, EPN 4038, 6130 Executive Boulevard, Bethesda, MD 20892-7337, tel.: (301) 496-8584, http://www.cancer.gov/cancertopics/smoking, http://www.tobaccocontrol.cancer.gov, http://www.smokefree.gov

Office on Smoking and Health, Centers for Disease Control and Prevention, Mailstop K-50, 4770 Buford Highway, NE, Atlanta, GA 30341, tel.: (770) 488-5705; 1-800-CDC-INFO (1-800-232-4636), http://www.cdc.gov/tobacco

Suggested Reading

Centers for Disease Control and Prevention (CDC). *Best Practices for Comprehensive Tobacco Control Programs—2007.* Atlanta, GA: U.S. Department of Health and Human Services, Centers for Disease Control and Prevention, Office on Smoking and Health (2007).

Fiore, M.C., C.R. Jaen, T.B. Baker, et al. *Treating Tobacco Use and Dependence Clinical Practice Guidelines, 2008 Update.* Rockville, MD: U.S. Department of Health and Human Services, Public Health Service (2008).

Orleans, C.T., and J. Slade, editors. *Nicotine Addiction; Principles and Management.* New York: Oxford University Press (1993).

Task Force on Community Preventive Services. Tobacco. In: Zaza, S., P.A. Briss, and K.W. Harris, editors, *The Guide to Community Preventive Services: What Works to Promote Health?* New York: Oxford University Press (2005).

U.S. Department of Health and Human Services (USDHHS). *Reducing Tobacco Use: A Report of the Surgeon General.* Washington, D.C.: U.S. Department of Health and Human Services, Centers for Disease Control and Prevention, Office on Smoking and Health (2000).

U.S. Department of Health and Human Services (USDHHS). *The Health Benefits of Smoking Cessation: A Report of the Surgeon General.* Atlanta, GA: U.S. Department of Health and Human Services, Centers for Disease Control and Prevention, Office on Smoking and Health (1990). DHHS Publication (CDC) 90–8416.

U.S. Department of Health and Human Services (USDHHS). *The Health Consequences of Smoking: A Report of the Surgeon General.* Atlanta, GA: U.S. Department of Health and Human Services, Centers for Disease Control and Prevention, Office on Smoking and Health (2004).

U.S. Department of Health and Human Services (USDHHS). *The Health Consequences of Involuntary Exposure to Tobacco Smoke. A Report of the Surgeon General.* Atlanta, GA: U.S. Department of Health and Human Services, Centers for Disease Control and Prevention, Office on Smoking and Health (2006).

U.S. Department of Health and Human Services (USDHHS). *Preventing Tobacco Use Among Young People: A Report of the Surgeon General.* Atlanta, GA: U.S. Department of Health and Human Services, Public Health Service, Centers for Disease Prevention and Control, National Center for Chronic Disease Prevention and Health Promotion, Office on Smoking and Health (1994).

U.S. Department of Health and Human Services (USDHHS). *The Health Consequences of Smoking—Nicotine Addiction: A Report of the Surgeon General.* Rockville, MD: U.S. Department of Health and Human Services, Public Health Service, Centers for Disease Prevention and Control, Office on Smoking and Health (1988).

References

Allen, D.R., N.L. Browse, D.L. Rutt, et al. The Effect of Cigarette Smoke, Nicotine, and Carbon Monoxide on the Permeability of the Arterial Wall. *J Epidemiol Community Health* (1988):39:286–293.

American Lung Association (ALA). *State Employee Health Plans Should Cover Cessation Treatments.* 2009. Available at: http://www.lungusa.org/atf/cf/%7B7a8d42c2-fcca-4604-8ade-7f5d5e762256%7D/CESSATION_DB_PDF_5.PDF. Accessed May 21, 2009.

American Lung Association (ALA). *State Legislated Actions on Tobacco Issues 2005.* 2008. Available at http://slati.lungusa.org/reports/SLATI_2008_final_online.pdf. Accessed May 21, 2009.

American Nonsmokers' Rights Foundation. 2009. Available at: http://www.no-smoke.org/pdf/mediaordlist.pdf. Accessed May 21, 2009.

Americans for Nonsmokers' Rights. *Smokefree Transportation Chronology.* 2005. Available at http://www.no-smoke.org/document.php?id=334. Accessed May 21, 2009.

Attorneys General Statement Agreement. 1997. Available at: http://stic.neu.edu/LIGGETTSETTLE.htm. Accessed May 21, 2009.

Backinger, C.L., P. McDonald, D.J. Ossip-Klein, et al. Improving the Future of Youth Smoking Cessation. *Am J Health Behav* (2003):27(Suppl):S170–S184.

Baker, F., S.R. Ainsworth, J.T. Dye, et al. Health Risks Associated with Cigar Smoking. *JAMA* (2000):284:735–740.

Beck, G.J., C.A. Doyle, and E.N. Schachter. Smoking and Lung Function. *Am Rev Respir Dis* (1981):123:149–155.

Behan, D.F., M.P. Eriksen, and Y. Lin. *Economic Effects of Environmental Tobacco Smoke.* Cambridge, MA: Society of Actuaries (2005).

Benowitz, N.L., and S.G. Gourlay. Cardiovascular Toxicity of Nicotine: Implications for Nicotine Replacement Therapy. *J Am Coll Cardiol* (1997):29:1422–1431.

Bolinder, G.M., B.O. Ahlborg, and J.H. Lindell. Use of Smokeless Tobacco: Blood Pressure Elevation and Other Health Hazards Found in a Largescale Population Survey. *J Intern Med* (1992):232:327–334.

Borland, R., H.H. Yong, K.M. Cummings, A. Hyland, S. Anderson, and G.T. Fong. Determinants and Consequences of Smoke-Free Homes: Findings from the International Tobacco Control (ITC) Four Country Survey. *Tob Control* (2006):15(Suppl 3):iii42–iii50.

California Department of Health Services, Tobacco Control Section. *California Tobacco Control Update, 2000.* 2000. Available at http://www.dhs.ca.gov/tobacco/documents/pubs/CTCUpdate.pdf. Accessed April 15, 2007.

California Department of Health Services. *California Department of Health Services: Fact Sheets.* 2005. Available at http://www.dhs.ca.gov/tobacco/html/factsheets.htm. Accessed August 11, 2005.

California Department of Health Services. *California Tobacco Control Update 2006: The Social Norm Change Approach.* Sacramento, CA: California Department of Health Services. Tobacco Control Section. 2006. Available at: http://ww2.cdph.ca.gov/programs/tobacco/Documents/CTCUpdate2006.pdf. Accessed May 21, 2009.

Campaign for Tobacco-Free Kids (CTFK). *A Broken Promise to Our Children: The 1998 State Tobacco Settlement Eight Years Later.* Washington, D.C.: Campaign for Tobacco-Free Kids (2006).

Campaign for Tobacco-Free Kids (CTFK). *State Cigarette Excise Tax Rates and Rankings.* Washington, D.C.: Campaign for Tobacco-Free Kids. 2009a. Available at http://www.tobaccofreekids.org/research/factsheets/pdf/0097.pdf. Accessed May 21, 2009.

Campaign for Tobacco-Free Kids (CTFK). *New Federal Tobacco Product Tax Rate Increases.* Washington, D.C.: Campaign for Tobacco-Free Kids. 2009b. Available at http://www.tobaccofreekids.org/research/factsheets/pdf/0343.pdf. Accessed May 21, 2009.

Campaign for Tobacco-Free Kids (CTFK). *A Decade of Broken Promises: The 1998 State Tobacco Settlement Ten Years Later.* Washington, D.C.: Campaign for Tobacco-Free Kids. 2009c. Available at: http://www.tobaccofreekids.org/reports/settlements/2009/fullreport.pdf. Accessed May 21, 2009.

Capehart, T. *Tobacco Situation and Outlook Yearbook.* Washington, D.C.: U.S. Department of Agriculture (2004). Publication no. TBS-2004.

Capehart, T. *Tobacco Outlook.* Washington, D.C.: U.S. Department of Agriculture (2007). Publication TBS-262.

Celermajer, D.S., K.E. Sorensen, D. Georgakopoulos, et al. Cigarette Smoking is Associated with Dose-Related and Potentially Reversible Impairment of Endothelium-Dependent Dilation in Healthy Young Adults. *Circulation* (1993):88(5 Pt 1):2149–2155.

Centers for Disease Control and Prevention (CDC). Guidelines for School Health Programs to Prevent Tobacco Use and Addiction. *MMWR* (1994):43(RR-2):1–18.

Centers for Disease Control and Prevention (CDC). Addition of Prevalence of Cigarette Smoking as a Nationally Notifiable Condition—June 1996. *MMWR* (1996a):45:537.

Centers for Disease Control and Prevention (CDC). *Making Your Workplace Smokefree: A Decision Maker's Guide.* Atlanta, GA: U.S. Department of Health and Human Services, Centers for Disease Control and Prevention, Office on Smoking and Health (1996b).

Centers for Disease Control and Prevention (CDC). Response to Increases in Cigarette Prices by Race/Ethnicity, Income, and Age Groups—United States, 1976–1993. *MMWR* (1998): 47:605–609.

Centers for Disease Control and Prevention (CDC). Effect of Ending an Antitobacco Youth Campaign on Adolescent Susceptibility to Cigarette Smoking—Minnesota, 2002–2003. *MMWR* (2004a):53:301–304.

Centers for Disease Control and Prevention (CDC). Indoor Air Quality in Hospitality Venues Before and After Implementation of a Clean Indoor Air Law—Western New York, 2003. *MMWR* (2004b):53:1038–1041.

Centers for Disease Control and Prevention (CDC). *Telephone Quitlines: A Resource for Development, Implementation, and Evaluation.* Atlanta, GA: U.S. Department of Health and Human Services, Centers for Disease Control and Prevention, Office on Smoking and Health (2004c).

Centers for Disease Control and Prevention (CDC). Cigarette Smoking Among Adults—United States, 2000. *MMWR* (2005):51:642–645.

Centers for Disease Control and Prevention (CDC). Cigarette Use Among High School Students—United States, 1991–2005. *MMWR* (2006):55:724–726.

Centers for Disease Control and Prevention (CDC). *Best Practices for Comprehensive Tobacco Control Programs—2007.* Atlanta, GA: U.S. Department of Health and Human Services, Centers for Disease Control and Prevention, Office on Smoking and Health (2007).

Centers for Disease Control and Prevention (CDC). Cigarette Smoking Among Adults—United States, 2007. *MMWR* (2008a):57:1221–1226.

Centers for Disease Control and Prevention (CDC). Smoking-Attributable Mortality, Years of Potential Life Lost, and Productivity Losses—United States, 2000–2004. *MMWR* (2008b):57:1226–1228.

Centers for Disease Control and Prevention (CDC). Smoking-Attributable Mortality, Morbidity, and Economic Costs (SAMMEC). 2008c. Available at http://apps.nccd.cdc.gov/sammec. Accessed June 17, 2009.

Centers for Disease Control and Prevention (CDC). Tobacco Use Among Middle and High School Students—United States, 2006. *MMWR* (in press).

Centers for Disease Control and Prevention (CDC). State Medicaid Coverage for Tobacco-Dependence Treatments—United States, 2007. *MMWR* (2009a):58(43):1199–1204.

Centers for Disease Control and Prevention (CDC). *State Tobacco Activities Tracking and Evaluation (STATE) System.* 2009b. Available at http://apps.nccd.cdc.gov/statesystem. Accessed May 21, 2009.

Centers for Disease Control and Prevention (CDC). State-Specific Prevalence and Trends in Adult Cigarette Smoking—United States, 1998–2007. *MMWR* (2009c):58:221–226.

Centers for Medicare and Medicaid Services. *Smoking Cessation.* 2007. Available at: http://www.cms.hhs.gov/SmokingCessation. Accessed May 21, 2009.

Cesaroni, G., F. Forastiere, N. Agabiti, P. Valente, P. Zuccaro, and C. Perucci. Effect of the Italian Smoking Ban on Population Rates of Acute Coronary Events. *Circulation* (2008):117:1183–1188.

Chao, A., M.J. Thun, J. Henley, et al. Cigarette Smoking, Use of Other Tobacco Products, and Stomach Cancer Mortality in U.S. Adults: The Cancer Prevention Study II. *Int J Cancer* (2002):101:380–389.

Cokkinides, V.E., E. Ward, A. Jemal, and M.J. Thun. Under-Use of Smoking Cessation Treatments: Results from the National Health Interview Survey, 2000. *Am J Prev Med* (2005):28:119–122.

Committee on Reducing Tobacco Use: Strategies, Barriers, and Consequences. In: Bonnie, R.J., K. Stratton, and R.B. Wallace, editors, *Ending the Tobacco Problem: A Blueprint for the Nation.* Institute of Medicine. Washington, D.C.: National Academies Press. 2007. Available at: http://www.nap.edu/catalog.php?record_id=11795. Accessed May 21, 2009.

Connolly, W., Director, Massachusetts Tobacco Control Program, Joint Hearing of the Pennsylvania House of Representatives Committee on Health and Human Services and the Pennsylvania Senate Committee on Public Health and Welfare, June 22, 1999. *Campaign for Tobacco-Free Kids (CTFK) Fact Sheet, Harm Caused by Pregnant Women Smoking or Being Exposed to*

Secondhand Smoke. Available at http://tobaccofreekids.org/research/factsheets/pdf/0007.pdf. Accessed May 21, 2009.

Cromwell, J., W.J. Bartosch, M.C. Fiore, et al. Cost-Effectiveness of the Clinical Practice Recommendations in the AHCPR Guideline for Smoking Cessation. *JAMA* (1997):278:1759–1766.

Cummings, S.R., S.M. Rubin, and G. Oster. The Cost-Effectiveness of Counseling Smokers to Quit. *JAMA* (1989):261:75–79.

Dalton, M., J. Sargent, M. Beach, et al. Effect of Viewing Smoking in Movies on Adolescent Smoking Initiation: A Cohort Study. *Lancet* (2003):362:281–285.

Delnevo, C.D., M. Hrywna, J. Foulds, et al. Cigar Use Before and After a Cigarette Excise Tax Increase in New Jersey. *Addict Behav* (2004):29:1799–1807.

Distefan, J., J.P. Pierce, and E.A. Gilpin. Do Favorite Movie Stars Influence Adolescent Smoking Initiation? *Am J Public Health* (2004):94:1239–1244.

Eisner, M.D., A.K. Smith, and P.D. Blanc. Bartenders' Respiratory Health After Establishment of Smoke-Free Bars and Taverns. *JAMA* (1998):280:1909–1914.

England, L.J., R.J. Levine, J.L. Mills, et al. Adverse Pregnancy Outcomes in Snuff Users. *Am J Obstet Gynecol* (2003):189:939–943.

Eriksen, M.P., L.W. Green, C.G. Husten, L.L. Pedersen, and T.F. Pechacek. Thank You for Not Smoking: The Public Health Response to Tobacco-Related Mortality in the United States. In: Ward, J.W., and C. Warren, editors, *Silent Victories: The History and Practice of Public Health in Twentieth-Century America.* New York: Oxford University Press (2007).

Evans, N., A. Farkas, E. Gilpin, et al. Influence of Tobacco Marketing and Exposure to Smokers on Adolescent Susceptibility to Smoking. *J Natl Cancer Inst* (1995):87:1538–1545.

Farrelly, M., K.C. Davis, M.L. Haviland, et al. Evidence of a Dose–Response Relationship Between "Truth" Antismoking Ads and Youth Smoking Prevalence. *Am J Public Health* (2005):95: 425–431.

Farrelly, M., T. Pechacek, and F. Chaloupka. The Impact of Tobacco Control Program Expenditures on Aggregate Cigarette Sales: 1981–2000. *J Health Econ* (2003):22:843–859.

Farrelly, M.C., C.G. Healton, K.C. Davis, et al. Getting to the Truth: Evaluating National Tobacco Countermarketing Campaigns. *Am J Public Health* (2002):92:901–907.

Farrelly, M.C., J.M. Nonnemaker, R. Chou, et al. Changes in Hospitality Workers' Exposure to Secondhand Smoke Following the Implementation of New York's Smoke-Free Law. *Tob Control* (2005):14:236–241.

Federal Trade Commission (FTC). *Report to Congress for 1995: Pursuant to the Federal Cigarette Labeling and Advertising Act.* Washington, D.C.: Federal Trade Commission (1997).

Federal Trade Commission (FTC). *Federal Trade Commission Cigarette Report for 2004 and 2005.* Washington D.C.: Federal Trade Commission (2007a).

Federal Trade Commission (FTC). *Federal Trade Commission Smokeless Tobacco Report for the Years 2002–2005.* Washington, D.C.: Federal Trade Commission (2007b).

Fichtenberg, C.M., and S.A. Glantz. Associations of the California Tobacco Control Program with Declines in Cigarette Consumption and Mortality from Heart Disease. *N Engl J Med* (2000):343:1772–1777.

Fiore, M.C., R.T. Coyle, S.J. Curry, et al. Preventing Three Million Premature Deaths and Helping Five Million Smokers to Quit. A National Action Plan for Tobacco Cessation. *Am J Public Health* (2004):94:205–210.

Fiore, M.C., C.R. Jaen, T.B. Baker, et al. *Treating Tobacco Use and Dependence Clinical Practice Guideline, 2008 Update.* Rockville, MD: U.S. Department of Health and Human Services, Public Health Service (2008).

Florida Department of Health. Monitoring Program Outcomes in 2002. *Florida Youth Tobacco Survey* (2002):5(1):1–23.

Friedman, G.D., A.B. Siegelaub, C.C. Seltzer, et al. Smoking Habits and the Leukocyte Count. *Arch Environ Health* (1973):26:137–143.

Fusegawa, Y., S. Goto, S. Handa, et al. Platelet Spontaneous Aggregation in Platelet-Rich Plasma is Increased in Habitual Smokers. *Thromb Res* (1999):93:271–278.

Gajalakshmi, C.K., P. Jha, K. Ranson, and S. Nguyen. Global Patterns of Smoking and Smoking-Attributable Mortality. In: Jha, P., and F. Chaloupka, editors, *Tobacco Control in Developing Countries.* New York: Oxford University Press (2000).

Givel, M.S., and S.A. Glantz. Tobacco Lobby Political Influence on U.S. State Legislatures in the 1990s. *Tob Control* (2001):10:124–134.

Glantz, S.A., K.A. Kacirk, and C. McCulloch. Back to the Future: Smoking in Movies in 2002 Compared with 1950 Levels. *Am J Public Health* (2004):94:261–263.

Goldman, L.K., and S.A. Glantz. Evaluation of Antismoking Advertising Campaigns. *JAMA* (1998):279:772–777.

Gupta, R., H. Gurm, and J.R. Bartholomew. Smokeless Tobacco and Cardiovascular Risk. *Arch Intern Med* (2004):164:1845–1849.

Halpern, M.T., R. Shikiar, A.M. Rentz, et al. Impact of Smoking Status on Workplace Absenteeism and Productivity. *Tob Control* (2001):10:233–238.

Henley, S.J., M.J. Thun, A. Chao, et al. Association between Exclusive Pipe Smoking and Mortality from Cancer and Other Disease. *J Natl Cancer Inst* (2004):96:853–861.

Henley, S.J., M.J. Thun, C. Connell, et al. Two Large Prospective Studies of Mortality among Men Who Use Snuff or Chewing Tobacco (United States). *Cancer Causes Control* (2005):16:347–358.

Henriksen, L., A.L. Dauphinee, Y. Wang, and S.P. Fortmann. Industry Sponsored Anti-Smoking Ads and Adolescent Reactance: Test of a Boomerang Effect. *Tob Control* (2006):15:13–18.

Holly, E.A., N.L. Petrakis, N.F. Friend, et al. Mutagenic Mucus in the Cervix of Smokers. *J Natl Cancer Inst* (1986):76:983–986.

Hoyert, D.L., M.P. Heron, S.L. Murphy, and H.C. Kung. *Deaths: Final Data for 2003: National Vital Statistics Report 54 No. 13.* Hyattsville, MD: U.S. Department of Health and Human Services, Centers for Disease Control and Prevention, National Center for Health Statistics (2006):1–119.

Institute of Medicine (IOM). *Clearing the Smoke: Assessing the Science Base for Tobacco Harm Reduction.* Washington, D.C.: National Academy Press (2001).

International Agency for Research on Cancer (IARC). Tobacco Habits Other than Smoking; Betel-Quid and Areca-Nut Chewing; and Some Related Nitrosamines. *IARC Monographs on the Evaluation of Carcinogenic Risks to Humans,* Vol. 37. Lyon, France: IARC (1985).

International Agency for Research on Cancer (IARC). Smoking and Tobacco Control Monograph No. 9. Tobacco Smoke and Involuntary Smoking. *IARC Monographs on the Evaluation of Carcinogenic Risks to Humans,* Vol. 83. Lyon, France: IARC (2004).

International Agency for Research on Cancer (IARC). Smokeless Tobacco and Some Related Nitrosamines. *IARC Monographs on the Evaluation of Carcinogenic Risks to Humans,* Vol. 89. Lyon, France: IARC (2005).

Jacobs, E.J., M.J. Thun, and L.F. Apicella. Cigar Smoking and Death from Coronary Heart Disease in a Prospective Study. *Arch Intern Med* (1999):159:2413–2418.

Johnston, L.D., P.M. O'Malley, J.G. Bachman, and J.E. Schulenberg. *More Good News on Teen Smoking: Rates at or Near Record Lows.* Ann Arbor, MI: University of Michigan News Service [Online] (December 11, 2008). Available: www.monitoringthefuture.org. Accessed May 21, 2009.

Juster, H.R., B.R. Loomis, T.M. Hinman, et al. Declines in Hospital Admissions for Acute Myocardial Infarction in New York State After Implementation of a Comprehensive Smoking Ban. *Am J Public Health* (2007):97:2035–2039.

Kenkel, D., and L. Chen. Consumer Information and Tobacco Use. In: Jha, P., and F. Chaloupka, editors, *Tobacco Control in Developing Countries.* New York: Oxford University Press (2000).

King, C., and M. Siegel. The Master Settlement Agreement with the Tobacco Industry and Cigarette Advertising in Magazines. *N Engl J Med* (2001):345:504–511.

Kropp, R.Y., and B.L. Halpern-Felsher. Adolescents' Beliefs about the Risks Involved in Smoking "Light" Cigarettes. *Pediatrics* (2004):114:445–451.

Kuller, L.H., R.P. Tracy, J. Shaten, et al. Relation of C-Reactive Protein and Coronary Heart Disease in the MRFIT Nested Case-Control Study. Multiple Risk Factor Intervention Trial. *Am J Epidemiol* (1996):144:537–547.

Kuratsune, M., S. Kohchi, and A. Horie. Carcinogenesis in the Esophagus. I. Penetration of Benzo[a]pyrene and other Hydrocarbons into the Esophageal Mucosa. *Gann* (1965):56:177–187.

Lange, P., J. Nyboe, M. Appleyard, et al. Relationship of the Type of Tobacco and Inhalation Pattern to Pulmonary and Total Mortality. *Eur Respir J* (1992):5:1111–1117.

Lee, A.M., C. Jepson, E. Hoffmann, et al. CYP2B6 Genotype Alters Abstinence Rates in a Bupropion Smoking Cessation Trial. *Biol Psychiatry* (2007):62:635–641.

Lerman, C., and W. Berrettini. Elucidating the Role of Genetic Factors in Smoking Behavior and Nicotine Dependence. *Am J Med Genet B Neuropsychiatr Genet* (2003):118B:48–54.

Loomis, B.R., M.C. Farrelly, and N.H. Mann. The Association of Retail Promotions for Cigarettes with the Master Settlement Agreement, Tobacco Control Programmes and Cigarette Excise Taxes. *Tob Control* (2006):15:458–463.

Lynch, B.S., and R.J. Bonnie, editors. *Growing Up Tobacco Free: Preventing Nicotine Addiction in Children and Youths*. Washington, D.C.: National Press (1994).

Maciosek, M.V., A.B. Coffield, N.M. Edwards, et al. Priorities among Effective Clinical Preventive Services: Results of a Systematic Review and Analysis. *Am J Prev Med* (2006):31:52–61.

Malarcher, A.M., S.L. Thorne, K. Jackson, V.J. Rock, J. Kahende, and R.K. Merritt. Surveillance for Selected Tobacco Use Behaviors—United States, 1900–2005. *MMWR.* (in press).

Maroney, C.L., A. Sesko, E.M. Whelan, and A. Dunston. *Tobacco and Women's Health: A Survey of Popular Women's Magazines: August 1999–August 2000*. New York: American Council on Science and Health (2001).

Marshall, L., M. Schooley, H. Ryan, et al. Youth Tobacco Surveillance—United States, 2001–2002. *MMWR CDC Surveill Summ* (May 19, 2006):55(SS-3):1–60.

Martin J.A., B.E. Hamilton, P.D. Sutton, et al. Births: Final Data for 2005. *National Vital Statistical Reports* (2007):56(6):1–104.

Maryland Attorney General. *Landmark Settlement of "Kool Mixx" Tobacco Lawsuits*. 2007. Available at http://www.oag.state.md.us/Press/2004/1006c04.htm. Accessed May 21, 2009.

Massachusetts Department of Health. *Smokeless Tobacco Advertising Expenditures Before and After the Smokeless Tobacco Master Settlement Agreement*. Boston, MA: Massachusetts Department of Health, Massachusetts Tobacco Control Program. 2002. Available at http://tobaccofreekids.org/pressoffice/release503/smokeless.pdf. Accessed May 21, 2009.

McDonald, P., B. Colwell, C.L. Backinger, et al. Better Practices for Youth Tobacco Cessation: Evidence of Review Panel. *Am J Health Behav* (2003):27(Suppl 2):S144–S158.

Murphy-Hoefer, R., A. Hyland, and C. Higbee. Perceived Effectiveness of Tobacco Counter-Marketing Advertisements among Young Adults. *Am J Health Behav* (2008):32(6):725–34.

National Cancer Institute (NCI). *The Impact of Cigarette Excise Taxes on Smoking Among Children and Adults: Summary Report of a National Cancer Institute Expert Panel*. Washington, D.C.: National Cancer Institute (1993).

National Cancer Institute (NCI). *Cigars: Health Effects and Trends*. Bethesda, MD: U.S. Department of Health and Human Services, National Institutes of Health, National Cancer Institute (1998).

National Cancer Institute (NCI). The Role of the Media in Promoting and Reducing Tobacco Use. Bethesda, MD: U.S. Department of Health and Human Services, National Institutes of Health, National Cancer Institute (2008).

National Institutes of Health (NIH). Consensus Development Panel. National Institutes of Health Consensus Statement: Health Implications of Smokeless Tobacco Use. *Biomed Pharmacother* (1988):42:93–98.

Nelson, D.E., R.M. Davis, J.H. Chrismon, et al. Pipe Smoking in the United States, 1965–1991: Prevalence and Attributable Mortality. *Prev Med* (1996):25:91–99.

North American Quitline Consortium. Mission and Background. 2009. Available at http://www. naquitline.org/index.asp?dbid=2&dbsection=about. Accessed May 21, 2009.

Nyboe, J., G. Jensen, M. Appleyard, et al. Smoking and the Risk of First Acute Myocardial Infarction. *Am Heart J* (1991):122:438–447.

Office of Disease Prevention and Health Promotion, and Centers for Disease Control and Prevention. *For a Healthy Nation: Returns on Investment in Public Health.* Washington, D.C.: Office of Disease Prevention and Health Promotion, and Centers for Disease Control and Prevention (1994).

Office of the New York State Attorney General. *Attorneys General and R.J. Reynolds Reach Historic Settlement to End the Sale of Flavored Cigarettes.* 2007. Available at http://www.oag.state.ny.us/media_center/2006/oct/oct11a_06.html. Accessed May 21, 2009.

Ohsfeldt, R.L., R.G. Boyle, and E. Capilouto. Effects of Tobacco Excise Taxes on the Use of Smokeless Tobacco Products in the USA. *Health Econ* (1997):6:525–531.

Ono, Y., and B. Ingersoll. RJR Retires Joe Camel, Adds Sexy Smokers. *Wall Str J* (July 11, 1997):B1.

Partnership for Prevention. *Why Invest: Recommendations for Improving Your Prevention Investment.* Washington, D.C.: Partnership for Prevention (2007).

Pechacek, T., M. Farrelley, K. Thomas, and D. Nelson. The Impact of Tobacco Control Programs on Adult Smoking. *Am J Public Health* (2008):98:304–309.

Pechman, C., and S. Ratneshawr. The Effects of Antismoking and Cigarette Advertising on Young Adolescents' Perceptions of Peers Who Smoke. *J Consum Res* (1994):21:236–251.

Pickett, M.S., S.E. Schober, D.J. Brody, et al. Smoke–Free Laws and Secondhand Smoke Exposure in U.S. Non-Smoking Adults, 1999–2000. *Tob Control* (2006):15:302–307.

Pierce, J.P., W.S. Choi, E.A. Gilpin, A.J. Farkas, and C.C. Berr. Tobacco Industry Promotion of Cigarettes and Adolescent Smoking. *JAMA* (1998):279:511–515.

Pierce, J.P., T.P. Gilmer, L. Lee, E.A. Gilpin, J. de Beyer, and K. Messer. Tobacco Industry Price-Subsidizing Promotions May Overcome the Downward Pressure of Higher Prices on Initiation of Regular Smoking. *Health Econ* (2005):14:1061–1071.

Pierce, J.P., L. Lee, and E.A. Gilpin. Smoking Initiation by Adolescent Girls, 1944–1988. An Association with Targeted Advertising. *JAMA* (1994):271:608–611.

Polansky, J.R., and S.A. Glantz. First-Run Smoking Presentations in U.S. Movies 1999–2003. Available at http://repositories.cdlib.org/cgi/viewcontent.cgi?article=1047&context=ctcre. Accessed May 21, 2009.

Pollay Tobacco Ad Collection. Available at: http://tobaccodocuments.org/pollay_ads/True01.08. html. Accessed May 21, 2009.

Pollay, R., S. Siddarth, M. Siegel, et al. The Last Straw? Cigarette Advertising and Realized Market Shares Among Youths and Adults, 1979–1993. *J Mark* (1996):60:1–16.

Prokopczyk, B., J.E. Cox, D. Hoffmann, et al. Identification of Tobacco Specific Carcinogen in the Cervical Mucus of Smokers and Nonsmokers. *J Natl Cancer Inst* (1997):89:868–873.

Quindlen, A. Quid Pro Quo. *New York Times* (October 8, 1994).

Repace, J. Respirable Particles and Carcinogens in the Air of Delaware Hospitality Venues Before and After a Smoking Ban. *J Occup Environ Med* (2004):46:887–905.

Repace, J.L. Tobacco Smoke Pollution. In: Orleans, C.T., and J. Slade, editors, *Nicotine Addiction: Principles and Management.* New York: Oxford University Press (1993):129–142.

Ribisi, K.M., R.S. Williams, and A.E. Kim. Internet Sales of Cigarettes to Minors. *JAMA* (2003):290:1356–1359.

Romer, D., and P. Jamieson. Do Adolescents Appreciate the Risks of Smoking? Evidence from a National Survey. *J Adolesc Health* (2001):29:12–21.

Saffer, H., and F. Chaloupka. *Tobacco Advertising: Economic Theory and International Evidence.* Cambridge, MA: National Bureau of Economic Research (1999).

Sargent, J.D., M.L. Beach, A. Adachi-Mejia, et al. Exposure to Movie Smoking: Its Relation to Smoking Initiation among U.S. Adolescents. *Pediatrics* (2005):116:1183–1191.

Sargent, J.D., S.E. Tanski, and J. Gibson. Exposure to Movie Smoking Among U.S. Adolescents Aged 10 to 14 Years: A Population Estimate. *Pediatrics* (2007):119:1167–1176.

Schauffler, H.H., and T. Rodriguez. Availability and Utilization of Health Promotion Programs and Satisfaction with Health Plan. *Med Care* (1994):32:1182–1196.

Schroeder, S. Tobacco Control in the Wake of the 1998 Master Settlement Agreement. *N Eng J Med* (2004):350:293–301.

Scientific Committee on Tobacco and Health. *Report of the Scientific Committee on Tobacco and Health.* London: The Stationery Office (1998).

Scollo, M., A. Lal, A. Hyland, et al. Review of the Quality of Studies on the Economic Effects of Smoke-Free Policies on the Hospitality Industry. *Tob Control* (2003):12:13–20.

Shapiro, J.A., E.J. Jacobs, and M.J. Thun. Cigar Smoking in Men and Risk of Death from Tobacco-Related Cancers. *J Natl Cancer Inst* (2000):92:333–337.

Shiao, Y.H., J.M. Rice, and L.M. Anderson. von Hippel Lindau Gene Mutations in *N*-Nitrosodimethylamine-Induced Rat Renal Epithelial Tumors. *J Natl Cancer Inst* (1998):90:1720–1723.

Siegel, M. Counteracting Tobacco Motor Sports Sponsorship as a Promotional Tool: Is the Tobacco Settlement Enough? *Am J Public Health* (2001):91:1100–1106.

Siegel, M., A.B. Albers, D.M. Cheng, L. Biener, and N.A. Rigotti. Effect of Local Restaurant Smoking Regulations on Progression to Established Smoking among Youths. *Tob Control* (2005):14:300–306.

Sloan, F.A., J. Ostermann, C. Conover, D.H. Taylor, and G. Picone. *The Price of Smoking.* Cambridge, MA: MIT Press (2004).

Sorensen, G., K. Emmons, A.M. Stoddard, L. Linnan, and J. Avrunin. Do Social Influences Contribute to Occupational Differences in Quitting Smoking and Attitudes Toward Quitting? *Am J Health Promot* (2002):16:135–141.

Stead, L.F., R. Perera, and T. Lancaster. Telephone Counselling for Smoking Cessation. *Cochrane Database Syst Rev.* 2006. Available at http://www.cochrane.org/reviews. Accessed May 21, 2009.

Substance Abuse and Mental Health Services Administration (SAMHSA). Center for Substance Abuse Prevention. *Tobacco/SYNAR.* 2008. Available at http://prevention.samhsa.gov/tobacco/default.aspx. Accessed May 21, 2009.

Tauras, J.A., F. Chaloupka, M. Farrelly, et al. State Tobacco Control Spending and Youth Smoking. *Am J Public Health* (2005):95:338–344.

The Public Health Cigarette Smoking Act of 1969. U.S. Public Health Law. 91–222.

Tobacco Free Mass. *New Data Show Disturbing Reversal of Progress on Reducing Smoking in Massachusetts.* 2005. Available at http://www.tobaccofreekids.org/documents/MA_program_rpt-4-9-07.pdf. Accessed May 21, 2009.

Tomar, S.L. Is Use of Smokeless Tobacco a Risk Factor for Cigarette Smoking? The U.S. Experience. *Nicotine Tob Res* (2003):5:561–569.

Tomar, S.L., C.G. Husten, and M.W. Manley. Do Dentists and Physicians Advise Tobacco Users to Quit? *J Am Dent Assoc* (1996):127:259–265.

U.S. Department of Health and Human Services (USDHHS). *The Health Consequences of Smoking: Chronic Obstructive Lung Disease.* Rockville, MD: U.S. Department of Health and Human Services, Public Health Service, Office on Smoking and Health (1984).

U.S. Department of Health and Human Services (USDHHS). *The Health Consequences of Using Smokeless Tobacco. A Report of the Surgeon General.* Bethesda, MD: U.S. Department of Health and Human Services, Public Health Service (1986). DHHS Publication 86-2874.

U.S. Department of Health and Human Services (USDHHS). *The Health Consequences of Smoking—Nicotine Addiction: A Report of the Surgeon General.* Rockville, MD: U.S. Department of Health and Human Services, Centers for Disease Control, Office on Smoking and Health (1988). DHHS Publication (CDC) 88-8406.

U.S. Department of Health and Human Services (USDHHS). *Reducing the Health Consequences of Smoking: 25 Years of Progress: A Report of the Surgeon General*. Atlanta, GA: U.S. Department of Health and Human Services, Centers for Disease Control and Prevention, Office on Smoking and Health (1989).

U.S. Department of Health and Human Services (USDHHS). *The Health Benefits of Smoking Cessation: A Report of the Surgeon General*. Atlanta, GA: U.S. Department of Health and Human Services, Centers for Disease Control and Prevention, Office on Smoking and Health (1990). DHHS Publication (CDC) 90–8416.

U.S. Department of Health and Human Services (USDHHS). *Spit Tobacco and Youth*. Washington, D.C.: U.S. Department of Health and Human Services, Office of Inspector General (1992). DHHS Publication (OEI) 06-92-00500.

U.S. Department of Health and Human Services (USDHHS). *Preventing Tobacco Use among Young People: A Report of the Surgeon General*. Atlanta, GA: U.S. Department of Health and Human Services, Centers for Disease Control and Prevention, National Center for Chronic Disease Prevention and Health Promotion, Office on Smoking and Health (1994).

U.S. Department of Health and Human Services (USDHHS). *Tobacco Use Among U.S. Racial/Ethnic Minority Groups: A Report of the Surgeon General*. Atlanta, GA: U.S. Department of Health and Human Services, Centers for Disease Control and Prevention, Office on Smoking and Health (1998).

U.S. Department of Health and Human Services (USDHHS). *Healthy People 2010* (conference ed., 2 vols.). Washington, D.C.: U.S. Department of Health and Human Services (2000a).

U.S. Department of Health and Human Services (USDHHS). *Reducing Tobacco Use: A Report of the Surgeon General*. Washington, D.C.: U.S. Department of Health and Human Services, Centers for Disease Control and Prevention, Office on Smoking and Health (2000b).

U.S. Department of Health and Human Services (USDHHS). *Women and Smoking: A Report of the Surgeon General*. Rockville, MD: U.S. Department of Health and Human Services, Public Health Service, Office on Smoking and Health (2001).

U.S. Department of Health and Human Services (USDHHS). *The Health Consequences of Smoking: A Report of the Surgeon General*. Atlanta, GA: U.S. Department of Health and Human Services, Centers for Disease Control and Prevention, Office on Smoking and Health (2004).

U.S. Department of Health and Human Services (USDHHS). *The Health Consequences of Involuntary Exposure to Tobacco Smoke. A Report of the Surgeon General*. Atlanta, GA: U.S. Department of Health and Human Services, Centers for Disease Control and Prevention, Office on Smoking and Health (2006a).

U.S. Department of Health and Human Services (USDHHS). Substance Abuse and Mental Health Services Administration (SAMHSA). *Results from the 2005 National Survey on Drug Use and Health: National Findings*. Rockville, MD: Office of Applied Studies (2006b). NSDUH Series H-30, DHHS Publication SMA 06-4194.

U.S. Department of Health and Human Services (USDHHS). *HHS Announces National Smoking Cessation Quitline Network*. 2007. Available at http://www.hhs.gov/news/press/2004pres/20040203.html. Accessed May 21, 2009.

U.S. Department of Health and Humans Services (USDHHS). Substance Abuse and Mental Health Services Administration (SAMHSA). *FFY 2007 Annual Synar Reports: Youth Tobacco Sales*. Rockville, MD: SAMHSA. 2008. Available at http://prevention.samhsa.gov/tobacco/synarreportfy2007.pdf. Accessed May 21, 2009.

U.S. Department of Labor. *Consumer Price Index—All Urban Consumers. U.S. City Average, Cigarettes*. Washington, D.C.: U.S. Department of Labor, Bureau of Labor Statistics. 2007. Available at http://data.bls.gov. Accessed May 21, 2009.

U.S. Food and Drug Administration (FDA). Regulations Restricting the Sale and Distribution of Cigarettes and Smokeless Tobacco Products to Protect Children and Adolescents—Final Rule. *Fed Regist* (1996):61:(41):314–375.

U.S. Preventive Services Task Force (USPSTF). *Counseling and Interventions to Prevent Tobacco Use and Tobacco-Caused Disease in Adults and Pregnant Women: Clinical Summary of U.S, Preventive Services Task Force Recommendation.* Available at http://www.ahrq.gov/clinic/uspstf09/tobacco/tobaccosum2.htm. Accessed May 21, 2009.

Wagner, E.H., S.J. Curry, L. Grothaus, et al. The Impact of Smoking and Quitting on Health Care Use. *Arch Intern Med* (1995):155:1789–1795.

Wakefield, M., Y. Terry-McElrath, S. Emery, et al. Effect of Televised, Tobacco Company-Funded Smoking Prevention Advertising on Youth Smoking-Related Beliefs, Intentions, and Behavior. *Am J Public Health* (2006):95:2154–2160.

Wallace, L. Environmental Exposure to Benzene: An Update. *Environ Health Perspect* (1996): 104(Suppl 6):1129–1136.

Warner, K.E., R.J. Smith, D.G. Smith, et al. Health and Economic Implications of a Work-Site Smoking-Cessation Program: A Simulation Analysis. *J Occup Environ Med* (1996):38:981–992.

Weis, W.L. Can You Afford to Hire Smokers? *Pers Adm* (1981):26:71–73, 75–78.

White, V.M., M.M. White, K. Freeman, et al. Cigarette Promotional Offers: Who Takes Advantage? *Am J Prev Med* (2006):30:225–231.

World Health Organization (WHO). WHO Framework Convention on Tobacco Control. Geneva: World Health Organization (2003).

Yamasaki, E., and B.N. Ames. Concentration of Mutagens from Urine by Absorption with the Nonpolar Resin XAD-2: Cigarette Smokers Have Mutagenic Urine. *Proc Natl Acad Sci USA* (1977):74:3555–3559.

Zagorsky, J.L. The Wealth Effects of Smoking. *Tob Control* (2004):13:370–374.

Zaza, S., P.A. Briss, and K.W. Harris. Task Force on Community Preventive Services. Tobacco. In: Zaza, S., P.A. Briss, and K.W. Harris, editors, *The Guide to Community Preventive Services: What Works to Promote Health?* New York, NY: Oxford University Press (2005).

Zhu, B.P., G.A. Giovino, P.D. Mowery, et al. The Relationship Between Cigarette Smoking and Education Revisited: Implications for Categorizing Persons' Educational Status. *Am J Public Health* (1996):86:1582–1589.

CHAPTER 6

DIET AND NUTRITION
(ICD-10 E40–68)

Nasuh Malas, M.D., M.P.H., Kathleen M. Tharp, Ph.D., M.P.H., R.D.,
and Susan B. Foerster, M.P.H., R.D.

Introduction

Nutrition is critical for health and survival, yet we eat for more than sustenance. Foods are deeply connected to our cultures, memories, lifestyles, and emotions. Every sector of society influences food choices in some manner (Story et al. 2008). Families, schools, and employers create social norms through policies and environments that can either facilitate or hinder healthy eating. On the other hand, the food and beverage industry drives choice and consumption through marketing, portion sizes, food ingredients, disclosure of nutritional information, location of grocery stores, offerings in restaurants, and pricing (Wootan and Osborn 2006; Guadalupe et al. 2008; Satia, Galanko, and Siega-Riz 2004; Franco et al. 2008). Similarly, the entertainment and sports industries impact product placement, promotion, and availability of healthy foods at sport, movie, and other entertainment venues. In total, the food business employs over 15% of American workers, which directly affects the livelihood of many Americans (Frazao 1999). Health care providers and insurers also influence patient behavior through standards, practices, and incentives. Finally, federal, state, and local governments set priorities for prevention, provide incentives and funding for nutrition assistance programs, and stimulate efforts in planning, land use, and transportation.

Public health nutrition must take a population-based approach to simultaneously address food security, health promotion, and disease prevention. Poor nutrition is linked to most major chronic diseases, including obesity, type 2 diabetes, cardiovascular disease, hypertension, poor oral health, osteoporosis, and many cancers (Kushi et al. 2006; USDA DGA 2005; Gonzales CA 2006; CDC Burdenbook 2004). Seven of every ten U.S. deaths are due to chronic disease (CDC Burdenbook 2004). Nutrition is one of the major modifiable risk factors for chronic disease and could significantly impact global chronic disease burden (WHO 2003). The proportion of premature deaths attributable to poor diet and physical inactivity is second only to that for tobacco use (CDC Burdenbook 2004). The challenge for public health is to provide leadership across the public, nonprofit, and business sectors that will result in norms and environments where the healthiest food choices are also the most affordable and readily accessible to all segments of society. The purpose of this chapter is to describe and discuss the downstream consequences of poor nutrition, the upstream factors that cause poor nutrition, the groups at highest risk for poor nutrition, and the associated conditions and diseases related to poor nutrition (Figure 6.1).

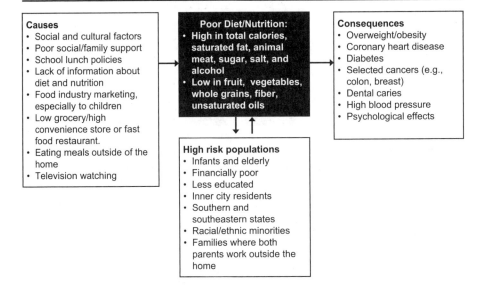

Causes
- Social and cultural factors
- Poor social/family support
- School lunch policies
- Lack of information about diet and nutrition
- Food industry marketing, especially to children
- Low grocery/high convenience store or fast food restaurant.
- Eating meals outside of the home
- Television watching

Poor Diet/Nutrition:
- High in total calories, saturated fat, animal meat, sugar, salt, and alcohol
- Low in fruit, vegetables, whole grains, fiber, unsaturated oils

Consequences
- Overweight/obesity
- Coronary heart disease
- Diabetes
- Selected cancers (e.g., colon, breast)
- Dental caries
- High blood pressure
- Psychological effects

High risk populations
- Infants and elderly
- Financially poor
- Less educated
- Inner city residents
- Southern and southeastern states
- Racial/ethnic minorities
- Families where both parents work outside the home

Figure 6.1. The causes, consequences, and populations affected by poor nutrition and diet.

Significance

As noted in other chapters in this text, cardiovascular disease and cancer are the two lead-ing causes of morbidity and mortality in the world, and type 2 diabetes is emerging as one of the most rapidly growing and costly. Cardiovascular disease and cancer together cause 42% of all deaths due to noncommunicable disease, and these chronic condi-tions are growing in importance in developed and developing countries alike (WHO Report 2002). Nutrition-related factors such as high blood pressure, high cholesterol, low fruit and vegetable intake, high Body Mass Index (BMI), and alcohol consump-tion are the leading contributors to chronic disease in developed countries (Ezzati et al. 2002). More than 130 million disability adjusted life-years (DALY) are lost each year to chronic disease, and nutrition-related factors contribute to nearly half of these DALYs (WHO 2000).

On the other hand, worldwide childhood and maternal underweight and micronu-trient deficiencies account for an additional 15% of disease burden (WHO 2000). The World Health Organization (WHO) has called for countries to come together to address the social determinants of poor health, including issues of social justice such as food, poverty, education, employment, environment, living conditions, and empowerment (WHO 2008).

In the United States, factors related to poor diet and physical activity are estimated to cause 15% of premature deaths each year, second only to tobacco use (Mokdad et al. 2004; Mokdad 2005). The *Global Strategy on Diet, Physical Activity, and Health*, as well as *Healthy People 2010*, were designed to help alleviate both global and national burdens of chronic disease (WHO 2004; USDHHS 2000). However, all available data show that we are falling far short of domestic and worldwide targets, including those outlined in the *Dietary Guidelines for Americans* (Table 6.1) (WHO 2003; FAO 2003).

Table 6.1. Dietary Guidelines for Americans, 2005

1. Eat a variety of highly nutritious foods and beverages within the basic food groups.
2. Eat two cups of fruit and 2 ½ cups of vegetables per day, selecting from all five vegetable groups (dark green, orange, legumes, starchy vegetables, and other vegetables).
3. Eat three or more ounce equivalents of whole grain foods per day, with at least half of all daily grain intake being from whole grains.
4. Eat leans meats with low fat content, like poultry and fish, and limit red meat.
5. Drink up to three cups per day of fat-free or low-fat milk or equivalent milk products, like low-fat cheese or yogurt.
6. Your caloric intake should only consist of 10% or less saturated fat, less than 300 mg per day of cholesterol, and no *trans* fatty acids.
7. Your total fat consumption should be between 25% and 30% of your total calories, and the majority of your daily fats should come from polyunsaturated or monounsaturated sources like fish, nuts, and vegetable oils.
8. Eat foods that are high in fiber.
9. Eat and drink foods with little added sugars or caloric sweeteners.
10. Use salt sparingly and do not consume more than 2,300 mg of salt per day.

Note: From the USDA Dietary Guidelines for Americans, 2005 Executive Summary.

Pathophysiology

There is a large body of evidence that explores diet–disease relationships. The most comprehensive to date is an international meta-analysis that examined the relationship of over 50 dietary constituents and associated factors such as physical activity, breastfeeding, abdominal girth, and television viewing to nearly 20 cancer sites (AICR 2007). It rated evidence of cancer causation on a seven-point scale, tempering the specific cancer prevention recommendations against consistency with other chronic diseases such as cardiovascular disease and diabetes. Given the amount and complexity of dietary research, only some of the most important relationships will be described below so as to illustrate ways that nutrition affects chronic disease biology.

Fruits and Vegetables

Increased consumption of fruits and vegetables has been associated with lower risk of many chronic diseases, including some cancers, type 2 diabetes, cardiovascular disease (CVD), and obesity (World Cancer Research Fund/American Institute for Cancer Research 2007; Liu et al. 2000; Van Duyn and Pivonka 2000; Rolls, Ello-Martin, and Tohill 2004). The protection appears to come from a variety of nutrients found in fruits and vegetables, including dietary fiber, vitamin C, vitamin E, folic acid, potassium, selenium, and phytochemicals such as terpenes, carotenoids, lycopene, isothiocyanates, dithiolthiones, and flavonoids.

One mechanism for the association between fruits and vegetables and reduced risk of CVD may be through antioxidants such as vitamin C, beta-carotene, and flavonoids. They may act by reducing oxidized cholesterol levels in the body, thereby protecting arteries from damage by slowing or inhibiting the development of atherosclerotic plaques made up of low-density lipoprotein (LDL) particles (Aviram 1993). Higher consumption of antioxidants such as vitamins E and C has also been associated with lower total and LDL cholesterol (Simon et al. 1993; Jacques et al. 1994). A second protective mechanism for CVD may be through a reduction of serum cholesterol caused by soluble fiber found in fruits and vegetables. A meta-analysis found both a reduction in coronary events and coronary deaths for each incremental increase in fiber consumption (Pereira et al. 2004).

Natural substances in fruits and vegetables may also be responsible for a decreased risk of some cancers. Antioxidants are theorized to protect cell membranes and DNA from oxidative damage (World Cancer Research Fund/American Institute for Cancer Research 2007). As yet, however, the lack of high quality studies exploring the role of antioxidants has provided inconclusive evidence of their effect on long-term disease prevention (NIH State-of-the-Art Conference Statement 2006). In addition, phytochemicals such as isothiocyanates, dithiolthiones, and indoles appear to induce enzymatic detoxification systems and block tumor production or growth. Isoflavones, found in soybeans and other legumes, may keep endogenous estrogens from binding to cell receptors which may reduce the risk of associated cancers. Phenols in fruits such as ellagic acid and delphinidin may inhibit activity of other receptors necessary for cancer development (Labreque et al. 2005; Lamy et al. 2006).

Fruits and vegetables are thought to influence body weight through a variety of mechanisms. Their high content of water and fiber, and low fat content, result in low energy density. Such foods have been associated with greater postmeal feelings of fullness or satiety and a reduction in the total calories eaten in a given meal (Rolls, Ello-Martin, and Tohill 2004). Nevertheless, studies examining an association between increased fruit and vegetable consumption and weight control are inconsistent (Rolls, Ello-Martin, and Tohill 2004; Tohill et al. 2004). This may be due at least in part to the inherent complexity and long-term nature of dietary research.

Dietary Fiber

Many studies have shown an association between higher consumption of dietary fiber and reduced incidence of coronary heart disease and some cancers. Several potential mechanisms for this association have been proposed. Insoluble dietary fiber speeds transit time and increases stool bulk, thereby decreasing exposure to and concentration of carcinogens in the gut (Key et al. 2002). It also binds bile acids that can potentially act as promoters of carcinogenesis. Production of short chain fatty acids, such as butyrate, occurs as dietary fiber is fermented in the colon. These short chain fatty acids may protect against cancer by promoting differentiation, inducing apoptosis or inhibiting secondary bile acid production (Nagengast, Grubben, and van Munster 1995). Many case-control studies have demonstrated a somewhat lower risk of cancer with high consumption of dietary fiber, yet large prospective studies have been largely inconsistent (Jacobs et al. 1998; Bueno De Mesquita, Ferrari, and Riboli 2002; Michels et al. 2000).

In terms of CVD, soluble fiber (β-glucan), such as in oat bran, has been shown to lower blood cholesterol levels, likely by binding bile acids, thereby preventing reabsorption (Chen et al. 2006; Naumann et al. 2006). Furthermore, dietary fiber appears to be inversely associated with blood insulin levels, which may have benefits for the prevention of insulin resistance and type 2 diabetes (Joint WHO/FAO Expert Consultation 2003).

Dietary Fat and Red Meat

Many studies underscore the importance of differentiating between different types of fat (Howard et al. 2006). Certain fats, such as *trans* fats or saturated fats have adverse affects on health, while others, like monounsaturated fats, have significant benefits. For example, women who consumed the lowest proportions of saturated fatty acids and *trans* fatty acids had reduced risk of coronary heart disease, cardiovascular disease, and stroke. An incremental decrease of 1% to 3% in dietary saturated fat was projected to lower primary heart attack rates by as much as 25% (Oster and Thompson 1996). Other studies find that a reduced intake of saturated fatty acids and cholesterol can reduce total cholesterol and LDL, leading to lower rates of atherosclerosis, ischemic stroke, and myocardial infarction (Lichtenstein et al. 2002; Jenkins et al. 2003; Obarzanek et al. 2001; Ginsberg et al. 1998). Replacing saturated fatty acids with polyunsaturated or monounsaturated fatty acids also results in decreased LDL cholesterol (Mensink et al. 2003).

Some fats are beneficial to a healthy diet, particularly omega-3 fatty acids and mono-unsaturated oils. Several studies show an inverse relationship between intake of omega-3 fatty acids and cancer. Omega-3 fatty acids are present in fish oils and in some vegetables. Among the hypotheses is that omega-3 fatty acids alter the immune response to cancer cells and influence transcription factor activity and gene expression (Larsson et al. 2004). Another hypothesis is that omega-3 fatty acids reduce circulating markers of inflammation, thus potentially protecting against heart disease, atherosclerosis, rheumatoid arthritis, and psychiatric disease (Lee et al. 2006). While some epidemiological studies have supported this hypothesis, clinical trials are not definitive. In some studies, monounsaturated oils, such as olive oil, have also reported a protective effect on health, particularly heart disease (Divisi et al. 2006).

Red meat has been associated with both positive and negative effects on diet. In moderation, red meat is a rich source of iron, folate, zinc, selenium, vitamins A and B12, and protein (Biesalski 2002). Diets that lack an adequate amount of red meat are deficient in bioavailable sources of iron (Zimmerman, Chaouki, Hurrell 2005). Diets in developing countries or lower-income communities are predominantly composed of cereal and legume-based foods with low bioavailable iron. The folate provided in red meat is of higher bioavailability than that provided in fruits and vegetables, which may explain the greater prevalence of iron deficiency anemia in these populations (Zimmerman, Chaouki, Hurrell 2005). Red meat is also a source of methyl donors, such as folate and B12, as well as the transfer factors methionine and choline (Biesalski 2002). It has been hypothesized that this lack of methylation can predispose one to a variety of cancers by altering the expression of genes important to tumor suppression (Biesalski 2002). Several studies have demonstrated that low folate intake leads to higher rates of colorectal cancer (Biesalski 2002).

However, high intake of red meat has been associated with some cancers, principally colorectal cancer (Kushi et al. 2006; Heidemann et al. 2008; Hu et al. 2008). The possible mechanisms include the polycyclic hydrocarbons and mutagenic amines that can be generated by cooking at high temperatures, the nitrites and other similar compounds found in salted, smoked, and processed meats that can be converted to toxic N-nitroso compounds within the colonic wall, and the high level of iron, which can lead to the formation of mutagenic free radicals in the gut wall (Gooderham et al. 1997; Kazerouni et al. 2001; Bingham et al. 1996; Lund et al. 1999). While associations exist, conclusive evidence supporting these associations is lacking.

Dairy Products and Milk

Dairy intake offers many benefits to a balanced diet. However, consumption can be precluded in many populations by lactose or milk protein intolerance. It is estimated that one in four Americans has lactose intolerance (Suarez et al. 1997).

Daily consumption of low fat milk products has been shown to be protective against some chronic diseases, including osteoporosis, CVD, and colon cancer (Houston et al. 2005; DGA 2005; DASH diet; AICR). Milk contains beneficial fatty acids, vitamins, minerals, and bioactive compounds that positively affect overall nutrition (Haug, Hostmark, and Harstad 2007). Calcium in dairy products directly inhibits lipid accumulation in cells and increases fecal excretion of lipids (Zemel 2004; Lorenzen et al. 2007). Conversely, calcium from food, but not supplements, preserves thermogenesis during calorie restriction (Zemel 2004). Theoretically, this should lead to accelerated weight loss yet data are conflicting regarding the role of dairy intake in weight loss (Zemel 2004; Fiorito et al. 2006; Barba and Russo 2006).

Despite the benefits of milk intake on nutrition, whole and 2% milk products contain a considerable amount of saturated fat and extra calories. The American Heart Association recommends all adults consume 1% or nonfat milk as a comprehensive approach to consuming a diet low in saturated fat without neglecting other necessary nutrients (Lichtenstein et al. 2006). A large prospective study of over 1,300 adults found no association between dairy or calcium intake and weight gain but did find a significant inverse relationship between low-fat dairy consumption and waist-to-hip ratio (Brooks et al. 2006). Nonetheless, public misconceptions about milk, coupled with heavy advertising for soft drinks, have led to significant declines in milk consumption (Haug, Hostmark, and Harstad 2007; DGA 2005).

Sugar-Sweetened Beverages

Over the past 30 years, the consumption of caloric sweeteners in the United States has increased markedly, totaling nearly 17% of daily energy intake (Lichtenstein et al. 2006; Vos et al. 2008). The standard definition used by researchers for caloric sweeteners includes all caloric carbohydrate sweeteners, such as table sugar, honey, and high fructose corn syrup, and excludes naturally occurring sugars and artificial sweeteners (Popkin and Nielsen 2003). The majority comes from soft drinks such as soda, juice drinks, sports drinks, sugar-sweetened coffee drinks, and iced tea (Guthrie and Morton 2000). Overconsumption of energy-dense, nutrient-poor beverages has been associated with chronic disease risk, particularly obesity and dental caries (Lichtenstein et al. 2006; DGA 2005; Malik, Schulze, and Hu 2006). The burden is especially significant for children due to their susceptibility to poor dentition (Marshall et al. 2003). It was previously hypothesized that the lack of satiety produced by sugar-sweetened beverages led to excessive consumption (Malik, Schulze, and Hu 2006), but high intake is now appreciated as being due to a myriad of factors (Drewnowski and Bellisle 2007).

Descriptive Epidemiology

High-Risk Populations

The U.S. population as a whole is considered at high risk of developing diet-related chronic disease. The American diet is energy-dense, high in saturated fats, red meat, and simple sugars with too few vegetables, fruits, and whole grains. International comparisons clearly indicate that typical dietary patterns in the United States, along with obesity, are associated with high rates of atherosclerotic disease (Labarthe 1998) and certain common cancers (World Cancer Research Fund/American Institute for Cancer Research 2007).

Sex

Dietary quality varies by sex. National data between 1999 and 2002 found that men had greater intakes of dairy and meat, and exhibited greater variety of choices. Women, on the other hand, tended to have greater consumption of fruit, vegetables, cholesterol, and salt (Ervin 2008). Women also generally place a greater importance on healthy eating (Warde et al. 2004). Concerns about weight control and beliefs about healthy eating explain much of the difference (Baker and Wardle 2003). By and large, men are less knowledgeable about the nutritional content of their diet, as well as the significance of the link between dietary intake and disease (Baker and Wardle 2003).

Age and Life Course

The extremes of age are particularly vulnerable for poor nutrition. In children and adolescents, taste preferences, family support for healthy foods, and food availability are strongly correlated with a healthy, balanced diet (Neumark-Stzainer et al. 2003; Shepherd et al. 2006). Youth gravitate to energy-dense foods, which are heavily marketed by the food industry, unless parents model healthy eating and set limits (AHA et al. 2006). Poor dietary habits that are established at an early age are often carried into adulthood and can be difficult to change (Guo et al. 2002).

Aging involves a variety of psychosocial, economic, and physiological changes. Physical activity and metabolism slow, chronic disease events occur, there is often less social support, and the sensory pleasure of eating may wane due to changes in taste and smell sensation (Drewnowski and Warren-Mears 2001; Westenhoefer 2005; de Graaf, Polet, and van Stavaren 1994). Consequently, it is not surprising that over 80% of older adults have diets that are either poor or need improvement, especially for meat, dairy, fruits, and vegetables (Ervin 2008).

Race and Ethnicity

Analysis of the National Health and Nutrition Examination Survey (NHANES) data between 1971 and 2002, which includes the period when rates of obesity began to rise, confirms that African American and white Americans increased their total energy intake and consumption of energy-dense foods (Kant, Graubard, and Kumanyika 2007). African Americans reported higher vitamin C intake and lower saturated fat intake but lower intakes of fruits, vegetables, potassium, calcium, and other essential nutrients. African Americans, as well as other racially diverse communities, face heavy barriers to obtaining nutritious food. These include limited access to fresh produce, high costs, decreased time to prepare home meals, and the lack of healthy culturally sensitive foods (Kim, Harrison, Kagawa-Singer 2007).

Non-Hispanic Whites have higher intakes of dairy, fruits, vegetables, and grains (Ervin 2008). Caucasians also have greater diet variety and overall quality than African Americans and Mexican Americans. On average, African Americans report diets with less variety and fewer nutrients. Mexican Americans do somewhat better, particularly in dairy, grains, and overall variety. Caucasians score poorest in saturated fat. The differences among the three racial groups are largely due to a variety of interlinked sociocultural, environmental, and behavioral factors (Ervin 2008).

Income

It is very clear that as the affluence of a given community decreases, the ability of that community to obtain healthy food also decreases (Morland, Wing, and Diez Roux 2002). On a given week, about 20% of low-income households do not purchase fruits and vegetables, twice the rate for higher-income homes (Blisard, Stewart, and Joliffe 2004). Energy-dense diets that are poor in nutritional value are more likely to be consumed by persons of lower economic means, while whole grains, lean meats, fish, low-fat milk products, and fresh fruits and vegetables are more likely to be consumed by those with greater means (Darmon and Drewnowski 2008). This relationship between income, and diet quality is true along a gradient of income levels and not only for extremes of income, indicating a strong positive relationship between low income and poor nutrition (Dynesen et al. 2003; Darmon and Drewnowski 2008).

Agricultural policy, food marketing, and grocery distribution support processed, high-fat meat production and provide ingredients for high-calorie processed foods. There are relatively few economic incentives or socially accepted behaviors that support production or marketing of nutrient-dense fresh foods, such as most fruits and vegetables. In many low-income urban areas, grocery stores that stock a wide variety of nutrient-dense foods can be scarce, which forces residents to use corner, convenience, and liquor stores that have few healthy choices (Baker et al. 2006). The same environmental stressors and poor social support that affect food choices within lower socioeconomic communities also contribute to poor health outcomes (Feldman and Steptoe 2004).

Education

Education and income are highly interrelated, and both have repeatedly been shown to strongly correlate to nutrition and chronic disease. For more than 30 years, higher consumption of fruits, vegetables, and foods with vitamins A and C, calcium, and potassium have been associated with higher levels of education (Kant and Graubard 2007). Maternal education is positively related to the nutritional content of home meals, with college-educated primary food providers spending the most per capita for fruits and vegetables (MacFarlane et al. 2007; Blisard, Stewart, and Joliffe 2004).

Geographic Distribution

Diets in Western, developed countries tend to be high in animal products and saturated fat, and rates of prostate, colorectal, and breast cancer are relatively high. Conversely, countries with diets rich in fruits, vegetables, starchy grains, fish, olive or other vegetable oils, and a lower intake of red meats, often have lower rates of diet-related cancers. Accordingly, studies have shown that high consumption of animal fats and polyunsaturated cooking oils, like safflower or corn oil, may increase the risk for breast and colorectal cancer (Divisi et al. 2006). Diets lower in saturated fat are associated with reduced risk of heart disease, stroke, cancer, diabetes, and osteoporosis (CDC Burden Book 2004).

Within the United States, there are important and long-standing regional differences in consumption of specific foods. For example, fish is consumed more frequently in coastal areas. Fruit and vegetable consumption is generally lower, and saturated fat consumption is higher, in regions that also have higher rates of obesity such as the South, Southeast, and lower Midwest. Sometimes described as the Stroke belt, many southern states consume diets high in sodium and saturated fat, and low in milk products, fresh fruits, and vegetables (Howard et al. 2004).

A growing body of research is revealing the relationship between chronic disease and local food availability and quality. In many inner-city neighborhoods, full-spectrum supermarkets that offer a wide variety of fresh produce and other foods have relocated to more affluent neighborhoods, translating into a reduction in healthy dietary options within those communities (Moore et al. 2008). People who live more than a mile away from a supermarket are 25% less likely to eat a healthy diet compared with those with a supermarket nearby (Moore et al. 2008).

Industrial Development and Immigration

Observational studies of populations that migrate from rural communities to city slums, or from countries with low rates of chronic disease, show that disease patterns of the acculturating migrants shift toward those of the new environment (IARC 1990). In developing countries, the nutrition transition from undernutrition to obesity with low-nutrient diets can occur in one generation. Thus, in transitional groups, it is important to preserve a positive dietary balance with fruits, vegetables, and whole grains and prevent the uptake of highly advertised, inexpensive low-nutrient foods, especially by children.

Time Trends

Since the National Health and Nutrition Examination Survey (NHANES) was first administered in 1971, there have been many changes in food consumption. The quantity of food and beverages consumed, the fraction of meals eaten outside the home, portion sizes, and energy density have increased significantly. Energy intake has increased by 196 kcal/day for men and 283 kcal/day for women, much of it from carbohydrates (Kant and Graubard 2006; Wright et al. 2004). Larger portion sizes have been observed both inside and outside the home, and portions for salty snacks, soft drinks, fruit drinks, and fast-foods have grown markedly (Nielsen and Popkin 2003).

Between 1965 and 2002, calories per capita from beverages increased by more than 200, rising from 12% to 21% of daily caloric intake (Duffey and Popkin 2007). In 2002,

30% of Americans were drinking 25% or more of their daily calories, with higher intakes coming from alcohol, soda, fruit drinks, sweetened tea, sweetened coffee, and other sweetened beverages.

Fruit and vegetable consumption is a common marker of individual diet quality. Between 1994 and 2005, the Behavioral Risk Factor Surveillance System (BRFSS) reported the frequency of fruit and vegetable consumption had declined from 3.43 times per day to 3.24 times per day (Blanck et al. 2008). Only 25% of adults ate the recommended minimum of five daily servings during that same period (Blanck et al. 2008). NHANES data reveals similar dietary trends (Casagrande et al. 2007).

Causes of Poor Nutrition

Barriers to Healthy Eating

Like any complex human behavior, the choice of one's diet is determined by multiple factors that work independently and concurrently. To fully understand what contributes to our dietary behaviors, one must understand influences that promote or barriers that inhibit healthy eating such as time, location, social relationships, culture, and environment (Caplan 1996; Swinburn et al. 1999). Barriers can be categorized as relating to one's personal or individual preferences, physical, sociocultural, or macro environment. This understanding can be used to design innovative interventions to combat barriers or build on strengths (Story et al. 2008).

Because these interacting factors each work on multiple levels, an ecological approach is the most inclusive model by which to address both barriers to and opportunities for healthy eating (IOM 2005, 2007; Story et al. 2008). Such a model (Figure 6.2, IOM 2007, p. 22) can help to assess forces, direct efforts, and positively influence the interactions within and among individuals; families, peers, and social groups; institutions and communities; businesses, nonprofits, and government programs; and larger forces of society and culture. As research expands and interventions grow more creative, it is this ecological approach that will serve to drive and help organize interventions at local, regional, state, and national levels.

Individual Preference

Self-efficacy, strong social support, and a good knowledge of nutritional benefits are strong predictors of fruit and vegetable intake (Shaikh et al. 2008). Other potential predictors of fruit and vegetable consumption include perceived barriers, strength of one's intentions, one's attitudes and beliefs about fruit and vegetable consumption, and autonomous motivation to consume a healthy diet. In addition, the nature and demands of an individual's lifestyle can affect one's ability to eat a healthy diet (Kapur et al. 2008).

Personal preference for certain qualities of foods, including taste, texture, and appearance, can vary considerably from person to person. Food preference can override the knowledge of nutritional benefits or risks and cause resistance to the adoption of a healthy diet. In the absence of economic barriers and low availability, personal preference can be the best predictor of food choice (Eertmans, Baeyens, and Van de Bergh 2001; Clark 1998; Furst et al. 1996; Rozin 2001). There is ample evidence that marketing and nutri-

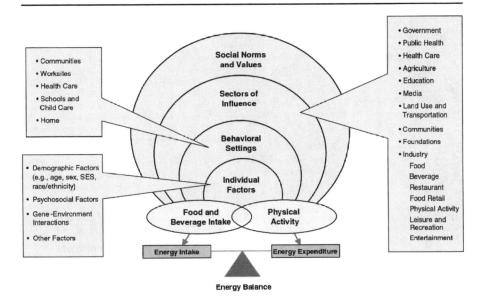

Figure 6.2. Comprehensive approach for preventing and addressing diet-related chronic diseases. Institute of Medicine (IOM). Progress in Preventing Childhood Obesity: How Do We Measure Up? Committee on Preventing Childhood Obesity (2007). Reprinted with permission from the National Academies Press. Copyright 2007. National Academy of Sciences.

tion education with taste testing of new foods, as well as introduction of healthy foods early in life, can alter population taste preferences.

Community and Family Environments

It is easier for an individual to make healthy dietary choices when supported by a physical environment with easy access to affordable, varied, nutritious foods (USDHSS 2001). The cost of food is considered second only to taste in its effect on dietary choice (Glanz et al. 1998). Costs are influenced by supply and demand factors such as consumer preferences, government subsidies and regulations, food advertising, and the geographic distribution of supermarkets, restaurants, and other food outlets. Many of the foods that are lowest in cost are also the least nutritious and most energy-dense, as shown in Figure 6.3 (Drewnowski 2004). The cost of food can be negatively associated with dietary quality, and the perception of high cost can lead to diets high in sodium, calories, and dietary fat, and lower in fiber (Bowman and Vinyard 2004; Beydoun and Wang 2008). Food prices have a much more significant affect on the food choices of individuals at lower socioeconomic strata than individuals at higher socioeconomics levels (Beydoun and Wang 2008).

The physical food environment strongly affects access to healthy food options (Glanz and Yaroch 2004; Glanz et al. 1995). Access to large supermarkets with a variety of competitively priced nutritious foods has been associated with better dietary practices in those communities (Larson, Story, and Nelson 2009). As the number of supermarkets

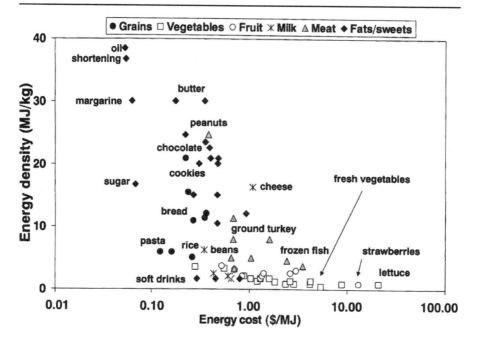

Figure 6.3. A graphical depiction of energy density (MJ/kg) compared with energy cost (dollars/ MJ). The x axis is depicted in logarithmic scale. Reprinted from Drewnowski, A. Obesity and the Food Environment: Diet Energy Density and Diet Costs. *Am J Prev Med* (2004:S3):27:S154- S162, with permission from Elsevier.

in a given community increases, the fruit and vegetable consumption proportionally in- creases (Morland, Wing, and Diez Roux 2002). Over the past 30 years, there has been a mass departure of grocery stores from lower socioeconomic areas, coinciding with an influx of fast-food and convenience stores. Communities of color and communities with lower socioeconomic status are disproportionately affected (Pothukuchi 2005; Powell et al. 2007). In such areas, shopping may be limited to nearby convenience stores tending to stock foods high in fat, salt, and sugar with little produce, whole grains, or lean meat (Larson, Story, Nelson, and 2009; Sloane et al. 2003; Glanz et al. 2005). This shift has been a major contributor to the growing divide in nutrition standards for low-income, racially diverse communities.

Americans are eating a greater proportion of their meals and snacks away from home. Between 1987 and 2000, the reported mean number of away-from-home meals eaten each week significantly increased from 2.48 to 2.77 (Kant and Graubard 2004). Forecasts for 2009 restaurant sales are expected to reach $566 billion dollars and total over 50% of the average American household food budget (Nat Res Assoc 2008). This forecast in- cludes a nearly twofold increase in sales at fast-food restaurants as compared with dine-in restaurants.

Studies have reported a high association between fast-food restaurant density in a location and the nutrition of the population in that location (Prentice and Jebb 2003; Mehta and Chang 2008). As the ratio of fast-food to dine-in restaurants increases, the dietary quality of a given population decreases (Mehta and Chang 2008). The public is largely unaware that foods consumed outside of the home tend to have fewer nutrients, more calories and saturated fat, and be served in larger portions (Briefel and Johnson 2004; Burton et al. 2006). Populations with lower socioeconomic status are more likely to have a greater density of fast-food restaurants within their communities and limited healthy eating options (Cummins, McKay, and MacIntyre 2005). As restaurant and fast-food consumption has grown, dietary quality has not improved and obesity rates have risen, disproportionately affecting disadvantaged communities.

Schools are environments that influence dietary behavior at formative ages, where often children may consume two school meals and several snacks each day (Brug and van Lenthe 2005). Most food at school is provided through U.S. Department of Agriculture (USDA) child nutrition programs, which must meet federal standards. Competitive private foods sold at school do not fall under these standards. Child nutrition programs, like the School Breakfast Program and National School Lunch Program, were mandated but have not yet been funded to comply with the 2005 *Dietary Guidelines*.

Pressure has come from Congress, some states, and school boards to regulate all foods and beverages sold at schools and reduce competitive foods that are high in fat and sugar (USGAO Report 2005). The influence of private vendors has caught national attention. The Institute of Medicine (IOM) recently released a statement in support of limiting private vendors and establishing federal meal programs as the primary source of school nutrition (IOM 2007). Currently, the IOM has been commissioned to make further recommendations in 2009 and 2010.

Near school grounds, there can be significant clustering of fast-food establishments, especially in low-income communities (Austin et al. 2005; Carter and Swinburn 2004). In coming years, school nutrition will likely be an area of much change, given public concern about childhood obesity and the current magnitude of influence flexed by private vendors. The 2009 reauthorization of the Child Nutrition and WIC Act that governs many of USDA's major nutrition programs is expected to upgrade the alignment of these programs with public health concerns.

As children transition to adulthood, they also move from school to work environments. Just as the school provides a captive audience of hungry minds and mouths, worksite modifications can have real impacts on dietary habits (Matson-Koffman et al. 2005). The Working Well Trial in the late 1990's was implemented at over 100 work sites, where physical and social attributes were adjusted to improve employee eating habits (Biener et al. 1999). Using employee surveys and interviews, significant changes were seen in dietary behaviors including increased access to nutritious foods, improved perception of healthy eating, and enhanced knowledge regarding nutrition. These results have been corroborated by other studies that secured positive changes following alterations in both access and availability to healthy food (Block et al. 2004). Even improving workplace social networks and social norms showed significant improvements in dietary choice (Sorensen et al. 2007). Social and cultural influence are important because dietary changes are rarely maintained if social and cultural support is weak or inconsistent (Holm 1993).

Families provide considerable social and cultural influence on dietary habits, through learned behavior, parent modeling, household food purchasing, and the regularity of family meals (Rankinen and Bouchard 2006; Corella et al. 2007; van der Horst et al. 2006; Utter et al. 2008; Gillman et al. 2000). As more families have multiple members working long hours outside the home, the amount of family meals can become limited and replaced by unhealthy snacking, missed meals, or fast-food. Adolescents particularly resort to low cost, energy-dense foods when there is little parental oversight (Grimm, Harnack, and Story 2004). Strong parental modeling and enforcement of home rules for healthy eating are promising strategies to improve nutrition (Story et al. 2008).

Outer Spheres of Influence

On the broadest level, economics, mass media, and public policy modulate the complexities of food choice. Food companies are the second largest advertiser on television, spending billions of dollars and competing vigorously to entice retailers and consumers to select their products and brands (Lake and Townshend 2006). Worldwide, for every dollar spent by the WHO to promote good nutrition, more than $500 is spent by the food industry to market processed foods (Lang and Millstone 2002). In the United States, over 80% of the $30 billion spent annually on food advertising is for sugar-laden foods, convenience foods, or fast-foods rather than fruits, vegetables, dairy, meats, poultry, or fish (Harrison and Marske 2005). Adults and children exposed to advertisements for high calorie, high fat, high sugar foods are also more likely to consume those foods (Wiecha et al. 2006; Thomson et al. 2008). One study found that children consumed an additional 167 kcal/day for each hour of television viewed, an amount that, over time, can lead to considerable weight gain and chronic disease (Wiecha et al. 2006).

Food marketing has a strong influence on children's dietary behaviors and preferences (Hastings et al. 2003). The number of advertisements per hour on children's television correlates with poor nutrition (Lobstein and Dibb 2005). Children from the ages of eight to 12 years were found to watch the most television advertisements, most of which were for high-sugar and fast-foods, with few for fruits and vegetables (Gantz et al. 2007). To put this into context, the bombardment of unhealthy food advertising, coupled with longer work hours for parents, can translate to fewer and fewer family meals and a growing proportion eaten away from home or composed of energy-dense processed foods, thereby promoting unhealthy eating in children (IOM 2005).

Prevention and Control

Primary Prevention Policy

Since 1980, the U.S. Department of Health and Human Services (USDHHS) and the USDA have updated the *Dietary Guidelines for Americans (Dietary Guidelines)* in line with new public health science on a five-year basis. The *Dietary Guidelines* are targeted to meet the dietary needs of Americans aged two years and older (USDA DGA 2005). The nine focus areas of the full policy are adequate nutrients within calorie needs, weight management, physical activity, food groups to encourage, fats, carbohydrates, sodium and potassium, alcoholic beverages, and food safety. The nutrition recommendations are summarized in Table 6.1.

The *Dietary Guidelines* emphasize eating a balanced diet with the majority of food coming from fruits, vegetables, whole grains, legumes, and low-fat or fat-free milk or milk equivalent. They encourage limiting saturated fats, *trans* fats, added sugars, salt, and alcohol. Weight maintenance, regular physical activity, and attention to food safety are also stressed. Recommendations for special population groups such as children and adolescents, pregnant and breastfeeding women, and older adults are added when applicable.

The *Dietary Guidelines* form the basis of MyPyramid, an interactive food guide developed by USDA. It was introduced in 2005 and is a revision of the Food Guide Pyramid. MyPyramid is intended as a graphic display to help all Americans know what to eat and how much physical activity to get every day. MyPyramid is USDA's interactive food guide. At the website (www.MyPyramid.gov) people can enter their age, sex, weight, height, and level of physical activity to calculate personalized diet and exercise recommendations based on the *Dietary Guidelines*. The output details the grains, vegetables, fruits, milk, meat and beans, oils, discretionary calories, and physical activity the individual needs on a daily basis. A pictorial representation of the food pyramid, developed by Willet et al., is shown in Figure 6.4.

Federal food and nutrition education programs such as the Special Supplemental Nutrition Program for Women, Infants, and Children (WIC), Child Nutrition Programs, and the Supplemental Nutrition Assistance Program (SNAP) (formerly the Food Stamp Program) use the *Dietary Guidelines* as the foundation for their programs. Other target audiences include policymakers, health care providers, nutritionists, nutrition educators, and the food industry.

The *Dietary Guidelines* have been modified over time to reflect the most current evidence. For example, early results of the long-term trial, Dietary Approaches to Stop

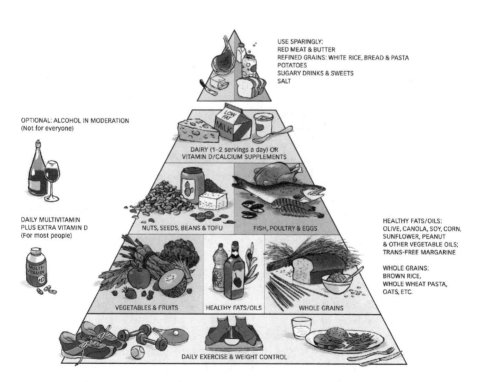

Figure 6.4. The healthy eating pyramid. Copyright © 2008. For more information about The Healthy Eating Pyramid, please see The Nutrition Source, Department of Nutrition, Harvard School of Public Health, http://www.thenutritionsource.org, and Eat, Drink, and Be Healthy, by Walter C. Willet, M.D. and Patrick J. Skerrett (2005), Free Press/Simon & Schuster Inc.

Hypertension (DASH), showed reductions in blood pressure, LDL-cholesterol, and CVD events and mortality (Appel et al. 1997; Obarzanek et al. 2001; Fung et al. 2008). The DASH Eating Plan also is low in saturated fat, cholesterol, sodium, and total fat, and it promotes whole grains, fish, poultry, and nuts. It encourages less frequent consumption of lean red meat, sweets, added sugars, and sugar-containing beverages. The positive study findings influenced the new recommendations in the 2005 *Dietary Guidelines* to nearly double fruits and vegetables and increase low-fat milk by half.

Surveillance

Public health practitioners can find nutrition surveillance data in the national surveys that together make up the National Nutrition Monitoring System surveys (IOM 2007, Appendix C). Cross-sectional and longitudinal surveys include measures of diet; physical activity; biological measures such as weight, anemia, CVD risk factors, and diabetes; school food; school health policies and programs; and youth media. Surveys with state-specific data include the Behavioral Risk Factor Surveillance System, Pediatric Nutrition Surveillance, the Youth Risk Factor Behavioral Surveillance System, School Health Policies and Programs, and the National Survey of Children's Health. Similarly, state-specific data about participation in USDA nutrition assistance programs that are available annually can be calculated at the county level (FRAC 2008; CFPA 2009). A growing number of states, counties and cities are conducting their own surveys and developing new approaches, such as Geographic Information Systems, to map and evaluate factors contributing to dietary, physical activity, and obesity risks.

Food disappearance data provide information about quantities of foods and nutrients in retail food distribution each year. The data are calculated by adding all foods produced in the United States, inventories from the previous year, and imported food, then subtracting year-end inventories, exported foods, and foodstuffs used for nonfood purposes. The final result is the quantity and nutrient value of food available for human consumption. Since the data are for foods available for purchase but not necessarily eaten, they overestimate food actually consumed. However, since the USDA Economic Research Service (ERS) has been tracking data on agricultural commodities since 1909, the statistics allow analysis of trends in food availability.

U.S. food consumption data are collected through the national food survey, What We Eat in America (WWEIA). WWEIA involves obtaining two 24-hour dietary recalls for each participant in NHANES. Its inaugural year was 2002, when two formerly separate surveys from two federal agencies combined their efforts. The former surveys were NHANES and USDA's Continuing Survey of Food Intakes by Individuals (CSFII). Before 2002, data were collected for each survey in discrete intervals with no surveillance in off-years. Now, fewer individuals are sampled, but surveillance is continuous. Data available include types and amounts of foods consumed as well as information on the food nutrients and energy.

Several instruments have been developed to assess overall dietary quality. Short term recall and diet record methods have traditionally been unrepresentative of dietary intake, time-intensive, and costly (Willet 1998). Therefore, epidemiologists have sought other means of measuring food intake. Food frequency questionnaires (FFQs) are the most popular form of assessing dietary quality in public health practice (see examples at http://riskfactor.cancer.gov/diet/screeners/fruitveg/instrument.html, http://riskfactor. cancer.gov/diet/screeners/fat/percent_energy.pdf, and http://riskfactor.cancer.gov/DHQ/

forms). The basic food frequency questionnaire consists of two parts: a food list and a section to mark the frequency of intake. The underlying principle behind the FFQ is that dietary intake over long periods, such as weeks or months, is more important than sampling data from a few specific days (Willet 1998). Although sampling data on specific days may be more exact, the crude data collected over longer periods is more essential to assessing dietary quality. In addition, individuals can often easily recall the consumption frequency of certain foods, as opposed to tabulating specific food items over the course of a few days (Willet 1998).

Many other dietary instruments have been designed for the purpose of assessing the quantity and quality of dietary intake. These include such instruments as food frequency screeners, 3-day recalls, food diaries, food records, and other variations of the aforementioned instruments.

Table 6.2. Healthy Eating Index, 2005 Components and Scoring System

Component	Minimum Score of Zero	Maximum Score	Maximum Score
Total fruit (including 100% fruit juice)	No fruit	5	≥0.8 cups per 1,000 kcal
Whole fruit	No whole fruit	5	≥0.4 cups per 1,000 kcal
Total vegetables	No vegetables	5	≥1.1 cups per 1,000 kcal
Dark green vegetables and legumes	No dark green vegetables or legumes	5	≥0.4 cups per 1,000 kcal
Total grains	No total grains	5	≥3.0 oz per 1,000 kcal
Whole grains	No whole grains	5	≥1.5 oz per 1,000 kcal
Milk	No milk	10	≥1.3 cups per 1,000 kcal
Meat and beans	No meat or beans	10	≥2.5 oz per 1,000 kcal
Oils	No oil	10	≥12 g per 1,000 kcal
Saturated fat	≥15% of energy	10	≤7 % of energy
Sodium	≥2.0 g per 1,000 kcal	10	≤0.7 g per 1,000 kcal
Calories from solid fats, alcoholic beverages, added sugars	≥50 % energy	20	≤20% of energy

Note: From the Nutrition Policy and Promotion Fact Sheet, June 2008.

One such instrument, the Healthy Eating Index, is depicted in Table 6.2. Developed by the USDA, the Healthy Eating Index (HEI-2005) assesses 12 aspects of dietary consumption (Table 6.2) and provides a validated tool for public health practitioners to track population characteristics and help modulate interventions (Guenther et al. 2008; Kennedy et al. 1995; USDA 2008). Such tools have helped reveal associations between population characteristics and nutrition.

Examples of Public Health Interventions

Economic concerns and a growing awareness of the role of social determinants are accelerating the pressure to use social marketing, environmental change, and policy as affordable and effective large-scale approaches for populations. They are seen as powerful complements to traditional educational and community organizing techniques (Contento et al. 1995; Glanz et al. 1995, McAlister 1995; Story et al. 2008).

Large-Scale Initiatives

Historically, the drive to use large-scale approaches for healthy nutrition promotion started with the National Cancer Institute/Kelloggs Campaign in the early 1980s. The then-controversial partnership between government and industry used a marketing approach that included mass media advertising, information on cereal boxes, in-store merchandising, and other commercial techniques to reach the general adult market and health professionals. The campaign increased consumer awareness of diet/cancer relationships and extended beyond the Kelloggs brand to a wide range of bran products (Levy and Stokes 1987).

The largest and longest-running partnership for nutrition and chronic disease prevention is the National 5 a Day Program, now renamed the National Fruit and Vegetable Program. In 1991, the National Cancer Institute and the Produce for Better Health Foundation entered into a partnership based on the California 5 a Day—for Better Health! Campaign (Foerster et al. 1995). The National 5 a Day Program used a social marketing approach to focus on specific market segments with a carefully designed communications campaign delivered in multiple channels (Heimendinger and Chapelsky 1996).

To assess the effectiveness of the National 5 a Day Program, an external evaluation and two large national randomized phone-based surveys were conducted (Stables et al. 2002). The external evaluation concluded that the low-cost effort should be continued and expanded, while the phone surveys found significant increases in fruit and vegetable consumption, a higher percentage of individuals reporting they ate at least five servings of fruit and vegetables a day, and a greater number meeting the then-current *Dietary Guidelines* (23% in 1991 to 26% in 1997). Additionally, awareness of the 5 a Day message increased (7% to 19%), correlating again with greater fruit and vegetable consumption.

In March 2007, the 5 a Day message was transitioned to *Fruits & Veggies—More Matters* in accord with the near-doubling of recommended levels of fruits and vegetables in the 2005 *Dietary Guidelines.* Governmental leadership as the national health authority shifted to the Centers for Disease Control and Prevention (CDC), and the Produce for Better Health Foundation continued to provide a single point of contact for the estimated 1,000 fruit and vegetable industry licensees. Leadership expanded to include other members of the National Fruit and Vegetable Alliance steering committee, namely the USDA, the National Cancer Institute, the California Department of Public Health, the National Council of Fruit and Vegetable Nutrition Coordinators, the National Alliance for Nutrition and Activity, the American Cancer Society, the American Diabetes Association, the Produce Marketing Association, the United Fresh Produce Association, the Canned Food Alliance, the Frozen Food Institute, and the American Heart Association. As with 5 a Day, state agencies are licensed by CDC, or the Produce for Better Health Foundation, to serve as health authorities, implement interventions, and assure conformity among public and nonprofit partners.

An example of another successful large-scale campaign is the 1% or Less Campaign. The 1% or Less Campaign sought to shift consumption from whole milk, 2% milk, or high-fat milk products to 1%, skim milk, or low-fat milk products, thereby increasing milk consumption and reduced saturated fat intake (Maddock et al. 2007; Reger, Wootan, and Booth-Butterfield 2000; Reger et al. 1998). It showed dramatic short-term sales increases by using paid advertising and public relations, with and without community-level programming, with the combination of both approaches being more effective, reaching more people, and therefore being more cost effective than community programming alone (Reger, Wootan, Booth-Butterfield 1999; Booth-Butterfield and Reger 2004). Similar effects on high fat milk intake have been reported in ethnically diverse communities, which were sustained far beyond the conclusion of the intervention (Maddock et al. 2007).

Site-Based Interventions

Worksites. The rising cost of health care benefits, together with lost work productivity due to obesity and other chronic diseases, is driving employer and policy interest in worksite modifications and programs that can reach employed adults in venues where they spend over half their waking hours. A 2005 review illustrated the promise of worksite interventions (Engbers et al. 2005). The review showed that among 13 predominantly multicenter trials exploring the effects of adapting work environment, there were statistically significant changes in dietary attitudes and behaviors (Jeffery et al. 1994). Even the simple dissemination of information about the benefits of healthy eating via email has been shown to improve employee fruit, vegetable, and dietary fat intake (Block et al. 2004).

Schools. Schools offer a venue to reach virtually all children and youth through education, skill-building, environmental change, and social support. Most large interventions in schools have shown a positive affect on both dietary attitudes and the consumption of a healthy diet (Knai et al. 2006).

The Gimme 5 Program in Alabama was designed to increase fruit and vegetable consumption among high school students as they progressed from the 9th to 12th grade (Nicklas et al. 1997). The program used the PRECEDE-PROCEED model, which addresses predisposing, enabling, and reinforcing factors for dietary behavior in a high school setting through schoolwide media, marketing, meal and snack modification, classroom workshops, and direct parent involvement. This comprehensive approach was successful in improving knowledge about nutrition ($p<.0001$), self-efficacy ($p<.0001$), and the reported consumption of fruits and vegetables (14% increase, +0.35 servings, $p<.001$) (O'Neil and Niklas 2002).

Minnesota's 5 a Day Power Plus Program served children, ages 8–11 years, and included four components: parental involvement and education, altered school food offerings, industry support, and basic nutritional instruction geared toward the children (Perry et al. 1998). The result of the intervention was a 0.4 serving per day increase in fruit and vegetable consumption (Perry et al. 1998). California's 5 a Day—*Power Play! Campaign*, which also targeted children nine to 11 years old in school, community, and media channels, found a direct, positive dose–response relationship in fruit and vegetable intake among the school, school and community, and comparison schools (Foerster et al. 1998).

Faith-based organizations. Comprehensive interventions supported by respected spiritual leaders and using approaches such as peer advisors, workshops, courses, motivational interviewing, and printed material as part of established religious infrastructures have been shown to be effective (Pomerleau et al. 2005). While many faith-based organizations are receptive to providing dietary information and interventions for their members, those given monetary backing and technical assistance offered, on average, three dietary interventions compared with none by control groups (*p*<.5) (Hannon et al. 2008). Programs based within religious centers have demonstrated increased consumption of fruits and vegetables by as much as 1.4 servings per day (Pomerleau et al. 2005).

Interventions Focusing on Specific Populations

Emerging community approaches. Increasing access to a diverse array of nutritious foods is needed to ensure population improvements in nutrition, particularly in low-income communities (CDC 2008). Increasingly, advocates, public health departments, and occasionally urban planning committees are working to bring full-service supermarkets into low-income communities, increase healthy foods stocked by small food stores, support community and school gardens, start farmers' markets, expand community-supported agriculture (CSAs), organize farm-to-institution networks, and stimulate other direct marketing opportunities for locally grown foods (Koc et al. 2008; Rayner, Barling, and Lang 2008; Hamm 2008). Retailers in low-income areas have offered free transportation and innovative, cost-saving technologies to provide products in a more customer-friendly, efficient manner (Pothukuchi 2005). The availability of a mix of nutritious foods not only requires expanding product offerings at grocery and convenience stores but also working with food preparers, restaurants, and fast-food entities to replace unhealthy meal choices with more nutritious options. Food policy councils in cities, counties, and states have emerged as a cross-cutting political response to bring diverse stakeholders together.

The Federal safety net. USDA's 16 nutrition assistance programs are designed to work together to provide healthy food to all schoolchildren and a nutrition safety net for America's low-income families. USDA programs serve one in six Americans everyday with a budget exceeding $60 billion dollars. The 30-year old Special Supplemental Nutrition Program for Women, Infants, and Children (WIC) starts at the beginning of life by providing high-risk pregnant and breastfeeding women with incomes less than 185% Federal Poverty Level (FPL) and their children up to age five years with nutrition education, links to health care, and grocery store vouchers for specific foods that are rich in nutrients needed for pregnancy, growth, and development. In 2005, federal funding totaled about $6 billion and reached about eight million women and children (IOM 2007). In 2009, the WIC food package will be updated to also provide, among other things, fresh fruits and vegetables, whole grains, and low-fat milk products. These changes enhance the chronic disease prevention component of its health promotion mission. As a discretionary program, WIC's funding level must be reappropriated by Congress each year. In most states, the department of public health administers the federal program and provides WIC services through a network of local public and nonprofit agencies.

The National School Lunch Program (NSLP) is USDA's largest program for America's schoolchildren. In most states, it is administered through the State Education Agency to local education agencies such as school districts, and the great majority of public schools participate to serve about 30 million students every school day with federal funds totaling approximately eight billion dollars (IOM 2007). The School Lunch Program subsidizes but does not fully pay the school's cost of free, reduced-price, and full-priced lunches. The amount of federal subsidy is based on the students' family income, where the divisions are as follows: less than 130% FPL (free), 130%–185% FPL (reduced-price), or greater than 185% FPL (full-priced). Some states and localities augment the federal reimbursements, while most schools make up the difference by charging students for reduced-price and full-priced meals. The percentage of free, reduced-price lunch enrollment is a criterion of child and community poverty used in many community, state, and national statistics. While federal regulations specify that the meals must be consistent with current *Dietary Guidelines*, standards have not yet been updated, nor are federal funds available, to pay the higher costs for more nutritious, fresh, and whole foods. Nutrition education of students is not a federal requirement.

The Supplemental Nutrition Assistance Program, formerly known as Food Stamps, is an entitlement program considered the centerpiece of the U.S. food security safety net. It uses Electronic Benefit Transfer cards rather than vouchers to provide households having gross incomes less than 130% FPL with a monthly cash allotment for food. The value of the food benefit is based on the cost of USDA's Thrifty Food Plan. All foods, except hot, ready-to-eat items, qualify. Even liquor and convenience stores may be certified by the USDA, if the food they carry meets minimum federal requirements. Complex means testing to determine eligibility typically is administered through state and local social services departments. It includes household income, the number of qualifying household members, specific types of expenses, documentation of U.S. citizenship or residency, and regular recertification. In 2005, Supplemental Nutrition Assistance Program served over 25 million persons, over half of whom were children, and it provided about $100 per month per person for food (IOM 2007). Increasingly, this program serves working poor, elderly, and newly unemployed families, but just 60% of eligible Americans are estimated to participate.

Supplemental Nutrition Assistance Program nutrition education (SNAP-Ed) is reimbursed as an optional administrative activity that requires detailed documentation of in-kind state share funds from nonfederal sources. Budgets and activities require annual federal approval of a SNAP-Ed state plan. While the amount per state depends on the matching funds a state can identify, all states now offer some SNAP-Ed. In 2005, states qualified for $225M in matching federal reimbursement. SNAP-Ed and WIC are the two largest sources of nutrition education funding in the United States.

Additional federal nutrition assistance programs at USDA include the School Breakfast Program, the Child and Adult Care Food Programs, and Afterschool Snacks. They are updated by Congress approximately every five years through the Child Nutrition and

WIC reauthorization. SNAP and other, more agriculturally based programs, such as the Fresh Fruit and Vegetable Snack Program, the WIC Farmer's Market Nutrition Program, and the Senior Farmer's Market Nutrition Program, and some commodity and emergency food programs, are reauthorized about every five years in a statute commonly known as the Farm Bill.

Eliminating racial disparities. Programming aimed at ethnic minority groups has lagged even though these groups bear a disproportionate burden of chronic disease, much of it due to poor nutrition (Flegal et al. 2002). A review of 23 ethnically inclusive, population-based interventions from the 1970s to 2003 found social marketing principles and a wide variety of information channels, like television and radio, were used in all interventions, regardless of racial demographics. Among ethnically diverse populations, greater focus was spent on building strong community partnerships, providing more tailored, culturally sensitive messages, seeking out populations in everyday life settings, and empowering social networks (Yancey et al. 2004a).

Early approaches aimed at promoting healthy nutrition within ethnically diverse communities directed efforts primarily toward mass media campaigns, changing community norms, altering environmental conditions, and coalition building (Yancey et al. 2004b). The Stanford Three Community Study advocated for the consumption of foods low in cholesterol and dietary fat by several modes of mass media in communities with large Latino communities (Fortmann et al. 1982). After three years, the study was able to elicit statistically significant reductions in dietary saturated fat intake in Latinos without reductions in their Caucasian counterparts.

In the early 1990s, the Heart to Heart Program brought together mass media, local speaker groups, community-based activities, enhanced restaurant labeling, and cooking seminars to provide a comprehensive, community-inclusive approach to nutrition in a predominantly African American community (Goodman, Wheeler, and Lee 1995). After four years, the intervention demonstrated a significant protective effect on weight gain and cholesterol levels compared with a matched control population.

The Salud Para Su Corazon community intervention targets the prevention of heart disease through nutrition and education in predominantly Latino populations in the Washington, D.C., area (Alcalay et al. 1999). Bilingual messages are presented via radio, brochure, recipe booklets, motivational videos, and culturally sensitive telanovelas. Although there was increased awareness of cardiovascular disease and its risk factors among Latinos, there was no significant behavioral change seen in the intervention. Regardless, interventions targeting communities of color have generally been sparse, and outcome data are limited.

Policy Approaches

While federal policies focus most directly on nutrition for women, children, and those with lesser means, the effects of poor nutrition on health have far reaching effects on nearly everyone. Policies that shape the supply, production, distribution, and promotion of food can have significant clout in shaping population dietary behavior.

Agriculture policy. Food and agricultural policy helps determine which crops farmers will produce and the prices they will get, thereby influencing the food products that retailers, foodservices, and restaurants offer the public. Federal agriculture policy has supported particular crop production through funding for research, enhancement of infrastructure, and subsidies (Schoonover 2007). Long-standing policy promoting the production of grains, corn, and soybeans has been driven harder by recent economic pressures for alternative fuels and commodity trading (Schoonover 2007).

Such crops can be converted to energy-dense food products laden with either simple sugars or saturated fats. Individuals often make choices about nutrition by their pocketbooks and not health benefits (Schoonover 2007; Drewnowski 2004). Therefore, current food and agricultural policy is seen as artificially lowering the costs of nutritionally deficient food products, making them more attractive to price-conscious food processors and consumers. Conversely, fruits and vegetables receive no price supports, and their prices have increased nearly 120% from 1985 to 2000, while the costs for oils increased only 35% and costs of high-sugar foods increased 46% (Putnam 2000).

Approximately every five years, there is the opportunity to change federal agricultural policy through the Farm Bill. The Farm Bill governs several domestic food policies, including SNAP, the Emergency Food Assistance Program, and the Commodity Food Assistance Program (Schoonover 2007). A much more diverse set of stakeholders became engaged in the 2008 Farm Bill, many of whom sought better alignment of agriculture policy with public health policies in nutrition, conservation, sustainable local food systems, climate change, the preservation of agricultural land, and economic development.

Nutrition right-to-know. Consumption of food from restaurants continues to grow. Unlike food in grocery stores, there are no federal requirements for restaurants or volume food packaging used by commercial or school food services to carry Nutrition Fact labels. Any information that is provided is typically piecemeal and scattered (Wootan and Osborn 2006). Most companies that provide nutrient information do so through the internet, making it inaccessible or inconvenient at the point of purchase.

Advocacy groups have attempted to rectify this lack of public information. One such attempt has been pursued by a private, nonprofit advocacy group called the Keystone Center whose purpose is to consider what can be done, given what is currently known, to support consumers' ability to manage calories (Keystone Center 2006). Unwilling to wait, in 2008, New York City became the first city to require restaurants to post the calorie content of their menu. California became the first state to do so. With a dozen states and a number of municipalities having proposed different approaches to menu labeling, while most of the restaurant industry lies in opposition, this policy area is likely to remain contentious.

School wellness policies. Policy within the public school system has also received rigorous review and criticism. In 2006, Congress mandated that schools develop wellness policies to improve the physical activity and nutrition of children. Although some schools have implemented policies, many gaps still exist (Action for Healthy Kids Network, Report 2008). Recently, the IOM made clear recommendations for federally funded school meal programs and the sale of competitive foods in schools (IOM 2007). Although there was no call for dismissal of private food vendors, the report urged that healthy food choices be used as an adjunct to federal meal programs.

Shortly thereafter advocates issued a School Foods Report Card stressing the need for collaboration by state and national agencies to provide a more cohesive, clear set of guidelines for private foods within schools (CSPI Report 2007). Since then, research has shown that a comprehensive approach to school wellness policy that marries self-assessment, nutrition education, nutrition policy, social marketing, and parent outreach resulted in a 50% reduction in overweight among 4th through 6th grade students in low-resource urban schools (Foster et al. 2008). Strengthening of school wellness policies is likely to be advanced at the national, state, and local levels, particularly in lower socioeconomic areas.

Advertising to children. The significant and detrimental effect that food marketing can have on dietary choice, particularly in children, has been refuted by advertisers and food producers. However, in 2006 an expert committee found a clear connection between advertising, adverse dietary choices, and overall declining childhood nutrition; concluding that television advertising has significant influence on the food preferences, purchase requests, and dietary choices of children (IOM 2006). The committee made strong recommendations for a more balanced approach to food marketing, including more emphasis on promoting fruits and vegetables.

The Federal Trade Commission, the USDHHS, and the American Academy of Pediatrics have echoed these recommendations and issued similar statements (Story et al. 2008). The Federal Communications Commission (FCC) has created a task force to address the effects of mass media on childhood nutrition and obesity (statement by Patti Miller 2007). In December 2006, several of the top food producers and marketers in the United States developed the Children's Food and Beverage Advertising Initiative to include more advertising for healthier foods, better dietary practices, and improved physical activity (Story et al. 2008). The impact of this initiative on children's advertising remains unknown.

Areas of Future Research and Demonstration

In the United States, the chronic disease challenge of the 1990s was to run aggressive efforts to prevent and control tobacco use. Tangible reductions in tobacco use and tobacco-related chronic disease were apparent within a decade. In this decade, the priority in regards to tobacco is to take prevention to scale, sustain urgency, and maintain earmarks for public resources.

Much like the issue of tobacco in the 1990s, the promotion of healthy eating is likely to assume a much more important role in this millennium and seems on a similar course with other public health movements that resulted in social change (USDHSS 2001; Economos et al. 2001). While the field of dietary change is bigger and more complex than tobacco control, there are better opportunities to develop cooperative, not solely confrontational, relationships with the food industry.

A large fraction of the more than $30 billion now spent annually on food advertising and promotion could be redirected toward the promotion of good nutrition and physical activity, as well as the reformulation of food products. Communities, schools, and workplaces could advocate for healthier food options and greater nutrition education. However, until healthy eating becomes normative and a routine part of organizational budgets, a massive reorientation of public health-related effort will be required, with redirection of funds and identification of new funding streams. Public health agencies will need new skills, new infrastructure, and new partnerships to support the work of the many stakeholders engaged in dietary improvement efforts. Much is still to be learned, but the literature suggests room for cautious optimism.

This chapter has introduced issues and trends in public health nutrition. It has illustrated that while vast areas of intervention research and theory should be explored, there are many proven effective solutions in the public health literature, and broad-based solutions are percolating within communities. The disparities in nutrition between socioeconomic, racial, and geographic divides that lead to chronic disease are being exposed, and concern about vulnerable groups who live in environments that promote poor nutrition, especially low-income families, children and the elderly, is creating urgency. Understanding the gaps and interconnections in policy and environmental information, built environment, community intervention, and surveillance systems increases clarity about opportunities for change. As the burden of poor nutrition grows, so has the willingness to find solutions. These solutions have been increasingly brokered by broad-based partnerships, multilevel interventions, public policy and collaborative efforts between health care, mass media, communities, and the producers of food.

Intervention resources and research for dietary change are needed in proportion to the magnitude of the problem. Much is to be learned through experience operating and evaluating programs, and much will be gained by adopting common, preferably, validated measures of environmental influence (Glanz et al. 2005). The focus must be on advancing research and interventions in parallel that focus on the many environmental and individual factors that affect food choice (Story et al. 2008). For public health applications, priorities include delineating the elements of sector- and population-specific interventions, understanding marketplace factors such as economic incentives and disincentives, sponsoring effective mass communications, and understanding how organizations on the national, state, regional, and local levels can complement and gain synergy from each others' efforts.

To date, there have been efforts to compose a unifying framework for organizing large-scale, complex dietary campaigns. One uses approaches found successful in large-scale antitobacco campaigns where mass communications conveys information that causes the public to question the status quo. Community programs are thus supported through media in multiple sectors, and are better able to drive new social norms. Public awareness and initiatives are later reinforced by policy and environmental change. Figure 6.5 (Ammerman et al. 2002) displays a logic model that provides a place for many different stakeholders in large-scale, multicomponent campaigns and suggests realistic evaluation metrics in line with the scope, complexity, and duration of intervention (IOM 2007).

Typically, social marketing interventions start with identifying the priority behavior changes or policy targets, the demographic or lifestyle segments to target, and the channels with the greatest reach and feasibility for conducting interventions. Formative research with consumers and intermediaries then defines the wants, needs, benefits, and barriers specific to each channel to guide development of the message and execution of the campaign. Planners must then systematically determine the following:

- Which media outlets and community channels reach the segment in the most persuasive manner (and can the industry marketing messages be countered)?
- What environmental influences modulate dietary behavior, how, and by whom might they be modified?

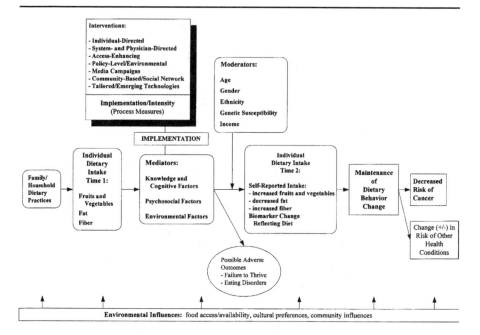

Figure 6.5. Evaluation framework for comprehensive nutrition programs and policies to prevent chronic diseases. Reprinted from Ammerman, A.S., C.H. Lindquist, K.N. Lohr, and J. Hersey. The Efficacy of Behavioral Interventions to Modify Dietary Fat and Fruit and Vegetable Intake: A Review of the Evidence. *Prev Med* (2002):35:25–41, with permission from Elsevier.

- What program services, including information and interactive interventions, would stimulate the desired behaviors?
- What institutional policies help or hinder behavior, and how they might be modified?
- What is the most current ongoing research with consumers, intermediaries, and intervention channels that would be needed?
- How can the campaign or intervention be delivered simply and in a user-friendly way?
- What are the metrics that partners look for as evidence of success?
- What are the potential positive and negative outcomes of the intervention?

From a systems perspective, two expert reports that examined the childhood obesity epidemic provide instructive, holistic guidance for chronic disease nutrition programs going forward (IOM 2005, 2007). The first report defined childhood obesity and its drivers as an epidemic, thereby placing the issue high on the public health priority list. In the second report, a committee was charged with assessing progress in America, and in so doing, identified gaps that can be seen as cutting across the entire field of nutrition and chronic disease. The report found that, while there appears to be considerable response to childhood obesity across the country, it is not clear what is working, and it is unclear what resources get the most return on investment. The resulting policy recommendations focused on four areas:

- Stronger leadership that will set policy, commit, and mobilize resources is needed at the national, state, and local levels.
- Across the United States, a more rigorous, organized approach to evaluation is needed.
- Monitoring and surveillance systems, together with research on the impacts of interventions, are inadequate and need to be developed or expanded.
- Information sharing and dissemination is needed to guide and scale-up effective efforts

Given the scope of the food system, it is not surprising that large-scale, comprehensive initiatives that require a mix of professional disciplines and stakeholders are needed to increase access to healthy food, collaborate with other stakeholders, generate resources, and deliver communication programs. Specialists needed at the table include those in the fields of public health nutrition, health education, marketing, epidemiology, mass communications and public relations, health care providers and insurers, policy, community organizing, schools, business, design and creative arts, culinary arts and retail merchandising, public health law, resource development, applied research, evaluation, and administration. While some of the specialties may be available through public/private partnerships, public health agencies need dedicated resources for these functions. The challenges in nutrition are large, but the growing interest and innovation is equally large. As public health interventions become more multifaceted, wider-reaching, and creative, the prospect of a healthier global diet grows more promising.

Resources

American Cancer Society, 1599 Clifton Road, NE, Atlanta, GA 30329-4251, +1-800-ACS-2345, http://www.cancer.org.

American Diabetes Association, 1701 N. Beauregard Street, Alexandria, VA 22311, +1-800-342-2383, http://www.diabetes.org.

American Dietetic Association, 120 South Riverside Plaza, Suite 2000, Chicago, IL 60606-6995, +800-877-1600, http://www.eatright.org.

American Heart Association, 7272 Greenville Avenue, Dallas, TX 75231-4596, 800-242-8721, http://www.americanheart.org.

Association of State and Territorial Public Health Nutrition Directors, P.O. Box 1001, Johnstown, PA 15907, www.astphnd.org.

California Food Policy Advocates, 436 14th Street #1220, Oakland, CA 94612, +510-433-1122, www.cfpa.net.

Center for Food Safety & Applied Nutrition, Food and Drug Administration, 5100 Paintbranch Parkway, College Park, MD 20740-3835, http://vm.cfsan.fda.gov/list.html.

Center for Nutrition Policy and Promotion, U.S. Department of Agriculture, 3101 Park Center Drive, 10th Floor, Alexandria, VA 22302-1594, +703-305-7600, http://www.cnpp.usda.gov.

Center for Science in the Public Interest, 1875 Connecticut Avenue, NW, Suite 300, Washington, DC 20009, +202-332-9110, http://www.cspinet.org.

Community Food Security Coalition, 3820 SE Division Street, Portland, OR 97202, +503-954-2970, www.foodsecurity.org.

Feeding America (formerly America's Second Harvest), 35 East Wacker Drive, Suite 2000, Chicago, IL 60601, 800-771-2303, www.feedingamerica.org.

Food and Nutrition Service, U.S. Department of Agriculture, 3101 Park Center Drive, Alexandria, VA 22302-1594, http://www.fns.usda.gov/fns.

Food Research and Action Center, 1875 Connecticut Avenue NW #540, Washington, DC 20009, +202-986-2200, http://www.frac.org.

National Association of WIC Directors, 2001 S St NW #580, Washington, DC 20009, +202-232-5492, www.nwica.org.

National Center for Chronic Disease Prevention and Health Promotion, Centers for Disease Control and Prevention, 4770 Buford Highway, NE, MS K-40, Atlanta, GA 30341-3717, +404-639-3534, http://www.cdc.gov/nccdphp.

Produce for Better Health Foundation, 5301 Limestone Road, Wilmington, DE, +302-235-1012, www.fruitsandveggiesmorematters.org and www.pbhcatalog.com.

School Nutrition Association, 2175 K Street NW, Washington, DC 20437, +202-653-2404, http://www.schoolnutrition.org.

Supplemental Nutrition Assistance Program—Nutrition Education (SNAP-Ed), www.snap.nal.usda.

Strategic Alliance Promoting Healthy Food and Activity Environments, 221 Oak Street, Oakland, CA 94607, +510-444-7738, www.preventioninstitute.org.

Trust for America's Health, 1707 H St NW, Washington, DC, +202-223-9870, healthyamericans.org.

Department of Nutrition for Health and Development (NHD), World Health Organization (WHO), Avenue Appia 20, 1211 Geneva 27, Switzerland, http://www.who.int/nutrition.

Suggested Reading

Byers, T. The role of epidemiology in developing nutritional recommendations: past, present, and future. *Am J Clin Nutr* (1999):69: S1304–S1308.

Joint WHO/FAO Expert Consultation on Diet Nutrition and the Prevention of Chronic Diseases. *Diet, Nutrition, and the Prevention of Chronic Diseases: Report of a Joint Who/Fao Expert Consultation.* Geneva, Switzerland, 2003.

Kushi, L.H., T. Byers, C. Doyle, F.V. Bandera, M. McCullough, T. Gansler, K.S. Andrews, M.J. Thun, and the American Cancer Society 2006 Nutrition and Physical Activity Guidelines Advisory Committee. American Cancer Society Guidelines on Nutrition and Physical Activity for Cancer Prevention: Reducing the Risk of Cancer With Healthy Food Choices and Physical Activity. *CA Cancer J Clin* (2006):56: 254–281.

Story, M., K.M. Kaphingst, R. Robinson-O'Brien, and K. Glanz. Creating Healthy Food and Eating Environments: Policy and Environmental Approaches. *Annu Rev Public Health* (2008):29:253–272.

U.S. Department of Health and Human Services and U.S. Department of Agriculture. *Dietary Guidelines for Americans*, 2005. Washington, D.C.: U.S. Government Printing Office, 2005.

World Cancer Research Fund/American Institute for Cancer Research. *Food, Nutrition, Physical Activity, and the Prevention of Cancer: A Global Perspective.* Washington, D.C.: AICR, 2007.

World Health Organization (WHO). *Global strategy on diet, physical activity, and health: Fifty-Seventh World Health Assembly. Resolution WHA56.17.* Geneva, Switzerland: WHO, 2004.

References

Action for Healthy Kids Network. *Progress or Promises? What's Working for and Against Healthy Schools* (2008). Available at http://www.actionforhealthykids.org/pdf/Progress%20or%20Promises.pdf. Accessed December 24, 2008.

Alcalay, R., M. Alvarado, H. Balcazar, E. Newman, and E. Huerta. Salud Para Su Corazon: A Community-Based Latino Cardiovascular Disease Prevention and Outreach Model. *J Community Health* (1999):24:359–379.

American Heart Association (AHA), S.S. Gidding, B.A. Dennison, L.L. Birch, S.R. Daniels, M.W. Gilman, A.H. Lichtenstein, K.T. Rattay, J. Steinberger, N. Stettler, and L. Van Horn. Dietary Recommendations for Children and Adolescents: A Guide for Practitioners. *Pediatrics* (2006):177:544–559.

Ammerman, A.S., C.H. Lindquist, K.N. Lohr, and J. Hersey. The Efficacy of Behavioral Interventions to Modify Dietary Fat and Fruit and Vegetable Intake: A Review of the Evidence. *Prev Med* (2002):35:25–41.

Appel, L.J., T.J. Moore, E. Obarzanek, et al. A Clinical Trial of the Effects of Dietary Patterns on Blood Pressure: Dash Collaborative Research Group. *N Engl J Med* (1997):336:1117–1124.

Austin, S.B.,S.J. Melly, B.N. Sanchez, A. Patel, S. Buka, and S.L. Gortmaker. Clustering of Fast-Food Restaurants Around Schools: A Novel Application of Spatial Statistics to the Study of Food Environments. *Am J Public Health* (2005):95:1575–1581.

Aviram, M. Modified Forms of Low Density Lipoprotein and Atherosclerosis. *Atherosclerosis* (1993):98:1–9.

Baker, E.A., M. Schootman, E. Barnidge, and C. Kelly. The Role of Race and Poverty in Access to Foods that Enable Individuals to Adhere to Dietary Guidelines. *Prev Chron Dis* (2006):3(A76):1–11.

Baker, A.H., and J. Wardle. Sex Differences in Fruit and Vegetable Intake in Older Adults. *Appetite* (2003):40:269–275.

Barba, G., and P. Russo. Dairy Foods, Dietary Calcium and Obesity: A Short Review of the Evidence. *Nutr Metab Cardiovasc Dis* (2006):16:445–451.

Beydoun, M.A., and Y. Wang. How Do Socio-Economic Status, Perceived Economic Barriers and Nutritional Benefits Affect Quality of Dietary Intake among US Adults? *Eur J Clin Nutr* (2008):62:303–313.

Biener, L., K. Glanz, D. McLerran, G. Sorensen, B. Thompson, K. Basen-Enquist, L. Linnan, and J. Varnes. Impact of the Working Well Trial on the Worksite Smoking and Nutrition Environment. *Health Educ Behav* (1999):26:478–494.

Biesalski, H.K. Meat and Cancer: Meat as a Component of a Healthy Diet. *Eur J Clin Nutr* (2002):56(1 Suppl):S2–S11.

Bingham, S.A., B. Pignatelli, J.R. Pollock, et al. Does Increased Endogenous Formation of N-nitroso Compounds in the Human Colon Explain the Association between Red Meat and Colon Cancer? *Carcinogenesis* (1996):17:515–523.

Blanck, H.M., C. Gillespie, J.E. Kimmons, J.D. Seymour, and M.K. Serdula. Trends in Fruit and Vegetable Consumption among U.S. Men and Women, 1994–2005. *Prev Chronic Dis* (2008):5(2). Available at http://www.cdc.gov/pcd/issues/2008/apr/07_0049.htm.

Blisard, N., H. Stewart, and D. Joliffe. Low-Income Households' Expenditures on Fruits and Vegetables. *Agric Econ Rep USDA* (2004):833.

Block, G., T. Block, P. Wakimoto, and C.H. Block. Demonstration of an E-mailed Worksite Nutrition Intervention Program. *Prev Chronic Dis* (2004):1A(06):1–13.

Booth-Butterfield, S., and B. Reger. The Message Changes Belief and the Rest is Theory: The 1% or Less Milk Campaign and Reasoned Action. *Prev Med* (2004):39:581–588.

Bowman, S.A., and B.T. Vinyard. Fast Food Consumption of US Adults: Impact on Energy and Nutrient Intakes and Overweight Status. *J Am Coll Nutr* (2004):23:163–168.

Briefel, R.R., and C.L. Johnson. Secular Trends in Dietary Intake in the United States. *Annu Rev Nutr* (2004):24:401–431.

Brooks, B.M., R. Rajeshwari, T.A. Nicklas, S.J. Yang, and G.S. Berenson. Association of calcium intake, dairy product consumption with overweight status in young adults (1995–1996): The Bogalusa Heart Study. *J Am Coll Nutr* (2006):25:523–532.

Brug, J., and F. van Lenthe, editors. *Environmental Determinants and Interventions for Physical Activity, Nutrition, and Smoking: A Review.* Netherlands: Rijksinstituut voor Volksgezondheid en Milieu (2005) pp. 378–389.

Bueno De Mesquita, H.B., P. Ferrari, and E. Riboli. Plant Foods and the Risk of Colorectal Cancer in Europe: Preliminary Findings. *IARC Sci Publ Ser* (2002):156:89–95.

Burton, S., E.H. Creyer, J. Kees, and K. Huggins. Attacking the Obesity Epidemic: The Potential Health Benefits of Providing Nutrition Information in Restaurants. *Am J Public Health* (2006):96:1669–1675.

Caplan, P. Why Do People Eat What They Do? Approaches to Food and Diet from a Social Science Perspective. *Clin Child Psychol Psychiatry* (1996):1:213–227.

Carter, M.A., and B. Swinburn. Measuring the 'Obesogenic' Food Environment in New Zealand Primary Schools. *Health Promotion Int* (2004):19(1):15–20.

Casagrande, S.S., Y. Wang, C. Anderson, and T.L. Gary. Have Americans Increased Their Fruit and Vegetable Intake? The Trends between 1988 and 2002. *Am J Prev Med* (2007):32(4):257–263.

Centers for Disease Control and Prevention (CDC). *The Burden of Chronic Disease and Their Risk Factors: National and State Perspectives* (2004). Available at http://www.cdc.gov/nccdphp/burdenbook2004/pdf/burden_book2004.pdf. Accessed December 3, 2088.

Centers for Disease Control and Prevention (CDC). State Nutrition, Physical Activity, and Obesity Program – Technical Assistance Manual. CDC Division of NPAO. Published January (2008):55–74.

Center for Science in the Public Interest. *School Foods Report Card.* Available at http://www.cspinet.org/2007schoolreport.pdf. Accessed December 24, 2008.

Chen, J., J. He, R.P. Wildman, K. Reynolds, R.H. Streiffere, and P.K. Whelton. A Randomized Controlled Trial of Dietary Fiber Intake on Serum Lipids. *Eur J Clin Nutr* (2006):60:62–68.

Clark, J.E. Taste and Flavour: Their Importance in Food Choice and Acceptance. *Proc Nutr Soc* (1998):57:639–643.

Contento, I., G.I. Balch, Y.L. Bronner, L.A. Lytle, S.K. Maloney, C.M. Olson, S.S. Swadender, and J.S. Randell. The Effectiveness of Nutrition Education and Implications for Nutrition Education Policy, Programs, and Research: A Review of the Research. *J Nutr Educ* (1995):27(6):277–418.

Corella, D., D.K. Arnett, M.Y. Tsai, et al. The –256t>C Polymorphism in the Apdolipoprotein a-Ii Gene Promoter Is Associated with Body Mass Index and Food Intake in the Genetics of Lipid Lowering Drugs and Diet Network Study. *Clin Chem* (2007):53:1144–1152.

Cummins, S.C.J., L. McKay, and S. MacIntyre. McDonald's Restaurants and Neighborhood Deprivation in Scotland and England. *Am J Prev Med* (2005):29:308–310.

Darmon, N., and A. Drewnowski. Does Social Class Predict Diet Quality? *Am J Clin Nutr* (2008):87:1107–1117.

de Graaf, C., P. Polet, and W.A. van Staveren. Sensory Perception and Pleasantness of Food Flavors in Elderly Subjects. *J Gerontol* (1994):49:93–99.

Divisi, D., S. Di Tommaso, S. Salvemini, M. Garramone, and R. Crisci. Diet and Cancer. *Acta Biomed* (2006):77:118–123.

Dixon, L.B., A.F. Subar, U. Peters, J.L. Weissfeld, R.S. Bresalier, A. Risch, A. Schatzkin, and R.B. Hayes. Adherence to the USDA Food Guide, DASH Eating Plan, and Mediterranean Dietary Pattern Reduces Risk of Colorectal Adenoma. *J Nutr* (2007):137:2443–2450.

Drewnowski, A. Obesity and the Food Environment: Diet Energy Density and Diet Costs. *Am J Prev Med* (2004; S3):27:S154–S162.

Drewnowski, A., and F. Bellisle. Liquid Calories, Sugar, and Body Weight. *Am J Clin Nutr* (2007):85:651–661.

Drewnowski, A., and V.A. Warren-Mears. Does Aging Change Nutrition Requirements? *J Nutr Health Aging* (2001):5:70–74.

Duffey, K.J., and B.M. Popkin. Shifts in Patterns and Consumption of Beverages between 1965 and 2002. *Obesity* (2007):15(11):2739–2747.

Dynesen, A.W., J. Haraldsdottir, L. Holm, and A. Astrup. Sociodemographic Differences in Dietary Habits Described by Food Frequency Questions–Results from Denmark. *Eur J Clin Nutr* (2003):57:1586–1597.

Economos, D., R. Brownson, M. DeAngelis, S. Foerster, C.T. Foreman, S. Kumanyika, R. Pate, and J. Gregson. What Lessons Have Been Learned from Other Attempts to Guide Social Change? *Nutr Reviews*, (March 2001):II:S40–S56.

Eertmans, A., F. Baeyens, and O. Van de Bergh. Food Likes and Their Relative Importance in Human Eating Behavior: Review and Preliminary Suggestions for Health Promotion. *Health Edu Research* (2001):16:443–456.

Engbers, L.H., M.N. van Poppel, A.P.M.J. Chin, and W. van Mechelen. Worksite Health Promotion Programs with Environmental Changes: A Systematic Review. *Am J Prev Med* (2005):29: 61–70.

Ervin, R.B. Healthy Eating Index Scores among Adults, 60 Years of Age and Over, by Sociodemographic and Health Characteristics: United States, 1999–2002. *Advance Data from Vital and Health Statistics*; vol. 395. Hyattsville, MD: National Center for Health Statistics (2008).

Ezzati, M., A.D. Lopez, A. Rodgers, S. Vander Hoorn, C.J.L. Murray, and Comparative Risk Assessment Collaborating Group. Selected Major Risk Factors and Global Regional Burden of Disease. *Lancet* (2002):360:1347–1360.

FAOSTAT Database. *Sources of Dietary Energy Consumption 2001–2003* (2003). Available at http:// faostat.fao.org/Portals/_Faostat/documents/pdf/sources_of_dietary_energy_consumption. pdf. Accessed December 1, 2008.

Feldman, P.J., and A. Steptoe. How Neighborhoods and Physical Functioning Are Related: The Roles of Neighborhood Socioeconomic Status, Perceived Neighborhood Strain, and Individual Health Risk Factors. *Ann Behav Med* (2004):27:91–99.

Fiorito, L.M., A.K. Ventura, D.C. Mitchell, H. Smicklas-Wright, and L.L. Birch. Girl's Dairy Intake, Energy Intake, and Weight Status. *J Am Diet Assoc* (2006):106:1851–1855.

Flegal, K.M., M.D. Carroll, C.L. Ogden, and C.L. Johnson. Prevalence and Trends in Obesity among U.S. Adults 1999–2000. *JAMA* (2002):288:1723–1727.

Foerster, S.B., J. Gregson, D.L. Beall, M. Hudes, H. Magnuson, S.A. Livingston, M.A. Davis, A.B. Joy, and T. Garbolino. The California Children's 5 a Day-Power Play! Campaign: Evaluation of a Large-Scale Social Marketing Initiative. *J Fam Community Health* (1998): 21(1):46–64.

Foerster, S.B., K.W. Kizer, L.K. Disogra, D.G. Bal, B.F. Krieg, and K.L. Bunch. California's 5 a Day—For Better Health! Campaign: An Innovative Population-Based Effort to Effect Large-Scale Dietary Change. *Am J Prev Med* (March–April 1995):11(2):124–131.

Fortmann, S.P., P.T. Williams, S.B. Hulley, N. Maccoby, and J.W. Farquhar. Does Dietary Health Education Reach Only the Privileged? The Stanford Three Community Study. *Circulation* (1982):66:77–82.

Foster, G.D., S. Sherman, K.E. Borradaile, K.M. Grundy, S.S. Vander Veur, J. Nachmani, A. Karpyn, S. Kumanyika, and J. Shults. A Policy-Based School Intervention to Prevent Overweight and Obesity. *Pediatrics* (2008):121:e794–e802.

Franco, M., A.V. Diez Roux, T.A. Glass, B. Caballero, and F.L. Brancati. Neighborhood Characteristics and Availability of Healthy Foods in Baltimore. *Am J Prev Med* (2008):35:561–567.

Frazao, E., editor. America's Eating Habits: Changes & Consequences. *Econ Res Serv Bull*. Washington, D.C.:U.S. Department of Agriculture (1999) p. 750.

Fung, T.T., S.E. Chiuve, M.L. McCullough, K.M. Rexrode, G. Logroscino, and F.B. Hu. Adherence to a Dash-Style Diet and Risk of Coronary Heart Disease and Stroke in Women. *Arch Intern Med* (2008):168:716–720.

Furst, T., M. Connors, C.A. Bisogni, J. Sobal, and L. Winter Falk. Food Choice: A Conceptual Model of the Process. *Appetite* (1996):26:247–266.

Gantz, W., N. Schwartz, J. Angelini, and V. Rideout. Food for Thought: Televisions Food Advertising to Children in the United States. *Kaiser Family Foundation Report* (2007). Available at http://www.kff.org/entmedia/upload/7618.pdf. Accessed December 27, 2008.

Gillman, M.W., S.L. Rifas-Shiman, A.L. Frazier, et al. Family Dinner and Diet Quality among Older Children and Adolescents. *Arch Fam Med* (2000):9:235–240.

Ginsberg, H.N., P. Kris-Etherton, B. Dennis, et al. Effects of Reducing Dietary Saturated Fatty Acids on Plasma Lipids and Lipoproteins in Healthy Subjects: The Delta Study, Protocol 1. *Arterioscler Thromb Vasc Biol* (1998):18:441–449.

Glanz, K., M. Basil, E. Maibach, J. Goldberg, and D. Snyder. Why Americans Eat What They Do: Taste, Nutrition, Cost, Convenience, and Weight Control Concerns as Influences on Food Consumption. *J Am Diet Assoc* (1998):98:1118–1126.

Glanz, K., B. Lankenau, S. Foerster, S. Temple, R. Mullis, and T. Schmid. Environmental and Policy Approaches to Cardiovascular Disease Prevention Through Nutrition: Opportunities for State and Local Action. *Health Educ Q* (1995):22(4):512–527.

Glanz, K., B. Lankenau, S. Foerster, S. Temple, R. Mullis, and T. Schmid. Environmental and Policy Approaches to Cardiovascular Disease Prevention Through Nutrition: Opportunities for State and Local Action. *Health Educ Q* (1995):22:441–449.

Glanz, K., J. Sallis, B. Saelens, and L. Frank. Healthy Nutrition Environments: Concepts and Measures. *Am J Health Promot* (2005):19:330–333.

Glanz, K., and A.L. Yaroch. Strategies for Increasing Fruit and Vegetable Intake in Grocery Stores and Communities: Policy, Pricing, and Environmental Change. *Prev Med* (2004):39 (2 Suppl):S75–S80.

Gonzalez, C.A. Nutrition and Cancer: The Current Epidemiological Evidence. *Br J Nutr* (2006):96(1 Supp):S42–S45.

Gooderham N.J., S. Murray, A.M. Lynch, et al. Assessing Human Risk to Heterocyclic Amines. *Mutation Res* (1997):375:53–60.

Goodman R.M., F.C. Wheeler, and P.R. Lee. Evaluation of the Heart To Heart Project: Lessons from a Community Based Chronic Disease Prevention Project. *Am J Health Promot* (1995):9:443–455.

Grimm, G.C., L. Harnack, and M. Story. Factors Associated with Soft Drink Consumption in School-Aged Children. *J Am Diet Assoc* (2004):104:1244–1249.

Guadalupe, X.A., M. Rogers, E.M. Arredondo, N.R. Campbell, B. Baquero, S.C. Duerksen, and J.P. Elder. Away-from-Home Food Intake and Risk for Obesity: Examining the Influence of Context. *Obesity* (2008):16:1002–1008.

Guenther, P.M., J. Reedy, S.M. Krebs-Smith, and B.B. Reeve. Evaluation of the Healthy Eating Index—2005. *J Am Diet Assoc* (2008):108:1854–1864.

Guo, S.S., W. Wu, W.C. Chumlea, and A.F. Roche. Predicting Overweight and Obesity in Adulthood from Body Mass Index Values in Childhood and Adolescence. *Am J Clin Nutr* (2002):76:653–658.

Guthrie, J.F., and J.F. Morton. Food Sources of Added Sweeteners in the Diets of Americans. *J Am Diet Assoc* (2000):100:43–51.

Hamm, M.W. Linking Sustainable Agriculture and Public Policy: Opportunities for Realizing Multiple Goals. *J Hunger Environ Nutr* (2/3, 2008):3:169–185.

Hannon, P.A., D.J. Bowen, C.L. Christensen, and A. Kuniyuki. Disseminating a Successful Dietary Intervention to Faith Communities: Feasibility of Using Staff Contact and Encouragement to Increase Uptake. *J Nutr Educ Behav* (2008):40:175–180.

Harrison, K., and A.L. Marske. Nutritional Content of Foods Advertised During the Television Programs Children Watch Most. *Am J Public Health* (2005):2005:1568–1574.

Hastings, G., M. Stead, L. McDermott, et al. Review of Research in the Effects of Food Promotion to Children. Food Standards Agency – Final Report. Glasgow: Centre for Social Marketing (2003).

Haug, A., A.T. Hostmark, and O.M. Harstad. Bovine Milk in Human Nutrition—A Review. *Lipids Health* (2007):Dis 6:6–25.

Healthy People 2010. Understanding and Improving Health. U.S. Department of Health and Human Services, U.S. Government Printing Office (2000).

Heidemann, C., M.B. Schulze, O.H. Franco, R.M. van Dam, C.S. Mantzoros, and F.B. Hu. Dietary Patterns and Risk of Mortality from Cardiovascular Disease, Cancer, and All Causes in a Prospective Cohort of Women. *Circulation* (2008):118:230–237.

Heimendinger, J., and D. Chapelsky. The National 5 a Day for Better Health Program. *Adv Exp Med Biol* (1996):401:199–206.

Holm, L. Cultural and Social Acceptability of a Healthy Diet. *Eur J Clin Nutr* (1993):47:592–599.

Houston, D.K., J. Stevens, J. Cai, and P.S. Haines. Dairy, Fruit, and Vegetable Intakes and Functional Limitations and Disability in a Biracial Cohort: The Atherosclerosis Risk in Communities Study. *Am J Clin Nutr* (2005):81:515–522.

Howard, V.J., J. Acker, C.R. Gomez, et al. Delta States Stroke Consortium. An Approach to Coordinate Efforts to Reduce the Public Health Burden of Stroke: The Delta States Stroke Consortium. *Prev Chronic Dis* (2004):4:A19.

Howard, B.V., L. Van Horn, J. Hsia, et al. Low-Fat Dietary Pattern and Risk of Cardiovascular Disease: The Women's Health Initiative Randomized Controlled Dietary Modification Trial. *JAMA* (2006):295:655–666.

Hu, J., C. La Vecchia, M. DesMeules, E. Negri, L. Mery, and Canadian Cancer Registries Epidemiology Research Group. Meat and Fish Consumption and Cancer in Canada. *Nutr Cancer* (2008):60:313–324.

Institute of Medicine (IOM). Food Marketing to Children and Youth: Threat or Opportunity? Committee on Food Marketing and the Diets of Children and Youth (2006).

Institute of Medicine (IOM). Nutrition Standards for Foods in Schools: Leading the Way Toward Healthier Youth. Report (2007).

Institute of Medicine (IOM). Preventing Childhood Obesity: Health in the Balance. Committee on Prevention of Obesity in Children and Youth (2005).

Institute of Medicine (IOM). Progress in Preventing Childhood Obesity: How Do We Measure Up? Committee on Preventing Childhood Obesity (2007).

International Agency for Research on Cancer. Cancer: Causes, Occurrence, and Control. IARC Scientific Publications (1990):100.

Jacobs, D.R.J., L. Marquart, J. Slavin, and L.H. Kushi. Whole-Grain Intake and Cancer: An Expanded Review and Meta-Analysis. *Nutr Cancer* (1998):30:85–96.

Jacques, P.F., S.I. Sulsky, G.A. Perrone, and E.J. Schaefer. Ascorbic Acid and Plasma Lipids. *Epidemiology* (1994):5:19–26.

Jeffery, R.W., S.A. French, C. Raether, and J.E. Baxter. An Environmental Intervention to Increase Fruit and Salad Purchases in a Cafeteria. *Prev Med* (1994):23:788–792.

Jenkins, D.J., C.W. Kendall, A. Marchie, et al. Effects of a Dietary Portfolio of Cholesterol-Lowering Foods vs Lovastatin on Serum Lipids and C-Reactive Protein. *JAMA* (2003):290:502–510.

Joint WHO/FAO Expert Consultation on Diet, Nutrition, and the Prevention of Chronic Diseases. Diet, Nutrition, and the Prevention of Chronic Diseases: Report of a Joint WHO/FAO Expert Consultation. Geneva, Switzerland (2003).

Kant, A.K., and B.I. Graubard. Eating Out in America, 1987–2000: Trends and Nutritional Correlates. *Prev Med* (2004):38:243–249.

Kant, A.K., and B.I. Graubard. Secular Trends in Patterns of Self-Reported Food Consumption of Adult Americans: NHANES 1971–1975 to NHANES 1999–2002. *Am J Clin Nutr* (2006):84:1215–1223.

Kant, A.K., and B.I. Graubard. Secular Trends in the Association of Socio-Economic Position with Self-Reported Dietary Attributes and Biomarkers in the US Population: National Health and Nutrition Examination Survey (NHANES) 1971–1975 to NHANES 1999–2002. *Public Health Nutr* (2007):10(2):158–167.

Kant, A.K., B.I. Graubard, and S.K. Kumanyika. Trends in Black–White Differentials in Dietary Intakes of U.S. Adults, 1971–2002. *Am J Prev Med* (2007):32(4):264–272.

Kapur, K., A. Kapur, S. Ramachandran, V. Mohan, S.R. Aravind, M. Badgandi, and M.V. Srishyla. Barriers to Changing Dietary Behavior. *J Assoc of Physicians of India* (2008):56: 27–32.

Kazerouni, N., R. Sinha, C.H. Hsu, A. Greenberg, and N. Rothman. Analysis of 200 Food Items for Benzo[a]pyrene and Estimation of its Intake in an Epidemiologic Study. *Food Chemistry and Toxicology* (2001):39:423–436.

Kennedy, E.T., J. Ohls, S. Carlson, and K. Fleming. The Healthy Eating Index: Design and Applications. *J Am Diet Assoc* (1995):95:1103–1108.

Key, T.J., N.E. Allen, E.A. Spencer, and R.C. Travis. The Effect of Diet on Risk of Cancer. *Lancet* (2002):360:861–868.

Kim, L.P., G.G. Harrison, and M. Kagawa-Singer. Perceptions of Diet and Physical Activity among California Hmong Adults and Youths. *Prev Chronic Dis* (2007):4:1–4.

Knai, C., J. Pomerleau, K. Lock, M. McKee. Getting Children to Eat More Fruit and Vegetables: A Systematic Review. *Prev Med* (2006):42:85–95.

Koc, M., R. MacRae, E. Desjardins, and W. Roberts. Getting Civil About Food: The Interactions between Civil Society and the State to Advance Sustainable Food Systems in Canada. *J Hunger Environ Nutr* (2/3,2008):3:122–144.

Kushi, L.H., T. Byers, C. Doyle, E.V. Bandera, M. McCullough, T. Gansler, K.S. Andrews, M.J. Thun, and the American Cancer Society 2006 Nutrition and Physical Activity Guidelines Advisory Committee. American Cancer Society Guidelines on Nutrition and Physical Activity for Cancer Prevention: Reducing the Risk of Cancer With Healthy Food Choices and Physical Activity. *CA Cancer J Clin* (2006):56:254–281.

Labarthe, D.R. Dietary Imbalance. In *Epidemiology and Prevention of Cardiovascular Diseases: A Global Challenge*. Gaithersburg, MD: Aspen Publishers (1998):133–165.

Labreque, L., S. Lamy, A. Chapus, S. Mihoubi, Y. Durocher, and B. Cass. Combined Inhibition of Pdgf and Vegf Receptors by Ellagic Acid, a Dietary-Derived Phenolic Compound. *Carcinogenesis* (2005):26:821–826.

Lake, A., and T. Townshend. Obesogenic Environments: Exploring the Built and Food Environments. *J of the Royal Society for the Prom of Health* (2006):126:261–267.

Lamy, S., M. Blanchette, J. Michaud-Levesque, R. Lafleur, Y. Durocher, and A. Moghrabi. Delphinidin, a Dietary Anothocyanidin, Inhibits Vascular Endothelial Growth Factor Receptor-2 Phosphorylation. *Carcinogenesis* (2006):27:989–996.

Lang, T., and E. Millstone, editors. *The Atlas of Food*. London, U.K.: Earthscan Publications Limited (2002).

Larson, N.I., M.T. Story, and M.C. Nelson. Neighborhood Environments—Disparities in Access to Healthy Foods in the U.S. *Am J Prev Med* (2009).

Larsson, S.C., M. Kumlin, M. Ingelman-Sundberg, and A. Wolk. Dietary Long-Chain N-3 Fatty Acids for the Prevention of Cancer: A Review of Potential Mechanisms. *Am J Clin Nutr* (2004):79:935–945.

Lee, S., K.M. Gura, S. Kim, D.A. Arsenault, B.R. Bistrian, and M. Puder. Current Clinical Applications of Omega-6 and Omega-3 Fatty Acids. *Nutr Clin Pract* (2006):4:323–341.

Levy, A.S., and R.C. Stokes. Effects of a Health Promotion Advertising Campaign on Sales of Ready-to-Eat Cereals. *Public Health Rep* (1987):102:398–403.

Lichtenstein, A.H., L.J. Appel, M. Brands, et al. Diet and Lifestyle Recommendations Revision 2006: A Scientific Statement from the American Heart Association Nutrition Committee. *Circulation* (2006):114:82–96.

Lichtenstein, A.H., L.M. Ausman, S.M. Jalbert, M. Vilella-Bach, M. Jauhiainen, S. McGladdery, A.T. Erkkila, C. Ehnholm, J. Frohlich, and E.J. Schaefer. Efficacy of a Therapeutic Lifestyle Change/Step 2 Diet in Moderately Hypercholesterolemic Middle-Aged and Elderly Female and Male Subjects. *J Lipid Res* (2002):43:264–273.

Liu, S., J.E. Manson, I.M. Lee, S.R. Cole, C.H. Hennekens, W.C. Willett, and J.E. Buring. Fruit and Vegetable Intake and Risk of Cardiovascular Disease: The Women's Health Study. *Am J Clin Nutr* (2000):72:922–928.

Lobstein, T., and S. Dibb. Evidence of a Possible Link between Obesogenic Food Advertising and Child Overweight. *Obes Rev* (2005):6:203–208.

Lorenzen, J.K., S. Nielsen, J.J. Holst, I. Tetens, J.F. Rehfeld, and A. Astrup. Effect of Dairy Calcium or Supplementary Calcium Intake on Postprandial Fat Metabolism, Appetite, and Subsequent Energy Intake. *Am J Clin Nutr* (2007):85:678–687.

Lund, E.K., S.G. Wharf, S.J. Fairweather-Tait, and I.T. Johnson. Oral Ferrous Sulfate Supplements Increase the Free Radical-Generating Capacity of Feces from Healthy Volunteers. *Am J Clin Nutr* (1999):16:250–255.

MacFarlane, A., D. Crawford, K. Ball, G. Savige, and A. Worsley. Adolescent Home Food Environments and Socioeconomic Position. *Asia Pac J Clin Nutr* (2007):16:748–756.

Maddock, J., C. Maglione, J.D. Barnett, C. Cabot, S. Jackson, and B. Reger-Nash. Statewide Implementation of the 1% or Less Campaign. *Health Educ Behavior* (2007):34:953–963.

Malik, V.S., M.B. Schulze, and F.B. Hu. Intake of Sugar-Sweetened Beverages and Weight Gain: A Systematic Review. *Am J Clin Nutr* (2006):84:274–288.

Marshall, T.A., S.M. Levy, B. Broffitt, J.J. Warren, J.M. Eichenberger-Gilmore, T.L. Burns, and P.J. Stumbo. Dental Caries and Beverage Consumption in Young Children. *Pediatrics* (2003):112:184–191.

Matson-Koffman, D.M., J.N. Brownstein, J.A. Neiner, and M.L. Greaney. A Site-Specific Literature Review of Policy and Environmental Interventions that Promote Physical Activity and Nutrition for Cardiovascular Health: What Works? *Am J Health Promot* (2005):19:167–193.

McAlister, A. Behavioral Journalism: Beyond the Marketing Model for Health Communication. *Am J Health Promot* (1995):9:417–420.

Mehta, N., and V. Chang. Weight Status and Restaurant Availability—A Multilevel Analysis. *Am J Prev Med* (2008):34:127–113.

Mensink, R.P., P.L. Zock, A.D. Kester, and M.B. Katan. Effects of Dietary Fatty Acids and Carbohydrates on the Ratio of Serum Total to Hdl Cholesterol and on Serum Lipids and Apolipoproteins: A Meta-Analysis of 60 Controlled Trials. *Am J Clin Nutr* (2003):77:1146–1155.

Michels K.B., G. Edward, K.J. Joshipura, et al. Prospective Study of Fruit and Vegetable Consumption and Incidence of Colon and Rectal Cancers. *J Natl Cancer Inst* (2000):92:1740–1752.

Miller, P. *Statement of Patti Miller, Vice President, Children Now FCC Task Force on Media and Childhood Obesity* (2007). Available at http://www.fcc.gov/obesity/march07meeting/Miller.pdf. Accessed January 20, 2009.

Mokdad, A.H. Correction: Actual Causes of Death in the United States, 2000. *JAMA* (2005):293(3):293–294.

Mokdad, A.H., J.S. Marks, D.F. Stroup, and J.L. Gerberding. Actual Causes of Death in the United States, 2000. *JAMA* (2004):291:1238–1245.

Moore, L.V., A.V. Diez Roux, J.A. Nettleton, and D.R. Jacobs. Associations of the Local Food Environment and Diet Quality—A Comparison of Assessments Based on Surveys and Geographic Information Systems. *Am J Epidemiol* (2008):167(8):917–924.

Morland, K., S. Wing, and A. Diez Roux. The Contextual Effect of the Local Food Environment on Residents' Diets: The Atherosclerosis Risk in Communities Study. *Am J Public Health* (2002):92:1761–1767.

Nagengast, F.M., M.J. Grubben, and I.P. van Munster. Role of Bile Acids in Colorectal Carcinogenesis. *Eur J Cancer* (1995):31A:1067–1070.

Naumann, E., A.B. vanRees, G. Onning, R. Oste, M. Wydra, and R.P. Mensink. Beta-Glucan Incorporated into a Fruit Drink Effectively Lowers Serum LDL-Cholesterol Concentrations. *Am J Clin Nutr* (2006):83:601–605.

Neumark-Sztainer, D., M. Wal, C. Perry, and M. Story. Correlates of Fruit and Vegetable Intake among Adolescents. Findings from Project EAT. *Prev Med* (2003):37:198–208.

Nicklas, T.A., C.C. Johnson, R. Farris, R. Rice, L. Lyon, and R. Shi. Development of a School-Based Nutrition Intervention for High School Students: Gimme 5. *Am J Health Promot* (1997):11:315–322.

Nielsen, S.J., and B.M. Popkin. Patterns and Trends in Food Portion Sizes. *JAMA* (2003):289(4):450–453.

National Institutes of Health (NIH). State-of-the-Science Conference Statement on Multivitamin/Mineral Supplements and Chronic Disease Prevention. *Ann Intern Med* (2006):145:364–371.

Obarzanek, E., F.M. Sacks, W.M. Vollmer, et al., and DASH Research Group. Effects on Blood Lipids of a Blood-Pressure–Lowering Diet: The Dietary Approaches to Stop Hypertension (DASH) Trial. *Am J Clin Nutr* (2001):74:80–89.

O'Neil, C.E., and T.A. Niklas. Gimme 5: An Innovative, School-Based Nutrition Intervention for High School Students. *J Am Diet Assoc* (2002):102.3:S93(4).

Oster, G., and D. Thompson. Estimated Effects of Reducing Dietary Saturated Fat on the Incidence and Costs of Coronary Heart Disease in the United States. *J Am Diet Assoc* (1996):96:127–131.

Pereira, M.A., E. O.'Reilly, K. Augustsson, et al. Dietary Fiber and Risk of Coronary Heart Disease: A Pooled Analysis of Cohort Studies. *Arch Intern Med* (2004):164:370–376.

Perry, C.L., D.B. Bishop, G. Taylor, D.M. Murray, R.W. Mays, B.S. Dudovitz, M. Smyth, and M. Story. Changing Fruit and Vegetable Consumption among Children: The 5-a-Day Power Plus Program in St. Paul, Minnesota. *Am J Pub Health* (1998):88:603–609.

Pomerleau, J., K. Lock, C. Knai, and M. McKee. Interventions Designed to Increase Adult Fruit and Vegetable Intake Can Be Effective: A Systematic Review of the Literature. *J of Nutr* (2005):135:2486–2495.

Popkin, B.M., and S.J. Nielsen. The Sweetening of the World's Diet. *Obes Res* (2003):11:1325–1332.

Pothukuchi, K. Attracting Supermarkets to Inner-City Neighborhoods: Economic Development Outside the Box. *Econ Dev Q* (2005):19:232–244.

Powell, L.M., S. Slater, D. Mirtcheva, Y. Bao, and F.J. Chaloupka. Food Store Availability and Neighborhood Characteristics in the United States. *Prev Med* (2007):44:189–195.

Prentice, A.M., and S.A. Jebb. Fast Foods, Energy Density, and Obesity: A Possible Mechanistic Link. *Obes Rev* (2003):4:187–194.

Putnam, J. Major Trends in the US Food Supply. *Food Rev* (2000):23:13.

Rankinen, T., and C. Bouchard. Genetics of Food Intake and Eating Behavior Phenotypes in Humans. *Annu Rev Nutr* (2006):26:413–434.

Rayner, G., D. Barling, and T. Lang. Sustainable Food Systems in Europe: Policies, Realities, and Futures. *J Hunger Environ Nutr* (2/3, 2008):3:145–168.

Reger, B., M. Wootan, and S. Booth-Butterfield. Using Mass Media to Promote Healthy Eating: A Community-Based Demonstration Project. *Prev Med* (1999):29:414–421.

Reger, B., M. Wootan, S. Booth-Butterfield, and H. Smith. 1% or Less: A Community Based Nutrition Campaign. *Public Health Rep* (1998):113:410–419.

Reger, B., M.G. Wootan, and S. Booth-Butterfield. A Comparison of Different Approaches to Promote Community-Wide Dietary Change. *Am J Prev Med* (2000):18:271–275.

Rolls, B.J., J.A. Ello-Martin, and B.C. Tohill. What Can Intervention Studies Tell Us About the Relationship between Fruit and Vegetable Consumption and Weight Management? *Nutr Rev* (2004):62:1–17.

Rozin, P. Food Preference. In: Smelser, N.J., and P.B. Baltes, editors, *International Encyclopedia of the Social and Behavioral Sciences*. Oxford: Elsevier (2001):5719–5722.

Satia, J.A., J.A. Galanko, and A.M. Siega-Riz. Eating at Fast-Food Restaurants Is Associated with Dietary Intake, Demographic, Psychosocial, and Behavioral Factors among African Americans in North Carolina. *Public Health Nutr* (2004):7:1089–1096.

Schoonover, H. *A Fair Farm Bill for Public Health. Inst. Agric. Trade Policy* (2007). Available at http://www.iatp.org/iatp/publications.cfm?accountID=258&refID=98598. Accessed December 27, 2008.

Simon, J.A., G.B. Schreiber, P.B. Crawford, M.M. Frederick, and Z.I. Sabry. Dietary Vitamin C and Serum Lipids in Black and White Girls. *Epidemiol* (1993):4:537–542.

Sloane, D.C., A.L. Diamant, L.B. Lewis, et al. Improving the Nutritional Resource Environment for Healthy Living Through Community-Based Participatory Research. *J Gen Intern Med* (2003):18:568–575.

Shaikh, R.A., A. Yaroch, L. Nebeling, M.C. Yeh, and K. Resnicow. Psychosocial Predictors of Fruit and Vegetable Consumption in Adults. *Am J Prev Med* (2008):34:535–543.

Shepherd, R. Influences on Food Choice and Dietary Behavior. *Diet Diversification and Health Promotion*. Forum Nutr. Basel, Karger (2005)57:36–43.

Shepherd, J., A. Harden, R. Rees, G. Brunton, J. Garcia, S. Oliver, and A. Oakley. Young People and Healthy Eating: A Systematic Review of Research on Barriers and Facilitators. *Health Edu Res* (2006):21:239–257.

Sorensen, G., A.M. Stoddard, T. Dubowitz, E.M. Barbeau, J. Bigby, K.M. Emmons, L.F. Berkman, and K.E. Peterson. The Influence of Social Context on Changes in Fruit and Vegetable Consumption: Results of the Healthy Directions Studies. *Am J Pub Health* (2007):97:1216–1227.

Stables, G.J., A.F. Subar, B.H. Patterson, K. Dodd, J. Heimendinger, M.A. Van Duyn, and L. Nebeling. Changes in Vegetable and Fruit Consumption and Awareness among U.S. Adults: Results of the 1991 and 1997 5 a Day for Better Health Program Surveys. *J Am Diet Assoc* (2002):102:809–817.

Story, M., K.M. Kaphingst, R. Robinson-O'Brien, and K. Glanz. Creating Healthy Food and Eating Environments: Policy and Environmental Approaches. *Annu Rev Public Health* (2008):29:253–272.

Suarez, F.L., D. Savaiano, P. Arbisi, and M.D. Levitt. Tolerance to the Daily Ingestion of Two Cups of Milk by Individuals Claiming Lactose Intolerance. *Am J Clin Nutr* (1997):65:1502–1506.

Swinburn, B., G. Egger, and F. Raza. Dissecting Obesogenic Environments: The Development and Application of a Framework for Identifying and Prioritizing Environmental Interventions for Obesity. *Prev Med* (1999):6 pt 1:563–570.

The Keystone Center. Final Report. May 2006. The Keystone Forum on Away From Home Foods: Opportunities for Preventing Weight Gain and Obesity. Available at http://www.keystone.org/spp/documents/Forum_Report_FINAL_5-30-06.pdf. Accessed December 24, 2008.

Thomson, M., J.C. Spence, K. Raine, and L. Laing. The Association of Television Viewing with Snacking Behavior and Body Weight of Young Adults. *Am J Health Promot* (2008):22:329–335.

Tohill, B.C., J.D. Seymour, M.K. Serdula, L. Kettel-Khan, and B.J. Rolls. What Epidemiologic Studies Tell Us About the Relationship between Fruit and Vegetable Consumption and Body Weight. *Nutr Rev* (2004):62:365–374.

U.S. Government Account Office. School Meal Programs: Competitive Foods Are Widely Available and Generate Substantial Revenues for Schools. *Report GAO—05–563* (2005).

U.S. Department of Agriculture (USDA). Mypyramid. Available at www.mypyramid.gov.

U.S. Department of Agriculture (USDA). *Factsheet on What We Eat in America NHANES* (2005–2006). Available at http://www.ars.usda.gov/Services/docs.htm?docid=17041. Accessed January 6, 2009.

U.S. Department of Agriculture (USDA), Center for Nutrition Policy and Promotion. *Healthy Eating Index* (2005). Available at http://www.cnpp.usda.gov/Publications/HEI/healthyeatingindex2005factsheet.pdf. Accessed January 3, 2009.

U.S. Department of Health and Human Services (USDHHS). *Healthy People 2010. Volume II. Conference Edition.* Washington, D.C.: U.S. Department of Health and Human Services (2000).

Utter, J., R. Scragg, D. Schaaf, and C.N. Mhurchu. Relationships between Frequency of Family Meals, BMI, and Nutritional Aspects of the Home Food Environment among New Zealand Adolescents. *Int J Behav Nutr Phys Act* (2008):5:50.

Van der Horst, K., A. Oenema, I. Ferreira, et al. A Systematic Review of Environmental Correlates of Obesity-Related Dietary Behaviors in Youth. *Health Educ Res* (2006):22:203–226.

Van Duyn, M.A., and E. Pivonka. Overview of the Health Benefits of Fruit and Vegetable Consumption for the Dietetics Professional: Selected Literature. *J Am Diet Assoc* (2000):100:1511–1521.

Vos, M.B., J.E. Kimmons, C. Gillespie, J. Welsh, and H.M. Blanck. Dietary Fructose Consumption among U.S. Children and Adults: The Third National Health and Nutrition Examination Survey. *Medscape J Med* (2008):10(7):160.

Westenhoefer, J. Age and Gender Dependent Profile of Food Choice. *Forum Nutr* (2005):57:44–51.

Wiecha, J.L., K.E. Peterson, D.S. Ludwig, J. Kim, A. Sobol, and S.L. Gortmaker. When Children Eat What They Watch: Impact of Television Viewing on Dietary Intake in Youth. *Arch Pediatr Adolesc Med* (2006):160:436–442.

Willett, W.C. *Nutritional Epidemiology* (2nd ed.). New York, NY: Oxford University Press (1998).

Wootan, M.G., and M. Osborn. Availability of Nutritional Information from Chain Restaurants in the United States. *Am J Prev Med* (2006):30:266–268.

World Cancer Research Fund/American Institute for Cancer Research. *Food, Nutrition, Physical Activity, and the Prevention of Cancer: A Global Perspective.* Washington, D.C.: AICR (2007).

World Health Organization (WHO). *World Health Report 2000.* Geneva, Switzerland: WHO (2000).

World Health Organization (WHO). *The World Health Report 2002. Reducing Risks, Promoting Healthy Life.* Geneva, Switzerland: WHO (2002).

World Health Organization (WHO). Global Strategy on Diet, Physical Activity, and Health: Fifty-Seventh World Health Assembly. Resolution WHA56.17. Geneva, Switzerland: WHO (2004).

World Health Organization (WHO). Diet, Nutrition, and the Prevention of Chronic Disease. Report of a Joint FAO/WHO Expert Consultation. WHO Technical Report Series No 916. Geneva, Switzerland: WHO (2003).

World Health Organization (WHO). Closing the Gap in a Generation: Health Equity Through Action on the Social Determinants of Death. Final Report of the Commission on the Social Determinants of Health (2008).

Wright, J.D., J. Kennedy-Stephenson, C.Y. Wang, M.A. McDowell, and C.L. Johnson. Trends in Intake of Energy and Macronutrients—United States, 1971–2000. *MMWR* (2004):53:80–82.

Yancey, A.K., S.K. Kumanyika, N.A. Ponce, W.J. McCarthy, J.E. Fielding, J.P. Leslie, and J. Akbar. Population-Based Interventions Engaging Communities of Color in Healthy Eating and Active Living: A Review. *Prev Chronic Dis* (2004a):1:1–18.

Yancey, A.K., A.M. Raines, W.J. McCarthy, et al. The Los Angeles Lift Off: A Sociocultural Environmental Change Intervention to Increase Workplace Physical Activity. *Prev Med* (2004b):38(6):848–856.

Zemel, M.B. Role of Calcium and Dairy Products in Energy Partitioning and Weight Management. *Am J Clin Nutr* (2004):79:907S–912S.

Zimmerman, M.B., N. Chaouki, and R.F. Hurrell. Iron Deficiency Due to Consumption of a Habitual Diet Low in Bioavailable Iron: A Longitudinal Cohort Study in Morroccan Children. *Am J Clin Nutr* (2005):81:115–121.

CHAPTER 7

PHYSICAL ACTIVITY
(ICD-10 Z72.3)

Barbara E. Ainsworth, Ph.D., M.P.H., F.A.C.S.M. and
Caroline A. Macera, Ph.D., F.A.C.S.M.

Introduction

The importance of being physically active has been repeatedly shown in countless studies of various populations. Physically active people have longer life expectancy and are less likely to be diagnosed with chronic diseases such as diabetes, heart disease, and some cancers. In 1996, the first Report of the Surgeon General on Physical Activity and Health summarized the many health benefits associated with physical activity and suggested that the minimum level of physical activity required to achieve health benefits was a daily expenditure of 150 kilocalories in moderate or vigorous activities (USDHHS 1996). This recommendation is consistent with a 1995 consensus statement issued by the Centers for Disease Control and Prevention (CDC) and American College of Sports Medicine recommending that every adult should accumulate at least 30 minutes of moderate activity most days of the week (Pate et al. 1995). In 2007, the American College of Sports Medicine and the American Heart Association issued an updated consensus statement that reaffirmed and clarified the minimal amount of physical activity needed to achieve health benefits (Haskell et al. 2007). The consensus panel recommended that all adults participate in 30 minutes of moderate-intensity (aerobic) physical activity for a minimum of 30 minutes for five days per week or vigorous-intensity physical activity for a minimum of 20 minutes per day for three days per week. A companion statement was issued for older adults that included recommendations for muscle-strengthening activity, reducing sedentary behavior, and risk management (Nelson et al. 2007).

The causes of physical inactivity, its consequences, and populations at high risk are summarized in Figure 7.1 and described in detail below.

Consequences

The consequences of physical inactivity are felt among many dimensions of health including physical, physiological, psychological, and societal. Regular physical activity performed on most days of the week reduces the risk of dying prematurely, developing coronary heart disease, diabetes, and colon cancer (USDHHS 1996). Regular activity also reduces blood pressure among people with hypertension (Ainsworth et al. 1991), promotes psychological well-being, and builds and maintains healthy bones, muscles, and joints so that older adults can avoid falls and maintain functional independence (USDHHS 1996).

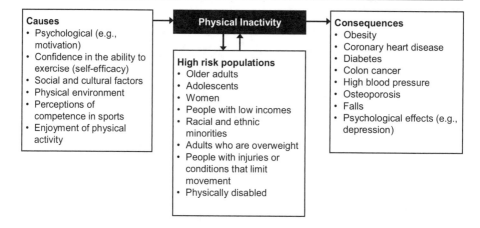

Figure 7.1. Physical inactivity: causes, consequences, and high-risk groups.

People who are not physically active are at twice the risk of dying from coronary heart disease than people who are physically active (Powell et al. 1987). This effect is similar to that of well-established risk factors such as cigarette smoking, increased systolic blood pressure, and elevated serum cholesterol. A study published in the *Journal of the American Medical Association* (*JAMA*) in 2004 estimated that 400,000 U.S. deaths in 2000 (16.6% of all U.S. deaths) were attributed to physical inactivity and poor nutrition (defined as obesity), while 435,000 (18.1%) were attributed to tobacco (Mokdad et al. 2004). One reason for the major impact this risk factor has on mortality is its prevalence. While less than 30% of adults use tobacco, twice that many are not physically active at levels necessary to obtain health benefits.

Using available estimates of the prevalence of physical inactivity and the coronary heart disease risk associated with physical inactivity, it has been suggested that approximately 35% of coronary heart disease mortality is due to physical inactivity (Macera and Powell 2001). This is particularly important because coronary heart disease is the leading cause of death in the United States, and for every person who dies of coronary heart disease, many others are disabled, often for many years.

The major economic impact of physical inactivity is felt through medical expenditures and loss of income and productivity associated with disease and disability. A study published in 2004 estimated that the burden of cardiovascular disease associated with physical inactivity was 23.7 billion dollars in direct medical expenditures in 2001 (Wang et al. 2004). These figures did not include associated costs of lost income.

The low prevalence of physical activity is a significant public health problem that affects various populations, multidimensional in its scope, and interdependent on other factors that may compound its effects. Actions are needed at the personal, social, economic, scientific, legal, and policy levels to reduce the prevalence of physical inactivity in the United States.

Pathophysiology

Several terms, shown in Table 7.1, are used to characterize human movement. *Physical activity* refers to any bodily movement that increases energy expenditure (Caspersen

Table 7.1. Definitions Used to Characterize Human Movement

Term	Definition
Physical activity (PA)	Bodily movement that is produced by the contraction of skeletal muscle and that substantially increases energy expenditure (Casperen 1989). • Occupational • Nonoccupational (leisure, family, transportation, household, other activities)
Exercise	Planned, structured, and repetitive bodily movement done to improve or maintain one or more components of physical fitness (Casperen 1989).
Physical fitness	A set of attributes that people have or achieve that relates to the ability to perform physical activity (Casperen 1989). The ability to carry out daily tasks with vigor and alertness, without undue fatigue, and with ample energy to enjoy leisure-time pursuits and to meet unforeseen emergencies (American College of Sports Medicine 1990). The ability to perform moderate to vigorous levels of physical activity without undue fatigue and the capability of maintaining such ability throughout life (Bouchard, Shepard, and Stephens 1994). Components of health-related fitness (deVries and Housh 1994). • *Cardiorespiratory*: submaximal exercise capacity, maximal aerobic power, heart and lung functions, blood pressure • *Muscular*: power, strength, endurance • *Metabolic*: glucose tolerance, insulin sensitivity, lipid and lipoprotein metabolism, substrate oxidation characteristics, motor • *Morphological*: body mass for height, body composition, subcutaneous fat distribution, abdominal visceral fat, bone density, flexibility • *Motor*: agility, balance, coordination, speed of movement, reaction time
Frequency	The times an activity is performed in a selected period (e.g., 1 week) (Ainsworth et al. 2000; Bouchard, Shepard, and Stephens 1994).
Duration	The minutes or hours one engages in physical activity (Ainsworth et al. 2000; Bouchard, Shepard, and Stephens 1994).
Intensity	The energy cost of performing an activity (Ainsworth et al. 2000; Bouchard, Shepard, and Stephens 1994). • *METs*: The activity metabolic cost divided by the resting metabolic rate • *MET-minutes*: The activity MET level × minutes of participation • *Kilocalories*: Met-minutes × (body weight in kilograms/60 kg) • *Light intensity*: Physical activities < 3 METs • *Moderate intensity*: Physical activities from 3 to 6 METs • *Vigorous intensity*: Physical activities > 6 METs

(continued on next page)

Table 7.1. (*continued*)

Term	Definition
Activity dose	A threshold for physical activity associated with health benefits. It is generally expressed in terms of energy expenditure, frequency, intensity, or duration (Ainsworth et al. 2000; Bouchard, Shepard, and Stephens 1994).
Leisure	Activities done in a setting that include the elements of free choice, freedom from constraints, intrinsic motivation, enjoyment, relaxation, personal involvement, and self-expression (Henderson et al. 1996).
Occupation PA	Activities done during paid employment.
Transportation PA	Physical activity performed when traveling to a destination.
Household PA	Activities performed for the care and maintenance of the home.
Family PA	Activities performed in the care for others.

1989). This is contrasted with the term *exercise*, which is planned, structured, and repetitive physical activity done to improve or maintain one or more of the components of physical fitness (American College of Sports Medicine 1990; Caspersen 1989). *Physical fitness* is a set of attributes that allows individuals to carry out daily tasks without undue fatigue. Components of health-related fitness include cardiorespiratory, muscular, metabolic, morphological, and motor (Bouchard, Shephard, and Stephens 1994). The terms *frequency, duration,* and *intensity* of an activity are used to measure the *activity dose* or the threshold level of physical activity associated with health benefits (Ainsworth et al. 2000; American College of Sports Medicine 1990; Bouchard, Shephard, and Stephens 1994; deVries and Housh 1994).

Another term that is often used concerning physical activity is *leisure*, as in leisure-time physical activity (also called recreational physical activity). This term applies to physical activities that include the elements of free choice, freedom from constraints, intrinsic motivation, enjoyment, relaxation, personal involvement, and self-expression (Henderson et al. 1996). Other domains for physical activity include *occupation, transportation, household,* and *family care* physical activity. Incorporating physical activity into all domains should be encouraged, as small amounts of activity accumulated throughout the day can have a positive impact for weight control (Levine et al. 2005). However, leisure-time physical activity is a behavior that should be encouraged, as these activities are likely to become habits that endure throughout life.

Physical activity affects all body systems associated with energy production, metabolism, and bodily movement. Table 7.2 shows the acute and chronic changes in body systems and associated disease risks following moderate amounts of physical activity. Acute changes refer to the immediate adaptations in body systems during a physical activity period. Chronic changes refer to long-term adaptations in body systems resulting from

Table 7.2. Acute and Chronic Changes Associated with Disease Risk Following Moderate Amounts of Physical Activity

System	Acute Changes	Chronic Changes
Cardiovascular	↑Heart rate ↓Resting heart rate ↑Stroke volume ↑Maximal stroke volume ↑Cardiac output ↑Maximal cardiac output ↑Systolic blood pressure ↑Hemoglobin ↑Blood volume ↓Blood pressure in hypertensives ↑Blood clot lysis ↓Thrombosis	↓CHD risk ↓Stroke risk ↑CHD rehabilitation ↓Symptoms of claudication
Pulmonary	↑Breath rate and depth ↓Breath rate for submax activity ↑Oxygen diffusion ↑Dilatation of airways	↑Pulmonary rehabilitation
Neuromuscular	↑Rate of nerve impulses ↑Mobility ↑Oxygen utilization ↑Mitochondria ↑Anaerobic enzymes ↑Aerobic enzymes	↑Size of motor nerves ↑Size of muscle fibers ↑Strength ↑Aerobic capacity ↑Functional independence ↑Fat and carbohydrate utilization ↑Muscle flexibility
Skeletal	↑Bone mass and density ↑Tendon and ligament strength	↓Osteoporosis bone loss ↓Risk of joint injury
Endocrine	↑Release of hormones from pituitary (most), adrenal, thyroid, parathyroid, kidney, ovaries, testes, pancreas (glucagon and insulin), endorphins ↓Release of glucose during activity ↓Adrenaline release during rest	↑Sensitivity of muscles to insulin ↓Diabetes ↑Psychological well-being
Metabolic	↓Body fat stores ↑Muscle mass ↑Ratio of lipid:carbohydrate oxidation ↑HDL-cholesterol ↓Triglycerides	↓Obesity ↓Cancer

(continued on next page)

Table 7.2. (*continued*)

System	Acute Changes	Chronic Changes
Immune	↑Resistance to illness ↑Leukocyte distribution ↑Lymphocyte proliferation ↑Innate immunity ↑Humoral immunity ↑Cytokines and cytotoxicity	↓Cancer ↓Acute illness ↓Atherosclerosis and CHD

Note: Data from Bouchard et al. (1994) and Ainsworth et al. (2000). CHD indicates coronary heart disease.

regular participation over time (Bouchard, Shephard, and Stephens 1994; deVries and Housh 1994). The time required for physical activity participation to produce chronic changes in the body may range from one week (in the neuromuscular system) to several years (some metabolic hormones and enzymes).

Regular physical activity reduces risk factors for coronary heart disease by raising high-density lipoprotein-cholesterol, lowering triglycerides, lowering resting and exercise blood pressures, and increasing blood clot dissolving mechanisms. Among people with coronary heart disease, regular physical activity can reduce the threshold for angina pectoris during physical activity and reduce the risks for sudden death. Regular physical activity is inversely associated with obesity and glucose-insulin intolerance and is positively associated with immune function, muscular strength, mobility, psychological well-being, and increased bone mass. Through modifications of these intermediate factors, regular physical activity can reduce the risks for diabetes mellitus, depression, injuries, osteoporosis, and some forms of cancer associated with immune deficiencies and excess body fat (USDHHS 1996).

The disease risk-reducing and health-enhancing effects of regular, moderate physical activity involve the integration of many body systems. Adaptations to body systems are specific to the imposed demands of the physical activity stress (deVries and Housh 1994). This is called the SAID principle (Specific Adaptations to Imposed Demands). Types of physical activities that impose the greatest stress on most systems simultaneously are aerobic (moderate or vigorous intensity), weight bearing, and resistance activities. These activities include brisk walking, gardening, home repair, most sports and conditioning activities, manual labor occupations, and vigorous house cleaning (Ainsworth et al. 2000).

Bouchard, Shepard, and Stephens (1994) describe the relationships among habitual physical activity, health-related fitness, and health status. Health-related fitness refers to changes in morphological, muscular, motor, cardiorespiratory, and metabolic systems due to regular physical activity. Components in the health-related fitness model are modified by levels of physical activity, health status, heredity, and other factors, such as lifestyle behaviors, personal attributes, and physical and social environments. Regular physical activity can provide a direct effect on health-related fitness, as observed in Table 7.2, or may indirectly modify health-related fitness levels through other changes in health status.

Distribution

Using a surveillance system can help to monitor the "distribution" of physical activity among the general population and to develop and evaluate interventions (Bauman et al. 2006). The national surveys already in place provide a framework from which to collect data regularly. However, physical activity surveillance systems must be updated regularly to provide sufficient information on a variety of physical activities to assure that prevalence data on activity patterns and trends are meaningful and complete. Previous surveillance systems focused on sports and conditioning activities, but many have been updated to provide more information on occupation, transportation, sex-, and ethnic-specific physical activities (NCHSa, CDCa, CDCb). Such activities may include walking, lifting and carrying activities during work, walking and cycling to and from work, family care and household activities, and activities relating to religious and cultural traditions.

Two major population-based surveys measure nonoccupational physical activity among U.S. adults. The *National Health Interview Survey* (NHIS) is a household interview conducted by the National Center for Health Statistics on a representative sample of noninstitutionalized adults aged 18 years and older (NCHSa). Questions on physical activity were included in 1985, 1990, 1991, and 1995. In 1997, the questions were modified and they have been included every year since. These questions include the frequency, self-assessed intensity, and duration of the activity over the past two weeks.

The Behavioral Risk Factor Surveillance System (BRFSS) is a telephone-administered survey conducted monthly by participating states in collaboration with the CDC (CDCa). National estimates are developed from state-specific data. The BRFSS included physical activity items from 1986 through 1992 and in even years from 1994 to 2000 and every odd year from 2001. Questions include the type, frequency, and duration of leisure-time physical activity during the past month. Intensity measures were estimated depending on the type of activity and the age of the respondent. In 2001, modifications to the questions focused on measuring lifestyle activities rather than specific sports. The intensity of the activities (housework, yard work, walking, etc.) was self-assessed as "moderate intensity" if it required an increase in heart rate or breathing or "vigorous intensity" if it required a large increase in heart rate or breathing. In addition to these questions, there has been one question assessing participation in any leisure-time physical activity (yes/no) that has been asked each year since 1984. In 2002, the BRFSS initiated the Selected Metropolitan/Micropolitan Area Risk Trends (SMART) project to analyze BRFSS data of 170 selected metropolitan and micropolitan statistical areas with 500 or more respondents. These data can be used to identify emerging health problems, establish and track health objectives, and develop and evaluate public health policies and programs within targeted areas of the United States (CDCb).

There a few national surveys designed to obtain information on the physical activity patterns of adolescents. The *Youth Risk Behavior Survey* (YRBS) is self-administered through schools (9th through 12th grade) and in odd years starting in 1991 included questions about moderate and vigorous physical activities done in the past seven days as well as participation in school-based physical education programs (CDCc). The question that assessed vigorous physical activity asked how many days in the past seven days did they exercise or take part in sports that made them sweat or breathe hard. The question to assess moderate physical activity asked how many days in the past seven days did they ride a bicycle or walk for 30 minutes at a time. There have been no changes in moderate or vigorous physical activity patterns during the time this survey has been administered (CDCd). Other surveys are conducted as needed; for example, the *Youth Media Campaign Longitudinal Survey* (YMCLS) was conducted in 2002 to assess the effectiveness of the Youth Media Campaign in increasing levels of physical activity among children and adolescents (CDCe). The YMCLS is a national random-digit-dialed telephone survey of children aged 9–13 years and their parents. Participation in organized and free-time physical activity was assessed for the seven days preceding the survey. Parents were asked about their perceptions of five potential barriers to the children's participation in physical activity.

To determine and monitor the prevalence of physical activity, surveillance definitions have been established to determine groups that are achieving health-related benefits associated with physical activity. For most surveys, physical activity is divided into three general groups as noted (CDCf).

Recommended physical activity. Reported moderate-intensity activities in a usual week (i.e., brisk walking, bicycling, vacuuming, gardening, or anything else that causes small increases in breathing or heart rate) for greater than or equal to 30 minutes per day, greater than or equal to 5 days per week; vigorous-intensity activities in a usual week (i.e., running, aerobics, heavy yard work, or anything else that causes large increases in breathing or heart rate) for greater than or equal to 20 minutes per day, greater than or equal to 3 days per week; or both. This can be accomplished through lifestyle activities (i.e., household, transportation, or leisure-time activities).

Insufficient physical activity. Doing more than 10 minutes total per week of moderate or vigorous-intensity lifestyle activities (i.e., household, transportation, or leisure-time activity) but less than the recommended level of activity.

Inactivity. Less than 10 minutes total per week of moderate or vigorous intensity lifestyle activities (i.e., household, transportation, or leisure-time activity).

High-Risk Groups

Results from the surveys described above consistently report that the prevalence of physical inactivity increases with age and is higher among women and ethnic minorities as compared with men and white populations (see Figure 7.1) (CDCa; NCHSa; USDHHS 1996). In Table 7.3, the prevalence of regular physical activity is shown for adult men and women by age. About 30% of men and women age 18 years and older participated in recommended levels of moderate or vigorous activity in 2007 (NCHSb). Among men, the prevalence of physical activity is highest among those between the ages of 18 and 24 years (41%) and lowest among those age 75 years and older (19%). Similarly, among women, the prevalence of physical activity was highest among those aged 18–24 years (34%) and lowest among those aged 75 years and older (14%).

Data from national surveys also identify U.S. adults who are at high risk for not achieving sufficient levels of physical activity. These are the physically disabled (CDC 2005a; USDHHS 1996) people with injuries (Carlson et al. 2006) or conditions that limit movement (Shih et al. 2006), older adults (Sapkota et al. 2005; USDHHS 1996), adolescents (Eaton et al. 2006), adults who are overweight (CDC 1996), women (CDC 2004a, 2005b, 2007; USDHHS 1996), ethnic minorities (CDC 2004b, 2005b), and people with low incomes (Eyler et al. 2003).

Although most of the national physical activity surveys focus on adults, physical inactivity among adolescents is of increasing concern. An expert panel, convened in 1994

Table 7.3. Percentage and 95% Confidence Interval of Self-Reported Regular Leisure-Time Physical Activity* by Age and Sex, Adults, United States, January to June 2007

Age (years)	Overall	Men	Women
18–24	37.0 (33.4–40.6)	40.6 (35.0–46.8)	33.5 (29.3–37.8)
25–64	31.9 (30.5–33.3)	31.6 (39.8–33.5)	32.2 (30.5–33.8)
65–74	24.5 (21.6–27.4)	28.7 (24.5–33.0)	20.9 (17.1–24.8)
75+	16.0 (13.2–18.8)	19.1 (14.5–23.8)	13.9 (11.0–16.9)
Total	30.7 (29.4–32.0)	31.8 (30.1–33.5)	29.8 (28.3–31.2)

Note: Adapted from National Center for Health Statistics, early release from the 2007 NHIS. (http://www.cdc.gov/nchs/data/nhis/earlyrelease/200712_07.pdf)
*Defined as engaging in light to moderate leisure-time physical activities for 30 or more minutes five or more times per week or engaging in vigorous leisure-time physical activities for 20 or more minutes, three or more times per week.

to examine physical activity requirements for adolescents, developed two guidelines: (1) adolescents should be physically active daily or nearly everyday as part of their lifestyles, and (2) adolescents should engage in three or more sessions per week of moderate vigorous activities that last at least 20 minutes (Sallis and Patrick 1994). While the detail necessary to assess adherence to these guidelines is not readily available, data from the 2005 YRBS indicates that more than 90% of children in grades nine through 12 participated in moderate or vigorous physical activity during the past seven days. Data from the 2002 YMCLS indicate that about 39% of children aged 9–13 years participate in organized physical activity, while 77% participate in free-time physical activity. Parents perceive expense to be a major barrier to their child's participation in physical activity (overall 47% report expense as a barrier), while lack of neighborhood safety was cited as a barrier for 16% of parents. These percentages significantly varied by income, education, and race/ethnicity (CDC 2003).

Geographic Distribution

Geographic variations in the prevalence of adults meeting recommended levels of physical activity in nonoccupational settings were found using data from the 2001 BRFSS (Reis et al. 2004). The prevalence was highest in the west (49%) and lowest in the south (43%). However, the area of the country may not be as important as the differences found in degree of urbanization (metro, large urban, small urban, and rural). In general, the highest prevalence of nonoccupational physical activity was found in large urban areas and the lowest prevalence was found in rural areas. However, further analysis of the data indicated that, even among urbanization levels, people living in the Midwest or the south were less active than people living in the west (Reis et al. 2004).

Another indication that geography may influence physical activity comes from studies relating characteristics of the physical environment (so-called built environment) to physical activity levels of the residents (Committee on Physical Activity, Health,

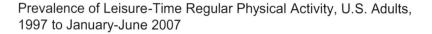

Transportation, and Land Use 2005). The built environment—the physical form of communities—includes land use patterns (the location of activities across space), large- and small-scale built and natural features (e.g., architectural details, quality of landscaping), and the transportation system (the facilities and services that link one location to another). A number of studies have shown that leisure walking and other leisure-time activities are positively associated with access to attractive open spaces and trails (Addy et al. 2004; Giles-Corti and Donovan 2003), availability of sidewalks, and satisfaction with the neighborhood environment (Ball et al. 2001; De Bourdeaudhuij, Sallis, and Saelens 2003), perceived personal safety (Giles-Corti et al. 2005; Wilson et al. 2004), and access to shopping malls for walking (Addy et al. 2004). Walking for transportation is higher in urban areas with street connectivity (Cevero and Duncan 2003; Giles-Corti et al. 2005; Greenwald and Boarnet 2001), in places where pedestrians are safe from traffic, and where one lives in a close proximity to destinations for shopping and work (Giles-Corti et al. 2005). Readers are directed to Saelens, Sallis, and Frank (2003), Owen et al. (2004), and Duncan, Spence, and Mummery (2005) for excellent reviews of this topic.

Time Trends

Although the benefits in physical activity have been well-known and promoted, the proportion of adults or adolescents who are regularly active has not changed over the

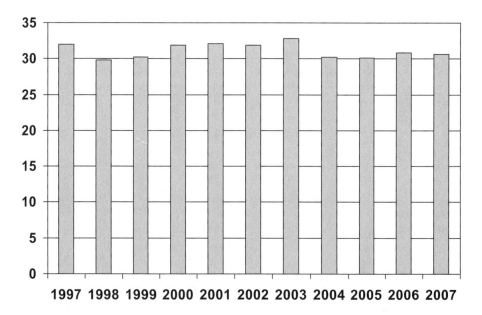

Figure 7.2. Trends in age-adjusted prevalence of regular leisure-time physical activity, adults, United States, 1997–2007. Source: http://www.cdc.gov/nchs/about/major/nhis/released200712.htm#7.

past few years (Brownson, Boehmer, and Luke 2005). As shown in Figure 7.2, the prevalence of regular activity increased slightly during the beginning of the decade but has gone back down to pre-2000 levels and has not changed much since 2004 (NCHSb). Based on available surveillance data, the trends are similar for adolescents (Eaton et al. 2006).

Causes

Modifiable Risk Factors

Identifying factors associated with a physically active lifestyle (also called determinants of physical activity) is important for the development of effective interventions. Although much work remains to be done, several investigators have suggested that correlates of behavior involve personal (i.e., age), psychological (i.e., motivation), confidence in the ability to exercise (self-efficacy), social and cultural factors, and the physical environment (Eyler et al. 2003). As for adults, correlates of physical activity behavior among youth and adolescents are not well identified but include confidence in one's ability to engage in exercise, perceptions of competence in sports, and enjoyment of physical activity (Heitzler et al. 2006; Van Der Horst et al. 2007).

Common barriers to physical activity are lack of time, motivation, social support, facilities, and knowledge of ways to become more physically active (CDC 2004b). Certain lifestyle characteristics may promote physical inactivity. These include commuting long distances to work (Zlot et al. 2006), sedentary jobs (Kruger et al. 2006), watching television (Koezuka et al. 2006), and using computers during leisure time (Zlot et al. 2006). However, more research is needed to understand lifestyle behaviors associated with physically inactive lifestyles.

Among women, fear of assault, cultural expectations, obligations to family care, and others are also cited as common barriers to being physically active. Women who work full-time and have home and family responsibilities report less physical activity than working women without family care responsibilities. Among minority women, additional barriers may include differences in native languages, acculturation issues, and economic status (CDC 2004b; Eyler et al. 2002).

Living in rural areas is associated with lower levels of leisure-time physical activity compared with living in urban areas (Parks, Housemann, and Brownson 2003; Reis et al. 2004; Wilcox et al. 2000). This may be due to differences in activity patterns that focus on activity patterns not captured on sport and recreation focused questionnaires (e.g., house, yard, and farm work, animal care) or not having environmental supports for leisure-time activity such as sidewalks, parks, and stores near one's home for transportation walking. More studies are needed to understand physical activity patterns of rural dwellers.

For some individuals, other health conditions may contribute to physical inactivity. Overweight status, chronic and infectious disease, injury, and physical disability may increase the energy cost of physical activity. The conditions may also prohibit being physically active. Often, inactivity due to existing health conditions or inaccessible facilities may create a positive feedback response by which the condition may worsen with decreased physical activity.

Population Attributable Risk

The proportion of physical inactivity attributable to the factors just described has not been estimated. Estimates could be made with more information about relative risks and the prevalence of exposure. For example, if 25% of adults live in communities without sidewalks and persons who live in a neighborhood without a sidewalk are twice as likely to be physically inactive, then about 20% of physical inactivity would be attributable to living in a neighborhood without sidewalks. See Chapter 2 for more information about population attributable risk.

Interventions

Prevention

As with any public health problem, prevention works best when operating at many levels: personal, medical, work site, school, and community. To guide prevention efforts and to measure the improvement in the risk profiles of the U.S. population, the government routinely develops national health objectives. The most recent document, *Healthy People 2010*, was published in 2000 and lists over 500 objectives in 28 focus areas (USDHHS 1991). These objectives provide baseline prevalence data and set 10-year targets for each objective. Table 7.4 shows the detail of Chapter 22, which relates to physical activity. Using data from the midcourse review, it appears as if these targets will not be met by the year 2010 (*Healthy People 2010 Midcourse Review*). Developing and modifying objectives for the next decade is an ongoing process. More information and opportunities for input are available at www.healthypeople.gov.

Strategies for improving physical activity among adults and children are summarized by U.S. Preventive Services Task Force (USPSTF) recommendations for clinical and community practice. *The Guide to Clinical Preventive Services* (the Clinical Guide, USPSTFa) provides updated counseling information for clinicians. This guide contains recommendations for prevention based on a review of evidence-based interventions to prevent 60 different illnesses and conditions. In the 2007 edition, it is concluded that there is insufficient evidence to recommend for or against behavioral counseling in primary care settings to promote physical activity. However, it is noted that multicomponent interventions combining provider advice in the form of patient goal setting, written exercise prescriptions, individually tailored physical activity regimes, with mailed or telephone follow-up assistance provided by specially trained staff are most effective in promoting physical activity behavior change. Further, the Clinical Guide notes that linking primary care patients to community-based physical activity programs provides the best setting to enhance primary care clinician counseling. Released in 2001, *The Guide to Community Preventive Services* (USPSTFb) provides evidence-based recommendations for programs and policies designed to promote population health in community settings. Reviewing intervention approaches for 16 behaviors and conditions, the guide is designed for use by public health professionals, legislators, and policymakers, community-based organizations, providers of health care services, researchers, and employers and other purchasers of health care services to promote public health. Recommended intervention approaches with sufficient to research show consistent and desired results. Intervention approaches with insufficient evidence are those that need more research showing consistent and

Table 7.4. Healthy People 2010 Risk Reduction Objectives Related to Physical Activity

	Objective	Baseline (%)	Target (%)
22-1	Reduce the proportion of adults who engage in no leisure-time physical activity	40	20
22-2	Increase the proportion of adults who engage in moderate physical activity for at least 30 minutes per day, five days or more per week or vigorous physical activity for at least 20 minutes per day, three days or days per week	32	50
22-3	Increase the proportion of adults who engage in vigorous physical activity that promotes the development and maintenance of cardiorespiratory fitness for at least 20 minutes per day, three days or more per week	23	30
22-4	Increase the proportion of adults who perform physical activities that enhance and maintain muscular strength and endurance	18	30
22-5	Increase the proportion of adults who perform physical activities that enhance and maintain flexibility	43	30
22-6	Increase the proportion of adolescents who engage in moderate physical activity for at least 30 minutes per day, five days or more per week	27	35
22-7	Increase the proportion of adolescents who engage in vigorous physical activity that promotes cardiorespiratory fitness, three days or more per week for 20 minutes or more per occasion	65	85
22-8a	Increase the proportion of the nation's public and private middle and junior high schools that require daily physical education for all students	6.4	9.4
22-8b	Increase the proportion of the nation's public and private high schools that require daily physical education for all students	5.8	14.5
22-9	Increase the proportion of adolescents who participate in daily school physical education	29	50
22-10	Increase the proportion of adolescents who spend at least 50% of school physical education class time being physically active	38	50
22-11	Increase the proportion of adolescents who view television two hours or fewer on a school day	57	75

(continued on next page)

Table 7.4. (*continued*)

	Objective	Baseline (%)	Target (%)
22-12	Increase the proportion of the nation's public and private schools that provide access to their physical activity spaces and facilities for all persons outside of normal school hours	35	50
22-13	Increase the proportion of work sites offering employer-sponsored physical activity and fitness programs	46	75
22-14a	Increase the proportion of trips made by walking (adults)	17	25
22-14b	Increase the proportion of trips made by walking (5–15 years)	31	50
22-15a	Increase the proportion of trips made by bicycling (adults)	0.6	2.0
22-15b	Increase the proportion of trips made by bicycling (5–15 years)	2.4	5.0

Note: Adapted from *Healthy People 2010 Midcourse Review,* http://www.healthypeople.gov/data/midcourse/pdf/FA22.pdf.

desired results. Recommended intervention approaches for physical activity are grouped into three areas: informational approaches, behavioral and social approaches, and environmental and policy approaches. A list of the types of recommended approaches and those with insufficient evidence for physical activity are highlighted in Table 7.5.

Environmental and Policy Factors

Understanding and modifying physical activity patterns is the first step in changing this behavior. Two public health approaches to increasing physical activity rely on environmental and policy strategies. Changes in public policy to promote physical activity often arise from grass roots community organizations designed to affect change at local, state, and national levels. However, in recent years, there have been increased coordinated efforts among public health, education, and advocacy groups to change policies for programs and facilities that promote regular physical activity in children and adults. Policy changes can be focused on removing environmental barriers for bicyclists and pedestrians, de-emphasizing automation, building more accessible facilities to enhance movement, requiring school physical education, redirecting the use of state or federal funds to support physical activity initiatives, or subsidizing parks and recreational facilities to provide physical activity programs for people of all ages (Schmid, Pratt, and Witmer 2006). An example of an environmental policy is to require architects to design buildings with open, well-lit, safe, and accessible stairways placed in visible locations, such as in the lobby of buildings. This provides an alternative to elevators and escalators. Other environmental interventions with policy implications can be developed at community levels, within work sites, at schools, and in recreation centers (Heath et al. 2006). For example, community developers and

Table 7.5. Guide to Community Preventive Services Physical Activity Intervention Recommendations

Approaches	Recommended Methods	Methods with Insufficient Evidence
Informational	Community-wide campaigns	Classroom-based health education focused on providing information
	Point-of-decision prompts	Mass media campaigns
Behavioral and social	School-based physical education	Classroom-based health education focused on reducing television viewing and video game playing
	Social support interventions in community settings	College-based health education and physical education
	Individually adapted health behavior change	Family-based social support
Environmental and policy	Creation of or enhanced access to places for physical activity combined with informational outreach activities	Transportation and travel policies and practices
	Point-of-decision prompts	
	Street-scale urban design and land use policies and practices	
	Community-scale urban design and land use policies and practice	

Note: Adapted from http://www.thecommunityguide.org/pa/default.htm.

city councils could be encouraged to install bicycle trails, walking trails, and sidewalks in new housing developments. Employers could provide safe and convenient exercise facilities as well as flexible work schedules to promote increased activity during the workday. Other examples of environmental opportunities for promoting physical activity include building bicycling paths and sidewalks along busy streets and providing access to shopping malls and schools as safe, heated, or air-conditioned walking and exercise spaces.

In the past five years, numerous state legislation and statutes have been introduced to state legislatures to increase access to and programs for physical activity (National Conference on State Legislators). In a review of the state legislation and statutes database for physical activity provided by the National Conference on State Legislators, nearly every state has introduced legislation to mandate state and local school boards to require school physical education with a focus on activities that can be practiced throughout life.

Similarly, legislation has been introduced in selected states to increase access to open space for recreation, ensure bicycle and pedestrian safety, assess fitness and fatness in school-age children, and to appropriate funding from various sources, such as deposits made on recyclable soda cans, for physical activity programs. Given the public health impact of physical inactivity in terms of personal health, the economy, and societal integration, policy and environmental approaches provide an effective way to increase opportunities for physical activity for people of all ages.

Examples of Public Health Interventions

Many programs conducted over the past decade provide insight as to strategies for behavior change through community interventions and initiatives (see Appendix 7.1). Within a social ecological model whereby activities are targeted at the individual, interpersonal, social and cultural, community, and policy levels, various theories of behavior change allow interventions to target groups with messages appropriate to their readiness to modify their behaviors. The Stages of Change Model, also called the Transtheoretical Model, describes five stages to behavior change: (1) *precontemplation*, one is not thinking about behavior change; (2) *contemplation*, one is thinking about changing a behavior but has not done anything about it; (3) *action*, one has adopted a new behavior for less than six months; (4) *maintenance*, one has practiced a new behavior for longer than six months; and (5) *relapse*, one has stopped the new behavior but plans to resume the behavior change (Marcus and Simkin 1994). The Stages of Change approach has been used to promote physical activity in individual and physician-based interventions.

Individual-based projects focus on the individual as the target for behavior change. Guided by the Social Cognitive Theory that focuses on one's belief in their ability to change their behavior, termed self-efficacy, Project Active (Dunn et al. 1997) is a classic lifestyle (home-based) exercise intervention versus a structured, traditional (a health club) exercise intervention that showed the value of lifestyle physical activity interventions in behavior change. The lifestyle exercise intervention consisted of advising each participant to accumulate at least 30 minutes of moderate intensity physical activity on most days of the week, in a way unique to each participant's lifestyle. The lifestyle participants also received information and skills needed to increase their self-efficacy for physical activity. The traditional exercise intervention offered structured exercise programs in a health club setting. Both activity programs received motivational messages targeted to participants based on their level of readiness to change their physical activity behaviors. After the six month intervention period, both groups had similar reductions in cardiovascular disease risk factors such as total cholesterol, the ratio of total to high-density lipoprotein cholesterol, diastolic blood pressure, and percentage body fat. At 24 months after the start of the study, declines in aerobic fitness, physical activity, and cardiovascular risk factors occurred in both groups; however, the lifestyle group showed smaller declines. This suggests that lifestyle and structured physical activity programs are equally effective in maintaining positive changes in aerobic fitness, physical activity, and cardiovascular risk factors (Dunn et al. 1999).

Physician-based programs have great potential for increasing physical activity among all age groups. A community study of white and African-American adults found that the strongest determinant for increasing physical activity after four years was whether or not a physician had recommended increasing physical activity (Macera et al. 1995). The problem is that very few physicians have specific training in physical activity promotion. Although guidelines for prescribing physical activity for patients are available (McInnis, Franklin, and Rippe 2003), this counseling takes valuable time and may not be appropriate for every patient.

Other important settings for physical activity intervention programs are work sites, schools, and assisted living facilities. Work site physical activity promotion can operate at many levels (Proper et al. 2003). Some companies are large enough to provide exercise facilities including showers and changing rooms. Other companies can support physical activity by allowing time off during the day for regular exercise. Still other companies may incorporate physical activity education into their health promotion program along with smoking cessation and nutritional education. Providing a supportive work site environment will help employees to recognize the importance of physical activity and to participate in social interaction as well as physical activity. Work site physical activity may be especially important for adults with family responsibilities that constrain physical activity at home.

Transdisciplinary partnerships among physical activity, public health, transportation, nonprofit, safety, government, and educational organizations are an effective approach to promoting physical activity in settings that involve multiple disciplines (National Safe Routes to School Task Force; Sallis et al. 2006; Sallis, Kraft, and Linton 2002). For example, in 2006, the U.S. Department of Transportation formed the National Safe Routes to School Task Force to develop strategies to assist communities in enabling and encouraging children to walk and bicycle safely to school in each state. The task force includes leaders in health, transportation, education, government, and nonprofit organizations (National Safe Routes to School Task Force).

An important approach to increasing physical activity in communities is the involvement of federal legislation to support environmental changes for physical activity. The Safe, Accountable, Flexible, and Efficient Transportation Equity Act (SAFETEA) is the Federal reauthorization of the Transportation Equity Act for the 21st Century (TEA-21) that authorizes surface transportation programs for highways, highway safety, and transit. Included in the legislation is funding to develop bicycle lanes and safety programs for bicycling, pedestrian walkways, and recreational hiking and bicycling trails (USDOT).

Other examples of public health approaches to promoting physical activity include several national and state campaigns as outlined below.

National Coalition for Promoting Physical Activity

The National Coalition for Promoting Physical Activity (NCPPA) coordinates the efforts of sports medicine, public health, and corporate agencies to increase physical activity in the United States. The goal of the coalition is to unite the strengths of public, private, and industry efforts into a collaborative partnership to inspire Americans to lead physically active lifestyles to enhance their health and quality of life. The NCPPA is open to nonprofit organizations that are membership-based and have identified physical activity and health as a primary mission.

President's Council on Physical Fitness and Sports

The President's Council on Physical Fitness and Sports (PCPFS) was established in 1956 to promote physical activity, fitness, and sports for all Americans. Members of the PCPFS are national leaders in physical activity, fitness, and sport. The PCPFS supports community, state, and national organizations to promote active lifestyles. Types of activities supported include holding physical activity and fitness clinics and campaigns and publishing a quarterly research digest that translates physical activity and fitness research into practice. In addition, the PCPFS provides grassroots support to educators, parents, physicians and health professionals, youth sport coaches and recreation workers, employers, public officials, and community leaders interested in promoting physical activity, fitness, and sport.

State Governor's Council on Physical Fitness

The State Governor's Council on Physical Fitness is an extension of the PCPFS at the state and community levels. The Chairs of Governors' Councils are generally employed by the State Health Department or the governor's office. Council members are state leaders in physical activity and are appointed to the council by the governor. Physical activity and fitness promotion efforts vary by state. However, they generally include regular meetings of the council, newsletters, awareness campaigns, conferences, and participation on policy decisions.

State Health Department Physical Activity Initiatives and Campaigns

Under the leadership of state and local health departments, physical activity initiatives and campaigns are designed to promote physical activity. Examples of initiatives are walking and bicycling events, work site challenges, and physical activity marketing efforts.

Areas of Future Research

The health effects of physical activity have been studied for nearly a half century. In the 1980s and 1990s, the emphasis shifted from performance and cardiorespiratory fitness benefits of exercise to understanding the myriad of health benefits that we now know accompany even small increases in moderate activity. Consensus conferences have been held to set a research agenda for physical activity, fitness, and health (Bouchard, Shephard, and Stephens 1994); recommendations have been written for health-enhancing physical activity for people of all ages (Physical Activity Guidelines Advisory Committee 2008; Haskell et al. 2007; Nelson et al. 2007; Pate et al. 1995; Sallis and Patrick 1994; USDHHS 1996); foundations, such as the Robert Wood Johnson Foundation, are supporting research and practice efforts to modify the environment, understand how policies can promote physical activity, increase physical activity in older adults (Sallis, Kraft, and Linton 2002); and the National Institutes of Health has sponsored research grants to advance the assessment of physical activity (USDHHS: *Improving Diet and Physical Activity Assessment*). Nevertheless, gaps still remain in understanding how to measure, translate research to public health practice, and to promote physical activity in underserved sectors of the population. The future directions for research are outlined next.

Measurement of Physical Activity

In the past 15 years, there has been considerable progress in the assessment of physical activity using questionnaires and objective measures in the field (LaMonte and

Ainsworth 2001). Most surveys now address moderate and vigorous physical activity based on the recommendations to accumulate at least 30 minutes of moderate activity, five days or more per week, or to perform 20 or more minutes of vigorous activity, three days or more per week (CDCa, CDCe, CDCf). Popular types of physical activity behaviors have also been measured, such as walking for transportation (Ham, Macera, and Lindley 2005) and walking the dog (Ham and Epping 2006). However, it is difficult to assess these behaviors by self-report with sufficient accuracy needed to track long-term trends and/or measure the success of intervention studies. Low-cost and nonobtrusive uses of integrated technology, such as pedometers, accelerometers, heart rate monitors, and electronic diaries, which identify the amount and type of activities that are performed, are needed for use in physical activity surveillance and intervention study settings (USDHHS: *Improving Diet and Physical Activity Assessment*). Further, these instruments need to be evaluated and used in diverse groups, including ethnic minorities, older adults, and children.

Adolescent Physical Activity

Adoption of guidelines to promote physical activity in schools (CDC 1997) and out of school settings (Sallis and Patrick 1994) provides a framework to address the decline in physical activity among adolescents. Despite recent research designed to test interventions to prevent declines in physical activity among adolescent girls (e.g., Stevens et al. 2005), additional research and demonstration projects are needed to identify effective strategies to encourage youth, especially girls and young women, to remain active during adolescence and to balance activity levels with adequate nutrition needed for growth and development.

Environmental and Policy Changes

There is increased awareness and action related to the importance of public policy change to increase physical activity at the population level. In 2004, the CDC and Prevention Research Centers (PRC) established the Physical Activity Policy Research Network to identify existing physical activity policies, and determinants of the policies, to describe the process of implementing policies, and to determine the outcomes of physical activity policies (PRC). Current projects are designed to understand policies related to active transport to and from school (Eyler et al. 2007), explore policy changes in the development of community trails, and to determine a policy and environmental research agenda (Brownson et al. 2008). Nevertheless, continued efforts are needed by community leaders, coalitions, legislators, public health experts, educators, and community residents to effect environmental and policy changes that promote physical activity among people of all ages (Bauman et al. 2006; Heath et al. 2006; King et al. 1995; Schmid, Pratt, and Witmer 2006). These efforts may take the form of working with neighborhood coalitions to adopt residential policies conducive to being physically active, writing letters to the editor of local newspapers, writing position statements for local agencies, and lobbying legislators and city planners to pass laws to require environmental changes that promote physical activity. Additional funding is needed for research into the effectiveness of environmental and policy changes in decreasing the prevalence of physical inactivity, especially in minority and disadvantaged community settings.

Community Physical Activity Promotion

In 1994, King presented a framework for community and public health approaches to promote physical activity (King 1994). Fifteen years after the publication of her article, physical activity is regarded as an important behavior for community health promotion (Lamarre and Pratt 2006). There have been systematic reviews of evidence-based interventions to increase physical activity, efforts to increase physical activity nationally (Dietz 2006), development of Pan-American partnerships to increase physical activity in Latin America (Gámez et al. 2006; Schmid et al. 2006), and collaborative initiatives have been implemented to increase physical activity globally (Bull et al. 2006; Craig et al. 2003; Kirsten, Bauman, and Pratt 2006). Guidelines also have been written on how to evaluate community-based physical activity programs (Martin and Heath 2006). In 2009, a national plan for promoting physical activity was introduced to provide the framework to support a broad and comprehensive national effort to increase physical activity throughout the population. Despite these activities, continued efforts are still needed to apply evidence-based approaches to increase physical activity in all sectors of the population, especially in older adults (Cress et al. 2005), adolescents (Brener et al. 2006), individuals with chronic diseases that can be minimized with regular physical activity (Brown et al. 2006; Imperatore et al. 2006) and in overweight individuals (Kruger, Blanck, and Gillespie 2006). Continued attention is needed to address physical activity disparities in underserved communities (Yancy, Ory, and Davis 2006).

Older Adults

In 2007, nearly 30% of the U.S. population was between the ages of 43 and 60 years. These "baby boomers" are the largest cohort of adults approaching retirement age ever in the United States, with nearly 8,000 adults turning 60 years old everyday (www.census. gov). There is an urgent need to understand more about the efficacy and effectiveness of community-wide physical activity programs designed to maintain physical function and to prevent physiological decline and disability in this aging cohort (Prohaska et al. 2006). Evidence-based, physical activity programs designed for younger adults and/or for older adults in clinical research settings need to be translated for use in older adults in community-wide settings. An example of such a program is *Active for Life—Increasing Physical Activity Levels in Adults Age 50 and Older*. Supported by the Robert Wood Johnson Foundation, Active for Life is designed to test the community translation of two empirically validated physical activity interventions (Active Choices and Active Living Every Day) created for midlife and older adults. To date, about 9,000 adults age 50 years and older from nine community-based programs in the United States have been recruited into the program. Following one year, increases in moderate-to-vigorous physical activity and total physical activity, decreases in depressive symptoms and stress, increases in satisfaction with body appearance and function, and decreases in body mass index provide evidence for the program's success (Wilcox et al. 2006). Similar programs are needed for use in community settings to maintain healthy and active lifestyles in adults as they age.

Resources

American Alliance for Health, Physical Education, Recreation and Dance (AAHPERD), http:// www.aahperd.org. AAHPERD is the largest organization of professionals supporting and assisting those involved in physical education, leisure, fitness, dance, health promotion, and education and all specialties related to achieving a healthy lifestyle.

American College of Sports Medicine, http://www.acsm.org//AM/Template.cfm?Section=Home_ Page. The American College of Sports Medicine promotes and integrates scientific research, education, and practical applications of sports medicine and exercise science to maintain and enhance physical performance, fitness, health, and quality of life.

Centers for Disease Control and Prevention (CDC), National Center for Chronic Disease Prevention and Health Promotion, Division of Nutrition and Physical Activity, http://www.cdc.gov. The CDC leads the Federal Government's programs to promote physical activity. Its website contains information and resources for individuals and organizations interested in physical activity.

National Association for Health and Fitness (NAHF), http://www.physicalfitness.org. The National Association for Health and Fitness is a nonprofit organization that exists to improve the quality of life for individuals in the United States through the promotion of physical fitness, sports, and healthy lifestyles, and by fostering and supporting State Governor's Councils on Physical Fitness and Sports in every state and U.S. territory.

National Coalition for Promoting Physical Activity (NCPPA), http://www.ncppa.org. The mission of the National Coalition for Promoting Physical Activity is to unite the strengths of public, private, and industry efforts into a collaborative partnership to inspire and empower all Americans to lead physically active lifestyles to enhance their health and quality of life.

National Center on Physical Activity and Disability (NCPAD), http://www.ncpad.org. The mission of the National Center on Physical Activity and Disability is to promote substantial health benefits that can be gained from participating in regular physical activity. This site provides information and resources that can enable people with disabilities to become as physically active as they choose to be.

National Recreation and Parks Association (NRPA), http://www.active.com/outdoors. The National Recreation and Park Association establishes new levels of service through partnerships that provide innovation programs, funding support, and public visibility for communities eager to showcase the benefits of parks and recreation.

President's Council for Physical Fitness and Sports, http://www.fitness.gov. The mission of the President's Council for Physical Fitness and Sports is to coordinate and promote opportunities in physical activity, fitness, and sports for all Americans.

World Health Organization (WHO), http://www.who.int/en. Founded in 1948, the World Health Organization leads the world alliance for Health for All. A specialized agency of the United Nations with 191 Member States, WHO promotes technical cooperation for health among nations, carries out programs to control and eradicate disease, and strives to improve the quality of human life.

Suggested Reading

Centers for Disease Control and Prevention (CDC). Guidelines for School and Community Programs to Promote Lifelong Physical Activity Among Young People. Promotion strategies to encourage young people to adopt and maintain a physically active lifestyle. Available at: http://www.cdc.gov/mmwr/preview/mmwrhtml/00046823.htm. Accessed June 28, 2009.

Centers for Disease Control and Prevention (CDC). Promoting Better Health for Young People through Physical Activity and Sports. A Report to the President From the Secretary of Health and Human Services and the Secretary of Education. Available at: http://www.cdc.gov/healthyyouth/physicalactivity/promoting_health. Accessed June 28, 2009.

U.S. Department of Health and Human Services (USDHHS). 2008 Physical Activity Guidelines for Americans. The Federal Government has issued its first-Ever Physical Activity Guidelines for Americans. They describe the types and amounts of physical activity that offer substantial health benefits to Americans. Available at: http://www.health.gov/paguidelines. Accessed June 28, 2009.

U.S. Department of Health and Human Services (USDHHS). Promoting Physical Activity: A Guide for Community Action. Centers for Disease Control and Prevention. National Center for Chronic Disease Prevention and Health Promotion. Division of Nutrition and Physical Activity. Available at: http://www.cdc.gov/nccdphp/dnpa/pahand.htm. Accessed June 28, 2009.

U.S. Department of Health and Human Services (USDHSS). Physical Activity and Health: A Report of the Surgeon General. 1996. Available at: http://www.cdc.gov/nccdphp/sgr/contents.htm. Accessed June 28, 2009.

References

Addy, C.L., D.K. Wilson, K.A. Kirtland, B.E. Ainsworth, P. Sharpe, and D. Kimsey. Associations of Perceived Social and Physical Environmental Supports with Physical Activity and Walking Behavior. *Aust J Polit Hist* (2004):94(3):440–443.

Ainsworth, B.E., W.L. Haskell, M.C. Whitt, et al. Compendium of Physical Activities: An Update of Activity Codes and MET Intensities. *Med Sci Sports Exerc* (2000):32(9)(Suppl):S498–S516.

Ainsworth, B.E., N.L. Keenan, D.S. Strogatz, J.M. Garrett, and S.A. James. Physical Activity and Hypertension in Black Adults: The Pitt County Study. *Aust J Polit Hist* (1991):81:1477–1479.

American College of Sports Medicine. The Recommended Quantity and Quality of Exercise for Developing and Maintaining Cardiorespiratory and Muscular Fitness in Healthy Adults. *Med Sci Sports Exerc* (1990):22:265–274.

Ball, K., A. Bauman, E. Leslie, and N. Owen. Perceived Environmental Aesthetics and Convenience and Company are Associated with Walking for Exercise among Australian Adults. *Prev Med* (2001):33(5):434–440.

Bauman, A.E., D.E. Nelson, M. Pratt, V. Matsudo, and S. Schoeppe. Dissemination of Physical Activity Evidence, Programs, Policies, and Surveillance in the International Public Health Arena. *Am J Prev Med* (2006):31:S57–S65.

Bouchard, C., R.J. Shephard, and T. Stephens. *Physical Activity, Fitness, and Health: International Proceedings and Consensus Statement.* Champaign, IL: Human Kinetics (1994).

Brener, N.D., L. Kann, S. Lee, et al. Secondary School Health Education Related to Nutrition and Physical Activity—Selected Sites, United States, 2004. *MMWR Morb Mortal Wkly Rep* (2006):55:821–824.

Brown, D.W., D.R. Brown, G.W. Heath, et al. Relationships Between Engaging in Recommended Levels of Physical Activity and Health-Related Quality of Life Among Hypertensive Adults. *J Phys Act Health* (2006):3:137–147.

Brownson, R.C., T.K. Boehmer, and D.A. Luke. Declining Rates of Physical Activity in the United States: What Are the Contributors? *Annu Rev Public Health* (2005):26:421–443.

Brownson, R.C., C.M. Kelly, A.A. Eyler, et al. Environmental and Policy Approaches for Promoting Physical Activity in the United States: A Research Agenda. *J Phys Act Health* (2008):5(4):488–503.

Bull, F.C., M. Pratt, R.J. Shephard, and B. Lankenau. Implementing National Population-Based Action on Physical Activity—Challenges for Action and Opportunities for International Collaboration. *Promot Educ* (2006):13(2):127–132.

Carlson, S.A., J.M. Hootman, K.S. Powell, et al. Self-Reported Injury and Physical Activity Levels: United States 2000 to 2002. *Ann Epidemiol* (2006):16:712–719.

Caspersen, C.J. Physical Activity Epidemiology: Concepts, Methods, and Applications to Exercise Science. *Exerc Sport Sci Rev* (1989):17:423–473.

Centers for Disease Control and Prevention (CDCa). *Behavioral Risk Factor Surveillance System.* Methods and Statistical Reports. Available at: http://www.cdc.gov/brfss. Accessed July 31, 2009.

Centers for Disease Control and Prevention (CDCb). *SMART: Selected Metropolitan/Micropolitan Area Risk Trends.* Available at: http://apps.nccd.cdc.gov/brfss-smart/index.asp. Accessed July 31, 2009.

Centers for Disease Control and Prevention (CDCc). *Youth Risk Behavior Survey.* Methods and Statistical Reports. Available at: http://www.cdc.gov/HealthyYouth/yrbs. Accessed July 31, 2009.

Centers for Disease Control and Prevention (CDCd). *Youth Risk Behavior Survey.* Prevalence and Trends. Available at: http://www.cdc.gov/HealthyYouth/yrbs/pdf/yrbs07_us_physical_activity_trend.pdf. Accessed July 31, 2009.

Centers for Disease Control and Prevention (CDCe). *Youth Media Campaign Longitudinal Survey.* Methods and Statistical Reports. Available at: http://www.cdc.gov/mmwr/preview/mmwrhtml/mm5233a1.htm. Accessed July 31, 2009.

Centers for Disease Control and Prevention (CDCf). Definitions for the BRFSS Physical Activity Categories. Available at: http://www.cdc.gov/nccdphp/dnpa/physical/stats/definitions.htm. Accessed July 31, 2009.

Centers for Disease Control and Prevention (CDC). Prevalence of Physical Inactivity during Leisure Time among Overweight Persons—Behavioral Risk Factor Surveillance System 1994. *MMWR* (1996):45(9):185–188.

Centers for Disease Control and Prevention (CDC). Guidelines for School and Community Programs to Promote Lifelong Physical Activity among Young People. *MMWR Recomm Rep* (1997):46:1–36.

Centers for Disease Control and Prevention (CDC). Physical Activity Levels among Children Aged 9–13 Years—United States, 2002. *MMWR Morb Mortal Wkly Rep* (2003):52(33):785–788.

Centers for Disease Control and Prevention (CDC). Prevalence of No Leisure-Time Physical Activity—35 States and the District of Columbia, 1988—2002. *MMWR* (2004a):53(4):82–86.

Centers for Disease Control and Prevention (CDC). REACH 2010 Surveillance for Health Status in Minority Communities—United States, 2001–2002. *MMWR Surveill Summ* (2004b):53(SS06):1–36.

Centers for Disease Control and Prevention (CDC). Physical Activity Among Adults with a Disability —United States. *MMWR* (2005a):56(39):1021–1024.

Centers for Disease Control and Prevention (CDC). Trends in Leisure-Time Physical Inactivity by Age, Sex, and Race/Ethnicity—United States, 1994–2004. *MMWR* (2005b):54(39):991–994.

Centers for Disease Control and Prevention (CDC). Prevalence of Regular Physical Activity Among Adults—United States, 2001 and 2005. *MMWR* (2007):56(46):1209–1212.

Cevero, R., and M. Duncan. Walking, Bicycling, and Urban Landscapes: Evidence from the San Francisco Bay Area. *Aust J Polit Hist* (2003):93(9):1478–1483.

Committee on Physical Activity, Health, Transportation, and Land Use. *Does the Built Environment Influence Physical Activity? Examining the Evidence.* Washington, D.C.: Transportation Research Board (2005).

Craig, C.L., A.L. Marshall, M. Sjöström, et al., and IPAQ Consensus Group, IPAQ Reliability and Validity Study Group. The International Physical Activity Questionnaire (IPAQ): A Comprehensive Reliability and Validity Study in Twelve Countries. *Med Sci Sports Exerc* (2003):35(8):1381–1395.

Cress, M.E., D.M. Buchner, T. Prohaska, et al. Best Practices for Physical Activity Programs and Behavior Counseling in Older Adult Populations. *J Aging Phys Act* (2005):13:61–74.

De Bourdeaudhuij, I., J.F. Sallis, and B.E. Saelens. Environmental Correlates of Physical Activity in a Sample of Belgian Adults. *Am J Health Promot* (2003):18(1):83–92.

deVries, H.A., and T.J. Housh. *Physiology of Exercise* (5th ed.). Dubuque, IA: Brown and Benchmark Publishers (1994).

Dietz, W.H. Canada on the Move: A Novel Effort to Increase Physical Activity among Canadians. *Can J Public Health* (2006):97:S3–S4.

Duncan, M.J., J.C. Spence, and W.K. Mummery. Perceived Environment and Physical Activity: A Meta-Analysis of Selected Environmental Characteristics. *Int J Behav Nutr Phys Act* (September 5, 2005):2:11.

Dunn, A.L., B.H. Marcus, J.B. Kampert, et al. Reduction in Cardiovascular Disease Risk Factors: 6-Month Results from Project Active. *Prev Med* (1997):26:883–892.

Dunn, A.L., B.H. Marcus, J.B. Kampert, et al. Comparison of Lifestyle and Structured Interventions to Increase Physical Activity and Cardiorespiratory Fitness—A Randomized Trial. *JAMA* (1999):281(4):327–334.

Eaton, D.K., L. Kann, S. Kinchen, et al. Youth Risk Behavior Surveillance—United States, 2005. *MMWR Surveill Summ* (June 9, 2006):55(SS05):1–108.

Eyler, A.A., R.C. Brownson, M.P. Doescher, et al. Policies Related to Active Transport to and from School: A Multisite Case Study. *Health Educ Res* (October 22, 2007) [Epub ahead of print].

Eyler, A.A., D. Matson-Koffman, J.R. Vest, et al. Environmental, Policy, and Cultural Factors Related to Physical Activity in a Diverse Sample of Women: The Women's Cardiovascular Health Network Project—Summary and Discussion. *Women Health* (2002):36(2):123–134.

Eyler, A.A., D. Matson-Koffman, D.R. Young, S. Wilcox, J. Wilbur, J.L. Thompson, B. Sanderson, and K.R. Evenson. Quantitative Study of Correlates of Physical Activity in Women from Diverse Racial/Ethnic Groups: The Women's Cardiovascular Health Network Project—Summary and Conclusions. *Am J Prev Med* (2003):25(3 Suppl 1):93–103.

Gámez, R., D. Parra, M. Pratt, and T. Schmid. Muévete Bogotá: Promoting Physical Activity with a Network of Partner Companies. *Promot Educ* (2006):13:138–143.

Giles-Corti, B., and R.J. Donovan. Relative Influences of Individual, Social Environmental, and Physical Environmental Correlates of Walking. *Aust J Polit Hist* (2003):93(9):1583–1589.

Giles-Corti, B., A. Timperio, F. Bull, and T. Pikora. Understanding Physical Activity Environmental Correlates: Increased Specificity for Ecological Models. *Exerc Sport Sci Rev* (2005):33(4):175–181.

Greenwald, M.J., and M.G. Boarnet. Built Environment as Determinant of Walking Behavior: Analyzing Nonwork Pedestrian Travel in Portland, Oregon. *Transp Res Rec* (2001):(1780):33–42.

Ham, S.A., and J. Epping. Dog Walking and Physical Activity in the United States. *Prev Chronic Dis* (2006):3:A47 [e-pub].

Ham, S.A., C.A. Macera, and C. Lindley. Trends in Walking for Transportation in the United States, 1995 and 2001. *Prev Chronic Dis* (2005):2:A14 [e-pub].

Haskell, W.L., I.M. Lee, R.R. Pate, et al. Physical Activity and Public Health: Updated Recommendation for Adults from the American College of Sports Medicine and the American Heart Association. *Med Sci Sports Exerc* (2007):39(8):1423–1434.

Healthy People 2010 Midcourse Review. Available at: http://www.healthypeople.gov/data/midcourse/default.htm#pubs.

Heath, G.W., R.C. Brownson, J. Kruger, et al., and the Task Force on Community Preventive Services. The Effectiveness of Urban Design and Land Use and Transport Policies and Practices to Increase Physical Activity: A Systematic Review. *J Phys Act Health* (2006):3:S55–S76.

Heitzler, C.D., S.L. Martin, J. Duke, and M. Huhman. Correlates of Physical Activity in a National Sample of Children Aged 9–13 Years. *Prev Med* (2006):42:254–260.

Henderson, K.A., M.D. Bialeschki, S.M. Shaw, and V.J. Freysinger. *Both Gains and Gaps: Feminist Perspectives on Women's Leisure.* State College, PA: Venture (1996).

Imperatore, G., Y.J. Cheng, D.E. Williams, J.E. Fulton, and E.W. Gregg. Physical Activity, Cardiovascular Fitness, and Insulin Sensitivity among U.S. Adolescents: The National Health and Nutrition Examination Survey, 1999–2002. *Diabetes Care* (2006):29:1567–1572.

King, A.C. Community and Public Health Approaches to the Promotion of Physical Activity. *Med Sci Sports Exerc* (1994):26:1405–1412.

King, A.C., R.W. Jeffery, F. Fridinger, et al. Environmental and Policy Approaches to Cardiovascular Disease Prevention through Physical Activity: Issues and Opportunities. *Health Educ Behav* (1995):22:499–511.

Kirsten, W., A. Bauman, and M. Pratt. Promoting Physical Activity Globally for Population Health. *Promot Educ* (2006):13(2):90–91.

Koezuka, N., M. Ko, K.R. Allison, et al. The Relationship between Sedentary Activities and Physical Inactivity among Adolescents: Results from the Canadian Community Health Survey. *J Adolesc Health* (2006):39(4):515–522.

Kruger, J., H.M. Blanck, and C. Gillespie. Dietary and Physical Activity Behaviors among Adults Successful at Weight Loss Maintenance. *Int J Behav Nutr Phys Act* (2006):3:17 [e-pub].

Kruger, J., M.M. Yore, B.E. Ainsworth, and C.A. Macera. Is Participation in Occupational Physical Activity Associated with Lifestyle Physical Activity Levels? *J Occup Environ Med* (2006):48(11):1143–1148.

Lamarre, M.C., and M. Pratt. Physical Activity and Health Promotion. *Promot Educ* (2006):3: 4–5.

LaMonte, M.J., and B.E. Ainsworth. Quantifying Energy Expenditure and Physical Activity in the Context of Dose Response. *Med Sci Sports Exerc* (2001):33(6 Suppl):S370–S378.

Levine, J.A., L.M. Lanningham-Foster, S.K. McCrady, et al. Interindividual Variation in Posture Allocation: Possible Role in Human Obesity. *Science* (2005):307:584–586.

Macera, C.A., and K.E. Powell. Population Attributable Risk: Implications of Physical Activity Dose. *Med Sci Sports Exerc* (2001):33(6 Suppl):S635–S639.

Macera, C.A., J.B. Croft, D.R. Brown, J. Ferguson, and M.J. Lane. Predictors of Adoption of Leisure-Time Physical Activity in a Biracial Community Sample. *Am J Epidemiol* (1995):142: 629–635.

Marcus, B.H., and L.R. Simkin. The Transtheoretical Model: Applications to Exercise Behavior. *Med Sci Sports Exerc* (1994):26:1400–1404.

Martin, S.L., and G.W. Heath. A Six-Step Model for Evaluation of Community-Based Physical Activity Programs. *Prev Chronic Dis* (2006):3:A24 [e-pub].

McInnis, K.J., B.A. Franklin, and J.M. Rippe. Counseling for Physical Activity in Overweight and Obese Patients. *Am Fam Physician* (2003):67(6):1249–1256.

Mokdad, A.H., J.S. Marks, D.F. Stroup, et al. Actual Causes of Death in the United States, 2000. *JAMA* (2004):291(10):1238–1245.

National Center for Health Statistics (NCHSa). *National Health Interview Survey.* Methods and Statistical Reports. Available at: http://www.cdc.gov/nchs/nhis.htm. Accessed July 31, 2009.

National Center for Health Statistics (NCHSb). Early release from the 2007 National Health Interview Study. Available at: http://www.cdc.gov/nchs/data/nhis/earlyrelease/200712_07.pdf. Accessed July 31, 2009.

National Conference on State Legislators. Legislation and Statue Database. Available at: http://www.ncsl.org/?tabid=17173. Accessed July 31, 2009.

National Safe Routes to School Task Force. Available at: http://www.saferoutesinfo.org/task_force.

Nelson, M.E., W.J. Rejeski, S.N. Blair, et al. Physical Activity and Public Health in Older Adults: Recommendation from the American College of Sports Medicine and the American Heart Association. *Med Sci Sports Exerc* (2007):39(8):1435–1445.

Owen, N., N. Humpel, E. Leslie, A. Bauman, and J.F. Sallis. Understanding Environmental Influences on Walking: Review and Research Agenda. *Am J Prev Med* (2004):27(1):67–76.

Parks, S.E., R.A. Housemann, and R.C. Brownson. Differential Correlates of Physical Activity in Urban and Rural Adults of Various Socioeconomic Backgrounds in the United States. *J Epidemiol Community Health* (2003):57:29–35.

Pate, R.R., M. Pratt, S.N. Blair, et al. Physical Activity and Public Health: A Recommendation from the Centers for Disease Control and Prevention and the American College of Sports Medicine. *JAMA* (1995):273:402–407.

Physical Activity Guidelines Advisory Committee. *Physical Activity Guidelines Advisory Committee Report, 2008.* Washington, DC: U.S. Department of Health and Human Services, 2008.

Powell, K.E., P.D. Thompson, C.J. Caspersen, and J.S. Kendrick. Physical Activity and the Incidence of Coronary Heart Disease. *Annu Rev Public Health* (1987):8:253–287.

Prevention Research Centers (PRC). Physical Activity Policy Research Network. Available at: http://prc.slu.edu/paprn.htm.

Prohaska, T., E. Belansky, B. Belza, et al. Physical Activity, Public Health, and Aging: Critical Issues and Research Priorities. *J Gerontol B Psychol Sci Soc Sci* (2006):61:S267–S273.

Proper, K.I., M. Koning, A. van der Beek, et al. The Effectiveness of Worksite Physical Activity Programs on Physical Activity, Physical Fitness, and Health. *Clin J Sport Med* (2003):13(2): 106–117.

Reis, J.P., H.R. Bowles, B.E. Ainsworth, K.D. Dubose, S. Smith, and J.N. Laditka. Nonoccupational Physical Activity by Degree of Urbanization and U.S. Geographic Region. *Med Sci Sports Exerc* (December 2004):36(12):2093–2098.

Saelens, B.E., J.F. Sallis, and L.D. Frank. Environmental Correlates of Walking and Cycling: Findings from the Transportation, Urban Design, and Planning Literatures. *Ann Behav Med* (2003):25(2):80–91.

Sallis, J.F., R.B. Cervero, W. Ascher, et al. An Ecological Approach to Creating Active Living Communities. *Annu Rev Public Health* (2006):27:297–322.

Sallis, J.F., K. Kraft, and L.S. Linton. How the Environment Shapes Physical Activity: A Transdisciplinary Research Agenda. *Am J Prev Med* (2002):22(3):208.

Sallis, J.F., and K. Patrick. Physical Activity Guidelines for Adolescents: Consensus Statement. *Pediatr Exerc Sci* (1994):6:302–314.

Sapkota, S., H.R. Bowles, S.A. Ham, and H.W. Kohl III. Adult Participation in Recommended Levels of Physical Activity—United States, 2001 and 2003. *MMWR Morb Mortal Wkly Rep* (2005):54:1208–1212.

Schmid, T.L., J. Librett, A. Neiman, M. Pratt, and A. Salmon. A Framework for Evaluating Community-Based Physical Activity Promotion Programs in Latin America. *Promot Educ* (2006):13(2):112–118.

Schmid, T.L., M. Pratt, and L. Witmer. A Framework for Physical Activity Policy Research. *J Phys Act Health* (2006):3:S20–S29.

Shih, M., J.M. Hootman, J. Kruger, and C.G. Helmick. Physical Activity in Men and Women with Arthritis: National Health Interview Survey, 2002. *Am J Prev Med* (2006):30:385–393.

Stevens, J., D.M. Murray, D.J. Catellier, et al. Design of the Trial of Activity in Adolescent Girls (TAAG). *Contemp Clin Trials* (2005):26(2):223–233.

U.S. Department of Health and Human Services (USDHHS). Public Health Service. *Healthy People 2000: National Health Promotion and Disease Prevention Objectives.* Washington, D.C.: U.S. Department of Health and Human Services, Public Health Service (1991). DHHS Publication 91-50212.

U.S. Department of Health and Human Services (USDHHS). *Physical Activity and Health: A Report of the Surgeon General.* Atlanta, GA: U.S. Department of Health and Human Services, Centers for Disease Control and Prevention, National Center for Chronic Disease Prevention and Health Promotion (1996).

U.S. Department of Health and Human Services (USDHHS). *Improving Diet and Physical Activity Assessment.* Available at: http://grants.nih.gov/grants/guide/pa-files/par-07-259.html.

U.S. Department of Transportation (USDOT). *SAFETEA. Description of the Safe, Accountable, Flexible and Efficient Transportation Equity Act.* Available at: http://www.fhwa.dot.gov/reauthorization/safetea.htm. Accessed July 31, 2009.

U.S. Preventive Services Task Force (USPSTFa). *The Guide to Clinical Preventive Services 2007.* Available at: http://www.ahrq.gov/Clinic/pocketgd.htm. Accessed July 31, 2009.

U.S. Preventive Services Task Force (USPSTFb). *The Guide to Community Preventive Services.* Available at: http://www.thecommunityguide.org/. Accessed July 31, 2009.

Van Der Horst, K., M.J. Paw, J.W. Twisk, and W. Van Mechelin. A Brief Review on Correlates of Physical Activity and Sedentariness in Youth. *Med Sci Sports Exerc* (2007):39(8): 1241–1250.

Wang, G., M. Pratt, C.A. Macera, Z.J. Zheng, and G. Heath. Physical Activity, Cardiovascular Disease, and Medical Expenditures in U.S. Adults. *Ann Behav Med* (2004):28(2):88–94.

Wilcox, S., C. Castro, A.C. King, R. Housemann, and R.C. Brownson. Determinants of Leisure Time Physical Activity in Rural Compared with Urban Older and Ethnically Diverse Women in the United States. *J Epidemiol Community Health* (2000):54:667–672.

Wilcox, S., M. Dowda, S.F. Griffin, et al. Results of the First Year of Active for Life: Translation of Two Evidence-Based Physical Activity Programs for Older Adults Into Community Settings. *Aust J Polit Hist* (2006):96:1201–1209.

Wilson, D.K., K. Kirtland, B.E. Ainsworth, and C.L. Addy. Socioeconomic Status and Perceptions of Access and Safety for Physical Activity. *Ann Behav Med* (2004):28(1):20–28.

Yancy, A.K., M.G. Ory, and S.M. Davis. Dissemination of Physical Activity Promotion Interventions in Underserved Populations. *Am J Prev Med* (2006):31(4 Suppl):S82–S91.

Zlot, A., J. Librett, D. Buchner, and T. Schmidt. Environmental, Transportation, Social, and Time Barriers to Physical Activity. *J Phys Act Health* (2006):1:15–21.

Appendix 7.1. Selected Websites with Focus on Physical Activity and Public Health

Topic	Name of Website	Website Address
Guidelines	Healthy People 2010	http://www.healthypeople.gov
	The Guide to Community Preventive Services	http://www.thecommunityguide.org/pa
	The Guide to Clinical Preventive Services	http://www.ahrq.gov/clinic/pocketgd/pocketgd.pdf
Surveillance	National Health Interview Survey	http://www.cdc.gov/nchs/nhis.htm
	Behavioral Risk Factor Surveillance System	http://www.cdc.gov/brfss
	Youth Risk Behavior Survey	http://www.cdc.gov/HealthyYouth/yrbs
	Youth Media Campaign Longitudinal Survey	http://www.cdc.gov/mmwr/preview/mmwrhtml/mm5233al.htm
Organizations and agencies	National Coalition for Promoting Physical Activity	http://www.ncppa.org/about.asp
	National Society of Physical Activity Practitioners in Public Health	http://www.nspapph.org
	Robert Wood Johnson Foundation	http://www.rwjf.org
	American College of Sports Medicine	http://www.acsm.org
	American Heart Association	http://americanheart.org
	Physical Activity and Health Branch, Centers for Disease Control and Prevention	http://www.cdc.gov/physicalactivity
	President's Council on Physical Fitness and Sports	http://www.fitness.gov
	National Association for Health and Fitness: A Network of State and Governor's Councils	http://www.physicalfitness.org

Appendix 7.1. (*continued*)

Topic	Name of Website	Website Address
	National Parks and Recreation Association	http://www.nrpa.org
Policy	University of South Carolina Prevention Research Center	http://prevention.sph.sc.edu
	Center for Science in the Public Interest	http://www.cspinet.org/ nutritionpolicy/ policy_options.html
	National Conference on State Legislators	http://www.ncsl.org/programs/ health/pp/healthpromo_srch. cfm
	Prevention Research Centers Physical Activity Policy Network	http://prc.slu.edu/paprn.htm
	National Center for Safe Routes to School	http://www.saferoutesinfo.org/ task_force
	Safe, Accountable, Flexible, Efficient Transportation Equity Act	http://www.fhwa.dot.gov/ reauthorization/safetea.htm
Environment	Active Living Research	http://www.activelivingresearch.org
	International Physical Activity and the Environment Network	http://www.ipenproject.org
	U.S. Environmental Protection Agency	http://www.epa.gov/aging/index.htm
	Association of State and Territorial Health Officials	http://www.astho.org/pubs/ BuiltEnvirofactsheet1-06.pdf

CHAPTER 8

ALCOHOL USE
(ICD-10 Z72.1, F10.2)

Mary C. Dufour, M.D., M.P.H., Rear Admiral, USPHS (Ret.)

Introduction

Consumption of alcoholic beverages has been a part of many societies since the dawn of prehistory. Ancient texts from Persia, Egypt, Babylon, and China as well as Biblical writers have documented that people have been aware of alcohol's beneficial and harmful effects for nearly as long as people have been drinking (Rubin and Thomas 1992). Like tobacco use, alcohol use has complex physiological, behavioral, social, and political interrelationships. Unlike tobacco use, however, alcohol use per se is clearly not considered to be harmful. Rather, alcohol consumption needs to be viewed on a continuum from abstinence to low-risk use to risky use, problem drinking, alcohol abuse, alcohol dependence, and other consequences (Saitz 2005).

The relationship between alcohol consumption and alcohol dependence is a complicated one. Clearly, a lifetime nondrinker cannot become alcohol dependent. And the more one drinks, the more likely one is to suffer negative consequences of their drinking; however, the relationship between the amount and duration of alcohol consumption and the risk of becoming alcohol dependent is not a linear one. Genetics, co-occurring conditions, and a whole host of other factors make some people more sensitive to the effects of alcohol than others. Drinking patterns and the settings in which drinking occurs are also important. The causes, consequences, and groups at high risk for alcohol misuse are summarized in Figure 8.1.

For those who choose to drink, the 2005 Dietary Guidelines for Americans recommend up to one drink a day for women and up to two drinks a day for men (USDHHS and USDA 2005). A drink is defined as 12 ounces of regular beer, five ounces of wine, or 1.5 ounces of 80-proof distilled spirits (USDHHS and USDA 2005). Drinking becomes problematic when it causes or elevates the risk for alcohol-related problems or complicates the management of other health problems. Epidemiological research suggests that men who drink more than four standard drinks in a day (or more than 14 per week) and women who drink more than three in a day (or more than seven per week) are at increased risk for alcohol-related problems (NIAAA 2005a).

Significance

Alcohol consumption is a part of contemporary life for many Americans. As a result, although most people drink moderately and without ill effect, alcohol abuse and alcohol

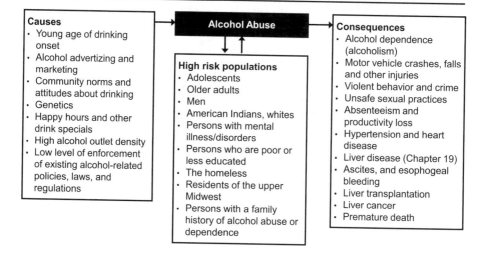

Figure 8.1. Alcohol misuse: causes, consequences, and high-risk groups.

dependence are major health problems in the United States. In 2001–2002, 17.6 million Americans aged 18 and older or 18.6% of the population met the criteria of the American Psychiatric Association's *Diagnostic and Statistical Manual of Mental Disorders*, 4th edition (DSM-IV) (APA 1994) for alcohol abuse and dependence (Grant et al. 2004). The Centers for Disease Control and Prevention (CDC) ranks alcohol as the third leading cause of preventable death in the United States (Mokdad et al. 2004). The World Health Organization (WHO) estimates that alcohol causes 1.8 million deaths (3.2% of total) and a loss of 58.3 million (4% of total) disability-adjusted life years (DALYS) each year (WHO 2004). Alcohol consumption is the leading risk factor for disease burden in low mortality developing countries and the third largest risk factor in developed countries (WHO 2004). Mortality from all causes is markedly elevated in alcoholics (Taylor, Combs-Orme, and Taylor 1983).

In economic terms, alcohol-related costs are estimated to have been $184.6 billion in 1998, the most recent year for which such estimates are available (NIAAA 2000). Of these costs, more than 70% are in the form of productivity losses due to premature mortality, excess morbidity, and crime attributed to alcohol, while only 10% are for medical treatment of alcohol abuse and dependence (NIAAA 2000). Alcohol dependence contributes to other health problems and thereby increases the use of health care services. Between 15% and 30% of patients in short-stay general hospitals have alcohol problems, regardless of their admitting diagnosis. Unfortunately, only a fraction of these alcohol diagnoses are reflected in discharge diagnoses (Umbricht-Schneiter, Santora, and Moore 1991). In addition, the families of alcoholics consume more health care services than do those of nonalcoholics (Holder 1987). Beyond its impact on health and economic productivity, alcohol misuse exacts an enormous toll in terms of human suffering. Failed marriages, anguished families, stalled careers, criminal records, and the pain of having loved ones killed or disabled in alcohol-related traffic crashes attest to its destructive power.

Although moderate alcohol use has been sanctioned in the United States for a long time, its objective physical health benefits have begun to be quantified only in the last 30 years. A substantial body of literature now exists describing the protective effects of low-level alcohol consumption against coronary heart disease (Rimm and Moats 2007).

The public has also become increasingly aware of alcohol's general risks, as well as benefits: News of grisly, alcohol-related, postprom car crashes shares the media spotlight with reports on the cardioprotective effects of low-level alcohol consumption. *Healthy People 2010*, the comprehensive, nationwide health promotion and disease prevention agenda for the first decade of the twenty-first century, has chosen substance abuse as one of ten leading health indicators—the major public health concerns in the United States (see the *Healthy People 2010* website at http://www.healthypeople.gov for more information). Within *Healthy People 2010*'s Substance Abuse section (Chapter 26) are 25 objectives, 18 of which are partly or entirely alcohol-related (USDHHS 2000). The overarching goal of the substance abuse chapter is to reduce substance abuse to protect the health, safety, and quality of life for all, especially children. Traffic statistics, news reports, and public health initiatives, however, do not necessarily delineate the health risks and benefits of alcohol consumption for a given individual.

The physical and mental health effects of alcohol use may range from beneficial to harmful. Other consequences, such as divorce or loss of a job, are not health-related per se, although they may negatively affect health indirectly through loss of income and concomitant access to health care.

Negative health consequences are of three broad types: (1) the acute consequences of ingesting large doses of alcohol in a short period of time, such as alcohol-related motor vehicle crash injuries and alcohol poisoning; (2) chronic disease consequences, such as alcoholic liver disease and alcoholic cardiomyopathy; and (3) the primary chronic disease of alcohol dependence or alcoholism. Individuals who suffer from alcohol dependence often experience other chronic and acute health effects as well. However, an individual need not be alcohol dependent to suffer other negative health consequences of alcohol consumption. For example, a teenager may die in an alcohol-related crash following his or her first drinking episode. It is also quite possible to drink enough to damage one's liver without being dependent on alcohol.

In the introductory portion of this chapter, numerous terms appeared, including *alcohol abuse, alcohol dependence, alcoholism, alcohol-related, alcohol problems, problem drinking, low-risk drinking, risky use, moderate alcohol use,* and *low-level alcohol consumption*. All of these terms have multiple interpretations. The lack of one standard, universally agreed on set of definitions has made alcohol epidemiology challenging. The issue of the diagnosis of alcohol use disorders is closely linked to the problems of nomenclature and classification.

Efforts to develop reliable and effective classification systems and well-founded diagnostic procedures have led to many modifications of the terms used to describe these disorders. The DSM-IV of the APA (1994) and the *International Classification of Diseases, 10th Revision* (ICD-10) of the WHO (1992) have emphasized the concept of "alcohol dependence" introduced by Edwards and Gross in 1976. Despite this diagnostic use of the term *alcohol dependence*, the term *alcoholism* continues to be widely used both among health professionals and the general public. The National Council on Alcoholism and Drug Dependency (NCADD) and the American Society of Addiction Medicine (ASAM) have formulated the following definition: "Alcoholism is a primary chronic disease with genetic, psychosocial, and environmental factors influencing its development and manifestations. The disease is often progressive and fatal. It is characterized by impaired control over drinking, preoccupation with the drug alcohol, use of alcohol despite adverse consequences, and distortions of thinking, most notably denial. Each of these symptoms may be continuous or periodic" (Morse and Flavin 1992). In this chapter, alcoholism and alcohol dependence are used interchangeably.

Pathophysiology

Alcohol affects every organ of the body, manifesting itself in a wide array of pathology. Most critical to alcohol dependence are the effects of alcohol on the brain itself. It has been known for millennia that alcohol ingestion creates a pleasurable state of mind. However, after extremely heavy drinking it leads to confusion, incoordination, sedation, and coma. How alcohol produces intoxication is only now beginning to be understood. The brain adapts to long-term exposure to alcohol and eventually functions more normally in its presence (tolerance). When alcohol is withdrawn suddenly, this adaptive state becomes nonadaptive and tremors, hallucinations, and convulsions may ensue (physical dependence).

With repeated drinking, susceptible individuals develop a craving for alcohol that becomes the dominating motivational force, sustaining long-term drinking in the face of loss of family, job, and personal dignity (psychological dependence). After years of heavy use, an alcoholic may suffer nutritional deficiency, repeated episodes of trauma, liver failure, and lesions of the brain due to the toxic effects of alcohol and its breakdown products. In some alcoholics, these accumulated insults result in social deterioration, inability to walk, and severely disabling disorders of memory and cognition and, with continued drinking, culminate in death (Charness 1990).

Alcohol abuse can lead to a variety of chronic health disorders. Liver disease, the most prominent of these disorders, is the leading cause of death in alcoholics (Dufour 2007). Not only is all-cause mortality elevated in alcoholics, but these deaths occur at younger ages (Taylor, Combs-Orme, and Taylor 1983). Heavy alcohol consumption and gallstones are the two leading causes of acute pancreatitis (Dufour and Adamson 2003). Approximately three-quarters of the patients with chronic pancreatitis have a history of heavy alcohol consumption (Dufour and Adamson 2003). Chronic alcohol consumption may also lead to degenerative changes of the heart and skeletal muscle. Reproductive disorders in both men and women are associated with alcohol. In women, they include anovulation, amenorrhea, and early menopause (Rubin 1989). Alcohol-related testicular atrophy may contribute significantly to sexual problems in male alcoholics (Rubin 1989). Alcohol consumption is a major risk factor for high blood pressure and contributes to a variety of neurological disorders (Rubin 1989). Alcohol abuse is associated with increased risk of cancer of the oral cavity, nasopharynx, larynx, esophagus, and liver (Corrao et al. 2004; Thakker 1998). For breast cancer in women, the risk rises relatively slowly but steadily with increasing alcohol consumption (Thakker 1998), although opinion remains divided on whether a causal relationship exists. It is clear that alcohol use is a risk factor for many of the chronic diseases discussed elsewhere in this text.

In keeping with the chronic disease epidemiology orientation of this book, this chapter focuses primarily on the chronic disease of alcohol dependence and the chronic disease consequences of alcohol consumption. However, the negative health consequences of acute excess alcohol consumption are serious and all too common. Alcohol-related traffic crashes, the largest single alcohol-related cause of death (Midanik et al. 2004), represent a public health problem of major proportions and some of the most effective alcohol policy measures relate to drinking and driving. Therefore, binge drinking and acute consequences are covered as well. Equally important but excluded from this chapter is discussion of the health impact of behavioral consequences of alcohol use. For example, alcohol consumption may lessen inhibitions and lead to a variety of risky behaviors including sexual risk taking, which, in turn, may result in pregnancy and sexually transmitted diseases, including HIV/AIDS.

Descriptive Epidemiology

In 2005, the most recent year for which data are currently available, the estimated alcohol consumption in the United States, based predominantly on alcoholic beverage sales and tax data, was as follows (Lakins et al. 2007):

Beer	6,354,809,000 gallons
Wine	662,255,000 gallons
Spirits	406,012,000 gallons

Beer, wine, and other alcoholic beverages differ in the amounts of alcohol they contain. In fact, the alcohol concentration in the same brand of beer bottled in different states may vary slightly. In order to be able to compare the amounts of alcohol consumed across a variety of alcoholic beverages, drinks are sometimes expressed in terms of the amount of ethanol (the type of alcohol in alcoholic beverages) they contain. This type of calculation results in an apparent per capita alcohol consumption in gallons of ethanol of 1.19 gallons for beer, 0.36 gallon for wine, and 0.70 gallon for distilled spirits (2.24 gallons ethanol total) for each individual aged 14 years and older. This is approximately equivalent to 282 twelve-ounce cans of beer, 71 five-ounce glasses of wine, and 145 shots (1.5 ounces) of 80-proof distilled spirits per person per year (Lakins et al. 2007). Although age 14 years is well below the legal drinking age, people aged 14 and older were included in the population used in this calculation because survey data suggest that many young people begin consuming alcohol about this age. Although quite robust, apparent per capita alcohol consumption is a crude measure because it assumes that everyone drinks. Clearly, this is not the case.

Data from national surveys provide more complete data on drinking prevalence, drinking patterns, and problems. Two large national surveys, the National Survey on Drug Use and Health (NSDUH) and the National Epidemiologic Survey on Alcohol and Related Conditions (NESARC), are two key sources of alcohol use and abuse in the United States. Prevalence estimates for some of the alcohol use outcomes differ somewhat between the surveys. Research suggests that a number of methodological differences are likely to account for these variations (Grucza et al. 2007). Nevertheless, taken together, these two surveys provide a valuable picture of alcohol use and abuse in this country.

NSDUH is a large annual survey sponsored by the Substance Abuse and Mental Health Services Administration (SAMHSA) and is one of the primary federal sources of information on the use of illicit drugs, alcohol, and tobacco in the civilian, noninstitutionalized population of the United States aged 12 years and older. This household survey has been conducted since 1971 and before 2002, was called the National Household

Survey on Drug Abuse (NHSDA). In recent years, the NSDUH has employed a state-based design with an independent, multistage area probability sample within each state and the District of Columbia. The survey interviews approximately 67,500 persons each year (SAMHSA 2007). In NSDUH, the following definitions are used:

- Current drinking—at least one drink in the 30 days before the survey
- Binge drinking—five or more drinks on the same occasion on at least 1 day in the past 30 days
- Heavy drinking—five or more drinks on the same occasion on each of 5 or more days in the past 30 days

According to the 2006 NSDUH, slightly more than half of Americans aged 12 years or older or approximately 125 million people reported being current drinkers, nearly one-quarter reported binge drinking and 6.9% reported heavy drinking. In 2006, 18.8 million persons aged 12 years or older were classified with alcohol abuse or dependence (7.6%) (SAMHSA 2007).

NESARC is a large, nationwide household survey of the civilian noninstitutionalized population of the United States, designed and conducted by the National Institute on Alcohol Abuse and Alcoholism (NIAAA) of the National Institutes of Health (NIH). This longitudinal survey is among the largest and most ambitious household surveys of alcohol and related comorbidity ever conducted. Wave 1 of this survey was conducted from 2001 to 2002 and consisted of interviews of 43,093 respondents 18 years and older. Categories of drinkers in the NESARC include:

- Lifetime abstainers—those respondents who never had one or more drinks in their life
- Former drinkers—those who had at least one drink in their life but not in the past year
- Current drinkers—those having at least one drink of any type of alcohol in the year before the survey (NIAAA 2006)

According to the 2001–2002 NESARC, two-thirds of the respondents were current drinkers, one-sixth were former drinkers, and the remaining one-sixth were lifetime abstainers. From the alcohol items collected in the NESARC, it is possible to calculate estimates of total ethanol consumption during the past year by summing beverage-specific volumes across the four individual beverage types. Dividing this annual total by 365 yields the average daily volume of ethanol intake, the key statistic used for "drinking level" classification. Drinkers are categorized as follows:

- Light—no more than 0.257 ounce of ethanol per day (i.e., three or fewer drinks per week)
- Moderate—more than 0.257 ounce and up to 1.2 ounces of ethanol per day (i.e., 3–14 drinks per week) for men and up to 0.6 ounce (i.e., 3–7 drinks per week) for women
- Heavier—more than 1.2 ounces of ethanol (i.e., more than two drinks) per day for men and more than 0.6 ounce (i.e., more than one drink) per day for women (NIAAA 2006).

According to the above information, 83% of adults age 18 years and older reported ever consuming alcohol and two-thirds reported drinking in the past year. However, only a fraction of drinkers are serious problem drinkers or drink sufficient quantities to suffer serious health consequences. The top 20% of current drinkers consume 80% of all alcohol, with the top 2.5% consuming 27% (Greenfield and Rogers 1999). According to the Wave 1 NESARC, using DSM-IV criteria, among individuals aged 18 years and older, the prevalence of lifetime and 12-month alcohol abuse was 17.8% and 4.7%, respectively, and prevalence of lifetime and 12-month alcohol dependence was 12.5% and 3.8%, respectively (Hasin et al. 2007). The distribution of current drinkers, heavier drinkers, men who consume five or more drinks in a day, women who consume four or more drinks in a day, and individuals suffering from alcohol use disorders among men and women by race/ethnicity and age is shown in Table 8.1.

High-Risk Groups

Adolescents

Alcohol continues to be the most widely used substance of abuse among America's youth, with a higher percentage of those aged 12–20 reporting the use of alcohol in the last 30 days (28.3%) than tobacco (22.4%) or illicit drugs (13.9%) (SAMHSA 2007). In 2007, 72.2% of 12th graders, 61.7% of 10th graders, and 38.9% of 8th graders reported consuming alcohol at some point in their lives (Johnston et al. 2007). In addition 55.1% of 12th graders, 41.2% of 10th graders, and 17.9% of 8th graders reported having been drunk at least once in their lives, and 28.7% of 12th graders, 18.1% of 10th graders, and 5.5% of 8th graders reported having been drunk in the past month (Johnston et al. 2007). Studies show that drinking often begins at very young ages. Data from recent surveys indicate that 10% of 9- to 10-year-olds have already started drinking (Donovan et al. 2004). More than one-fourth of underage drinkers begin before age 13 years (Eaton et al. 2006). The adverse consequences of underage drinking include alcohol-related motor vehicle crashes (the greatest single mortality risk for underage drinkers); increased risk for suicide and homicide; assault and rapes; unintentional injuries such as burns, falls, and drownings; potential brain impairment; an increased risk for developing an alcohol use disorder later in life; unwanted, unintended, and unprotected sexual activity; academic problems; various social problems; and physical problems, such as alcohol poisoning or medical illnesses. Persons aged 21 years or older who reported first use of alcohol before age 14 years were more than six times as likely to report past year alcohol dependence or abuse than persons who first used alcohol at age 21 years or older (SAMHSA 2007; Grant and Dawson 1997).

Older Americans

Alcohol abuse, dependence, and adverse consequences appear to be less prevalent among individuals aged 65 years and older compared with younger individuals (Dufour 2006). However, among older individuals who drink, the proportion of heavy drinkers is nearly as high as among younger age groups (NIAAA 2006). According to the 2001–2002 NESARC, among those aged 65 years and older, the 12-month prevalence estimates for alcohol abuse were 2.36% for men and 0.38% for women. The 12-month prevalence estimates for alcohol

Table 8.1. Percent Distribution of Current Drinkers, Drinking Levels, and Alcohol Use Disorder Status among Current Drinkers by Age, Sex, and Race/Ethnicity

Category	% Current Drinkers[a]	% Heavier Drinkers[b]	% 5+ for Men; 4+ for Women[c]		% Alcohol Use Disorders[d]
			1–11 Times	≥12 Times	
All age 18 and older	65.4	15.7	14.7	21.4	12.9
18–24	70.8	20.4	17.7	39.7	26.0
25–44	72.9	14.7	18.9	23.6	14.3
45–64	64.3	15.6	11.2	15.4	8.4
65+	45.1	13.9	3.9	6.1	3.2
White, not Hispanic					
18–24	77.1	22.5	18.3	43.7	27.2
25–44	78.5	15.3	21.0	24.1	15.1
45–64	69.0	15.7	11.8	15.1	8.4
65+	48.3	14.5	4.0	5.7	2.9
African American, not Hispanic					
18–24	60.1	14.9	12.1	22.0	19.5
25–44	61.2	16.2	9.2	20.2	12.2
45–64	49.6	18.6	7.9	16.1	10.9
65+	23.4	11.7	2.8*	9.6	7.0
American Indian/Alaska Native, not Hispanic					
18–24	70.7	38.7	21.1*	46.3	46.0
25–44	65.8	19.9	19.5	31.2	22.2
45–64	53.3	19.7	11.8	20.0	12.2
65+	37.9	15.6*	3.8*	9.7*	10.3*
Asian/Native Hawaiian/Pacific Islander					
18–24	59.1	17.8	18.2	34.2	22.2

Table 8.1. (*continued*)

Category	% Current Drinkers[a]	% Heavier Drinkers[b]	% 5+ for Men; 4+ for Women[c]		% Alcohol Use Disorders[d]
			1–11 Times	≥12 Times	
25–44	52.5	7.6	10.2	12.3	8.6
45–64	40.8	10.0*	2.2*	10.1*	3.3*
65+	32.7	2.8*	1.5*	1.7*	0.0
Hispanic					
18–24	60.4	14.0	18.7	36.3	24.1
25–44	65.7	10.9	17.8	25.7	12.3
45–64	54.4	12.3	10.4	19.0	6.7
65+	36.6	9.5	3.8	10.6	5.2*
All men age 18 years and older	71.8	17.8	15.3	27.6	17.2
White, not Hispanic men	74.3	18.5	15.9	27.5	17.3
African American, not Hispanic men	62.6	19.9	9.5	23.9	17.2
American Indian/ Alaska Native, not Hispanic men	65.5	21.6	14.2	31.7	24.2
Asian/Native Hawaiian/ Pacific Islander men	61.5	10.8	8.7	17.3	11.0
Hispanic men	69.9	13.8	17.7	33.2	17.3
All women age 18 years and older	59.6	13.3	14.1	14.6	8.2
White, not Hispanic women	65.1	13.9	14.9	14.5	8.1

(*continued on next page*)

Table 8.1. (*continued*)

Category	% Current Drinkers[a]	% Heavier Drinkers[b]	% 5+ for Men; 4+ for Women[c]		% Alcohol Use Disorders[d]
			1–11 Times	≥12 Times	
African American, not Hispanic women	45.9	12.7	8.5	13.5	8.3
American Indian/ Alaska Native, not Hispanic women	51.7	22.2	17.9	23.3	16.8
Asian/Native Hawaiian/ Pacific Islander women	36.1	8.2	10.1	12.1	6.8
Hispanic women	49.5	8.8	13.1	14.9	7.2

[a]A current drinker has had at least one drink of alcohol in the past year.
[b]Percent distribution of heavier drinkers among current drinkers. A heavier drinker is defined as a man who has had more than two drinks per day or a woman who has had more than one drink per day.
[c]Percent distribution of frequency of drinking five or more drinks for men and four or more drinks for women in a single day in the past year among current drinkers.
[d]Percent of current drinkers meeting DSM-IV criteria for alcohol use disorders in the past year.
*Relative standard error >0.3.

dependence were 0.39% for men and 0.13% for women (NIAAA 2006). One reason for the lower prevalence among older individuals may be underreporting. Instruments for detecting alcoholism were largely designed and validated on younger individuals. For example, a retired widower who is no longer driving will report no alcohol-related marital or job problems or arrests for drunk driving, regardless of how much alcohol he consumes.

Among clinical populations, estimates of alcohol abuse and dependence are substantially higher because problem drinkers of all ages are more likely to present themselves to health care settings. Rates of concurrent alcoholism range from 15% to 58% among older patients seeking treatment in hospitals, primary care clinics, and nursing homes for medical or psychiatric problems (Dufour 2006). Most older individuals with drinking problems began to abuse alcohol earlier in life. However, the risk for new cases continues through the later years even as overall prevalence declines. Late-onset heavy drinking may begin in response to stressful life experiences such as bereavement, poor health, economic changes, or retirement (Dufour 2006). Sensitivity to alcohol increases with age. In the United States, those aged 65 years and older use 30% of the prescription drugs and 40% of the over-the-counter medications. Alcohol interacts with more than 100 prescription and over-the-counter medications, including over half of the 100 most frequently pre-scribed drugs (Dufour 2006). Clearly, the older individual need not be alcohol dependent to get into trouble with alcohol use.

Sex

As shown in Table 8.1, men in the United States are more likely to be drinkers than are women (NIAAA 2006). Overall, the rates of DSM-IV alcohol use disorders are substan-tially higher for men than women, and the sex differences become more pronounced with increasing age (Grant et al. 2004). On the whole, women have fewer alcohol-related prob-lems and dependence symptoms than do men (Dawson, Grant, and Chou 1995; Wil-snack, Kristjanson, and Wilsnack 2006). However, among the heaviest drinkers, women equal or surpass men in the number of problems that result from their drinking.

Several factors appear to play a role in women's increased sensitivity to alcohol. First, because a woman has lower total body water content than a man of comparable size, she will achieve a higher concentration of alcohol in her blood than a man after consuming an equivalent amount of alcohol. Second, fluctuation in gonadal hormone levels during the menstrual cycle may affect the rate of alcohol metabolism, making women more suscep-tible to elevated blood alcohol concentrations at certain points in the cycle (Marshall et al. 1983). Finally, there is the issue of first-pass metabolism of ethanol and sex differences in the activity of an alcohol metabolizing enzyme found in the stomach—gastric alcohol de-hydrogenase (ADH). This topic is the subject of considerable interest and intense debate (Lee et al. 2006). Some research suggests that women have a lower first-pass metabolism of alcohol due to lower gastric ADH activity while other research shows no sex differences in gastric ADH activity or first-pass metabolism (Lee et al. 2006).

Race/Ethnicity

Differences in alcohol consumption and problems with and across race/ethnic minorities have become increasingly important as the proportion of race/ethnic minorities in the population of the United States has increased. Past studies of alcohol dependence and adverse consequences of drinking among racial and ethnic minorities have been criticized for assuming that a given group is homogeneous. Intraethnic variations, such as self-assessment of ethnic identification, culture retention, incorporation of mainstream cul-ture, and whether individuals are foreign- or native-born, are important to consider when examining alcohol-related questions.

According to NESARC, white and American Indian/Alaska Native men are least likely to report being lifetime abstainers and most likely to be current drinkers (NIAAA 2006). Asian/Native Hawaiian/Pacific Islander men are most likely to be lifetime abstain-ers. African American and American Indian/Alaska Native men are more likely to report being former drinkers. African American and Asian/Native Hawaiian/Pacific Islander men are least likely to be current drinkers with Hispanic men reporting intermediate levels of current drinking (NIAAA 2006).

Although women are less likely to drink than men, the distribution of drinking sta-tus and drinking levels are similar. Over half of Asian/Native Hawaiian/Pacific Islander women and about a third of African American and Hispanic women report being lifetime abstainers. While men of some race/ethnic groups are less likely to be drinkers, among those who are, the proportions drinking at the various levels are more similar. Asian/ Native Hawaiian/Pacific Islander men who drink are most likely to be light drinkers and least likely to be moderate or heavier drinkers. They are also much less likely to meet criteria for an alcohol use disorder (alcohol abuse or dependence). American Indian/Alaska Native men are slightly more likely to report heavier drinking and somewhat more likely to meet criteria for an alcohol use disorder. As shown in Table 8.1, the patterns of race/ ethnic distribution are similar for women. Compared with women as a whole, a slightly lower proportion of Asian/Native Hawaiian/Pacific Islander women meet criteria for an alcohol use disorder and nearly double the proportion of Native American/Alaska Native women meet criteria for an alcohol use disorder (NIAAA 2006).

Hispanic Americans are one of the fastest growing groups in the United States; however, Hispanics are not a homogeneous population. Nearly two-thirds of Hispanics in the United States trace their origins to Mexico (U.S. Census Bureau 2006). A number of older studies have compared alcohol use among Mexican Americans, Cuban Americans, and Puerto Ricans. Although Mexican-American men are more likely to abstain than other Hispanic men, they are also more likely to drink heavily and to have more alcohol-related problems. Cuban men are least likely to abstain or drink heavily and report the fewest problems. Puerto Rican and other Latin American men are intermediate on these measures. Among Hispanics, Cuban women are least likely to abstain, Mexican-American and Puerto Rican women are intermediate, and other Latin-American women are most likely to abstain. Few foreign-born women drink heavily. First-generation U.S.-born men and women drink more than other Hispanics, although they do not experience more alcohol-related problems (Randolph et al. 1998). A recent study of acculturation and drinking among Hispanics on the Texas–Mexico border found that acculturation has different effects on drinking for men and women. Acculturation was related to lower rates of alcohol use disorders among men and a higher frequency of heavy episodic drinking among women (Caetano et al. 2007). In 2006, nearly a quarter of Hispanic Americans traced their origins to Central and South America and other locations (U.S. Census Bureau 2006). Studies of drinking practices and problems among these groups are urgently needed.

According to the Indian Health Service (IHS), the alcohol-related death rate for American Indians and Alaska Natives (AI/AN) averaged over the years 1996–1998 was over seven times that of the U.S. all-race rate of 6.3 for 1997 (IHS 2002). The age-specific alcohol-related death rate for AI/AN men was higher for all age groups in comparison with AI/AN women. However, rates among AI/AN women were much higher than for women of all races in the U.S. population (IHS 2002). For those same years, the death rate for cirrhosis and other chronic liver disease was nearly five times that of the general population; for unintentional injuries (accidents), the rate was three times higher; for suicide, nearly twice as high; and for homicide, 1.8 times higher (IHS 2002). More recent alcohol-related death rates for AI/AN individuals are not available from the IHS; however, in 2004, the death rate for cirrhosis and chronic liver disease among AI/AN was 2.5 times higher than for the population as a whole; for unintentional injuries, 1.4 times higher; and nearly the same for homicide and suicide (NCHS 2007).

Homelessness

Thirty-eight percent of homeless individuals have mental health problems. Nearly one-half of homeless men (47%) and 16% of homeless women also experience alcohol use disorders (Johnson and Cnaan 1995). Homeless individuals who abuse alcohol and other drugs are quite susceptible to liver disease, gastrointestinal ailments, tuberculosis, seizures and other neurological disorders, hypertension, cardiopulmonary diseases/disorders, and HIV/AIDS infection (Johnson and Cnaan 1995). Furthermore, the combined chances of alcohol, drug, and mental health problems anytime in a homeless person's life are estimated at 30% (Burt et al. 1999). Because homeless populations are often hidden from view and therefore difficult to study, research on the homeless with alcohol disorders is not as abundant as it is with many other groups.

Personality

While no evidence suggests that alcohol-dependent individuals have a unique personality type, alcohol dependence and risk for alcohol dependence most consistently have been associated with two broad dimensions of personality (NIAAA 1997a). The first is behavioral disinhibition (also called behavioral undercontrol or deviance proneness), which refers to an individual's inability or unwillingness to inhibit behavioral responses to cues of impending punishment. Indicators include impulsivity, unconventionality, overactivity, and aggression. The second dimension, negative emotionality or neuroticism, refers to an individual's propensity to experience negative mood states or psychological distress. Indicators of this dimension include emotionality, neuroticism, depression, and anxiety. Current research is aimed at characterizing the process by which personality factors influence drinking behavior and ascertaining how the effects of these personality factors interact with other known risk factors for alcohol use disorders (NIAAA 1997a).

Genetics

The observation that alcoholism runs in families is an ancient one, but research to tease out the relative contributions of genetics and environment is much more recent. Studies have confirmed that identical twins, who share the same genes, are about twice as likely as fraternal twins, who share about half their genes, to resemble each other in terms of the presence of alcoholism. Recent research also reports that 50%–60% of the risk for alcoholism is genetically determined for both men and women. Genes alone, however, do not preordain that someone will become alcoholic; features in the environment and gene–environment interactions account for the remainder of the risk (NIAAA 2003). Dramatic progress is being made in understanding genetic vulnerability to the effects of alcohol. Unlike cystic fibrosis or sickle cell disease, alcohol dependence is a genetically complex disease—many genes play a role in shaping alcoholism risk. One well-characterized relationship between genes and alcoholism is the result of variation in the liver enzymes that metabolize alcohol. By speeding up the metabolism of alcohol to a toxic intermediate, acetaldehyde, or slowing down the conversion of acetaldehyde to acetate, genetic variants in the enzymes alcohol dehydrogenase or aldehyde dehydrogenase raise the level of acetaldehyde after drinking, causing symptoms that include flushing, nausea, and rapid heartbeat. The genes for these enzymes and the alleles or gene variants that alter alcohol metabolism have been identified. Genes associated with flushing are more common among Asian populations than other race/ethnic groups, and as mentioned earlier, the rates of drinking and alcoholism are correspondingly lower among Asian populations (NIAAA 2003).

Over recent years, there has been an exponential increase in research on the genetics of alcoholism. Several genetic variants linked to alcohol abuse and dependence have been discovered, and many more are expected to be identified in the near future (NIAAA 2003). Genetic differences in a patient's response to medications have also been discovered. For example, patients with a certain gene variant drank less and experienced better overall clinical outcomes than patients without the variant while taking the medication naltrexone (Anton et al. 2008). A separate issue is genetic vulnerability to organ damage. Approximately 10% of detoxified alcoholics are severely impaired as a result of alcohol-induced chronic brain disorders (Eckardt and Martin 1986). An abnormal form of a particular enzyme may play a role in causing this alcoholic brain damage. Studies are also under way to investigate the genetics of differential susceptibility to alcoholic liver disease.

Geographic Distribution

As mentioned earlier, apparent per capita consumption calculations are based on the total population of a given state or region. Such data underestimate average consumption for actual drinkers because the percentage of people who abstain varies considerably from state to state. Starting in 1999, the NSDUH sample was expanded to produce state-level estimates. The samples in each state are selected to represent proportionately the geography and demography of that state. The current practice is to base annual estimates on a two-year moving average of NSDUH data in order to enhance the precision for states with smaller samples (Wright, Sathe, and Spagnola 2007). NSDUH reports state estimates for 23 measures of substance use or mental health problems including several measures of alcohol use and dependence. In 2004–2005, the rate of past month alcohol use in states among all persons aged 12 or older ranged from a low of 30.1% in Utah to a high of 65.3% in Wisconsin (Table 8.2). Figure 8.2 presents the geographic distribution of current drinking by state. The highest rates of past month alcohol use occurred in the 18- to 25-year age group, with Wisconsin having the highest rate (75.7%) for this age group. Several states ranked in the top fifth for all three age groups (12–17 years, 18–25 years, and 26 years or older): Connecticut, North Dakota, Rhode Island, South Dakota, and Wisconsin (Wright, Sathe, and Spagnola 2007).

The Behavioral Risk Factor Surveillance System (BRFSS) conducted by individual states and coordinated by the Centers for Disease Control and Prevention (CDC) is the world's largest, ongoing telephone health survey system, tracking health conditions and risk behaviors in the United States yearly since 1984. Currently, data are collected monthly in all 50 states, the District of Columbia, Puerto Rico, the U.S. Virgin Islands, and Guam. State prevalence data are available for the following three alcohol consumption variables: (1) adults (aged 18 years and older) who have at least one drink of alcohol within the past 30 days, (2) heavy drinkers (adult men having more than two drinks per day and adult women having more than one drink per day), and (3) binge drinkers (men having five or more drinks on one occasion and women having four or more drinks on one occasion). The magnitude and distribution of BRFSS prevalence rates for past month alcohol consumption by state are roughly similar to those in NSDUH. For example, in 2005, the rates of alcohol use in the past month among adults aged 18 years and older ranged from a low of 27.3% in Utah to a high of 67.9% in Wisconsin. The BRFSS website (http://www.cdc.gov/brfss/) provides a number of features especially useful to public health professionals including interactive databases such as the State Prevalence Data

Table 8.2. Alcohol Use and Binge Alcohol Use in Past Month and Alcohol Dependence or Abuse (AUD) in Past Year by Age Group and State: Percentages, Annual Averages Based on 2004 and 2005 NSDUHs

	Total			Age Group (Years) 12–17			18–25			26 or Older		
State	Past Month Use	Past Month Binge	Past Year AUD	Past Month Use	Past Month Binge	Past Year AUD	Past Month Use	Past Month Binge	Past Year AUD	Past Month Use	Past Month Binge	Past Year AUD
Total	51.05	22.70	7.71	17.06	10.49	5.78	60.69	41.54	17.47	54.03	21.07	6.27
Alabama	42.07	19.11	6.55	15.97	10.03	5.47	52.63	33.61	12.67	43.69	17.76	5.61
Alaska	50.55	21.80	7.51	14.67	9.62	5.98	57.44	37.34	16.10	55.71	20.97	6.11
Arizona	55.43	24.11	9.00	18.01	11.54	7.08	61.27	44.03	17.77	59.73	22.31	7.69
Arkansas	39.63	19.23	6.63	16.45	10.23	5.12	53.21	36.63	15.63	40.31	17.33	5.23
California	50.14	20.02	7.77	16.20	9.99	6.08	55.02	35.42	16.74	54.37	18.73	6.39
Colorado	59.43	24.28	9.23	20.52	12.63	7.45	69.30	48.57	20.70	62.99	21.59	7.46
Connecticut	61.28	25.82	8.49	20.94	12.05	6.31	71.44	48.69	22.04	65.07	24.16	6.71
Delaware	49.71	20.60	7.02	16.41	9.82	5.00	63.20	42.95	18.56	51.59	18.09	5.28
District of Columbia	58.44	27.46	9.83	12.70	6.79	3.95	68.93	46.30	18.69	60.90	26.03	8.80
Florida	52.04	21.52	8.02	17.01	9.26	5.76	58.59	38.69	16.94	55.35	20.44	6.96

(continued on next page)

Table 8.2. (*continued*)

| State | Total | | | Age Group (Years) | | | | | | | | |
| | | | | 12–17 | | | 18–25 | | | 26 or Older | | |
	Past Month Use	Past Month Binge	Past Year AUD	Past Month Use	Past Month Binge	Past Year AUD	Past Month Use	Past Month Binge	Past Year AUD	Past Month Use	Past Month Binge	Past Year AUD
Georgia	44.11	19.55	5.97	14.52	8.43	4.31	52.16	32.81	11.87	46.88	18.72	5.13
Hawaii	47.08	21.66	6.84	13.74	9.34	5.37	57.77	42.88	17.51	49.63	19.94	5.38
Idaho	46.43	22.09	7.82	15.88	10.52	7.05	53.80	39.11	16.34	49.53	20.36	6.19
Illinois	54.17	26.27	8.40	17.24	10.41	5.80	65.20	46.71	19.95	57.35	24.84	6.70
Indiana	49.94	21.99	7.87	17.12	10.80	5.93	61.34	42.03	18.26	52.50	19.92	6.26
Iowa	54.46	27.87	8.75	18.27	12.95	7.48	69.28	52.50	23.30	56.28	25.19	6.23
Kansas	51.81	26.18	8.86	19.45	13.98	7.61	65.35	48.64	20.55	53.68	23.50	6.76
Kentucky	42.61	21.91	6.78	17.01	11.24	6.10	55.60	39.12	14.16	43.66	20.34	5.62
Louisiana	46.76	24.06	7.61	17.59	10.48	5.09	58.80	38.73	14.21	48.61	23.09	6.64
Maine	51.49	20.99	7.31	19.14	11.59	6.72	64.01	42.52	16.57	53.51	18.80	5.94
Maryland	53.05	19.96	6.84	15.71	9.13	5.05	62.88	37.26	15.13	56.69	18.65	5.74

Massachusetts	6.43	23.56	62.71	19.42	52.78	70.60	5.32	12.06	19.11	7.96	26.15	59.55
Michigan	6.28	22.88	57.36	18.89	45.85	66.30	5.57	10.43	17.09	7.88	24.59	54.17
Minnesota	7.14	25.67	64.99	19.60	47.63	69.71	6.10	12.94	19.18	8.76	27.42	60.99
Mississippi		18.45	38.87		34.41	49.04		8.72	15.43		19.76	37.84
Missouri	7.03	21.82	49.71	20.95	47.07	65.63	7.04	12.84	19.96	8.93	24.35	48.83
Montana	7.21	25.51	59.44	25.60	53.81	70.43	9.01	15.55	21.22	9.94	28.47	57.20
Nebraska	6.99	24.41	57.61	23.63	51.31	71.30	7.47	13.05	18.63	9.47	27.17	55.60
Nevada	6.86	21.39	50.95	19.68	39.38	57.33	6.23	10.60	16.56	8.39	22.50	48.17
New Hampshire	5.84	21.33	62.54	21.19	48.94	71.84	6.04	11.71	18.09	7.76	23.74	59.07
New Jersey	5.29	19.69	58.06	15.51	42.19	62.41	5.68	10.47	18.77	6.52	21.35	54.48
New Mexico	6.93	19.46	50.94	18.67	37.74	57.15	6.65	12.17	18.09	8.57	21.27	48.21
New York	5.42	21.12	56.88	16.95	43.43	63.30	5.38	11.21	18.75	6.90	23.00	53.92
North Carolina	5.87	19.48	45.49	14.66	37.21	55.48	5.29	8.98	14.92	6.94	20.67	43.62
North Dakota	7.03	28.24	61.15	24.19	58.05	74.56	8.23	14.24	20.04	9.80	31.52	59.32
Ohio	5.64	20.66	53.49	18.05	45.05	63.71	5.41	10.63	16.37	7.26	22.86	51.00

(continued on next page)

Table 8.2. (*continued*)

| State | Total | | | Age Group (Years) | | | | | | | | |
| | | | | 12–17 | | | 18–25 | | | 26 or Older | | |
	Past Month Use	Past Month Binge	Past Year AUD	Past Month Use	Past Month Binge	Past Year AUD	Past Month Use	Past Month Binge	Past Year AUD	Past Month Use	Past Month Binge	Past Year AUD
Oklahoma	42.37	21.42	7.88	17.41	11.83	6.25	55.52	39.75	18.55	43.19	19.17	6.04
Oregon	56.61	20.70	7.74	18.32	11.57	6.31	64.13	40.23	17.94	60.22	18.55	6.19
Pennsylvania	52.86	24.67	7.57	16.69	10.33	5.65	64.85	46.57	19.03	55.55	22.91	5.93
Rhode Island	60.38	27.96	8.26	19.79	12.69	5.89	73.05	51.94	19.99	63.25	25.56	6.44
South Carolina	42.98	20.18	7.79	13.67	8.34	4.61	52.79	35.70	13.60	45.24	19.04	7.20
South Dakota	59.71	27.18	9.35	22.03	13.59	8.15	72.36	52.23	22.59	62.45	24.10	6.89
Tennessee	40.85	17.79	6.67	14.34	7.68	4.81	55.11	34.76	14.83	41.76	16.20	5.54
Texas	48.62	24.00	7.72	16.91	10.26	5.25	57.65	39.70	16.28	51.73	23.02	6.41

Utah	30.05	16.33	12.08	8.67	5.23	34.91	26.66	14.15	31.82	14.82	5.71
Vermont	59.19	23.63	18.63	12.45	6.43	71.40	49.21	22.71	62.26	20.67	6.55
Virginia	51.24	22.44	13.93	8.71	5.01	64.16	44.41	18.27	54.07	20.63	5.89
Washington	56.48	21.74	15.78	9.44	5.74	62.85	39.18	18.78	60.74	20.34	6.77
West Virginia	35.95	18.67	16.47	10.77	6.49	53.83	40.49	18.18	35.33	16.13	5.28
Wisconsin	65.30	31.42	22.59	14.69	8.05	75.72	55.47	24.12	69.11	29.31	7.90
Wyoming	53.00	23.87	19.17	12.90	8.10	66.67	47.04	20.31	54.84	20.89	7.43

"Binge alcohol use" is defined as drinking five or more drinks on the same occasion (i.e., at the same time or within a couple of hours of each other) on at least 1 day in the past 30 days.

Dependence or abuse is based on definitions found in the 4th edition of the DSM-IV.

Complete table for past month alcohol use can be found at http://www.oas.samhsa.gov/2k5State/AppB.htm#TabB.9.

Complete table for past month binge alcohol use can be found at http://www.oas.samhsa.gov/2k5State/AppB.htm#TabB.10.

Complete table for alcohol dependence or abuse in past year can be found at http://www.oas.samhsa.gov/2k5State/AppB.htm#TabB.16.

Note: Estimates are based on a survey-weighted hierarchical Bayes estimation approach.

Source: SAMHSA, Office of Applied Studies, NSDUH (2004, 2005).

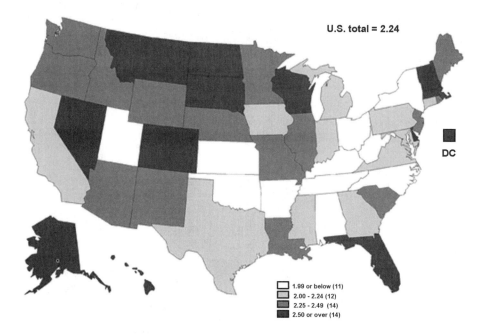

Figure 8.2. Geographic distribution of current drinking by state.

Charts and BRFSS Maps (GIS), which make it possible to view specific alcohol variables by state and map them. The Web Enabled Analysis Tool permits researchers to create cross-tabulation reports and perform logistic analysis of BRFSS data.

As mentioned earlier, in the NSDUH, binge alcohol use is defined as drinking five or more drinks on the same occasion on at least 1 day in the 30 days before the survey. Nationally, 22.7% of all persons aged 12 years or older reported binge alcohol use in 2004–2005 (Table 8.2). For that same period, past month rate of binge use ranged from 16.3% in Utah to 31.5% in North Dakota. Five states ranked in the top fifth in all three age groups in binge drinking: Iowa, Montana, Nebraska, North Dakota, and Wisconsin (Wright, Sathe, and Spagnola 2007). According the BRFSS, nationally 14.4% of all persons aged 18 years and older reported binge alcohol use in 2005. Past month rate of binge alcohol use ranged from 8.3% in Utah to 22.1% in Wisconsin.

According to NSDUH, nationally in 2004–2005, 7.7% of the population aged 12 years or older met criteria for alcohol use disorders (alcohol abuse or dependence) in the past year with the rate among those aged 18–25 years being highest (17.5%) (Table 8.2). Wisconsin had the highest rate (10.1%) and Georgia the lowest rate (6.0%) of alcohol abuse or dependence. Three states—Montana, North Dakota, and Wisconsin—ranked in the top fifth for all three age groups for alcohol abuse or dependence (Wright, Sathe, and Spagnola 2007).

Another useful resource is Chronic Disease Indicators (CDI), a collaborative effort of the Council of State and Territorial Epidemiologists, the National Association of Chronic Disease Directors, and the National Center for Chronic Disease Prevention and Health

Promotion at the CDC, which allows public health officials in states and territories to uniformly define, collect, and report chronic disease data that are important to public health practice (Pelletier et al. 2005; CDC 2004). This cross-cutting set of 90 indicators is divided into seven categories, one of which is tobacco and alcohol use. Included in this category are the following alcohol items:

- Alcohol use among youth
- Binge drinking among youth
- Binge drinking among adults aged 18 years and older
- Binge drinking among women of childbearing age
- Heavy drinking among adult women aged 18 years and older
- Heavy drinking among adult men aged 18 years and older
- Mortality from chronic liver disease

Data for the indicators are derived from nine sources including the BRFSS. The CDI website (www.cdc.gov/nccdphp/cdi) is interactive and allows comparisons between states on the different categories of indicators. The website also serves as a gateway with hyperlinks to additional information and resources such as BRFSS and Alcohol and Public Health.

Time Trends

Beginning in 1934, following Prohibition, per capita alcohol consumption generally increased (excluding fluctuations during and immediately following World War II), reaching a peak of 2.76 gallons of ethanol in 1980 and 1981, and declining during the remainder of the 1980s. After a slight increase in 1990, per capita alcohol consumption decreased slightly from 1991 to 1998. From 1999 to 2005, per capital alcohol consumption has gradually increased reaching 2.24 gallons of ethanol in 2005. Beer consumption has remained relatively stable over the past 40 years, peaking in 1981 and gradually decreasing since that time (Lakins et al. 2007). In 2005, beer comprised approximately 53% of the per capita alcohol consumption from all alcoholic beverages combined. Wine consumption increased throughout the 1980s, peaked in 1986, and then decreased until 1996. Since then wine consumption has gradually increased reaching 1.36 gallons of ethanol in 2005, the same level as in 1988. In 2005, wine represented about 16% of the per capita alcohol consumption from all alcoholic beverages (Lakins et al. 2007). In 1997, spirits consumption reached its lowest level in 56 years. Since that time, it has gradually increased. In 2005, spirits comprised approximately 31% of per capita alcohol consumption (Lakins et al. 2007). Total per capita ethanol consumption as well as per capita consumption by beverage type in the United States from 1977 to 2005 is shown in Figure 8.3.

Long-term time trends in the prevalence of alcohol abuse and dependence in the United States are difficult to assess. Since the early 1980s, large-scale U.S. and international surveys have produced a range of rates of the prevalence of current and lifetime alcohol abuse and dependence utilizing a range of diagnostic criteria (DSM-III, DSM-IIIR, DSM-IV). Given the range of rates over time, location, and diagnostic criteria, it is very difficult to tease out true time trends from methodological differences. The 1991–1992 National Longitudinal Alcohol Epidemiologic Survey and the 2001–2002 NESARC are two large national surveys conducted approximately ten years apart both of which use

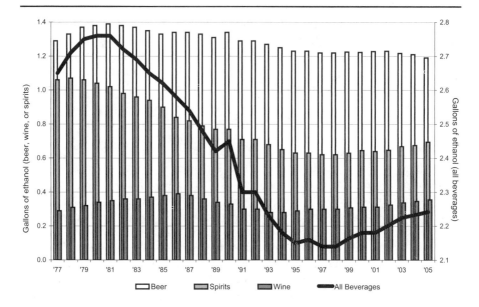

Figure 8.3. Total per capita ethanol consumption by beverage type, United States, 1977–2005.

DSM-IV diagnostic criteria (Grant et al. 2004). Therefore, for the first time, it is possible to present accurate trends in the prevalence of alcohol abuse and dependence across these years. During this time, the prevalence of alcohol dependence significantly declined from 4.38% to 3.81%. The prevalence of alcohol dependence decreased among men while remaining stable among women resulting in a somewhat smaller sex difference than had been found previously. Dependence also decreased among whites and Hispanics. In contrast, there was a significant increase in the prevalence of alcohol abuse, from 3.03% to 4.56%. This increase was seen in both men and women and was especially marked among young black and Hispanic men and young Asian women (Grant et al. 2004).

Long-term time trend data for all-cause alcohol-related mortality do not exist. Utilizing the Alcohol Related Disease Impact (ARDI) system, recently revised by the CDC (http://www.cdc.gov/alcohol/ardi.htm), it is now possible to calculate the alcohol-attributable deaths in the United States or in individual states. ARDI estimates alcohol-attributable deaths by multiplying the number of deaths from a particular alcohol-related condition by its alcohol-attributable fraction. Certain conditions (e.g., alcoholic cirrhosis of the liver) are, by definition, 100% alcohol attributable. For the majority of the chronic conditions profiled in ARDI, the system calculates alcohol-attributable fractions by using relative risk estimates from meta-analyses and prevalence data on alcohol use from the BRFSS. In 2001, ARDI estimates that there were 75,766 alcohol-attributable deaths out of a total of 2,416,425 deaths in the United States (Midanik et al. 2004). The National Center for Health Statistics has also begun to report number of deaths and death rates from "alcohol-induced" causes (Kung et al. 2008). The category "alcohol-induced" includes not only deaths from dependent and nondependent use of alcohol, but also accidental poisoning by alcohol and a number of other causes such as alcoholic polyneuropathy, alcoholic liver disease, and others. Alcohol-induced causes exclude accidents, homicides, and other causes indirectly related to alcohol use. Among the exclusions are alcohol-related motor vehicle crashes—a significant cause of death. In 2006, 42,642 people were killed in motor vehicle traffic crashes, 17,602 of which were alcohol-related (NHTSA 2007). Alcohol-induced death data are available for 1999–2005 (Kung et al. 2008). In 1999, there were 19,469 deaths compared with 21,634 in 2005. Age-adjusted mortality rates have shown very little variation over these years: 7.1 per 100,000 in 1999 and 7.0 in 2005 (Kung et al. 2008).

Causes

Modifiable Risk Factors

The risks of adverse health outcomes resulting from alcohol abuse are well known. In contrast, the epidemiology of alcohol use is relatively unknown. For many areas of interest, baseline data remain to be collected. The state of the art is such that at present it is impossible to quantify the magnitudes of particular risk factors except in the broadest terms.

The influence of alcohol advertising on young people continues to be the subject of much debate. A recent review of the literature indicates that while many econometric studies suggest little effect, more focused consumer studies, especially recent ones with sophisticated designs, are beginning to show clear links between advertising and behavior (Hastings et al. 2005). Most studies of outlet density have used ecological designs, which are considered problematic for drawing causal inferences about individual drinking. Current studies attempting to identify associations between alcohol outlets and problem drinking and other health problems, including clinical measures, using individual level data will contribute substantially to our knowledge in this area.

Age of onset of drinking is a modifiable risk factor in that early onset of drinking poses an increased risk for lifetime alcohol-related problems. Individuals aged 21 years and older who reported first use of alcohol before age 14 years were more than six times as likely to report past-year alcohol dependence or abuse as people who first used alcohol at age 21 years or older (Grant and Dawson 1997).

As mentioned earlier, children of alcoholics are at extremely high risk for developing alcohol use disorders themselves. At this point in time genetic predisposition is not a modifiable risk factor; however, not all of these children develop alcohol use disorders. Therefore, knowledge of this increased risk can be protective in that it allows children of alcoholics to modify their own drinking behavior accordingly.

Population-Attributable Risk

Estimates of the proportion of alcohol use in the population related to various modifiable risk factors are difficult to make. Generally these estimates are not possible because precise relative risk estimates for these factors are not available, and no data are available on the proportion of the population exposed to many of these risk factors.

Estimates of relative risk of adverse health outcomes from alcohol misuse are available. For example, estimates of fatal motor vehicle crash by blood alcohol concentration (BAC) have been produced (Zador, Krawchuk, and Voas 2000). Examining relative risk across six age and sex groups, at a BAC of 0.035%, the relative risk ranged from 2.6 to 4.6; at a BAC of 0.065%, from 5.8 to 17.3; at a BAC of 0.09%, from 11.4 to 52; at a BAC of

Table 8.3. Psychosocial and Environmental Risk Factors for Alcohol Use

Policies regulating alcohol behavior

Price of alcoholic beverages

Happy hours and other drink specials

Other alcohol sales and service practices

Alcohol advertising

Outlet density

Alcohol availability

Community norms and attitudes about drinking

Positive alcohol expectancies

Level of enforcement of existing alcohol-related policies, laws, and regulations

---

0.125%, from 29.3 to 240.9; and at a BAC of 0.220%, from 382 to 15,560. Compared with other drivers, drivers aged 16–20 years had an increased relative risk of fatal crashes with no alcohol involvement. Among these young drivers, relative risk increased substantially even at BACs under 0.02%. The relative risk curve increased fastest with increasing BAC among males 16–20 years (Zador, Krawchuk, and Voas 2000).

Other studies have estimated the population-attributable risk of hypertension from heavy drinking in the United States (3%–12%; Larbi et al. 1984) and breast cancer in white women (0.0%–6.1% (Clark, Purdie, and Glaser 2006). No studies of the population-attributable risk for alcohol abuse and dependence currently exist.

The above-mentioned statistics highlight the risk of adverse outcomes of alcohol use. Also of interest are risk factors for alcohol use and alcohol abuse. Psychosocial risk factors for underage drinking include parents' and siblings' drinking behavior and favorable attitudes about drinking; lack of parental support, monitoring, and communication; peer drinking and peer acceptance of drinking; positive alcohol expectancies; and alcohol advertising (NIAAA 1997c). Psychosocial and environmental risk factors for alcohol use among the general population are shown in Table 8.3. Most studies of these risk factors focus on particular alcohol-related outcomes such as violence or traffic fatalities.

Prevention and Control

Prevention

Prevention measures aim to reduce alcohol abuse, dependence, and other alcohol-related consequences through multiple strategies employed at the individual and community level. Such measures include policies regulating alcohol-related behavior on the one hand

and community and educational interventions seeking to influence drinking behavior on the other. Most programs are focused on immediate goals, such as decreasing binge drinking among youth or preventing driving after drinking. If successful, however, these programs could also affect longer-term health consequences such as alcoholic liver disease or alcohol dependence and mortality. Research has demonstrated that alcohol consumption, intoxication, and drinking/driving rates are sensitive to the price of alcoholic beverages. Underage individuals and young adults are particularly affected by the cost of alcohol. Studies show that increases in price significantly reduce the number of drinks consumed by this population. Happy hours, drinking contests, "all-you-can-drink" specials and other promotions encourage overconsumption by reducing prices, a potent inducement to drinking large amounts of alcohol in short time periods. As of January 1, 2003, 27 states had provision expressly prohibiting excessive drinking practices or "happy hour" types of promotions. In addition, many communities have passed local ordinances prohibiting these practices (NHTSA 2005). Almost no literature exists on enforcement and adjudication of these laws.

Nearly every state prohibits sales and service of alcohol to obviously intoxicated people (NHTSA 2005). Again, little research is available to determine how these laws are enforced, the extent with which they are complied with, and the impact enforcement and compliance might have on public health outcomes (NHTSA 2005). Multiple examples of prevention efforts are included later in this chapter in the section on Public Health Interventions.

Screening

Preventive health services include early intervention programs that focus on identifying people who are drinking in unhealthy ways or are beginning to experience adverse consequences of their alcohol use. Screening all patients for alcohol problems, particularly in primary health care settings, is a medical necessity. The U.S. Preventive Services Task Force (USPSTF) recommends routine screening of adults for alcohol misuse in the primary care setting as well as brief counseling interventions for individuals with nondependent alcohol misuse (USPSTF 2004). Such brief counseling has been shown to reduce alcohol consumption and alcohol-related harms (USPSTF 2004).

Structured interviews and self-report instruments are useful for screening. Both are rapid, inexpensive, noninvasive, and relatively accurate tools. A number of screening instruments are available. A specific screening instrument should be selected on the basis of staff experience and training, available testing time, and characteristics of the patient population.

The CAGE questionnaire (Table 8.4) derives its name from a mnemonic for attempts to *c*ut down on drinking, *a*nnoyance with criticisms about drinking, *g*uilt about drinking, and using alcohol as an *e*ye-opener (Mayfield, McLeod, and Hall 1974). It is popular for screening in the primary care setting because it is short, simple, easy to remember, and has been proven effective for detecting a range of alcohol problems (NIAAA 2005b). The CAGE questionnaire can be self-administered or asked by a clinician; it poses four overt yes–no questions. Since it takes less than a minute to administer, the CAGE can be woven into a standard, brief clinical history.

The Michigan Alcoholism Screening Test (MAST) is a formal 25-item questionnaire that requires approximately 25 minutes to complete. The MAST focuses on the

Table 8.4. CAGE Questions

1. Have you ever felt you should <u>c</u>ut down on your drinking?

2. Have people <u>a</u>nnoyed you by criticizing your drinking?

3. Have you ever felt bad or <u>g</u>uilty about your drinking?

4. Have you ever taken a drink first thing in the morning (<u>e</u>ye opener) to steady your nerves or get rid of a hangover?

Data from Mayfield, McLeod, and Hall (1974).

consequences of problem drinking and on the subjects' own perceptions of their alcohol problems. Recent studies have reported that a cutoff score of 12 or 13 achieves balanced rates of false-positives and false-negatives. Two shortened forms of the MAST, a 13-item Short MAST (SMAST) and a 10-item brief MAST (b-MAST), have been constructed using items from the original test that are highly discriminating for alcoholism. A cutoff score of 3 is suggested for the SMAST; a cutoff score of 6 is suggested for the b-MAST (NIAAA 1990). A geriatric version of the instrument (MAST-G) has several elder-specific items such as "after drinking have you ever noticed an increase in your heart rate or beating in your chest?" and "does alcohol make you so sleepy that you often fall asleep in your chair?" The MAST-G has high sensitivity and specificity among older adults recruited from a wide range of settings, including primary care clinics, nursing homes, and older adult congregate housing locations. The instrument, which requires about 10 minutes, can be given as a paper-and-pencil self-administered assessment or by interview (SAMHSA 1998).

The Alcohol Use Disorders Identification Test (AUDIT) is a ten-question instrument that includes questions about the quantity and frequency of alcohol use, as well as binge drinking, dependency symptoms, and alcohol-related problems The AUDIT, which was developed by the WHO, takes about five minutes to complete, has been tested internationally in primary care settings, and found to be highly valid and reliable (NIAAA 2005a; Babor et al. 2001). It is especially useful in screening women and minorities. It also shows promise in screening adolescents and young adults. Although it has not been extensively tested in older individuals, some studies suggest that it may be less accurate in that population.

NIAAA has produced an updated edition of *Helping Patients Who Drink Too Much: A Clinician's Guide* (NIAAA 2005a) with guidance from physicians, nurses, advanced practice nurses, physician assistants, and clinical researchers. The guide is intended for primary care and mental health clinicians and features guidelines on screening and brief intervention. The guide is available in English and Spanish and comes with a variety of supporting materials including downloadable versions of the AUDIT in both English and Spanish, preformatted progress notes and templates, training materials, and patient education materials. The guide and related materials are available at http://www.niaaa. nih.gov/Publications/EducationTrainingMaterials/guide.htm.

Several clinical laboratory tests may be useful in detecting harmful alcohol use. Increased activity of serum gamma glutamyl transferase (GGT) is a relatively sensitive index of liver damage in heavy drinkers. However, this test lacks diagnostic specificity because all types of liver damage and a wide variety of diseases also cause elevated serum activity of this enzyme. Results may be more discriminating when interpreted in conjunction with additional tests, such as mean corpuscular volume (MCV). MCV, an index of red blood cell volume, increases with excessive alcohol intake. The liver enzyme aspartate aminotransferase (AST) can be a useful marker for alcohol abuse. The ratio of levels of mitochondrial AST to total AST has been found to be effective in differentiating alcoholics from other patients and in detecting chronic excessive drinking (Peterson 2004/2005).

In recent years, carbohydrate-deficient transferrin (CDT) has begun to be used to screen for heavy alcohol consumption. Although it is a highly specific measure of alcohol consumption, CDT is difficult to measure accurately. Recently, researchers have made several improvements in measuring CDT (Peterson 2004/2005). Some studies have also examined the usefulness of combining the CDT and GGT tests finding that, at least in men, using both tests is more sensitive than using either marker alone (Hietala et al. 2006).

Several new markers for assessing alcohol intake and alcohol abuse are at various stages of research and development (Peterson 2004/2005). None of these tests are commercially available yet but some look promising. Until more sensitive and specific markers become available, self-report interviews and questionnaires remain more sensitive and specific than routine blood tests. Laboratory tests may be used most effectively in conjunction with self-report instruments to enhance objectivity.

Treatment

Unlike traditional specialty alcoholism treatments that are designed for people who are alcohol dependent, brief interventions—short one-on-one counseling sessions—are very effective for people who drink in ways that are harmful or abusive. Brief interventions generally aim to moderate a person's drinking to sensible levels and to eliminate harmful drinking practices like binge drinking (NIAAA 2005c). Brief interventions differ from most other treatments for alcohol problems because they are generally restricted to four or fewer sessions; are usually performed in a treatment setting not specific for alcoholism, typically a primary care context; and are commonly performed by personnel who have not specialized in addiction treatment. Brief interventions are inexpensive, can readily be incorporated into many settings, and are reasonably effective. Brief interventions in no way preclude subsequent application of more intensive intervention. People who do not respond well can be referred for further treatment.

Despite evidence that brief interventions are useful and effective in the primary care setting, they are not yet a routine practice. One survey of primary care physicians found that although most (88%) reported asking their patients about alcohol use, only 13% used standard screening instruments. A survey of primary care patients revealed that more than half said their physician did nothing about their substance abuse and nearly as many said their physician never diagnosed their condition (NIAAA 2005c). New technology such as computerized interventions may offer an effective alternate means of implementing brief interventions, particularly in settings in which time constraints or lack of resources or training in intervention techniques are factors (NIAAA 2005c).

Alcohol dependence is a complex disorder, not a single straightforward entity. Clinicians and researchers have long recognized the heterogeneity of individuals with alcohol dependence. In order to improve clinical management and to understand the complexity of genetic and environmental influences on the disorder, efforts have been made to classify alcoholic individuals into subtypes (Moss, Chen, and Yi 2008). NIAAA researchers, who recently analyzed the large national sample of individuals with alcohol dependence available in NESARC, report five distinct subtypes of the disease: young adult, young antisocial, functional, intermediate familial, and chronic severe subtype (Moss, Chen, and Yi 2008). These findings clearly show that there is no such thing as a "typical alcoholic." Since these data are derived from the general population rather than from alcoholics in treatment, they provide a broader and more accurate picture of the true heterogeneity of alcohol use disorders (Moss, Chen, and Yi 2008).

A number of treatments are available within the specialized alcohol treatment system. In many cases, the beginning phase of treatment is detoxification, the set of interventions aimed at managing acute intoxication and alcohol withdrawal. Abstinence from alcohol may lead to the alcohol withdrawal syndrome, the cluster of symptoms observed in people who stop drinking alcohol following continuous heavy consumption. Milder manifestations of alcohol withdrawal include tremulousness, seizures, and hallucinations, typically occurring within 6–48 hours after the last drink. Much more serious is delirium tremens, which includes profound confusion, hallucinations, and severe autonomic nervous system overactivity, typically beginning 48–96 hours after the last drink. Many withdrawal symptoms appear to result in part from overactivity of the sympathetic nervous system. Thus, the preferred medications are benzodiazepines that help to dampen the racing sympathetic nervous system while also preventing seizures. Ongoing research indicates that repeated, unmedicated alcohol withdrawal episodes may increase the risk of seizures and other complications during detoxification (NIAAA 1997b). Third-party payers sometimes prefer to manage payment for detoxification separately from other phases of alcohol treatment. This unbundling of services may result in fragmentation of care. In addition, reimbursement for detoxification may not cover counseling, which is an integral part of alcohol treatment (SAMHSA 1997).

No single definition of treatment exists and no standard terminology describes the different dimensions and elements of treatment. Describing a facility as providing inpatient care or ambulatory services characterizes only one aspect of treatment—the setting. The continuum of treatment settings, from most to least intensive includes inpatient hospitalization, residential treatment, intensive outpatient treatment, and outpatient treatment. All specialized alcohol treatment programs have three broad goals: (1) reducing alcohol abuse or achieving an alcohol-free life, (2) maximizing multiple aspects of life functioning, and (3) preventing or reducing the frequency and severity of relapse. Within each treatment approach, a variety of treatment services are provided to achieve specific goals (SAMHSA 1997). The emphasis may change, from pharmacological intervention to treat withdrawal to behavioral therapy, mutual-help support, and relapse prevention efforts during the initial care and stabilization phase and continued Alcoholics Anonymous (AA) participation after discharge from formal treatment. The principal elements of most treatment programs include:

- Pharmacotherapies that discourage alcohol use, suppress withdrawal symptoms, block or diminish cravings, or treat coexisting psychiatric problems
- Psychosocial or psychological interventions that modify destructive interpersonal feelings, attitudes, and behaviors through individual, group, marital, and/or family therapy

- Behavioral therapies that lessen or extinguish undesirable behaviors and encourage desired ones, and
- Self-help groups, sometimes called mutual-help groups, for support and encouragement to become or remain abstinent before, during, and after formal treatment (SAMHSA 1997)

Clinical trials have demonstrated that behavioral approaches such as motivational enhancement therapy, cognitive behavioral therapy, and 12-step facilitation are effective in treating alcohol dependence (Project MATCH Research Group 1997). When used in conjunction with behavioral therapies, medications have been shown to improve the likelihood of recovery (Anton et al. 2008; Donovan et al. 2008). The choice of medication depends on clinical judgment and patient preference (NIAAA 2005a). Each has a different mechanism of action and some patients may respond better to one type of medication than another. Several medications are currently FDA-approved for treating alcoholism and other promising candidates are in the pipeline (Johnson et al. 2007).

The availability of alcoholism treatment services varies, with more services available in urban areas. Where available, assessment and referral services can provide a recommendation for treatment intensity and location. The ASAM Patient Placement Criteria (ASAM PPC-2R) is the most widely used and comprehensive national guidelines for placement, continued stay, and discharge of patients with alcohol and other drug problems. It provides two sets of guidelines—one for adults and the other for adolescents—across five broad levels of care for each group.

SAMHSA's online Substance Abuse Treatment Facility Locator (http://dasis3.samhsa.gov/) is a convenient and comprehensive resource that provides an up-to-date list of private and public facilities that are licensed, certified, or otherwise approved for inclusion by their state substance abuse agency as well as treatment facilities administered by the Department of Veterans Affairs, the IHS, and the Department of Defense. Also available on this website is a list of state substance abuse agencies including names, contact information (e-mail, phone, and address), and links to individual state agency websites. Information and guidance can also be obtained by calling the Referral Helpline run by the SAMHSA Center for Substance Abuse Treatment at 1-800-622-HELP.

Alcoholism is a chronic disease with all the attendant relapses and patient compliance issues. A recent review of seven large studies of alcoholism treatment found that about one-third of the patients either were abstinent or drank moderately without negative consequences or dependence in the year following treatment. Although the other two-thirds had some bouts of heavy drinking, on average, they reduced consumption and alcohol-related problems by half. These reductions appeared to last at least 3 years. This substantial improvement in patients who do not attain complete abstinence or problem-free reduced drinking should not be ignored. These individuals may require additional treatment and their chances of benefiting the next time do not appear to be compromised significantly by having had previous treatments. Like patients with other chronic diseases, individuals with more severe forms of alcohol dependence may require long-term management (Miller, Walters, and Bennett 2001).

A significant proportion of alcohol-dependent individuals eventually change their drinking without specific help from alcoholism treatment providers or mutual-help groups (Dawson et al. 2005; Venner et al. 2006). Recovery outside of formal treatment is more likely to occur in those having fewer symptoms of dependence, fewer comorbid psychiatric disorders, less pressure to quit drinking, and more social capital (Venner et al. 2006). Although alcohol dependent individuals who maintain abstinence generally have the best outcomes, emerging evidence suggests that some alcohol dependent individuals are able to return to low-risk drinking without recurrence of alcohol dependence at least in the short term (Dawson, Goldstein, and Grant 2007). Long-term follow-up of such individuals is clearly a research priority. Not only is abstinence important for recovery from alcoholism itself, but it also has a significant positive impact on other chronic health consequences of alcohol consumption. For example, although cirrhosis is an irreversible condition, abstinence plays a key role in length and quality of life. In cirrhosis patients without serious complications, 5-year survival was 89% for patients who abstained compared with 68% for those who continued to drink. In cirrhosis patients with serious complications, 5-year survival was 60% for abstainers versus 34% for continuing drinkers (Dufour 2007).

Examples of Public Health Interventions

Multiple successful prevention and intervention strategies that could serve as effective components of a public health effort are outlined here. Examples of policy measures relating to alcohol include regulation of the price of beverages, a minimum legal drinking age of 21 years, 0.08% BAC limits for drivers ages 21 years and older, zero-tolerance laws (laws that make it illegal for drivers younger than age 21 years to drive after drinking alcohol, typically setting the BAC at 0.00%–0.02%), administrative license revocation laws, server liability, warning labels, and limitations on numbers, types, hours of operation, and locations of outlets that sell alcoholic beverages.

Underage youth obtain alcohol from friends, coworkers, parents, siblings, and strangers. Polices that address youth social access to alcohol include beer keg registration, alcohol use restrictions on public property, alcohol restrictions at community events, and social host liability. Underage youth also obtain alcohol from licensed alcohol establishments such as bars, convenience stores, liquor stores, grocery stores, and restaurants. Policies that address reducing commercial access include compliance checks, administrative penalties, responsible beverage service training, checking age identification, regulations or bans on home delivery of alcohol, minimum age of seller requirements, and alcohol warning posters. Restrictions on alcohol advertising and on alcohol sponsorship can be instituted through local ordinances or state laws, or can be implemented voluntarily by a business, event, or organization (Toomey and Wagenaar 2002).

Maintaining the minimum legal drinking age at 21 years and zero tolerance laws continue to be effective in reducing the proportion of fatal crashes involving young drinking drivers (Voas, Tippetts, and Fell 2003). By July of 2004, all states and the District of Columbia had enacted laws mandating BAC levels of 0.08% for motor vehicle drivers age 21 years and older in order to further reduce alcohol-related traffic crashes. A recent meta-analysis of 0.08 BAC laws in 19 jurisdictions showed a statistically significant decline of 14.8% ($p < .005$) in the rate of drinking drivers in fatal crashes after the 0.08 law was introduced. The reductions were greater in states that also had an administrative license suspension/revocation law and implemented frequent sobriety checkpoints (Tippetts et al. 2005). Extensive information on other alcohol policies can be found at the NIAAA Alcohol Policy Information System (APIS) at http://www.alcoholpolicy.niaaa.nih.gov/.

The Task Force on Community Preventive Services produces *The Community Guide*, which provides evidence-based recommendations for programs and policies to promote population health. Interventions directed to the general population recommended in *The Community Guide* include outlet density and zoning restrictions. Interventions directed to underage drinkers include enhanced enforcement of laws prohibiting the sale of alcohol to minors (CDC). *The Community Guide* can be accessed at http://www.thecommunityguide.org.

Many successful community interventions have been implemented. One example is the Communities Mobilizing for Change on Alcohol (CMCA), a community organizing program designed to reduce teen (13–20 years of age) access to alcohol by changing community policies and practices. CMCA seeks both to limit youth access to alcohol and to communicate a clear message to the community that underage drinking is inappropriate and unacceptable. The program involves community members in seeking and achieving changes in local public policies and the practices of community institutions that can affect youth access to alcohol. CMCA is based on established research that has demonstrated the importance of the social and policy environment in facilitating or impeding drinking among youth. CMCA was first implemented and evaluated in a fully randomized 5-year trial across 15 U.S. communities. Since that initial trial in the early 1990s, numerous communities in the United States, Sweden, and other countries have implemented interventions based closely on the CMCA model (Wagenaar, Murray, and Toomey 2000a; Wagenaar et al. 2000b). Materials, training, and resources are available (see http://nrepp.samhsa.gov/). Additional examples of rigorously evaluated programs can be found at the SAMHSA National Registry of Evidence-Based Programs and Practices at http://www.nrepp.samhsa.gov/.

Education of primary health care providers is an evolving public health intervention. Tobacco, alcohol, and other drug use must become a standard part of every medical history. The American Medical Association (AMA) has established guidelines that allow physicians to fulfill their responsibility to meet the needs of alcohol and other drug abuse patients by providing care at one of three levels: (1) diagnosis and referral (designated as the minimum acceptable level of care); (2) acceptance of limited responsibility for treatment (i.e., restoring the patient to a point of being capable of participating in a long-term treatment program); or (3) acceptance of responsibility for long-term treatment and follow-up care. The guidelines further specify the actions and knowledge required at each level of involvement (Wilford 1989).

Health care providers for population subgroups at high risk should be made more aware of the need for routine use of alcohol abuse screening and intervention. Hospitalized trauma patients represent one such population. The AMA and the ASAM recommend that BACs be ascertained in all such patients and, when positive, that individuals be evaluated and treated for their alcohol problems as well as the traumatic injury.

Public health officials strengthen and magnify their impact in addressing alcohol problems when they work in collaboration with other health care professionals, designated public officials, and community groups dedicated to the prevention and treatment of alcohol abuse. All too often, public health practitioners in chronic disease control and alcohol and drug abuse professionals are located in different state or local agencies and may not even know each other.

Areas of Future Research and Demonstration

Research on alcohol epidemiology and control is progressing at an unprecedented pace. Exciting advances in neuroscience are contributing significant new insights. The neural basis of alcohol dependence is being clarified, thanks in part to new imaging techniques and technologies. Research showing that drinking is influenced by multiple neurotransmitter systems, neuromodulators, hormones, and intracellular networks points to a number of potential target sites for which new medications may be developed. Treatment research is focused not only on discovering the most effective pharmacotherapies and psychosocial therapies, but also on clinical trials to ascertain the best combinations of psychosocial and pharmacotherapy.

Progress in the genetics of alcoholism has been explosive. As genes are identified and their functions explicated, not only will we be in a better position to identify individuals at increased genetic risk, but we will also be in a better position to clarify environmental factors that further increase risk or that confer protection. Important advances are being made in our understanding of exactly how alcohol damages the body, particularly understanding of the mechanisms involved in alcoholic liver damage. We are also gaining a much clearer understanding of alcohol's protective effects against coronary artery disease. Results of this research will more fully inform public health policy makers and practitioners. Issues under investigation of particular interest to public health professionals include:

- Improving the quantification of the magnitude and modifiability of specific risk and protective factors, including the risks and benefits of various levels of alcohol consumption across the life span
- Identifying effective community-based interventions to prevent alcohol abuse among at-risk populations
- Improving the identification of individuals susceptible to alcohol abuse and dependence and specific alcohol-related chronic health consequences in order to prevent these negative outcomes or, failing that, to intervene as early in the disease process as possible
- Developing additional, even more effective pharmacologic agents to diminish craving or other factors that result in relapse
- Determining the most effective, cost-effective, and user-friendly screening procedures, and further refining screening tools for special populations, including women, minorities, adolescents, and older individuals
- Identifying barriers to implementing alcohol screening in primary care practice, and explore the acceptability of new screening technologies, such as computer assisted interviewing
- Pursuing the development, and assessment of dimensional or quantitative criteria as an improved indicator of alcohol use disorders, for both categorization and severity determination
- Developing biomarkers for chronic alcohol use, for example, through the exploration of the effects of alcohol on glycoproteomics and lipidomics
- Determining if expression of alcohol use disorders differs by age, sex, and race/ethnicity variables and establish criteria for identifying alcohol use disorders that take such differences into consideration
- Defining the full range of pharmacodynamic effects of alcohol on central nervous system function and the variability associated with unique genetic and gene–environment profiles
- Continuing to investigate how changes in brain structure and function arise from alcohol use by utilizing the newest imaging technologies
- Applying new techniques for quantifying neurotransmitters, receptors, and transporters to obtain a more complete understanding of alcohol's effects on these systems

- Continuing to identify genes associated with vulnerability for alcohol dependence by employing new and emerging technologies, particularly on samples from study populations previously recruited for genetic research on alcohol dependence (e.g., the Collaborative Study on the Genetics of Alcoholism)
- Identifying alcohol's effects on developing brain structures and behavioral regulatory systems
- Identifying the relationship among reproductive hormones, stress hormones, and sex differences in alcohol use and dependence that unfolds during late puberty, through longitudinal studies of hormonal, electrophysiological, and other biological factors over the course of puberty

Resources

Recent Surveillance Reports

Yoon, Y.H., and H.Y. Yi. *Liver Cirrhosis Mortality in the United States, 1970–2004*. August 2007. Bethesda, MD: National Institute on Alcohol Abuse and Alcoholism (NIAAA), National Institutes of Health. Surveillance Report #79. Available at http://pubs.niaaa.nih.gov/publications/surveillance79/Cirr04.pdf.

Chen, C.M., and H.Y. Yi. *Trends in Alcohol-Related Morbidity Among Short-Stay Community Hospital Discharges, United States, 1979–2005*. August 2007. Bethesda, MD: National Institute on Alcohol Abuse and Alcoholism (NIAAA), National Institutes of Health. Surveillance Report #80. Available at http://pubs.niaaa.nih.gov/publications/surveillance80/HDS05.pdf.

Newes-Adeyi, G., C.M. Chen, G. D. Williams, and V.B. Faden. *Trends in Underage Drinking in the United States, 1991–2005*. October 2007: Bethesda, MD: National Institute on Alcohol Abuse and Alcoholism (NIAAA), National Institutes of Health. Surveillance Report #81. Available at http://pubs.niaaa.nih.gov/publications/surveillance81/Underage05.pdf.

Lakins, N.E., G.D. Williams, and H.Y. Yi. *Apparent Per Capita Alcohol Consumption: National, State, and Regional Trends, 1977–2005*. August 2007. Bethesda, MD: National Institute on Alcohol Abuse and Alcoholism (NIAAA), National Institutes of Health. Surveillance Report #82. Available at http://pubs.niaaa.nih.gov/publications/surveillance82/CONS05.pdf.

Useful Websites

National Institute on Alcohol Abuse and Alcoholism (NIAAA), National Institutes of Health, http://www.niaaa.nih.gov

NIAAA-Sponsored websites (accessible through the NIAAA website or at the following URLs:
- The Coolspot, http://www.thecoolspot.gov
- National Epidemiologic Survey on Alcohol and Related Conditions (NESARC), http://niaaa.census.gov
- College Drinking Prevention, http://www.collegedrinkingprevention.gov
- Leadership to Keep Children Alcohol Free, http://www.alcoholfreechildren.org
- Alcohol Policy Information System (APIS), http://www.alcoholpolicy.niaaa.nih.gov

Substance Abuse and Mental Health Services Administration (SAMHSA), http://www.samhsa.gov

Links to resources on the SAMHSA website:
- Preventing and Reducing Underage drinking, http://www.samhsa.gov/underagedrinking/index.aspx
- Statistics, http://www.oas.samhsa.gov. This link provides access to reports and data from all of the SAMHSA major national databases, including NSDUH, mentioned in this chapter.

- National Registry of Evidence-based Programs and Practices (NREPP), http://www.nrepp. samhsa.gov
- Screening, Brief Intervention, Referral and Treatment (SBIRT), http://sbirt.samhsa.gov
- SAMHSA's Substance Abuse Treatment Facility Locator, http://dasis3.samhsa.gov

The Referral Helpline run by SAMHSA's Center for Substance Abuse Treatment (CSAT) can be reached by calling 1-800-622-HELP.

Centers for Disease Control and Prevention (CDC), http://www.cdc.gov

- Chronic Disease Indicators, http://www.cdc.gov/nccdphp/cdi
- Alcohol and Public Health, http://www.cdc.gov/alcohol/index.htm and http://apps.nccd. cdc.gov/ardi/Homepage.aspx (an interactive tool that calculates alcohol-attributable deaths and years of potential life lost due to alcohol for the United States as a whole or for specific states.
- Behavioral Risk Factor Surveillance System, http://www.cdc.gov/brfss
- National Center for Health Statistics (NCHS), http://www.cdc.gov/nchs. The NCHS homepage provides a link to an alphabetical list of topics including "alcohol use" (http:// www.cdc.gov/nchs/fastats/alcohol.htm), which provides information on the prevalence of alcohol use, alcohol-induced mortality, and other alcohol information.

Other Resources

Alcohol Epidemiologic Data System, CSR, Incorporated, 2107 Wilson Boulevard, Suite 1000, Arlington, VA 22201, tel.: 703-312-5220, http://www.csrincorporated.com.

American Society of Addiction Medicine, 4601 N. Park Avenue, Upper Arcade #101, Chevy Chase, MD 20815, tel.: 301-656-3920, e-mail: email@asam.org, http://www.asam.org.

National Association of State Alcohol and Drug Abuse Directors, 808 17th Street, NW Suite 410, Washington, DC 20006, tel.: 202-293-0090, e-mail: dcoffice@nasadad.org, http://www. nasadad.org.

National Council on Alcoholism and Drug Dependence, 224 East 58th Street, 4th Floor, New York, NY 10022, tel.: 212-269-7797, e-mail: national@ncadd.org, http://www.ncadd.org.

Suggested Reading

Recent issues of *Alcohol Research and Health* (a quarterly peer-reviewed scientific publication for educated lay readers) (available at http://www.niaaa.nih.gov/Publications/AlcoholResearch):
Volume 30(1) 2007—Alcohol Metabolism Part II: A Key to Unlocking Alcohol's Effects
Volume 29(4) 2006—Alcohol Metabolism Part I: Mechanisms of Action
Volume 29(3) 2006—Alcohol and Tobacco: An Update
Volume 29(2) 2006—National Epidemiologic Survey on Alcohol and Related Conditions
Helping Patients Who Drink Too Much: A Clinician's Guide (2005)
(http://pubs.niaaa.nih.gov/publications/Practitioner/ClinicianGuide2005/guide.pdf)—a 34-page booklet including pocket screening guide and a variety of other resources. Continuing Medical Education (CME) credits available for physicians.

References

American Psychiatric Association (APA). *Diagnostic and Statistical Manual of Mental Disorders: DSM-IV* (4th ed.). Washington, D.C.: American Psychiatric Association (1994).

Anton, R.F., G. Oroszi, S. O'Malley, et al. An Evaluation of the μ-Opioid Receptor (OPRM1) as a Predictor of Naltrexone Response in the Treatment of Alcohol Dependence. *Arch Gen Psychiatry* (2008):65(2):135–144.

Babor, T.F., J. Higgins-Biddle, J. Saunders, and M. Monteiro. *AUDIT: The Alcohol Use Disorders Identification Test Guidelines for Use in Primary Care* (2nd ed.). Geneva: World Health Organization (2001).

Burt, M., L. Aron, T. Douglas, J. Valente, E. Lee, and B. Iwen. Homelessness: Programs and the People They Serve. Summary Report: Findings of the National Survey of Homeless Assistance Providers and Clients. Washington, D.C.: The Urban Institute (1999).

Caetano, R., S. Ramisetty-Mikler, L.S. Wallisch, C. McGrath, and R.T. Spence. Acculturation, Drinking, and Alcohol Abuse and Dependence among Hispanics in the Texas–Mexico Border. *Alcohol Clin Exp Res* (2008):32(2):314–321.

Centers for Disease Control and Prevention (CDC). Indicators for Chronic Disease Surveillance. *MMWR* (2004):53(RR-11).

Charness, M.E. Alcohol and the Brain. *Alcohol Health Res World* (1990):14:85–89.

Clark C.A., D.M. Purdie, and S. Glaser. Population Attributable Risk of Breast Cancer in White Women Associated with Immediately Modifiable Risk Factors. *BMC Cancer* (2006):6:170–181.

Corrao, G., V. Bagnardi, A. Zambon, and C. La Vecchia. A Meta-Analysis of Alcohol Consumption and the Risk of 15 Diseases. *Prev Med* (2004):38:613–619.

Dawson, D.A., B.F. Grant, and P.S. Chou. Gender Differences in Alcohol Intake. In: Hunt, W.A., and S. Zakhari, editors, *Stress, Gender, and Alcohol-Seeking Behavior,* Research Monograph No. 29. Bethesda, MD: National Institute on Alcohol Abuse and Alcoholism (1995). NIH Publication 95-3893.

Dawson, D.A., B.F. Grant, F.S. Stinson, P.S. Chou, B. Huang, and W.J. Ruan. Recovery from DSM-IV Alcohol Dependence: United States, 2001–2002. *Addiction* (2005):100:281–292.

Dawson, D.A., R.B. Goldstein, and B.F. Grant. Rates and Correlates of Relapse Among Individuals in Remission from DSM-IV Alcohol Dependence: A 3-Year Follow-Up. *Alcohol Clin Exp Res* (2007):31:2036–2045.

Donovan, D.M., R.F. Anton, W.R. Miller, et al. Combined Pharmacotherapies and Behavioral Interventions for Alcohol Dependence (the COMBINE Study): Examination of Posttreatment Drinking Outcomes. *J Stud Alcohol Drugs* (2008):69:5–9.

Donovan, J., S. Leech, R. Zucker, et al. Really Underage Drinkers: Alcohol Use among Elementary Students. *Alcohol Clin Exp Res* (2004):28:341–349.

Dufour, M.C. *Chapter 15: Alcohol Use and Abuse.* In: Pathy, M.S.J., A.J. Sinclair, and J.E. Morley, editors, *Principles and Practice of Geriatric Medicine* (4th ed.), Vol. 1. Chichester, England: Wiley and Sons (2006):157–168.

Dufour, M.C. Alcoholic Liver Disease. In: Talley, N.J., G.R. Locke III, and Y.A. Saito, editors, *GI Epidemiology*. Malden, MA: Blackwell (2007):231–237.

Dufour, M.C., and M.D. Adamson. The Epidemiology of Alcohol-Induced Pancreatitis. *Pancreas* (2003):27:286–290.

Eaton, D.K., L. Kann, S. Kinchen, et al. Youth Risk Behavior Surveillance—United States, 2005. *MMWR* (2006):55:(SS-5):1–108.

Eckardt, M.J., and P.R. Martin. Clinical Assessment of Cognition in Alcoholism. *Alcohol Clin Exp Res* (1986):10:123–127.

Edwards, G., and M.M. Gross. Alcohol Dependence: Provisional Description of a Clinical Syndrome. *BMJ* (1976):1:1058–1061.

Grant, B.F., and D.A. Dawson. Age at Onset of Alcohol Use and its Association with DSM-IV Alcohol Abuse and Dependence. Results from the National Longitudinal Alcohol Epidemiologic Survey. *J Subst Abuse* (1997):9:103–110.

Grant, B.F., D.A. Dawson, F.S. Stinson, S.P. Chou, M.C. Dufour, and R.P. Pickering. The 12-Month Prevalence and Trends in DSM-IV Alcohol Abuse and Dependence: United States, 1991–1992 and 2001–2002. *Drug Alcohol Depend* (2004):74(3):223–234.

Greenfield, T.K., and J.D. Rogers. Who Drinks Most of the Alcohol in the U.S.? The Policy Implications. *J Stud Alcohol* (1999):60:78–89.

Grucza, R.A., A.M. Abbacchi, T.R. Przybeck, and J.C. Gfroerer. Discrepancies in Estimates of Prevalence and Correlates of Substance Use and Disorders between Two National Surveys. *Addiction* (2007):102(4):623–629.

Hasin, D.S., F.S. Stinson, E. Ogburn, and B.F. Grant. Prevalence, Correlates, Disability, and Co-morbidity of DSM-IV Alcohol Abuse and Dependence in the United States. *Arch Gen Psychiatry* (2007):64:830–842.

Hastings, G., S. Anderson, E. Cooke, and R. Gordon. Alcohol Marketing and Young People's Drinking: A Review of the Research. *J Public Health Policy* (2005):26:296–311.

Hietala, J., H. Koivisto, P. Anttila, and O. Niemela. Comparison of the Combined Marker GGT–CDT and the Conventional Laboratory Markers of Alcohol Abuse in Heavy Drinkers, Moderate Drinkers and Abstainers. *Alcohol Alcohol* (2006):41:528–533.

Holder, H.D. Alcoholism Treatment and Potential Health Care Cost Savings. *Med Care* (1987):25:52–71.

Indian Health Service (IHS). *Trends in Indian Health 2000–2001.* Rockville, MD: Division of Public Health, Indian Health Service (2002). Available at: http://www.ihs.gov/NonMedicalPrograms/IHS_Stats/files/trends00-01_Part4.pdf.

Johnson, A.K., and R.A. Cnaan. Social Work Practice with Homeless Persons: State of the Art. *Res Social Work Prac* (1995):5:340–382.

Johnson, B.A., N. Rosenthal, J.A. Capece, et al. for the Topiramate for Alcoholism Advisory Board and the Topiramate for Alcoholism Study Group. Topiramate for Treating Alcohol Dependence: A Randomized Controlled Trial. *JAMA* (2007):298:1641–1651.

Johnston, L.D., P.M. O'Malley, J.G. Bachman, and J.E. Schulenberg. *Overall, Illicit Drug Use by American Teens Continues Gradual Decline in 2007.* National Press Release. Ann Arbor, MI: University of Michigan News Service (2007). Press Release, Data Tables, and Figures Available at http://monitoringthefuture.org/pressreleases/07drugpr_complete.pdf.

Kung, H.C., D.L. Hoyert, J. Xu, and S.L. Murphy. *Deaths: Final Data for 2005.* National Vital Statistics Reports, Vol. 56, No. 10. Hyattsville, MD: National Center for Health Statistics, Centers for Disease Control and Prevention (2008).

Lakins, N.E., G.D. Williams, and H. Yi. *Apparent Per Capita Alcohol Consumption: National, State, and Regional Trends, 1977–2005.* Bethesda, MD: National Institute on Alcohol Abuse and Alcoholism, Alcohol Epidemiologic Data System (2007). Surveillance Report no. 82. Available at http://pubs.niaaa.nih.gov/publications/surveillance82/CONS05.pdf.

Larbi, E.B., J. Stamler, A. Dyer, et al. The Population Attributable Risk of Hypertension from Heavy Alcohol Consumption. *Public Health Rep* (1984):99:316–319.

Lee, S., G. Chau, C. Yao, C. Wu, and S. Yin. Functional Assessment of Human Alcohol Dehydrogenase Family in Ethanol Metabolism: Significance of First-Pass Metabolism. *Alcohol Clin Exp Res* (2006):30(7):1132–1142.

Marshall, A.W., D. Kingstone, M. Boss, and M. Morgan. Ethanol Elimination in Males and Females: Relationships to Menstrual Cycle and Body Composition. *Hepatology* (1983):3(5):701–706.

Mayfield, D., G. McLeod, and P. Hall. The CAGE Questionnaire: Validation of a New Alcoholism Instrument. *Am J Psychiatry* (1974):131:1121–1123.

Midanik, L.T., F.J. Chaloupka, R. Saitz, et al. Alcohol-Attributable Deaths and Years of Potential Life Lost—United States, 2001. *MMWR* (2004):53(37):866–870.

Miller, W.R., S.T. Walters, and M.E. Bennett. How Effective is Alcoholism Treatment in the United States? *J Stud Alcohol* (2001):62:211–220.

Mokdad, A.H., J.S. Marks, D.F. Stroup, and J.L. Gerberding. Actual Causes of Death in the United States, 2000. *JAMA* (2004):291:1238–1245.

Morse, R.M., and D.K. Flavin. The Definition of Alcoholism. *JAMA* (1992):268:1012–1014.

Moss, H B., C.M. Chen, and H. Yi. DSM-IV Criteria Endorsement Patterns in Alcohol Dependence: Relationship to Severity. *Alcohol Clin Exp Res* (2008):32:306–313.

National Center for Health Statistics (NCHS). *Health United States, 2007 with Chartbook on Trends in the Health of Americans.* Hyattsville, MD: National Center for Health Statistics (2007). Available at: http://www.cdc.gov/nchs/data/hus/hus07.pdf.

National Highway Traffic Safety Administration (NHTSA). *Research Report: Preventing Over-Consumption of Alcohol-Sales to the Intoxicated and "Happy Hour" (Drink Special) Laws.* Washington, D.C.: National Highway Traffic Safety Administration (2005). DOT HS 809 878.

National Highway Traffic Safety Administration (NHTSA). *2006 Traffic Safety Annual Assessment—Alcohol-Related Fatalities.* Traffic Safety Facts Research Note. Washington, D.C.: National Highway Traffic Safety Administration, National Center for Statistics and Analysis (2007). DOT HS 810 821.

National Institute on Alcohol Abuse and Alcoholism (NIAAA). Screening for Alcoholism. *Alcohol Alert* (1990):8.

National Institute on Alcohol Abuse and Alcoholism (NIAAA). Genetic, Psychological, and Sociocultural Influences on Alcohol Use and Abuse. In: *Ninth Special Report to Congress on Alcohol and Health.* Bethesda, MD: National Institute on Alcohol Abuse and Alcoholism (1997a). NIH Publication 97-4017.

National Institute on Alcohol Abuse and Alcoholism (NIAAA). Treatment of Alcoholism and Related Problems. In: *Ninth Special Report to Congress on Alcohol and Health.* Bethesda, MD: National Institute on Alcohol Abuse and Alcoholism (1997b). NIH Publication 97-4017.

National Institute on Alcohol Abuse and Alcoholism (NIAAA). Youth Drinking: Risk Factors and Consequences. *Alcohol Alert* (1997c):37.

National Institute on Alcohol Abuse and Alcoholism (NIAAA). *Updating Estimates of the Economic Costs of Alcohol Abuse in the United States: Estimates, Update Methods, and Data.* Bethesda, MD: National Institute on Alcohol Abuse and Alcoholism (2000).

National Institute on Alcohol Abuse and Alcoholism (NIAAA). The Genetics of Alcoholism. *Alcohol Alert* (2003):60.

National Institute on Alcohol Abuse and Alcoholism (NIAAA). *Helping Patients Who Drink Too Much: A Clinician's Guide.* Bethesda, MD: National Institute on Alcohol Abuse and Alcoholism, National Institutes of Health (2005a). Available at http://pubs.niaaa.nih.gov/publications/Practitioner/Clinicians Guide2005/guide.pdf.

National Institute on Alcohol Abuse and Alcoholism (NIAAA). Screening for Alcohol Use and Alcohol-Related Problems. *Alcohol Alert* (2005b):65.

National Institute on Alcohol Abuse and Alcoholism (NIAAA). Brief Interventions. *Alcohol Alert* (2005c):66.

National Institute on Alcohol Abuse and Alcoholism (NIAAA). *Alcohol Use and Alcohol Use Disorders in the United States: Main Findings from the 2001–2002 National Epidemiologic Survey on Alcohol and Related Conditions (NESARC).* U.S. Alcohol Epidemiologic Data Reference Manual, Vol. 8, No. 1. Bethesda, MD: National Institute on Alcohol Abuse and Alcoholism (2006).

Pelletier, A.R., P.Z. Siegel, M.S. Baptiste, and C. Maylahn. Revisions to Chronic Disease Surveillance Indicators, United States, 2004. *Preventing Chronic Disease Public Health Research, Practice, and Policy* (2005):2:1–5.

Peterson, K. Biomarkers of Alcohol Use and Abuse. *Alcohol Res Health* (2004/2005):28:30–37.

Project MATCH Research Group. Matching Alcoholism Treatments to Client Heterogeneity: Project MATCH Posttreatment Drinking Outcomes. *J Stud Alcohol* (1997):58:7–29.

Randolph, W.M., C. Stroup-Benham, S.A. Black, and K.S. Markides. Alcohol Use among Cuban-Americans, Mexican-Americans, and Puerto Ricans. *Alcohol Health and Research World* (1998):22(4):265–269.

Rimm, E.B., and C. Moats. Alcohol and Coronary Heart Disease: Drinking Patterns and Mediators of Effect. *Ann Epidemiol* (2007):17:S3–S7.

Rubin, E. How Alcohol Damages the Body. *Alcohol Health Res World* (1989):13:322–333.

Rubin, E., and A.P. Thomas. Effects of Alcohol on the Heart and Cardiovascular System. In: Mendelson, J.H., and N.K. Mello, editors, *Medical Diagnosis and Treatment of Alcoholism.* New York: McGraw-Hill (1992):263–287.

Saitz, R. Unhealthy Alcohol Use. *N Engl J Med* (2005):352:596–607.

Substance Abuse and Mental Health Services Administration (SAMHSA). *TIP 24: A Guide to Substance Abuse Services for Primary Care Clinicians.* Rockville, MD: Center for Substance Abuse Treatment (1997). DHHS Publication No. (SMA) 97-3139.

Substance Abuse and Mental Health Services Administration (SAMHSA). *TIP 26: Substance Abuse among Older Adults.* Rockville, MD: SAMHSA, Center for Substance Abuse Treatment (1998). DHHS Publication No. (SMA) 98-3179.

Substance Abuse and Mental Health Services Administration (SAMHSA). *Results from the 2006 National Survey on Drug Use and Health: National Findings.* Rockville, MD: Office of Applied Studies (2007). NSDUH Series H-32, DHHS Publication No. SMA 07-4293. Available at: http://www.oas.samhsa.gov/nsduh/2k6nsduh/2k6Results.pdf.

Taylor, J.R., T. Combs-Orme, and D.A. Taylor. Alcohol and Mortality: Diagnostic Considerations. *J Stud Alcohol* (1983):44:17–25.

Thakker, K.D. An Overview of Health Risks and Benefits of Alcohol Consumption. *Alcoholism Clin Exp Res* (1998):22:285S–298S.

Tippetts, A.S., R.B. Voas, J.C. Fell, and J.L. Nichols. A Meta-Analysis of .08 BAC Laws in 19 Jurisdictions in the United States. *Accident Anal Prev* (2005):37:149–161.

Toomey, T.L., and A.C. Wagenaar. Environmental Policies to Reduce College Drinking: Options and Research Findings. *J Stud Alcohol* (2002):(Suppl 14):193–205.

Umbricht-Schneiter, A., P. Santora, and R.D. Moore. The Impact of Alcohol-Associated Morbidity in Hospitalized Patients. *Subst Abuse* (1991):12:145–155.

U.S. Census Bureau. U.S. Hispanic Population: 2006 from the Current Population Survey, Annual Social and Economic Supplement 2006. Available at http://www.census.gov/population/www/socdem/hispanic/cps2006/CPS_Powerpoint_2006.pdf.

U.S. Department of Health and Human Services (USDHHS). *Healthy People 2010* (2nd ed.). With Understanding and Improving Health and Objectives for Improving Health. 2 Volumes. Washington, D.C.: U.S. Government Printing Office (2000).

U.S. Department of Health and Human Services and U.S. Department of Agriculture. *Dietary Guidelines for Americans 2005.* Washington D.C.: U.S. Department of Health and Human Services and U.S. Department of Agriculture (2005). Available at http://www.health.gov/dietaryguidelines/dga2005/document/pdf/DGA2005.pdf.

U.S. Preventive Services Task Force (USPSTF). Screening and Behavioral Counseling Interventions in Primary Care to Reduce Alcohol Misuse: Recommendation Statement. *Ann Intern Med* (2004):140:554–556.

Venner, K.L., H. Matzger, A.A. Forcehimes, et al. Course of Recovery from Alcoholism. *Alcohol Clin Exp Res* (2006):30(6):1079–1090.

Voas, R.B., A.S. Tippetts, and J.C. Fell. Assessing the Effectiveness of Minimum Legal Drinking Age and Zero Tolerance Laws in the United States. *Accid Anal Prev* (2003):35:579–587.

Wagenaar, A.C., D.M. Murray, and T.L. Toomey. Communities Mobilizing for Change on Alcohol (CMCA): Effects of a Randomized Trial on Arrests and Traffic Crashes. *Addiction* (2000a):95:209–217.

Wagenaar, A.C., D.M. Murray, J.P. Gehan, et al. Communities Mobilizing for Change on Alcohol: Outcomes from a Randomized Community Trial. *J Stud Alcohol* (2000b):61:85–94.

Wilford, B.B. Stopping Silent Losses: The American Medical Association Responds. *Alcohol Health Res World* (1989):13:169–172.

Wilsnack, R.W., A.F. Kristjanson, and S.C. Wilsnack. Are U.S. Women Drinking Less (or More)? Historical and Aging Trends, 1981–2001. *J Stud Alcohol* (2006):67:341–348.

World Health Organization (WHO). *The International Classification of Diseases, 10th Revision: Clinical Descriptions and Diagnostic Guidelines*. Geneva: World Health Organization (1992).

World Health Organization (WHO). *Global Status Report on Alcohol 2004*. Geneva: World Health Organization, Department of Mental Health and Substance Abuse (2004), Available at http://whqlibdoc.who.int/publications/2004/9241562722_(425KB).pdf.

Wright, D., N. Sathe, and K. Spagnola. *State Estimates of Substance Use from the 2004–2005 National Surveys on Drug Use and Health*. Rockville, MD: Office of Applied Studies, SAMHSA (2007). NSDUH Series H-31, DHHS Publication No. SMA 07-4235.

Zador, P.L., S.A. Krawchuk, and R.B. Voas. Alcohol-Related Relative Risk of Driver Involvement in Fatal Crashes in Relation to Driver Age and Sex: An Update Using 1996 Data. Washington, D.C.: National Highway Traffic Safety Administration (2000). DOT HS 809 050.

CHAPTER 9

OBESITY AND OVERWEIGHT (ICD-10 E66)

Deborah A. Galuska, Ph.D., M.P.H. and William H. Dietz, M.D., Ph.D.

Introduction

Obesity is defined as the accumulation of excess fat. In clinical and public health settings, it is most often assessed by the body mass index (BMI). BMI is a measure of weight that accounts for height and is estimated as weight (in kilograms)/ height (in meters)^2. For adults, an absolute value of BMI is used to define weight status as follows: overweight—BMI 25.0–29.9; obese—BMI greater than or equal to 30. The obese category can be subdivided into three classes: Class 1—BMI 30.0–34.9; Class 2— BMI 35.0–39.9; and Class 3 (also called extreme obesity)—BMI greater than or equal to 40 (NIH 1998).

For children and adolescents, because of their growth patterns, the classification of weight status is relative; BMI is compared to age- and sex-specific percentiles on the Centers for Disease Control and Prevention (CDC) growth charts (CDC 2007a) and has been classified as follows: at risk for overweight—BMI 85 to less than 95 percentile for age and sex; overweight—BMI 95th percentile for age and sex. A recent expert panel recommended renaming the BMI 85 to less than 95 percentile for age and sex as overweight and BMI greater than or equal to 95th percentile for age and sex as obese (Barlow et al. 2007).

Significance

The public health burden from obesity and overweight in the United States is significant (Figure 9.1). In 2005–2006, more than a third of adults (34%) in the United States were obese (Ogden et al. 2007a). In 2003–2006, one-sixth of children and adolescents, aged 2–19 years (16%), had a BMI greater than or equal to 95 percentile (Ogden, Carroll, and Flegal 2008). Overweight and obesity are associated with an increased risk of a multitude of deleterious health outcomes that can be grouped into four major categories: (1) psychosocial, (2) risk factors for chronic disease, (3) morbidity, and (4) mortality. The relationship of these outcomes with obesity has been extensively reviewed for both adults (NIH 1998; WHO 1999) and children (Dietz 1998; Must and Strauss 1999) and is summarized below.

Psychosocial

Obesity may affect how a person feels about him/herself as well as how others in society feel about them. Some, but not all, studies show an association between obesity and lower

Disclaimer: The findings and conclusions of this chapter are those of the authors and do not necessarily represent the views of the Centers for Disease Control and Prevention.

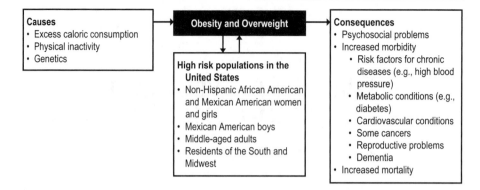

Figure 9.1. Obesity and overweight: causes, consequences, and high-risk groups.

self-esteem (French, Story, and Perry 1995; Wardle and Cooke 2005). Obese people may be perceived negatively by others and be the target of discrimination (NIH 1998; Fabricatore and Wadden 2004; Latner and Stunkard 2003). Obesity also appears to be correlated with lower levels of socioeconomic achievement, in particular for women (Puhl, Henderson, and Brownell 2005; Gortmaker et al. 1993). For example, a study of adolescents followed up for seven years found that compared to those not overweight, those who were overweight were less educated, more likely to be unmarried, had lower incomes, and had higher rates of household poverty (Gortmaker et al. 1993).

The relation between obesity and mood disturbances is unclear. Cross-sectional studies have demonstrated a positive, albeit small, association between obesity and mental disorders including depressive disorders and anxiety disorders. These associations may be modified by sex, level of obesity, age (Scott et al. 2008), education (Scott et al. 2008; Simon et al. 2006), and race/ethnicity (Simon et al. 2006). Whether obesity causes the disturbances or is a result of the disturbances remains uncertain (Fabricatore and Wadden 2004).

Risk Factors for Chronic Disease

The positive association between excess weight and risk factors for chronic disease, in particular cardiovascular disease (CVD) and type 2 diabetes, has been documented in a number of reviews for both adults (NIH 1998; WHO 1999) and children (WHO 1999; Dietz 1998; Must and Strauss 1999; Steinbeck 2005). These risk factors include elevated blood pressure, dyslipidemias, and insulin resistance. Obesity is also associated with higher levels of inflammatory markers such as C-reactive protein (Ford 1999; Ford et al. 2001). These chronic disease risk factors are more likely to cluster in overweight and obese persons than normal weight persons (Freedman et al. 1999; Must et al. 1999). Childhood adiposity is associated with adult adiposity (Freedman et al. 2005; Juonala et al. 2006), and through this mechanism may influence the risk of obesity-related conditions in adulthood (Juonala et al. 2006).

Morbidity

Obesity, either directly or indirectly, impacts multiple organ systems, and is thus associated with greater morbidity from a number of chronic conditions including some of the leading causes of death. A 1998 review documented that among adults, obesity increased the risk of serious health conditions. These are cardiovascular conditions such as coronary heart disease, ischemic stroke and congestive heart failure, diabetes, and some cancers including colon cancer, endometrial cancer, and postmenopausal breast cancer. This review also documented an association between obesity and less serious health conditions that could still affect quality of life. These include sleep disturbances, gallbladder disease, gastroesophageal reflux, and osteoarthritis (NIH 1998). Since the review, obesity has been linked to several other conditions including dementia (Barett-Connor 2007) and nonalcoholic fatty liver disease (Angulo 2007). Table 9.1 documents the relative risks for the association of obesity and overweight with select outcomes.

Among women, obesity can negatively affect menstrual function and fertility (NIH 1998; Sarwer et al. 2006). Obese women experience both complications during pregnancy including hypertension (NIH 1998) and gestational diabetes (NIH 1998; Sarwer et al. 2006; Chu et al. 2007a), as well as complications during labor and delivery (NIH 1998) including an increased risk of cesarean section (Sarwer et al. 2006; Chu et al. 2007b) and stillbirths (Chu et al. 2007c). Obesity during pregnancy may also affect the developing fetus manifested by an increased risk of neural tube defects (Shaw, Velie, and Schaffer 1996).

Children also experience morbidities associated with their weight, many of them similar to adults. These include respiratory problems such as sleep apnea, orthopedic problems such as Blount's disease (a growth disorder of the tibia that causes the bowing of legs) and slipped capital femoral epiphysis (a separation of the ball of the hip joint from the thigh bone), and gastrointestinal problems such as hepatic steatosis and gallbladder disease (Dietz 1998; Steinbeck 2005). Severe obesity in childhood is also a risk factor for the incidence of type 2 diabetes in childhood (Weiss et al. 2005).

Mortality

Among adults, obesity is associated with greater all-cause and CVD-specific mortality (NIH 1998; WHO 1999; McGee 2005; Troiano et al. 1996). A recent meta-analysis estimated that compared to persons with a BMI of 18.5–25.0, those with a BMI of 30 (obese) or higher had a relative risk of 1.22 for all-cause mortality, 1.48 for CVD, and 1.07 for cancer (McGee 2005). In contrast, this study found little evidence for an association between overweight and mortality. The association between obesity and mortality may be modified by age; a recent study of National Health and Nutrition Examination Survey data found no association among adults aged 70 years and older (Flegal et al. 2005). Among children, overweight also appears to be associated with increased overall and CVD mortality in adulthood (Must and Strauss 1999; Freedman, Serdula, and Khan 2002). Whether this association is independent of adult obesity is unclear.

These health conditions pose economic costs for society. For example, among adults one study estimated that direct medical costs of overweight and obesity in 1998 was $78.5 billion with approximately half of these costs paid for by Medicare or Medicaid (Finkelstein, Fiebelkom, and Wang 2003). Another study estimated the direct and indirect medical costs at $117 billion in 2000 (USDHHS 2001). Because the more serious consequences of weight appear in adulthood, the costs of obesity for children are smaller but not insignificant and are increasing. One study found the hospital costs of obesity-associated conditions increased from $35 million during 1979–1981 to $127 million in 1997–1999 (Wang and Dietz 2002).

Table 9.1. Relative Risks for the Association Between Body Mass Index (BMI) and Select Health Outcomes as Estimated by Meta-Analyses

Health Outcome	Relative Risk[a]	Comparison	Source
Cancer—Colon	1.15	BMI 25.0–29.9 vs. BMI 20.0–24.9	Bergström et al. (2001)
	1.33	BMI ≥30 vs. BMI 20.0–24.9	
Cancer—Postmenopausal Breast	1.12	BMI 25.0–29.9 vs. BMI 20.0–24.9	Bergström et al. (2001)
	1.25	BMI ≥30 vs. BMI 20.0–24.9	
Cancer—Endometrial	1.59	BMI 25.0–29.9 vs. BMI 20.0–24.9	Bergström et al. (2001)
	2.52	BMI ≥30 vs. BMI 20.0–24.9	
Cardiovascular Disease	1.32	BMI 25.0–29.9 vs. BMI 18.5–24.9 (unadjusted for blood pressure and cholesterol level)	Bogers et al. (2007)
	1.17	BMI 25.0–29.9 vs. BMI 18.5–24.9 (adjusted for blood pressure and cholesterol level)	
	1.81	BMI ≥30 vs. BMI 18.5–24.9 (unadjusted for blood pressure and cholesterol levels)	
	1.49	BMI ≥30 vs. BMI 18.5–24.9 (adjusted for blood pressure and cholesterol levels)	
Diabetes	1.87	Standard deviation of BMI (4.3 units)	Vazquez et al. (2007)

[a]Variables adjusted for vary by study.

Pathophysiology

The factors contributing to excessive weight gain are considered later in this chapter. The adverse effects of obesity are directly mediated by the link of obesity with body size, and less directly by the effects of excess weight and body fat distribution on a variety of metabolic functions.

The direct effects of obesity can be divided into two groups: those linked to the visibility of body size to others and those linked to biomechanical changes caused by large body size. The visibility of obesity may account for its stigmatization as well the discrimination directed at obese persons (Fabricatore and Wadden 2004; Gortmaker et al. 1993). For example, for more than 40 years, young children have ranked obese children as those that they least liked (Latner and Stunkard 2003; Richardson et al. 1961). Discrimination is one hypothesis for the association between lower levels of social and economic achievement for women (Puhl, Henderson, and Brownell 2005; Gortmaker et al. 1993). Because it is a chronic stressor, discrimination may contribute to mood disorders experienced by the obese.

Increased body weight is hypothesized to account for the adverse orthopedic effects in childhood, such as slipped capital femoral epiphysis and Blount's disease (Dietz 1998; Steinbeck 2005). In adults, increased body weight may contribute to the increased frequency of osteoarthritis, potentially through increasing stress on joints or by altering alignment of joints (Felson et al. 2000). Increased peripharyngeal fat increases the risk of sleep apnea, and increased abdominal fat reduces diaphragmatic excursion and contributes to the Pickwickian syndrome (a syndrome characterized by the clustering of obesity, sleepiness, hypoventilation, and red face; Koenig 2001).

Obesity's adverse metabolic effects appear to be mediated by total body fat in children, and by both total body fat and visceral fat in adults. Increased free fatty acid release by visceral adipose tissue may produce insulin resistance and increased triglyceride synthesis in the liver (Albu and Pi-Sunyer 2007). Insulin resistance accounts for glucose intolerance, the eventual development of type 2 diabetes mellitus, and may contribute to polycystic ovary syndrome. The release of inflammatory factors by visceral adipose tissue may contribute to insulin resistance (Albu and Pi-Sunyer 2007) as well as nonalcoholic fatty liver disease (Tilg and Hotamisligil 2006). Although obesity-associated hypertension is associated with abdominal obesity and hyperinsulinemia, the mechanism that mediates these associations remains unclear. Together, these risk factors increase the risk of CVD. How increased body fat resets the body mechanisms that tend to maintain weight at increased levels remains uncertain.

Both obese children and adults report an overall lower quality of life than those of normal weight. This appears to be mediated through both the social and medical consequences of obesity (Schwimmer, Burwinkle, and Varni 2003; Doll, Petersen, and Stewart-Brown 2000).

Descriptive Epidemiology

High-Risk Populations

Data from the National Health and Nutrition Surveys provide evidence that obesity and overweight differentially affects certain demographic subgroups of the population characterized by sex, race/ethnicity, age (Ogden et al. 2006; Ogden, Carroll, and Flegal 2008), and socioeconomic status (Ogden et al. 2007b). Among adults in 2003–2004, the prevalence of obesity was approximately the same between the two sexes (33.2% versus 31.3%), whereas the prevalence of extreme obesity was higher among women than men (6.9% versus 2.8%). Racial/ethnic distributions vary by sex. Among men, the prevalence of obesity was approximately the same for non-Hispanic whites (31.1%), non-Hispanic African Americans

(34.0%), and Mexican Americans (31.6%). In contrast, among women, non-Hispanic African Americans (53.9%) had a 60% higher rate than non-Hispanic whites (30.2%) and a 25% higher rate than Mexican Americans (42.3%). For both men and women, obesity was highest among those aged 40–59 years, and lowest among those aged 20–39 years. For extreme obesity, there was relatively little difference by age for men, whereas for women those 20–39 years (8.0%) and 40–59 years (7.9%) have more than double the rates of those 60 years and older (3.3%) (Ogden et al. 2006). The association of income with obesity is complex (Ogden et al. 2007b). Household income poverty threshold was inversely associated with obesity in non-Hispanic white women and positively associated with obesity in Mexican-American men. No significant associations were observed for other demographic subgroups.

Among children and adolescents aged 2–19 years in 2003–2006, the prevalence of obesity was slightly higher for males than females (17.1% versus 15.5%). Among males, Mexican Americans had the highest prevalence (23.2%), followed by non-Hispanic African Americans (17.4%) and non-Hispanic whites (15.6%), a pattern different from adults. In contrast, the racial/ethnic pattern in female children and adolescents was the same as adults; non-Hispanic African Americans had the highest rate (24.1%), followed by Mexican Americans (18.5%), and non-Hispanic whites (13.6%). For both males and females, the prevalence is approximately 5% lower in children aged 2–5 years than those aged 6–11 and 12–19 years (Ogden, Carroll, and Flegal 2008). Unlike adults, household income poverty threshold was not associated with obesity in children in any demographic subgroups of children (Ogden et al. 2007b).

Geographic Distribution

In 2007, the state-specific prevalence of adult obesity based on self-report ranged from 18.7% to 32.0% across the 50 states and the District of Columbia. In general, the prevalence of obesity was lowest among states in the West and Northeast, in particular western mountain states and highest among states in the Midwest and South (Galuska et al. 2008) (Figure 9.2). Similar geographic patterns are observed for the prevalence of obese adolescents (Eaton et al. 2008).

Time Trends

Over the past three decades in the United States, the prevalence of obesity for adults and for children has more than doubled. For adults aged 20–74 years, the age-adjusted prevalence of obesity doubled from 15.0% to 32.2% between 1976–1980 and 2003–2004 (Ogden et al. 2006; Flegal et al. 2002). Between 1976–1980 and 2003–2006, as illustrated in Figure 9.3, the prevalence increased from 5.0% to 12.4% for children aged 2–5 years, from 6.5% to 17.0% for children aged 6–11 years, and from 5.0% to 17.6% for adolescents 12–19 years old (Ogden, Carroll, and Flegal 2008; Ogden et al. 2002). Although the magnitude of the increase varies, the increase is observed for both males and females; among non-Hispanic whites, non-Hispanic African Americans, and Mexican Americans and across all states in the United States. (Ogden, Carroll, and Flegal 2008; Ogden et al. 2006; Flegal et al. 2002; Ogden et al. 2002; Densmore et al. 2006; Galuska et al. 2008). The population distribution in weight has not been uniform over time; larger increases have been observed in the highest percentiles of the distribution (Ogden et al. 2007b).

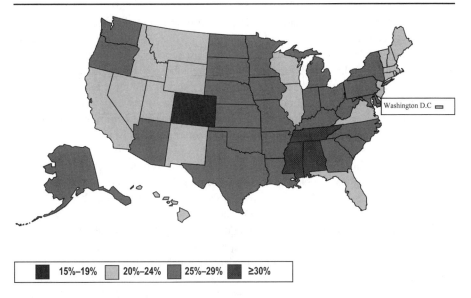

Figure 9.2. The prevalence of obesity (BMI ≥30) based on self-report among U.S. adults, 2007. Source: Behavioral Risk Factor Surveillance System, CDC.

Causes

The principal causes of obesity and overweight result from an imbalance of caloric intake and expenditure (see Figure 9.1).

Modifiable Risk Factors

Excessive weight gain is ultimately caused by an imbalance between energy intake and energy expenditure. Thus, interventions to reduce excessive weight gain need to identify

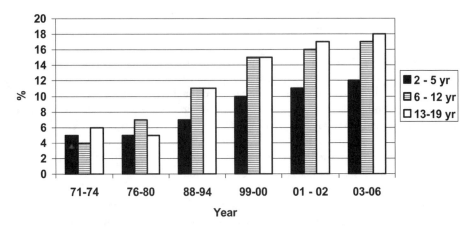

Figure 9.3. Proportion of U.S. children and adolescents with BMI >95 percentile (percentile value based on sex and age percentile on CDC growth charts) by age and year. Source: National Health and Nutrition Examination Surveys.

and target modifiable factors related to the overconsumption of calories or related to reduced energy expenditure.

Calories are obtained from four dietary sources: carbohydrates, proteins, fats, and alcohol. The energy density of fats (9 kcal/g) and alcohol (7 kcal/g) are approximately twice that of carbohydrates (4 kcal/g) and proteins (4 kcal/g) (National Research Council 1989). Interventions to alter caloric intake are challenged by the complex relationships between an individual's physiological triggers and responses to food intake, their beliefs and attitudes about food, their environmental exposure to certain foods, and characteristics of food such as satiety and palatability (Blundell and Stubbs 2007).

One public health intervention strategy related to diet is to focus on dietary patterns or practices that lead to excessive calorie consumption and thus weight gain. However, the risks associated with various dietary patterns are not well established. A recent review examined the evidence as to how 28 dietary factors contribute to obesity for adults and children based on an evaluation of four types of evidence: studies of secular trends, mechanistic/experimental studies, observational/epidemiologic studies, and prevention trials. Based on these criteria, the authors identified 11 factors for which there was moderately consistent evidence of a relationship with lower levels of adiposity (Woodward-Lopez et al. 2006). These 11 factors are: (1) decreased dietary fat intake; (2) increased total percent carbohydrate intake; (3) increased dietary fiber intake; (4) increased calcium intake; (5) increased dairy intake; (6) increased vegetable and fruit intake; (7) decreased sweetened beverage intake; (8) decreased consumption of restaurant prepared foods; (9) total dietary patterns characterized by a high intake of lower-fat foods, whole grains, fruits, vegetables, and legumes; (10) breakfast consumption; and (11) breast-feeding. The authors cautioned that even among these factors, there are substantial gaps in the literature, particularly related to the lack of prevention trial evidence and the limited number of studies in children.

Total daily energy expenditure consists of three components: basal and resting metabolic expenditure, the thermic effect of eating, and physical activity (Bouchard and Shepard 1994; USDHHS 1996). Prospective studies of the impact of reduced metabolic rate on weight gain are equivocal (Bandini et al. 2004; Tataranni et al. 2003). Because physical activity is modifiable, it is the target of interventions to alter energy expenditure. Among adults, epidemiologic studies have demonstrated a relation between physical activity and obesity in cross-sectional studies (USDHHS 1996; Erlichman, Kerbey, and James 2002), and a relationship between increases in physical activity and less weight gain in longitudinal studies (Erlichman, Kerbey, and James 2002; Fogelholm and Kokkonen-Harjula 2000). Similar findings have been observed for children (Strong et al. 2005).

Another modifiable risk factor for obesity, television viewing, has received attention in children. Hypothesized mechanisms for the influence of television viewing on adiposity include the replacement of more intense physical activities, poor dietary patterns while watching television, and the influence of television commercials on the foods consumed in the house (Woodward-Lopez et al. 2006). A recent synthesis of the observational and experimental evidence for the relationship between television viewing and adiposity in children found a significant, albeit small, association between increased television viewing and obesity (Marshall et al. 2004). Some, but not all, television reduction interventions result in weight change. Two studies performed on school-age children—one a curriculum-based intervention to reduce time spent on television, video, and video games (Robinson 1999) and the other a multicomponent intervention that included recommendations to limit television viewing (Gortmaker et al. 1999)—found a reduction in adiposity status related to a reduction in television viewing for the population and for girls, respectively. In contrast, an intervention conducted in preschools did not change the weight status of the children (Dennison et al. 2004).

Population-Attributable Risk

The state of the science in obesity research precludes the estimation of population-attributable risk (PAR) for most proposed risk factors for obesity because either the assumptions of the PAR cannot be met or the estimates needed for the calculation are not available. This is particularly true for dietary risk factors. The limitations in the literature include: (1) the lack of consensus on the causal link between many hypothesized risk factors and obesity; (2) limited number of longitudinal studies that have addressed the incidence of obesity (as compared to weight change); (3) difficulty in establishing an independent effect of different dietary behaviors that are often highly correlated; and (4) difficulty in disentangling caloric intake from caloric expenditure, which are interdependent in weight control.

Prevention and Control

Prevention

The goal for the primary prevention of obesity is to prevent unhealthy weight gain. A World Health Organization consultation identified two strategies to achieve this goal: (1) increasing the knowledge and skills of the population related to diet, physical activity, or weight; or (2) reducing population exposure to an obesity-promoting environment (WHO 1999). The evidence that specific strategies and/or interventions either targeted at individuals or populations prevent unhealthy weight gain is limited, in part because this area of research is relatively new.

Among adults, only a few interventions to specifically prevent weight gain have been evaluated. These interventions were carried out in young adult men and women (Jeffery and French 1999), young women (Levine et al. 2007), middle-aged women (Simkin-Silverman et al. 2003), parent/child pairs (Rodearmel et al. 2006), and college students (Hivert et al. 2007). They used knowledge and skill-building approaches delivered either in person (Levine et al. 2007; Simkin-Silverman et al. 2003; Rodearmel et al. 2006; Hivert et al. 2007) or through the mail (Jeffery and French 1999; Levine et al. 2007). Results have been equivocal, with some interventions showing significant positive changes in at least one measure of adiposity (Simkin-Silverman et al. 2003; Rodearmel et al. 2006; Hivert et al. 2007), whereas others showed no change (Jeffery and French 1999; Levine et al. 2007). No single intervention component distinguished successful interventions from those that were not. Community-level interventions focusing on weight gain prevention are rare. However, a number of community interventions carried out during the 1970s and 1980s designed to address CVD risk factors, but not weight specifically, demonstrated minimal impact on weight (WHO 1999).

The effectiveness of primary prevention for obesity has been more widely studied in children than in adults and has been summarized in a number of recent reviews (Doak et al. 2006; Flynn et al. 2006; Summerbell et al. 2005). As with results observed in adults, findings have been mixed. For example, a recent Cochrane review summarized the findings from 22 intervention studies. These studies were done across a variety of venues including families, after/school community programs, and day care with the majority done in schools (Summerbell et al. 2005). Interventions focused on diet only (9%), physical activity only (27%), or combined diet and physical activity (64%). Most interventions included an educational or behavioral change component such as classroom instruction, physical education classes, or group learning sessions. A number combined these informational interventions with environmental change such as changes in food service or vending machines. Based on the results of these 22 studies, the authors concluded that "the interventions employed to date, have largely not impacted on weight status of children to any significant degree" (Summerbell et al. 2005). However, the authors indicated that most interventions result in diet and/or physical activity behavior change, a necessary first step in altering weight status. They also identified two good quality interventions that did impact weight through reductions in television viewing (Gortmaker et al. 1999; Robinson 1999). These two interventions were previously described (see section on modifiable risk factors). Based on results from two recent studies, community-level interventions may be a promising area for children. Shape Up Somerville, a multicomponent intervention designed to change the options and environment for diet and physical activity across multiple venues in Somerville, MA, found a small but significant decline in BMI z-score for children in the intervention community as compared to the control communities (Economos et al. 2007). The Apple Project was an intervention implemented in New Zealand designed to enhance opportunities for a more healthful diet and noncurricular physical activity in schools and the community. The project reported a significant mean reduction in BMI for normal-weight, but not overweight, children in intervention schools when compared to control schools (Taylor et al. 2007).

In the absence of a body of interventions that are effective and the need to initiate prevention strategies for obesity, public health practitioners have begun to heed the advice of the 2005 Institute of Medicine (IOM) and implementing interventions "based on the best available evidence—as opposed to waiting for the best possible evidence" (IOM 2005). For example, two behaviors, increased fruit and vegetable consumption and increased breast-feeding are obesity prevention strategies in a number of public health programs (CDC 2007b). Neither behavior has been shown to prevent unhealthy weight gain in randomized controlled trials. However, both are linked to weight in observational studies (Woodward-Lopez et al. 2006), both have plausible explanations of why they would prevent unhealthy weight gain (Woodward-Lopez et al. 2006), and both have some effective interventions for behavior change (Shealy et al. 2005; Ammerman et al. 2002). As such, the best available evidence supports their use. Similarly, environmental and policy interventions to change physical activity have not been demonstrated to change weight in the population. However, the best available evidence indicates that physical activity is linked to weight (USDHHS 1996), and physical activity can be changed through strategies such as improving access combined with information or changing street-scale or community-scale urban design and land use policies (Heath et al. 2006; Kahn et al. 2002).

Screening

Among adults, a number of clinical committees have recommended clinical screening in combination with counseling and/or behavioral interventions. The U.S. Preventive Services Task Force (USPSTF) recommended that clinicians screen all adult patients for obesity and offer intensive counseling and behavioral interventions to promote sustained weight loss for obese patients (USPSTF 2003). High-intensity counseling was defined as more than one person-to-person session per month for at least the first three months of the intervention. The task force found that interventions combining education and counseling about diet and physical activity with the discussion of behavioral strategies to help patients achieve these behaviors was the most effective intervention. The task force also recommended that screening be done using the BMI.

The NIH Clinical Guidelines on the Identification, Evaluation, and Treatment of Overweight and Obesity in Adults recommended that clinicians assess their adult patients' candidacy for weight loss therapy through three measures: the patient's BMI, waist circumference, and the presence of concomitant CVD risk factors or comorbidities. High waist circumference measures were defined as greater than 88 cm for women and greater than 102 cm for men. Patients with a BMI greater than or equal to 30, or patients with BMI 25–29.9 or high waist circumference combined with two or more risk factors or comorbidities are candidates for weight loss treatment. Treatment should minimally address diet, physical activity, and behavioral modification (NIH 1998).

For children, there is no consensus on whether to screen in clinical settings for the purpose of identifying and subsequently treating overweight children. A recent expert committee recommended yearly assessment of weight and height; those children with age- and sex-specific BMI over the 85th percentile are to be followed up with a more comprehensive clinical assessment that includes measurement of pulse, blood pressure, and fasting lipids as well as family history (Barlow et al. 2007). In addition, based on the level of BMI, these children should also receive interventions of varying intensities.

In contrast, the USPSTF found insufficient evidence to recommend for or against routine screening for overweight in children and adolescents as a means to prevent adverse health outcomes (USPSTF 2005). The primary limitation in the evidence was the lack of effective interventions available for the primary care settings.

For children, whether to screen in the school setting is also being debated. A recent systematic review to address the question as to whether primary school children should be routinely screened concluded that screening could not be justified because of both the lack of information on the benefits and harms of screening as well as the limited information on effective treatments (Westwood et al. 2007). Nihiser and colleagues, based on a review of the literature and existing practices as well as the input of an expert panel convened by CDC, concluded that "BMI screening meets some but not all the criteria established by the American Academy of Pediatrics for determining whether screening for specific health conditions should be implemented in schools" (Nihiser et al. 2007). In contrast, the IOM recommended that schools should "routinely measure weight, height, and gender- and age-specific BMI percentile and make this information available to parents and to the student (when age appropriate)" on the basis that many children do not have routine physicals and their parents may not recognize a weight problem (IOM 2005). However, the IOM recognized concerns regarding student privacy and stigmatization, and the ability of schools and parents to link children to effective interventions.

Treatment

Among adults, weight loss in the range of 5–10% of the baseline weight appears to positively impact health. A review of clinical trials documented an association between weight loss and positive changes in blood pressure, lipid profiles, and blood glucose (NIH 1998). Weight loss also appears to improve function in persons suffering from osteoarthritis (Miller et al. 2006) and is associated with lowered depression and improved self-esteem (Blaine, Rodman, and Newman 2007). There is increasing evidence that weight loss, particularly when it is achieved as part of a lifestyle intervention, can reduce the risk of diabetes (Knowler et al. 2002; Tuomilehto et al. 2001). For example, the U.S. Diabetes Prevention Program intervention found a lifestyle intervention that recommended a 7% weight loss and 150 min of physical activity per week resulted in a reduced incidence of type 2 diabetes in individuals with prediabetes (Knowler et al. 2002). Among overweight children, weight loss also results in improvements in cardiovascular risk factors such as lipid profile, blood pressure, and insulin resistance (Epstein et al. 1998; Berkowitz et al. 2006).

For adults and children alike, a variety of approaches can be used to facilitate weight loss. These include dietary modification, physical activity, behavioral modification, pharmacotherapy, and surgery. The effectiveness and appropriateness of each modality have been extensively reviewed and are summarized below.

Dietary Modification

The goal of dietary modification is to reduce energy intake. For adults, based on evidence from randomized control weight loss trials, calorie reductions in the range of 500–1,000 calories per day are recommended to facilitate weight losses in the range of 1–2 lb per week (NIH 1998). A recent clinical trial indicated that a variety of dietary approaches can lead to caloric reduction and subsequent weight loss over a 12-month period (Dansinger et al. 2005). These included diets that target a reduction in portion size and calorie restriction, limit fat intake, limit carbohydrate intake without fat restriction, and promote macronutrient balance.

Current recommendations for weight loss among children focus on changing dietary patterns over the reduction of a specific number of calories (Barlow et al. 2007; Barlow and Dietz 1998). An example of this approach is the Traffic Light Diet. In this diet, children are guided in their dietary choices by the designation of foods as red, yellow, or green light foods on the basis of their caloric content (Epstein et al. 1998). The use of this diet when provided in the context of a behavior modification program results in weight loss.

Physical Activity

Because it increases energy expenditure, physical activity has a role in weight loss. Even in the absence of weight loss, however, physical activity appears to improve the risk profile of obese persons (NIH 1998; Shaw et al. 2006; van Baak and Saris 2005). As a sole weight loss strategy, the use of physical activity results in modest weight loss for both adults (NIH 1998; Shaw et al. 2006) and children (Strong et al. 2005), although the effect is smaller than that of dietary restriction alone (NIH 1998; Shaw et al. 2006). For adults, physical activity combined with diet improves weight loss more than diet or physical activity alone (NIH 1998; Shaw et al. 2006).

The amount of physical activity needed for weight loss is not known and, in part, depends on the reductions in caloric intake. Current recommendations suggest that obese adults initially aim for 30–45 min of moderate-intensity physical activity per day (NIH 1998; Jakicic et al. 2001), and children aim for one hour or more of daily physical activity (Bandini et al. 2004).

Behavioral Therapies

Weight loss appears to be enhanced when persons develop strategies to address the day-to-day challenges of changing their diet or physical activity habit (NIH 1998), and thus are a recommended component of weight loss therapies for both adults (NIH 1998; Glenny et al. 1997) and children (Epstein et al. 1998). Examples of these strategies include tracking the amount of food consumed and frequency of types of physical activity, limiting one's exposure to calorie-dense foods or situations in which they are served, setting realistic and specific goals and rewarding oneself for achieving them, and seeking social support from friends and family (NIH 1998).

Clinical Therapies

Pharmacological and surgical therapies can be used to facilitate weight loss in select individuals. Sibutramine and orlistat are approved by the U.S. Food and Drug Administration (FDA) for the long-term treatment of obesity (Atkinson 2005). A reduced-strength form of orlistat has recently been approved for over-the-counter sale (USFDA 2007). Sibutramine is an appetite suppressant whose action is caused by the inhibition of serotonin and noradrenaline reuptake (Atkinson 2005). In contrast, orlistat acts by blocking the digestion and absorption of fat by inhibiting gastric lipases (Atkinson 2005). Clinical trials lasting more than 1 year found an average weight loss of 4.3 kg for sibutramine and 2.7 kg for orlistat (Padwal, Li, and Lau 2003). The NIH Clinical Guidelines on the Identification, Evaluation, and Treatment of Overweight and Obesity in Adults concluded that FDA-approved weight loss drugs should only be used in patients who are obese (BMI greater than or equal to 30) or those who have a BMI of 27 with other comorbidities, and that they should be used as an adjunct to diet and physical activity and only after the patient has not achieved weight loss through dietary and physical activity interventions (NIH 1998).

The use of surgical interventions to treat obesity has increased substantially in recent years for both adults and children (Davis et al. 2006). The purpose of surgical intervention is to reduce caloric intake by changing the structure of the gastrointestinal tract. This can be done in two ways: changes that limit the intake of food (restrictive) and changes that limit the absorption of nutrients (malabsorptive) (DeMaria 2007). Procedures include gastric stapling, adjustable gastric banding, proximal Roux-en-Y gastric bypass, and biliopancreatic diversion. These surgeries result in substantial weight loss and are associated with a reduction in comorbidities (NIH 1998; Maggard et al. 2005) and reduced all-cause mortality (Adams et al. 2007; Sjöström et al. 2007). However, these procedures are associated with medical complications (DeMaria 2007) and require a major lifestyle change related to food consumption. For both adults and adolescents, surgical interventions are recommended only for select persons with severe obesity who have been unsuccessful in using less invasive methods of weight loss and who are at high risk for obesity-related morbidity and mortality (NIH 1998; Inge et al. 2004).

Weight Loss Maintenance

An important component of weight control is the long-term maintenance of weight loss. Limited information exists on the proportion of population who achieve long-term success. One proposed definition of success is "individuals who have intentionally lost at least 10% of their body weight and kept it off for at least one year" (McGuire, Wing, and Hill 1999). Based on this definition, one population-based study found that about 20% of overweight people successfully maintained their weight losses (McGuire, Wing, and Hill 1999). Limited information also exists on the methods used to achieve long-term success. The National Weight Loss Registry, a volunteer registry of persons who have lost at least 30 lb and kept it off for a year, identified six strategies associated with long-term success at weight loss. These include: (1) engaging in high levels of physical activity (60 min/day), (2) eating low calorie/low fat diets, (3) eating breakfast, (4) regularly monitoring weight, (5) having a consistent dietary pattern, and (6) addressing small regains early (Wing and Phelan 2005). A recent review indicated that physical activity in the range of 40–90 min may be needed to maintain weight loss (Goldberg and King 2007).

Examples of Evidence-Based Interventions

Public health is defined as "the approach to medicine that is concerned with health of the community as a whole" (MedicineNet 2007) and as such focuses on population-based interventions. For obesity prevention and control, population-based interventions include behavioral interventions aimed at groups of people, as well as environmental and policy interventions designed to provide more supportive environments for diet and physical activity or to provide incentives for the treatment of obesity. Some examples follow.

As the lead federal public health agency, CDC supports public health interventions to address overweight and obesity or its related risk factors through three different programs. The Nutrition and Physical Activity Program to Prevent Obesity and Other Chronic Diseases in 2007 funded 28 state public health departments to help reduce the risk of obesity and other chronic disease by addressing physical inactivity and poor diet (CDC 2007b). State health departments worked toward these goals by developing a state-wide comprehensive plan, establishing and leveraging partnerships, and implementing science-based interventions designed to increase physical activity and improve nutrition. These interventions were implemented across multiple settings. For example, a community-based intervention in Moses Lake, WA, implemented changes to increase access to fruits and vegetables through community gardens, improve access to physical activity opportunities by changing streets and sidewalks, and improve breast-feeding by providing supportive community environments. In North Carolina, an intervention in child care settings seeks to identify and address environmental barriers to healthy eating and physical activity. In 2008, 23 states were funded to continue addressing nutrition and physical activity with a focus on addressing environmental and policy supports for these behaviors.

Through a second public health program, the STEPS program, CDC provides funding to communities nationwide to implement evidence-based community interventions to reduce the burden of diabetes, asthma, and obesity (CDC 2007d). Communities work across multiple sectors in the community including schools, the medical setting, and workplaces. One example of a STEPS intervention to address obesity is Mission Melt-away. This intervention, implemented in Broome County, NY, is a collaborative effort with the Office for Aging and the local YMCA. Mission Meltaway, conducted over an eight-week period, uses a group approach to weight management. A trained facilitator leads support groups on topics such as nutrition, physical activity, and mental health (CDC 2007d).

In a third program, CDC funds about half of the state education agencies to implement coordinated school health programs (CDC 2007e). These programs address eight components: health education, physical education, health services, nutrition services, counseling and psychological services, health school environments, health promotion for staff, and family/community involvement. As a result of this program, two of the risk factors for overweight and obesity, poor diet and physical activity, are addressed in school settings.

Legislative bodies, recognizing the impact of obesity on health and costs, have implemented another type of public health intervention to address the issue of obesity: legislative actions. In a recent paper, Boehmer et al. (2007) documented the increased number of proposed and enacted bills in state legislatures related to childhood obesity and its risk factors between 2003 and 2005. Examples include legislation for schools addressing nutrition and physical education standards, and legislation for communities addressing the creation of walking paths or farmer's markets (Boehmer et al. 2007). A case study that illustrates how legislation can lead to more widespread activities is the state of Arkansas (Ryan et al. 2005). In 2003, the Arkansas General Assembly passed Arkansas Act 1220. The goals of this legislation were to "improve the environment within which children go to school and learn health habits, to engage the community to support parents and to build a system that encourages health, and to increase awareness of childhood obesity" (Ryan et al. 2005). As a result of this legislation, a statewide advisory board was formed, standardized policies related to nutrition and physical activity rules in schools were implemented, and a statewide program to annually access BMI and report findings to parents was implemented. The impact of this initiative is being evaluated.

Areas of Future Research

Given the magnitude of the obesity problem, a number of research areas need to be further addressed. Because of the limited body of existing research, prevention research is a critical need. Topics for further development include better characterization of the specific dietary, activity, and behavioral components of weight gain prevention, as well as an evaluation of the effectiveness and efficacy of individual and multicomponent interventions implemented across different settings. Of particular interest is the impact of policy and environmental interventions singly and in combination with behavioral interventions.

Translation research is another need. One type of research should examine how to facilitate the wide-scale implementation of interventions determined to be effective in research settings. This research should work with decisions-makers and public health practitioners to identify the most efficient and effective ways to adopt, adapt, and maintain use of effective interventions over time. Another type of research should identify effective communication strategies for translating scientific information about physical activity, diet, and obesity to the lay public.

Another area that merits further development is research that addresses the disparities in obesity levels, particularly for African American and Mexican American women and girls, and Mexican-American boys. Researchers should work with affected groups to better characterize the cultural, behavioral, and environmental barriers to diet and physical activity, and to develop and evaluate interventions addressing these barriers.

At least four areas of weight loss and treatment also merit further attention. First, as more adults become morbidity obese, identification of effective treatment strategies for this group is needed. These efforts could include understanding the unique barriers to diet and physical activity in this group, identifying more aggressive therapies for weight loss such as medications and surgeries, and understanding how to best clinically manage the obesity-related comorbidities. A second gap is the limited information on the appropriate timing and the most effective weight loss strategies for children and adolescents. Third, among adults and children who successfully lose weight, the health impact of this loss could be enhanced by identifying the strategies to maintain this weight loss in the long term. Fourth, few well-documented, effective, and sustainable public health approaches to weight loss and maintenance have been identified.

Finally, policymakers and decision-makers would benefit from research that better informs their decision-making. This research includes studies of the cost and cost-effectiveness of various options to address the problem of obesity.

Resources

American Academy of Pediatrics (AAP) (http://www.aap.org/obesity/index.html)
General information about childhood overweight and obesity.
The American Society of Bariatric Physicians (ASBP) (http://www.asbp.org)
ASBP offers information on the problem of obesity, tips on weight loss, and a referral program to
    bariatric physicians (specializing in obesity treatment) for professional consultation.
Centers for Disease Control and Prevention (CDC) (http://www.cdc.gov/obesity)
General information about overweight and obesity among adults and youth, and general informa-
    tion on healthy eating and physical activity.
Federal Trade Commission (FTC), Weight Loss and Fitness Consumer Information (http://www.
    ftc.gov/bcp/menus/consumer/health/weight.shtm)
Consumer information on topics such as finding the right weight loss program and avoiding decep-
    tion.
Federal Citizen Information Center (http://www.pueblo.gsa.gov/cic_text/health/works4you/weightloss.
    htm)
Booklet designed to help consumers ask the right questions to choose a safe and effective weight loss
    method and to determine if their weight puts them at risk for health problems.
National Institutes of Health (NIH), National Heart Lung and Blood Institute (NHLBI) (http://
    www.nhlbi.nih.gov/health/public/heart/obesity/lose_wt/patmats.htm)
Guidelines for the measurement of overweight and obesity and steps for safe and effective weight loss.
National Institute of Diabetes and Digestive and Kidney Diseases (NIDDK) (http://win.niddk.nih.
    gov/publications/choosing.htm)
Weight-control Information Network (WIN)
Fact sheet to help consumers make an informed decision about joining a weight-loss program.
United States Department of Agriculture (USDA), Food and Nutrition Information Center Reports
    and Studies on Obesity (http://fnic.nal.usda.gov/nal_display/index.php?tax_level=1&info_
    center=4&tax_subject=271)
See Chapters 6 and 7 for additional readings and resources.

References

Adams, T.D., R.E. Gress, S.C. Smith, et al. Long-Term Mortality after Gastric Bypass Surgery. *N Engl J Med* (2007):357:753–761.

Albu, J., and F.X. Pi-Sunyer. Obesity and Diabetes. In: Bray, G.A., and C. Bouchard, editors, *Handbook of Obesity*. New York, NY: Informa Healthcare (2007) pp. 899–917.

Ammerman, A.S., C.H. Lindquist, K.N. Lohr, and J. Hersey. The Efficacy of Behavioral Interventions to Modify Dietary Fat and Fruit and Vegetable Intake: A Review of the Evidence. *Prev Med* (2002):35:25–41.

Angulo, P. Obesity and Nonalcoholic Fatty Liver Disease. *Nutr Rev* (2007):65:S57–S63.

Atkinson, R.L. Management of Obesity: Pharmacotherapy. In: Kopelman, P.G., I.D. Caterson, and W.H. Dietz, editors, *Clinical Obesity in Adults and Children*, 2nd ed. Malden, MA: Blackwell (2005) pp. 380–393.

Bandini, L.G., A. Must, S.M. Phillips, E.N. Naumova, and W.H. Dietz. Relation of Body Mass Index and Body Fatness to Energy Expenditure: Longitudinal Changes from Preadolescence through Adolescence. *Am J Clin Nutr* (2004):80(5):1262–1269.

Barlow, S.E., and W.H. Dietz. Obesity Evaluation and Treatment: Expert Committee Recommendations. *Pediatrics* (1998):120:e29.

Barlow, S.E., and the Expert Committee. Expert Committee Recommendations Regarding the Prevention, Assessment, and Treatment of Child and Adolescent Overweight and Obesity: Summary Report. *Pediatrics* (2007):120:S164–S192.

Barrett-Connor, E. An Introduction to Obesity and Dementia. *Curr Alzheimer Res* (2007):4:97–101.

Bergström, A., P. Pisani, V. Tenet, A. Wolk, and H.O. Adami. Overweight as an Avoidable Cause of Cancer in Europe. *Int J Cancer* (2001):91(3):421–430.

Berkowitz, R.I., K. Fujioka, S.R. Daniels, et al. Effects of Sibutramine Treatment in Obese Adolescents: A Randomized Trial. *Ann Intern Med* (2006):145:81–90.

Blaine, B.E., J. Rodman, and J.M. Newman. Weight Loss Treatment and Psychological Well-Being: A Review and Meta-Analysis. *J Health Psychol* (2007):12:66–82.

Blundell, J.E., and R.J. Stubbs. Diet Composition and the Control of Food Intake in Humans. In: Bray, G.A., and C. Bouchard, editors, *Handbook of Obesity*. New York, NY: Informa Healthcare (2007) pp. 427–460.

Boehmer, T.K., R.C. Brownson, D. Haire-Joshu, and M.L. Dreisinger. Patterns of Childhood Obesity Prevention Legislation in the United States. *Prev Chronic Dis* (2007). Available at http://www.cdc.gov/pcd/issues/2007/jul06_0082.htm. Accessed September 18, 2007.

Bogers, R.P., W.J.E. Bemelmans, R.T. Hoogenveen, et al. Association of Overweight with Increased Risk of Coronary Heart Disease Partly Independent of Blood Pressure and Cholesterol Levels. *Arch Intern Med* (2007):167:1720–1728.

Bouchard, C., and R.J. Shepard. Physical Activity, Fitness, and Health: The Model and Key Concepts. In: Bouchard, C., R.J. Shepard, and T. Stephens, editors, *Physical Activity, Fitness, and Health: International Proceedings and Consensus Statement*. Champaign, IL: Human Kinetics Publishers (1994) pp. 77–88.

Centers for Disease Control and Prevention (CDC). *Division of Nutrition, Physical Activity, and Obesity. About BMI for Children and Teens* (2007a). Available at http://www.cdc.gov/nccdphp/dnpa/bmi/childrens_BMI/about_childrens_BMI.htm. Accessed September 18, 2007.

Centers for Disease Control and Prevention (CDC). *Division of Nutrition, Physical Activity, and Obesity. CDC's State-Based Nutrition and Physical Activity Program to Prevent Obesity and Other Chronic Diseases* (2007b). Available at http://www.cdc.gov/nccdphp/dnpa/obesity/state_programs/index.htm. Accessed September 18, 2007.

Centers for Disease Control and Prevention (CDC). *Steps Program* (2007c). Available at http://www.cdc.gov/steps/. Accessed September 18, 2007.

Centers for Disease Control and Prevention (CDC). Division of Adolescent and School Health. *Coordinated School Health Program* (2007d). Available at http://www.cdc.gov/healthyyouth/ CSHP. Accessed September 18, 2007.

Chu, S.Y., W.M. Callaghan, S.Y. Kim, et al. Maternal Obesity and Risk of Gestational Diabetes Mellitus. *Diabetes Care* (2007a):30(8):2070–2076.

Chu, S.Y., S.Y. Kim, C.H. Schmid, et al. Maternal Obesity and Risk of Cesarean Delivery: A Meta-Analysis. *Obes Rev* (2007b):8(5):385–394.

Chu, S.Y., S.Y. Kim, J. Lau, et al. Maternal Obesity and Risk of Stillbirth: A Meta-Analysis. *Am J Obstet Gynecol* (2007c):197(3):223–228.

Dansinger, M.L., J.A. Gleason, J.L. Griffith, H.P. Selker, and E.J. Schaefer. Comparison of the Atkins, Ornish, Weight Watchers, and Zone Diets for Weight Loss and Heart Disease Risk Reduction: A Randomized Trial. *JAMA* (2005):293:43–53.

Davis, M.M., K. Slish, C. Chao, and M.D. Cabana. National Trends in Bariatric Surgery, 1996–2002. *Arch Surg* (2006):141:71–74.

DeMaria, E.J. Bariatric Surgery for Morbid Obesity. *New Engl J Med* (2007):356:2176–2183.

Dennison, B.A., T.J. Russo, P.A. Burdick, and P.L. Jenkins. An Intervention to Reduce Television Viewing by Preschool Children. *Arch Pediatr Adolesc Med* (2004):158:170–176.

Densmore, D., H.M. Blanck, W.H. Dietz, et al. State-Specific Prevalence of Obesity among Adults—United States, 2005. *MMWR* (2006):55(36):985–988.

Dietz, W.H. Health Consequences of Obesity in Youth: Childhood Predictors of Adult Disease. *Pediatrics* (1998):101:518–524.

Doak, C.M., T.L.S. Visscher, C.M. Renders, and J.C. Seidell. The Prevention of Overweight and Obesity in Children and Adolescents: A Review of Interventions and Programmes. *Obes Rev* (2006):7:111–136.

Doll, H.A., S.E.K. Petersen, and S.L. Stewart-Brown. Obesity and Physical and Emotional Well-Being: Associations between Body Mass Index, Chronic Illness, and the Physical and Mental Components of the SF-36 Questionnaire. *Obes Res* (2000):8:160–170.

Eaton, D.K., L. Kann, S. Kinchen, et al. Youth Risk Behavior Surveillance—United States, 2007. *MMWR* (2008):57:1–131.

Economos, C.D., R.R. Hyatt, J.P. Goldberg, et al. A Community Intervention Reduces BMI *z*-Score in Children: Shape up Somerville First Year Results. *Obesity* (2007):15(5):1325–1336.

Epstein, L.H., M.D. Myers, H.A. Raynor, and B.E. Saelens. Treatment of Pediatric Obesity. *Pediatrics* (1998):101:554–570.

Erlichman, J., A.L. Kerbey, and W.P.T. James. Physical Activity and its Impact on Health Outcomes: Prevention of Unhealthy Weight Gain and Obesity by Physical Activity: An Analysis of the Evidence. *Obes Rev* (2002):3:273–287.

Fabricatore, A.N., and T.A. Wadden. Psychological Aspects of Obesity. *Clin Dermatol* (2004):22:332–337.

Felson, D.T., R.C. Lawrence, P.A. Dieppe, et al. Osteoarthritis: New Insights: Part 1. The Disease and its Risk Factors. *Ann Intern Med* (2000):133(8):635–646.

Finkelstein, E.A., I.C. Fiebelkorn, and G. Wang. National Medical Spending Attributable to Overweight and Obesity: How Much, and Who's Paying? *Health Aff* (2003):W3:219–226.

Flegal, K.M., M.D. Carroll, C.L. Ogden, and C.L. Johnson. Prevalence and Trends in Obesity among U.S. Adults, 1999–2000. *JAMA* (2002):288:1723–1727.

Flegal, K.M., B.I. Graubard, D.F. Williamson, and M.H. Gail. Excess Deaths Associated with Underweight, Overweight, and Obesity. *JAMA* (2005):293:1861–1867.

Flynn, M.A.T., D.A. McNeil, B. Maloff, et al. Reducing Obesity and Related Chronic Disease Risk in Children and Youth: A Synthesis of Evidence with "Best Practice" Recommendations. *Obes Rev* (2006):7:S7–S66.

Fogelholm, M., and K. Kokkonen-Harjula. Does Physical Activity Prevent Weight Gain—a Systematic Review. *Obes Rev* (2000):1:95–111.

Ford, E.S. Body Mass Index, Diabetes, and C-Reactive Protein among U.S. Adults. *Diabetes Care* (1999):22:1971–1977.

Ford, E.S., D.A. Galuska, C. Gillespie, J.C. Will, W.H. Giles, and W.H. Dietz. C-Reactive Protein and Body Mass Index in Children: Findings from the Third National Health and Nutrition Examination Survey, 1988–1994. *J Pediatr* (2001):138:486–492.

Freedman, D.S., W.H. Dietz, S.R. Srinivasan, and G.S. Berenson. The Relation of Overweight to Cardiovascular Risk Factors among Children and Adolescents: The Bogalusa Heart Study. *Pediatrics* (1999):103:1175–1182.

Freedman, D.S., L.K. Khan, M.K. Serdula, W.H. Dietz, S.R. Srinivasan, and G.S. Berenson. The Relation of Childhood BMI to Adult Adiposity: The Bogalusa Heart Study. *Pediatrics* (2005):115:22–27.

Freedman, D.S., M.K. Serdula, and L.K. Khan. The Adult Health Consequences of Childhood Obesity. In: Chen, C., and W.H. Dietz, editors, *Obesity in Childhood and Adolescence.* Nestle Nutrition Workshop Series, Pediatric Program, vol. 49. Philadelphia, PA: Lippincott Williams and Wilkins (2002) pp. 63–82.

French, S.A., M. Story, and C.L. Perry. Self-Esteem and Obesity in Children and Adolescents: A Literature Review. *Obes Res* (1995):3:479–490.

Galuska, D.A., C. Gillespie, S.A. Kuester, et al. State Prevalence of Obesity among Adults in the United States. *MMWR* (2008):57(28):765–768.

Glenny, A.M., S. O'Meara, A. Melville, T.A. Sheldon, and C. Wilson. The Treatment and Prevention of Obesity: A Systematic Review of the Literature. *Int J Obes* (1997):21:715–737.

Goldberg, J.H., and A.C. King. Physical Activity and Weight Management across the Lifespan. *Annu Rev Public Health* (2007):28:145–170.

Gortmaker, S.L., K. Peterson, J. Wiecha, et al. Reducing Obesity via a School-Based Interdisciplinary Intervention among Youth: Planet Health. *Arch Pediatr Adolesc Med* (1999):153:409–418.

Gortmaker, S.L., A. Must, J.M. Perrin, A.M. Sobol, and W.H. Dietz. Social and Economic Consequences of Overweight in Adolescence and Young Adulthood. *N Engl J Med.* (1993):329:1008–1012.

Heath, G.W., R.C. Brownson, J. Kruger, et al. The Effectiveness of Urban Design and Land Use and Transport Policies and Practices to Increase Physical Activity: A Systematic Review. *JPAH* (2006):3:S55–S76.

Hivert, M.F., M.F. Langlois, P. Berard, J.P. Cuerrier, and A.C. Carpentier. Prevention of Weight Gain in Young Adults through a Seminar-Based Intervention Program. *Int J Obes* (2007):31:1262–1269.

Inge, T.H., N.F. Krebs, V.F. Garcia, et al. Bariatric Surgery for Severely Overweight Adolescents: Concerns and Recommendations. *Pediatrics* (2004):114:217–223.

Institute of Medicine (IOM). *Preventing Childhood Obesity: Health in the Balance.* Koplan, J.P., C.T. Liverman, and V.I. Kraack, editors. Washington, D.C.: National Academies Press (2005).

Jakicic, J.M., K. Clark, E. Coleman, et al. American College of Sports Medicine Position Stand: Appropriate Intervention Strategies for Weight Loss and Prevention of Weight Regain for Adults. *Med Sci Sports Exerc* (2001):33:2145–2156.

Jeffery, R.W., and S.A. French. Preventing Weight Gain in Adults: The Pound of Prevention Study. *AJPH* (1999):89:747–751.

Juonala, M., M. Raitakari, J. Viikari, and O.T. Raitakari. Obesity in Youth is not an Independent Predictor of Carotid IMT in Adulthood. The Cardiovascular Risk in Young Finns Study. *Atherosclerosis* (2006):185:388–393.

Kahn, E.B., L.T. Ramsey, R.C. Brownson, et al. The Effectiveness of Interventions to Increase Physical Activity: A Systematic Review. *Am J Prev Med* (2002):22:73–107.

Knowler, W.C., E. Barrett-Connor, S.E. Fowler, et al. Reduction in the Incidence of Type 2 Diabetes with Lifestyle Intervention or Metformin. *N Engl J Med* (2002):346:393–403.

Koenig, S.M. Pulmonary Complications of Obesity. *Am J Med Sci* (2001):331:249–279.

Latner, J.D., and A.J. Stunkard. Getting Worse: The Stigmatization of Obese Children. *Obes Res* (2003):11:452–456.

Levine, M.D., M.L. Klem, M.A. Kalarchian, et al. Weight Gain Prevention among Women. *Obesity* (2007):15:1267–1277.

Maggard, M.A., L.R. Shugarman, M. Suttorp, et al. Meta-Analysis: Surgical Treatment of Obesity. *Ann Intern Med* (2005):142:547–559.

Marshall, S.J., S.J.H. Biddle, T. Gorely, N. Cameron, and I. Murdey. Relationships between Media Use, Body Fatness and Physical Activity in Children and Youth: A Meta-Analysis. *Int J Obes* (2004):28:1238–1246.

McGee, D.L., and the Diverse Populations Collaboration. Body Mass Index and Mortality: A Meta-Analysis Based on Person-Level Data from Twenty-Six Observational Studies. *Ann Epidemiol* (2005):15:87–97.

McGuire, M., R. Wing, and J. Hill. The Prevalence of Weight Loss Maintenance among American Adults. *Int J Obes* (1999):23:1314–1319.

MedicineNet. Available at http://www.medterms.com. Accessed September 18, 2007.

Miller, G.D., B.J. Nicklas, C. Davis, R.F. Loeser, L. Lenchik, and S.P. Messier. Intensive Weight Loss Program Improves Physical Function in Older Obese Adults with Knee Osteoarthritis. *Obesity* (2006):14:1219–1230.

Must, A., J. Spadano, E.H. Coakley, et al. The Disease Burden Associated with Overweight and Obesity. *JAMA* (1999):282:1523–1529.

Must, A., and R.S. Strauss. Risks and Consequences of Childhood and Adolescent Obesity. *Int J Obes* (1999):23:S2–S11.

National Institutes of Health (NIH). *Clinical Guidelines on the Identification, Evaluation, and Treatment of Overweight and Obesity in Adults: The Evidence Report.* Bethesda, MD: National Institutes of Health, U.S. Department of Health and Human Services (1998).

National Research Council. Committee on Diet and Health. Calories: Total Macronutrient Intake, Energy Expenditure, and Net Energy Stores. In: *Diet and Health: Implications for Reducing Chronic Disease Risk.* Washington, D.C.: National Academies Press (1989) pp. 139–158.

Nihiser A.J., S.M. Lee, H. Wechsler, et al. Body Mass Index Measurement in Schools. *J Sch Health* (2007):77:651–671.

Ogden, C.L., M.D. Carroll, and K.M. Flegal. High Body Mass Index for Age among U.S. Children and Adolescents, 2003–2006. *JAMA* (2008):299:2401–2405.

Ogden, C.L., M.D. Carroll, L.R. Curtin, et al. Prevalence of Overweight and Obesity in the United States, 1999–2004. *JAMA* (2006):295:1549–1555.

Ogden, C.L., K.M. Flegal, M.D. Carroll, and C.L. Johnson. Prevalence and Trends in Overweight among U.S. Children and Adolescents, 1999–2000. *JAMA* (2002):288:1728–1732.

Ogden, C.L., M.D. Carroll, M.A. McDowell, and K.M. Flegal. *Obesity among Adults in the United States—No Change Since 2003–2004.* NCHS Data Brief No 1. Hyattsville, MD: National Center for Health Statistics (2007a).

Ogden, C.L., S.Z. Yanovski, M.D. Carroll, and K.M. Flegal. The Epidemiology of Obesity. *Gastroenterology* (2007b):132:2087–2102.

Padwal, R., S.K. Li, and D.C. Lau. Long-Term Pharmacotherapy for Obesity and Overweight. *Cochrane Database Syst Rev* (2003):CD004094.

Puhl, R.M., K.E. Henderson, and K.D. Brownell. Social Consequence of Obesity. In: Kopelman, P.G., I.D. Caterson, and W.H. Dietz, editors, *Clinical Obesity in Adults and Children*, 2nd ed. Malden, MA: Blackwell (2005) pp. 29–45.

Richardson, S.A., N. Goodman, A.H. Hastorf, and S.M. Dornbusch. Cultural Uniformity in Reaction to Physical Disabilities. *Am Sociol Rev* (1961):26:241–247.

Robinson T.N. Reducing Children's Television Viewing to Prevent Obesity: A Randomized Controlled Trial. *JAMA* (1999):282:1561–1567.

Rodearmel, S.J., H.R. Wyatt, M.J. Barry, et al. A Family-Based Approach to Preventing Excessive Weight Gain. *Obesity* (2006):14:1392–1401.

Ryan, K.W., P. Card-Higginson, S.G. McCarthy, M.B. Justus, and J.W. Thompson. Arkansas Fights Fat: Translating Research into Policy to Combat Childhood and Adolescent Obesity. *Health Aff* (2005):25:992–1004.

Sarwer, D.B., K.C. Allison, L.M. Gibbons, J. Tuttman Markowitz, and D.B. Nelson. Pregnancy and Obesity: A Review and Agenda for Future Research. *J Women's Health* (2006):15(6):720–733.

Schwimmer, J.B., T.M. Burwinkle, and J.W. Varni. Health-Related Quality of Life of Severely Obese Children and Adolescents. *JAMA* (2003):289:1813–1819.

Scott, K.M., R. Bruffaerts, G.E. Simon, et al. Obesity and Mental Disorders in the General Population: Results from the World Mental Health Surveys. *Int J Obes* (2008):32:192–200.

Shaw, G.M., E.M. Velie, and D. Schaffer. Risk of Neural Tube Defect-Affected Pregnancies among Obese Women. *JAMA* (1996):275:1093–1096.

Shaw, K., H. Gennat, P. O'Rourke, and C. Del Mar. Exercise for Overweight or Obesity. *Cochrane Database of Syst Rev* (2006): Issue 4. Art. No. CD003817 (DOI: 10. 1002/14651858. CD003817.pub3). Available at http://www.cochrane.org/reviews/en/ab003817.html.

Shealy, K.R., R. Li, S. Benton-Davis, and L.M. Grummer-Strawn. *The CDC Guide to Breastfeeding Interventions*. Atlanta, GA: U.S. Department of Health and Human Services, Centers for Disease Control and Prevention, National Center for Chronic Disease Prevention and Health Promotion (2005).

Simkin-Silverman, L.R., R.R. Wing, M.A. Boraz, and L.H. Kuller. Lifestyle Intervention Can Prevent Weight Gain during Menopause. Results from a 5-Year Randomized Clinical Trial. *Ann Behav Med* (2003):26:212–220.

Simon, G.E., M. Von Korff, K. Saunders, et al. Association between Obesity and Psychiatric Disorders in the U.S. Adult Population. *Arch Gen Psychiatry* (2006):63:824–830.

Sjöström, L., K. Narbro, C.D. Sjöström, et al. Effects of Bariatric Surgery on Mortality in Swedish Obese Subjects. *N Engl J Med* (2007):357:741–752.

Steinbeck, K. Childhood Obesity. In: Kopelman, P.G., I.D. Caterson, and W.H. Dietz, editors, *Clinical Obesity in Adults and Children*, 2nd ed. Malden, MA: Blackwell (2005) pp. 231–248.

Strong, W.B., R.M. Malina, C.J. Blimkie, et al. Evidence-Based Physical Activity for School-Age Youth. *J Pediatrics* (2005):146:732–737.

Summerbell, C.D., E. Waters, L.D. Edmunds, et al. Interventions for Preventing Obesity in Children. *Cochrane Database of Syst Rev.* Issue 3 (2005):Art. No. CD001871 (DOI:10.1002/14651858. CD001871.pub2). Available at http://www.cochrane.org/reviews/en/ab001871.html.

Tataranni, P.A., I.T. Harper, S. Snitker, et al. Body Weight Gain in Free-Living Pima Indians: Effect of Energy Intake vs. Expenditure. *Int J Obes* (2003):27:1578–1583.

Taylor, R.W., K.A. McAuley, W. Barbezat, et al. Apple Project: 2-Year Findings of a Community-Based Obesity Prevention Program in Primary School Age Children. *Am J Clin Nutr* (2007):86:735–742.

Tilg, H., and G.S. Hotamisligil. Nonalcoholic Fatty Liver Disease: Cytokine–Adipokine Interplay and Regulation of Insulin Resistance. *Gastroenterology* (2006):131:934–945.

Troiano, R.P., E.A. Frongillo, Jr., J. Sobal, and D.A. Levitsky. The Relationship between Body Weight and Mortality: A Quantitative Analysis of Combined Information from Existing Studies. *Int J Obes Relat Metab Disord* (1996):20:63–75.

Tuomilehto, J., J. Lindstrom, J.G. Eriksson, et al. Prevention of Type 2 Diabetes Mellitus by Changes in Lifestyle among Subjects with Impaired Glucose Tolerance. *N Engl J Med* (2001):344:1343–1350.

U.S. Department of Health and Human Services (USDHHS). *Physical Activity and Health: A Report of the Surgeon General.* Atlanta, GA: U.S. Department of Health and Human Services,

Centers for Disease Control and Prevention, National Center for Chronic Disease Prevention and Health Promotion (1996).

U.S. Department of Health and Human Services (USDHHS). *The Surgeon General's Call to Action to Prevent and Decrease Overweight and Obesity 2001*. Rockville, MD: U.S. Department of Health and Human Services, Public Health Service, Office of the Surgeon General (2001).

U.S. Food and Drug Administration (USFDA). *Orlistat OTC (marketed as alli) Information*. Available at http://www.fda.gov/cder/drug/infopage/orlistat_otc. Accessed September 18, 2007.

U.S. Preventive Services Task Force (USPSTF). Screening for Obesity in Adults: Recommendations and Rationale. *Ann Intern Med* (2003):139:930–932.

U.S. Preventive Services Task Force (USPSTF). Screening and Interventions for Overweight in Children and Adolescents: Recommendations Statement. *Pediatrics* (2005):116:205–209.

van Baak, M.A., and W.H.M. Saris. Exercise and Obesity. In: Kopelman, P.G., I.D. Caterson, and W.H. Dietz, editors, *Clinical Obesity in Adults and Children*, 2nd ed. Malden, MA: Blackwell (2005) pp. 363–379.

Vazquenz, G., S. Duval, D.R. Jacobs, Jr., and K. Silventoinen. Comparison of Body Mass Index, Waist Circumference, and Waist/Hip Ratio in Predicting Incident Diabetes: A Meta-Analysis. *Epidemiol Rev* (2007):29:115–128.

Wang, G., and W.H. Dietz. Economic Burden of Obesity in Youths Aged 6 to 17 Years: 1979–1999. *Pediatrics* (2002):109:e81.

Wardle, J., and L. Cooke. The Impact of Obesity on Psychological Well-Being. *Best Pract Res Clin Endocrinol Metab* (2005):19:421–440.

Weiss, R., S.E. Taksali, W.V. Tamorlane, et al. Predictors of Changes in Glucose Tolerance in Obese Youth. *Diabetes Care* (2005):28:902–909.

Westwood, M., D. Fayter, S. Hartley, et al. Childhood Obesity: Should Primary School Children Be Routinely Screened? A Systematic Review and Discussion of the Evidence. *Arch Dis Child* (2007):92:416–422.

Wing, R.R., and S. Phelan. Long-Term Weight Loss Maintenance. *Am J Clin Nut* (2005):82:222S–225S.

Woodward-Lopez, G., L.D. Ritchie, D.E. Gerstein, and P.B. Crawford. *Obesity: Dietary and Developmental Influences*. Boca Raton, FL: CRC Press (2006).

World Health Organization (WHO). *Obesity: Preventing and Managing the Global Epidemic*. Geneva: World Health Organization (1999).

CHAPTER 10

DIABETES
(ICD-10 E10–E14)

*Donald B. Bishop, Ph.D., Patrick J. O'Connor, M.D., M.P.H.,
and Jay Desai, M.P.H.*

Introduction

D iabetes mellitus designates a group of diseases characterized by a myriad metabolic abnormalities including abnormal metabolism of glucose. Type 1 diabetes, which comprises 5%–10% of all diabetes cases, is caused by immune-mediated β-cell destruction, which leads to absolute insulin deficiency and a need for insulin treatment over time (CDC 2008; Atkinson and Maclaren 1994). Type 2 diabetes, which accounts for 90% to 95% of all diagnosed cases of diabetes (CDC 2008), is caused by resistance to insulin and is more common in elderly and persons who are overweight.

Approximately 23.6 million people in the United States have diabetes. Over a quarter of these, 5.7 million, are undiagnosed (CDC 2008), in part because symptoms develop gradually and it can take several years before severe symptoms occur. Between 1997 and 2003, the incidence of diagnosed diabetes in U.S. adults increased 41%—from 4.7 to 6.9 per 1,000 population (Geiss et al. 2006). The rise in obesity rates is the major factor in this increase, but the increase in incidence rate may be due, in part, to enhanced case detection among extremely obese (body mass index [BMI] greater than or equal to 35) people (Gregg et al. 2004). Because the incidence rate of diagnosed diabetes is rising and the relative risk (RR) of death for men is declining (Gregg et al. 2007), the current projection is that there will be over 48 million people in the United States with diabetes by 2050 (Narayan et al. 2006).

The prevalence rate for diagnosed cases of diabetes has risen steadily for decades, having increased from a rate of 0.37% in 1935 (Kenny, Aubert, and Geiss 1995; CDC 1997) to 7.8% in 2007 (CDC 2008). One and a half million new cases of diabetes were identified in 2005, double the annual rates from a decade ago (CDC 1997). The estimated prevalence of diabetes in adults 20 years and older is 10.7% and for adults 60 years and older 23.1% (CDC 2008). Adjusting for population age differences, the prevalence rates of diabetes among adults 20 years and older by race/ethnicity are 6.6% non-Hispanic whites, 7.5% Asian Americans, 10.4% Hispanics, 11.8% non-Hispanic African Americans, and 16.5% American Indians/Alaska Natives (CDC 2008).

For individuals born in 2000, the risk of developing diabetes during their lifetime is 32.8% for men and 38.5% for women (Narayan et al. 2003). If diagnosed at age 10 years, life expectancy declines by 19 years (Narayan et al. 2003). The incidence of diabetes among youth under 20 years old is 24 cases per 100,000 (Writing Group for the SEARCH for Diabetes in Youth Study Group 2007). Approximately 186,300 youth under 20 years old have diabetes (CDC 2008). As of 2001, about one in every 523 youth had physician-diagnosed diabetes (Minino et al. 2007). In data from the SEARCH for Diabetes in Youth Study, for children younger than 10 years old, the incidence rate for diabetes other than type 1 is exceedingly low, but this changes as they reach adolescence. Incidence rates for type 1 and type 2 diabetes presented in five year age groupings (0–4, 5–9, 10–14, and 15–19 years) for 100,000 person-years in 2002–2003 were 14.3, 22.1, 25.9, and 13.1 for type 1 and 0.0, 0.8, 8.1, and 11.8 for type 2, respectively. Broken down by race and ethnicity, non-Hispanic white youth was the only group to continue to show a higher rate for type 1 (15.1) than type 2 (5.6) in the 15–19 year age group. By comparison, American Indian youth in this same age bracket had the lowest incidence of type 1 (4.8) and highest incidence of type 2 (49.4) (Writing Group for the SEARCH for Diabetes in Youth Study Group 2007).

Significance

Diabetes has been ranked among the ten leading causes of death in the United States since 1932 (Harris 1993), and it is currently the sixth leading underlying cause of death, with 73,138 deaths directly attributed to diabetes in 2004 with the age-adjusted death rate for diabetes at 24.5 per 100,000. The age-adjusted death rates over time for men and women have proceeded in different directions: for men in 1950, 1980, and 2004, the rates per 100,000 were 18.8, 18.1, and 28.2, respectively; for women 27.0, 18.0, and 21.72, respectively (NCHS 2007). The age-adjusted death rates by race and Hispanic origin for 1990 and 2004 were as follows: white, not Hispanic, 18.3 and 21.5; black or African American, 40.5 and 48.0; American Indian or Alaska Native, 34.1 and 39.2; Asian or Pacific Islander, 14.6 and 16.6; and Hispanic, 28.2 and 32.1. The death rate from diabetes for African Americans in 1950 was 23.5, compared with 48.0 in 2004, while for all whites, the rate over the same period was essentially unchanged at 22.9 and 22.3 (NCHS 2007).

Mortality statistics alone clearly understate the impact of diabetes. Based on death certificate reports, diabetes contributed to 233,619 deaths in 2005 (CDC 2008). In data from the Multiple Risk Factor Intervention Trial (MRFIT) study, the 25-year age-adjusted death rate from cardiovascular disease (CVD) for those with diabetes without myocardial infarction (MI) at baseline was 144.2 per 20,000 person-years compared with 43.1 in those who had neither diabetes nor MI at baseline (Vaccaro et al. 2004). Because people die of the complications of diabetes rather than the disease itself, diabetes is underreported as the underlying or even contributing cause of death. Diabetes has been consistently listed on the death certificates of less than 40% of the decedents who actually have diabetes and only about 10% of the time as the underlying cause of death (McEwen et al. 2006). Death rates of middle-aged people with diabetes are twice that of people without diabetes (Geiss, Herman, and Smith 1995). A recent study examined the all-cause mortality rates based on diabetes status for participants in the National Health and Nutrition Examination Surveys (NHANES) I (1971–1980), NHANES II (1976–1992), and NHANES III (1998–2000) (Gregg et al. 2007). Across time, men with diabetes age-adjusted all-cause mortality rate declined from 42.6/1,000 to 24.4/1,000 while women with diabetes rose from 18.4/1,000 to 25.9/1,000.

Over the course of the disease, diabetes leads to a variety of disabling and life-threatening complications. Some of the major complications of diabetes include CVD (over 40% of all diabetes-related deaths) (Vaccaro et al. 2004; McEwen et al. 2007), blindness (12,000–24,000 new cases each year due to diabetes retinopathy) (CDC 2008), and kidney failure (47,000 new cases each year due to diabetes) (CDC 2008). Diabetes can also lead to inadequate circulation and sensation in peripheral tissues, which can result in infection, injury, and amputation (71,000 nontraumatic lower-limb amputations performed in 2002 due to diabetes) (CDC 2008). About 75% of adults with diabetes have high blood pressure (BP) and 60%–70% have mild to severe damage to the nervous system (neuropathy) (CDC 2008). Almost one-third of people with diabetes have periodontal disease, and in general, people with diabetes are more susceptible to severe complications during pregnancy, are vulnerable to life-threatening events such as diabetic ketoacidosis (DKA), and are more susceptible to other illnesses and will have a worse prognosis (CDC 2008). Approximately 30% of people with diabetes have symptoms of depression with 10% experiencing major depression (Anderson et al. 2001).

Largely because of these long-term complications, disability affects 20%–50% of the diabetic population. A much higher proportion of persons with diabetes than those without diabetes experience physical limitations (66% versus 29%); after adjusting for confounders, the odds ratio (OR) of physical limitation for adults with diabetes compared with those without diabetes is 1.9 (Ryerson et al. 2003). In data from the 1999 National Health Interview Survey (NHIS), the prevalence of functional disability for those with diabetes was 51%, and for those with diabetes and depression, 78%, compared with 24% in those not experiencing either diabetes or depression (Egede 2004).

The economic impact of diabetes is profound. The American Diabetes Association (ADA) estimated direct medical costs in 2007 at $116 billion and indirect costs at $58 billion, totaling approximately $174 billion (ADA 2008a). Over half (56%) of health care expenditures attributed to diabetes were incurred by people over 65. The per capita medical expenditures for people with diabetes were $11,744 compared with $2,935 for those without diabetes compared with what expected costs would be for the same population absent diabetes ($11,744 versus $5,095) (ADA 2008a). Adjusted for differences in age and sex, medical expenditures were approximately 2.3 times higher for those with diabetes. The number of prescription and nonprescription drugs recorded during physician office visits and outpatient department visits for patients who have diabetes has more than doubled between 1995–1996 and 2004–2005, while days of care in nonfederal short-stay hospitals has declined steadily from 1990 (NCHS 2007).

Up to half the economic burden of diabetes is due to long-term complications (Herman et al. 1997), especially coronary heart disease and end-stage renal disease (ESRD). Because of the aging and increasingly diverse U.S. population and continued rise in the overall level of obesity in all ages, the economic burden of diabetes on society will continue to rise rapidly, failing a strong public health effort to reduce the prevalence of obesity and physical inactivity in our population.

Pathophysiology

The etiology and pathophysiology of type 2 diabetes is complex. In general, people with type 2 diabetes have insulin resistance, which means they cannot make efficient use of insulin in the muscle or liver, despite sufficient insulin production early in the course of the disease. Obesity and hyperinsulinemia are characteristic of this early phase, and obesity accentuates the insulin resistance (Haffner et al. 1990). Over time, the pancreas fails to increase insulin secretion enough to compensate adequately for the insulin resistance and hyperglycemia begins. Type 2 diabetes is a progressive disease, and over time, the response to treatment varies (DeFronzo 1999). Specific genetic markers have been identified and offer promise of a better understanding of this disease (Chandalia et al. 2007).

The prevalence rate for gestational diabetes mellitus (GDM) has increased from 1.9% in 1989–1990 to 4.2% in 2003–2004 (Getahum et al. 2008). Although glucose tolerance typically reverts to normal after delivery, more than 60% of women with gestational diabetes will develop type 2 diabetes in future years. Gestational diabetes can result in significant adverse outcomes for the fetus, although these are largely preventable through appropriate screening and intervention (ADA 2003a).

Prediabetes includes two categories, impaired glucose tolerance (IGT) and impaired fasting glucose (IFG), and is associated with increased risk of cardiovascular events. About 40% of the population has prediabetes (CDC 2008), which progresses to overt diabetes and occurs at a rate of about 10% per year. Healthy lifestyle and pharmacological agents may delay progression by about 50%.

Diabetes complications may be classified as macrovascular or microvascular complications (Orchard, LaPorte, and Dorman 1992). Macrovascular complications include accelerated atherosclerosis resulting in MI, stroke, or peripheral vascular disease. Up to 65% of adults with diabetes will ultimately die of macrovascular events or their sequelae. Drivers of excess macrovascular complications in diabetes include high BP, high low-density lipoprotein (LDL) cholesterol, low high-density lipoprotein (HDL) cholesterol, increased fibrinogen levels, and plasminogen activator inhibitor levels, which increase the tendency of the blood to clot and a variety of other factors. Microvascular complications include disorders of the eye, kidney, and foot, which increase risk of blindness, renal failure, and amputation. The prevalence rates of macrovascular and microvascular complications are shown in Table 10.1.

Effective multifactorial therapy can substantially reduce complications of both type 1 and type 2 diabetes (Paterson et al. 2007; Cleary et al. 2006). In the aggregate, these data suggest that glucose, smoking cessation, aspirin use, BP control, and LDL control are important, and glucose control goals should be individualized for type 2 diabetes, including less intensive glycemic goals for patients with severe or frequent hypoglycemia (ADA 2008b). Recent clinical trials found that near-normal glycemic control achieved through pharmacological means over a 3.5- to five-year period reduced nonfatal cardiovascular events about 10%–15% but failed to reduce mortality (ADVANCE Collaborative Group 2008). Of particular concern in one of the studies is that more intensive glucose control was associated with increased risk of death (Dluhy and McMahon 2008; Action to Control Cardiovascular Risk in Diabetes Study Group 2008). A1c is a measure of a person's average blood glucose level over the past two to three months, shown as the percent of hemoglobin proteins attached to glucose. For someone without diabetes a typical level is about 5%, for those with diabetes the range is usually elevated (6.5% – 7.0% and higher). Although many patients fail to reach A1c, BP, or LDL goals, there has been impressive progress in diabetes care in the last 10 years, and the median A1c level nationally is now approaching 7%. With respect to the cost-effectiveness of diabetes treatment, a CDC analysis reported in 2002 indicated that the cost per quality-adjusted life year (QALY) of life saved by aggressive A1c control was $41,384 but increased with age at diagnosis and ranged from about $9,600 for 25- to 34-year-olds to $2.1 million for patients 85–94 years

Table 10.1. Prevalence With and Without Diabetes of Macrovascular and Microvascular Complications[a]

Complication	Normal Blood Sugar Levels (%)	Diagnosed Diabetes
Macrovascular		
Congestive heart failure	1.1	7.9
Chest pain	1.7	9.5
Heart attack	1.8	9.8
Coronary heart attack	6.1	27.8
Stroke	1.8	22.9
Microvascular		
Chronic kidney disease	6.1	27.8
Foot problems	10.0	22.9
Eye damage	N/A	18.9

[a]Adapted from State of Diabetes Complications in America (2007). Original data source: NHANES 1999–2004.

of age. By comparison, the cost-effectiveness ratio for intensive hypertension control was −$1,959 per QALY (i.e., cost-saving) and LDL control using statin is close to cost-saving if generic statin is used (CDC Diabetes Cost-Effectiveness Group 2002).

Descriptive Epidemiology

The U.S. National Diabetes Surveillance System (NDSS) relies primarily on national health survey data to monitor population and geographic disparities in diabetes, diabetes risk factors, and diabetes complications, as well as trends over time (CDCe). For the most part, these surveys do not distinguish between type 1 and type 2 diabetes and, with the exception of the NHANES, only capture persons with diagnosed diabetes. (In general for this section, unless specified, the term "diabetes" refers to a diagnosis of diabetes regardless of type.) Additional data sources, such as vital statistics and health care administrative data and population-based studies are also used to monitor the morbidity and mortality associated with diabetes, especially in special populations such as youth, women during pregnancy, older persons, and populations of color.

Type 2 diabetes accounts for 90%–95% of diabetes cases and is usually detected in older adults. Type 1 diabetes, however, is predominantly diagnosed in persons younger than 20 years (Soltesz, Patterson, and Dahlquist 2007). Internationally, the incidence of type 1 diabetes varies 60-fold (0.5–30.3 per 100,000) (Onkamo et al. 1999). From 1960 to 1996, the global annual increase in incidence was estimated at 3.0%. This sustained increase suggests an interaction between the environment and gene susceptibility (Gale 2002). Data on the prevalence and incidence of type 1 diabetes in the United States are limited. In 2001, the SEARCH for Diabetes in Youth Study found a diabetes prevalence of 0.79/1,000 in youth 0–9 years and 2.80/1,000 in those 10–19 years. Almost 91% of prevalent diabetes among non-Hispanic whites was type 1. This compares with 64% in African Americans, 74% in Hispanics, 58% in Asian/Pacific Islanders, and only 21% in American Indians. When restricted to children 0–9 years of age, 95% of cases were type 1 among non-Hispanic whites, African Americans, and Hispanics (SEARCH for Diabetes in Youth Study Group 2006). They were 87% for Asian/Pacific Islanders and 80% for American Indians. The same age, racial, and ethnic heterogeneity in diabetes type is observed for incident cases (Writing Group for the SEARCH for Diabetes in Youth Study Group 2007).

High-Risk Groups

Diabetes is not equally distributed in the population. Older Americans, racial/ethnic minorities, persons with lower socioeconomic status, and those with a family history of diabetes suffer disproportionately high rates of diabetes and its complications (Cowie et al. 2006; Engelgau et al. 2004; Valdez et al. 2007). Diabetes incidence and prevalence increase dramatically with age (Geiss et al. 2006; Cowie et al. 2006). In 2003, the age-adjusted incidence of self-reported diabetes was 2.5, 11.2, and 16.8 per 1,000 for persons 18–44, 45–64, and 65–79 years, respectively (Geiss et al. 2006). Similarly, in 1999–2002, diabetes prevalence (diagnosed and undiagnosed) was 2.4% in persons 20–39 years, 9.8% in persons 40–59 years, and 20.9% in persons 60 years and older. Diagnosed and undiagnosed diabetes both increase with age, with about 30% of cases being undiagnosed (Cowie et al. 2006). A slight decrease in the oldest age groups is likely due to selective mortality (CDCe; McBean et al. 2004; Selvin, Coresh, and Brancati 2006). Because of increasing prevalence with age, diabetes screening is recommended every three years in those 45 years and older (Ford et al. 2005). There is also growing concern that diabetes is rising in younger age groups (Mokdad et al. 2000; Acton et al. 2002; Koopman et al. 2005).

Several diabetes complications increase substantially with age (CDCe). CVD, ESRD, lower-extremity disease, eye disease, and disability are all highest among persons 65 years and older (CDCe; Selvin, Coresh, and Brancati 2006). For example, in 2003, the self-reported prevalence of any CVD in persons with diabetes was 27.8% in those 35–64 years, 48.0% in those 65–74 years, and 58.0% in those 75 years or older (CDCe). For diabetes-related ESRD, in 2005, the incidence per million population was 10.3, 106.5, 545.4, and 766.3 in persons 20–29, 40–49, 60–64, and 70–79 years old, respectively (U.S. Renal Data System 2007). In contrast, occurrences of DKA in 2003 were 39.7, 3.6, and 1.1 per 1,000 persons with diabetes 0–44, 45–64 years, and 65 years and older, respectively (CDCe).

The incidence and prevalence of diabetes tend to be higher in minority populations, with some of the highest rates observed in the Pima Indians (Geiss et al. 2006; Cowie et al. 2006; Schulz et al. 2006; Pavkov et al. 2007; Brancati et al. 2000; Burke et al. 1999). From 1991 to 2003, Pima Indians five years and older had a diabetes incidence of 25.3 per 1,000 patient-years and this is even higher in 25- to 64-year olds (Pavkov et al. 2007). In 2003, self-reported diabetes incidence in U.S. adults was 1.5 times greater among non-

Hispanic African Americans and Hispanics compared with non-Hispanic whites (9.1 and 9.9 versus 6.6 per 1,000 cases), yet all considerably lower than the Pima Indians (Geiss et al. 2006). Among the elderly in 2001, diabetes incidence per 1,000 persons was 52.3, 76.9, and 49.4 among African Americans, Hispanics, and Asians, respectively, and is significantly greater than the 34.3 per 1,000 found among whites (McBean et al. 2004).

Similar racial and ethnic disparities are seen with diabetes prevalence as for incidence. Again, diabetes prevalence is very high among the Pima Indians. In 1994, for adults 20 years and older, 34.2% of men and 40.8% of women had diabetes (Schulz et al. 2006). Throughout the United States, diagnosed diabetes among American Indian/Alaska Native persons 20 years and older are two to three times higher than among U.S. adults. In 2002, diabetes was 15.3% in American Indians and Alaska Natives compared with 7.3% in the U.S. population (Acton et al. 2003). However, these rates vary considerably by tribe (Acton et al. 2003). In 1999–2002, the diabetes prevalence in persons 20 years and older was almost two times higher in non-Hispanic African Americans and Mexican Americans (14.6% and 13.5%, respectively) compared with non-Hispanic whites (7.8%) (Cowie et al. 2006). Diabetes prevalence is consistently at least two times higher in Hispanics, African Americans, and American Indians compared with non-Hispanic whites (Burrow et al. 2004; Kurian and Cardarelli 2007; Liao et al. 2004). Diabetes prevalence in Asians 30 years and older is similar or slightly lower than whites (5.0% versus 6.9%); prevalence in Pacific Islanders is 13.8%. In the same study, diabetes prevalence was 12.0% in African Americans, 9.4% in Hispanics, and 11.8% in American Indians (McNeely and Boyko 2004). There is evidence that diabetes prevalence is growing quickly among Asians, especially in the elderly population. From 1993 to 2001, and in the 65 years and older Medicare population, diabetes prevalence increased 68% among Asians compared with a 36% increase among whites (McBean et al. 2004). Such strong increases may in part be due to the increased acculturation and environmental exposure to Western lifestyles such as seen with the Pima Indians (Schulz et al. 2006). Similar increases are likely to be occurring among many immigrant populations.

Lower socioeconomic status, as measured by income or education, is associated with increased risk of diabetes (Geiss et al. 2006; Robbins et al. 2001, 2005). Diabetes incidence in persons with less than a high school education was 9.8 per 1,000 in 2003 compared with 6.2 in persons with more than a high school education (Geiss et al. 2006). Similarly, diabetes prevalence increases as education and household income decrease (CDCa). Persons with lower SES may have elevated risk factors for diabetes and other chronic diseases (Brancati et al. 2000; Robbins et al. 2005), less access to care, higher levels of stress, and low levels of health literacy, all of which affect self-care and medical care (Berkman et al. 2004).

Having a family history of diabetes is a strong risk factor for diabetes. In a recent study, diabetes prevalence was 30% for persons with high familial risk, 14.8% for moderate risk, and 5.9% for average risk (Valdez et al. 2007). After adjustment, the odds of diabetes were 2.4 and 5.8 times greater for persons with moderate and high familial risk, respectively (Valdez et al. 2007). A review of diabetes family history studies found the risk of diabetes to be two to six times greater in persons with parents who had diabetes (Harrison et al. 2003). It is likely that the increased risk associated with a family history of diabetes is the combination of genetic predisposition and familial environmental influences.

Prediabetes is a strong risk factor for the future development of diabetes. It is defined as either IFG (glucose levels between 100 and 125 mg/dL) or IGT (glucose levels between

140 and 199 mg/dL) (ADA 2003a). Persons with isolated IGT or IFG have a 20%–30% risk of developing diabetes within five to seven years (Unwin et al. 2002). Individuals with IFG and IGT have a 5- to 7-year risk of about 40%. The Diabetes Prevention Program (DPP) found an annual diabetes incidence of 11% for persons with both IFG and IGT (Diabetes Prevention Program Research Group 2002). Persons with prediabetes are at increased risk of macrovascular and microvascular complications and death (ADA 2003a; Unwin et al. 2002; Barr et al. 2007; Williams et al. 2005). The prevalence of IGT and IFG increases with age. In 1988–1994, IGT was 20.7% among persons 60–74 years compared with 11.9% among persons 40–49 years (Harris et al. 1998). In 1999–2002, IFG was 37.9% in persons 60 years and older compared with 15.7% in persons 20–39 years (Cowie et al. 2006). Among U.S. adolescents 12–19 years, 7% had IFG (Williams et al. 2005). Men have higher rates of IFG compared with women (32.8% versus 19.5%). The components of prediabetes also vary by race/ethnicity. In 1988–1994 and among persons 40–74 years, the prevalence of IGT was 19.4% in Mexican Americans, 15.3% in non-Hispanic whites, and 13.1% in non-Hispanic African Americans (Harris et al. 1998). In 1999–2002, IFG was higher in non-Hispanic whites and Mexican Americans (26.1% and 31.6%, respectively) compared with non-Hispanic African Americans (17.7%). The explanation of differences by sex and race/ethnicity are unclear.

GDM mirrors type 2 diabetes in that the burden disproportionately impacts older women, minority women, obesity, and women with a family history of diabetes or previous gestational diabetes (Ferrara 2007; Dabelea et al. 2005; Thorpe et al. 2005; Devlin et al. 2008). GDM can cause complications during pregnancy, increase the mother's risk of developing type 2 diabetes, and may also increase the child's future risk of developing diabetes (Dabelea et al. 2005). Pregnancies complicated by GDM increase with age (Thorpe et al. 2005). Increases with age are observed across racial and ethnic populations (Gerstein 1994). Studies in New York City, California, Colorado, Montana, and Minnesota have all found GDM to be about two times higher in Hispanics, Asians, and American Indians (Thorpe et al. 2005). In general, GDM complicates 2%–5% of pregnancies and appears to be increasing over time, and women with GDM have a 17%–63% risk of developing diabetes within 5–16 years (Thorpe et al. 2005). Women with GDM are a high-risk population that can impact the future of diabetes in the United States. Increased efforts are needed to address this population before, during, and after pregnancy.

Geographic Distribution

There are clear geographic patterns for diabetes, its risk factors, and its complications. Diabetes prevalence is highest in the south and southeastern states (8% and higher) and lowest in the northern plains and mountain states (5%–5.9%) (Ford et al. 2005). These have been consistent differences from 1994 through 2005 and are likely driven by the underlying racial and ethnic makeup of the states and the state obesity rates (Ford et al. 2005). Geographic patterns in diabetes and obesity are similar. Regional differences in GDM likely mirror those observed for diabetes prevalence and diabetes risk factors (Ferrara 2007). No current data exist to examine state-level differences in prediabetes.

In the past, type 1 diabetes incidence appeared higher in northern, colder climates. However, this likely stems from early surveillance systems being established in northern countries such as Norway and Finland (Gale 2002). Over the past couple decades, type 1 diabetes has been examined in many diverse populations throughout the world, and incidence rates observed in Scandinavian countries are also being observed in countries such as Kuwait (Onkamo et al. 1999; Gale 2002). This suggests that susceptibility to type 1 diabetes may be similar across regions and racial and ethnic populations (Onkamo et al. 1999; Gale 2002).

Time Trends

Compared with other CVD risks of BP and blood cholesterol, only diabetes has continued to increase since the early 1960s (Gregg et al. 2005). Contributing to the growth of diabetes in the United States is that the population is aging, becoming more racially and ethnically diverse, and is getting heavier (Engelgau et al. 2004). Since 1958, the prevalence of diagnosed diabetes has risen from 0.9% to 5.6% in 2005 (CDCe; Engelgau et al. 2004). This is an increase from 1.6 to 16.2 million Americans yet remains an underestimate because another 30% are undiagnosed (Cowie et al. 2006). Similar trends are observed for total diabetes prevalence (diagnosed and undiagnosed). NHANES data from 1960–1962 through 1999–2000 show continuous increases in diabetes over the five measurement periods, particularly in diagnosed diabetes (Gregg et al. 2004; Cowie et al. 2006). Furthermore, the growth in diagnosed diabetes is in all age groups, men and women, all racial and ethnic groups, and across the United States (CDCe; Cowie et al. 2006). The substantial increase in obesity since the early 1980s is contributing to the diabetes epidemic (Ogden et al. 2004, 2006). The greatest changes in diagnosed diabetes are among Americans with a BMI greater than or equal to 35 kg/m^2 (Gregg et al. 2004). Increased survival and incidence of diabetes are also influencing diabetes prevalence (Geiss et al. 2006; Leibson et al. 1997).

National estimates and cohort studies indicate diabetes incidence is increasing in all demographic groups. From 1997 to 2003, the self-reported incidence of diabetes increased from 5.2 to 7.1 per 1,000 persons. Increases were seen by sex, race, ethnicity, BMI, education, and physical inactivity (Geiss et al. 2006). Among the elderly, incidence increased 37% from 1994 to 2001 (26.8–36.7 per 1,000) (McBean et al. 2004). Hispanic elderly had a 55% increase (McBean et al. 2004). The San Antonio Heart Study, the Framingham study, and the Rochester Epidemiological study all found increases in diabetes incidence over time (Burke et al. 1999; Fox et al. 2006). Among the Pima Indians, the already high incidence remained between 23 and 25 cases per 1,000 patient-years from 1965 to 2003 (Pavkov et al. 2007).

The incidence of type 1 diabetes is increasing in many regions of the world, including the United States (Onkamo et al. 1999; The DIAMOND Project Group 2006; Geiss et al. 2005). Pooled data from 37 populations have shown an increase of 3.0% per year (Onkamo et al. 1999). The increases have been observed in diverse populations ranging from Scandinavia to Kuwait to the United States (Onkamo et al. 1999; Gale 2002). In the United States, the Philadelphia and Allegheny Registries found stable incidence rates among youth through the mid-1980s, but then, an increase among the nonwhite populations, possibly due to misclassification of type 2 diabetes as type 1 diabetes. In Colorado, there was a 1.6-fold increase in type 1 diabetes incidence from 1978–1988 to 2002–2004 in Hispanics and non-Hispanic whites (The DIAMOND Project Group 2006). Although national trend data among youth are limited, the SEARCH study should improve our picture of type 1 and type 2 diabetes trends. IFG has not changed between 1988–1994 and 1999–2002, 24.7% compared with 26.0%, and recent data on IGT prevalence are not currently available (Cowie et al. 2006).

Although population-wide estimates are limited, increasing GDM in all populations is a public health concern (Ferrara 2007). In the United States, GDM and prepregnancy diabetes mellitus combined rose from 21.3 to 35.8 per 1,000 live births between 1990 and 2004 (Martin et al. 2006). In Colorado, GDM in a managed-care population doubled from 1994 to 2002, going from 2.1% to 4.1% (Dabelea et al. 2005). In New York City, GDM increased 46% (2.6%–3.8%) from 1990 to 2001, and in Minnesota, GDM increased from 25.6 to 34.8 per 1,000 live births from 1993 to 2003 (Thorpe et al. 2005; Devlin et al. 2008). Increases were seen by age, education, country of origin, and racial and ethnic groups. The largest increases were observed in Hispanics and Asians. Potentially accelerating these trends is the recurrence of GDM in from 30% to 84% of women, with the higher rates observed in minority populations (The DIAMOND Project Group 2006).

There is encouraging evidence that diabetes complications have been decreasing or at least leveling over the decade. Between 1997 and 2003, there have been no apparent changes in the age-adjusted CVD prevalence among persons 35 years and older (CDCe). Similarly, hospitalization for CVD, heart failure, and stroke have decreased or leveled off (CDCe; Geiss et al. 2005) (Table 10.2). Complications such as DKA, ESRD, and lower-extremity amputations all increased during the 1980s and into the 1990s but have since

Table 10.2. Age-Adjusted Hospital Discharge Rates for First-Listed Complications per 1,000 Population with Diabetes, United States, 1980 to 2003[a]

Complication	Hospital Discharge Rate (per 1,000)		
	1980	1995	2003
Ischemic heart disease	24.5 (46.2)[b]	36.0 (61.9)	21.5 (38.2)
Heart failure	7.1 (11.2)	19.5 (31.5)	18.5 (26.7)
Stroke	8.5 (13.8)	13.4 (21.5)	8.7 (12.8)
DKA	27.5 (11.1)	32.4 (11.6)	26.8 (8.3)
ESRD[c,d]	1.7 (1.2)	3.1 (3.6)	2.3 (3.2)
Peripheral arterial disease	3.6	7.4	3.3
Ulcer/inflammation/infection	5.4	7.7	6.9
Neuropathy	7.2	4.6	6.8
Lower-extremity amputation	4.4 (5.9)	7.6 (9.6)	4.4 (5.2)

[a]*Source:* National Diabetes Surveillance System. Diabetes Data and Trends. Available at http://www.cdc.gov/diabetes/statistics/index.htm.
[b]Crude rates are in parentheses when available.
[c]Years for ESRD are 1984, 1995, and 2002.
[d]Incidence of treatment for ESRD-DM.

begun leveling and are even decreasing across all sex and racial and ethnic populations (CDCe; Geiss et al. 2005). For the last decade, diabetes preventive care practices such as HbA1c tests, eye examinations, flu shots, and foot examinations, have been steadily improving among many populations, in a variety of care settings, and across the United States as a whole (CDCe; Landon et al. 2007; Mangione et al. 2006; Kerr et al. 2004; Saaddine et al. 2006). Improvements in risk factors such as BP, blood cholesterol, and HbA1c levels are mixed (Landon et al. 2007; Kerr et al. 2004; Imperatore et al. 2004; Saydah, Fradkin, and Cowie 2004a; Hoerger et al. 2008). However, since 1999, HbA1c levels have decreased (Hoerger et al. 2007). The efficacy of preventive care and risk factor reduction is well-established, yet there is still much room to improve, particularly ensuring persons with diabetes achieve all recommended care and risk factor levels (Narayan et al. 2000).

Despite improvements in diabetes care, diabetes incidence and prevalence continue to grow and, as a consequence, so will the overall human and economic burden (Chandalia et al. 2007; CDCe; Gilbertson et al. 2005). Considering the expected changes in population characteristics, estimates indicate that by 2050, 12.0% of Americans, or 48.3 million people, will have diagnosed diabetes (Narayan et al. 2006). Furthermore, for Americans born in 2000, 33% of men and 39% of women will develop diabetes during their lifetime (Narayan et al. 2003). This will be even greater for minorities and individuals who are obese (Narayan et al. 2003, 2007).

Causes

Modifiable Risk Factors

Type 1, Immune-Mediated Diabetes

Although few, if any, modifiable risk factors for type 1 diabetes have been clearly established, changes in incidence over time, geographic patterns, twin studies, and seasonality are all strongly indicative of major environmental determinants of type 1, immune-mediated diabetes (Orchard, LaPorte, and Dorman 1992; Krolewski et al. 1987). Genetic susceptibility to type 1 diabetes appears necessary but not sufficient to cause the disease (Dorman et al. 1995; Leslie and Elliott 1994). Nutrition and viruses may be important environmental triggers for those with genetic susceptibility. The most widely studied nutritional risk factors for type 1 diabetes are breast-feeding and exposure to cow's milk. A meta-analysis of selected studies found that patients with type 1 diabetes were 43% more likely to have been breast-fed for less than three months and 63% more likely to have consumed cow's milk before age three to four months (Gerstein 1994). Two recent studies suggest that the timing (less than 3 or greater than 7 months) of initial exposure to gluten or other cereal-driven proteins may place genetically vulnerable children at increased risk (Norris et al. 2003; Ziegler et al. 2003). Viruses that have been linked to development of type 1 diabetes include enteroviruses (especially the Coxsackie B4 virus), human cytomegalovirus, and the virus causing measles during pregnancy (Dorman et al. 1995). About 20% of people born with congenital rubella have diabetes later in life (Eisenbarth 1986). Other possible risk factors include stress, higher maternal or paternal age at birth (older than 35 years), birth order, birth weight, lower gestational age, childhood overnutrition, maternal autoimmunity, and negative stress events (Peng and Hagopian 2006; Baan, Bos, and van der Bruggen 2005).

Type 2 Diabetes

Conditions associated with increased insulin resistance are significant risk factors for type 2 diabetes (Table 10.3). The association between obesity and abnormal glucose tolerance is well recognized. Approximately 80% of people with type 2 diabetes are obese at the time of diagnosis (Orchard et al. 1992).

In a recent review of 29 studies that reported age-adjusted RR estimates for BMI on diabetes incidence, the RR estimates varied between 1.1 and 1.35 per unit of BMI (kg/m^2), with the effect being somewhat greater for men than women and decreasing for both with advancing age (Baan, Bos, and van der Bruggen 2005). The severely obese (BMI greater than or equal to 35) were at especially high risk.

Many studies have shown that the distribution of body fat, independent of obesity, is a risk factor for type 2 diabetes (Rewers and Hamman 1995). An increased central deposition of fat, often measured as an increased waist-to-hip ratio, appears to predict type 2 diabetes (Kaye et al. 1991). Duration or years of obesity is also a risk factor, as is a high-fat diet, even when adjusted for degree of obesity (Everhart et al. 1992).

In addition to obesity and physical activity, several dietary elements appear to either increase or decrease the risk for developing type 2 diabetes. Consumption of whole grains or cereal fiber (Schulze et al. 2007; Montonen et al. 2003), nuts and peanut butter (Jiang et al. 2002; Lovejoy 2005), magnesium (Schulze et al. 2007; Lopez-Ridaura et al. 2004), low-fat dairy products (Liu et al. 2006; Choi et al. 2005), coffee (unrelated to caffeine) (Pereira, Parker, and Folsom 2006; van Dam et al. 2006; van Dam and Hu 2005), and moderate consumption of alcohol (Howard, Arnsten, and Gourevitch 2004; Carlsson et al. 2005; Koppes et al. 2005) are all associated with reduced risk. The ratio of polyunsaturated to saturated fat has been associated with reduced risk in some studies (Harding et al. 2004). Consumption of red or processed meats (Song et al. 2004; Schulze et al. 2003; van Dam et al. 2002), heme iron from animal products (Rajpathak et al. 2006; Jiang et al. 2004), perhaps especially when consumed with alcohol (Lee, Folsom, and Jacobs 2004), and high-fat diets and saturated fat (Harding et al. 2004; Steyn et al. 2004) may increase risk.

The lack of physical activity is an independent risk factor for type 2 diabetes, distinct from diet and obesity (Helmrich et al. 1991; Manson et al. 1991a,b). Long-term prospective studies show a strong, linear relationship between frequency and intensity of exercise

Table 10.3. Modifiable Risk Factors for Type 2 Diabetes

Magnitude	Risk Factor
Strong (RR >4)	Obesity
Moderate (RR 2–4)	None
Weak (RR <2)	Physical inactivity Smoking High (saturated) fat/low fiber diet
Possible	Not breast-fed

and diminished risk of type 2 diabetes (Perry et al. 1995). Upon review of 13 publications that reported RR for physical activity, Baan, Bos, and van der Bruggen (2005) calculated weighted mean RRs for inactive versus active, adjusted for BMI, of 1.53 for men and 1.36 for women. In another review of ten prospective cohort studies of moderate-intensity physical activity (five studies focused on walking), the calculated summary RR for diabetes was 0.69 for active versus inactive (Jeon et al. 2007). In addition, women who regularly participated in vigorous physical activity before pregnancy had lower risk (RR 0.66) for gestational diabetes (Zhang et al. 2006). The prevalence of type 2 diabetes is consistently lower in populations where habitual physical activity is high (Rewers and Hamman 1995).

Smoking has been associated with increased risk for type 2 diabetes in several prospective studies (Rimm et al. 1993, 1995; Pettitt et al. 1997; Young et al. 2002; Nakanishi et al. 2000; Wannamethee, Shaper, and Perry 2001; Will et al. 2001; Lanting et al. 2005; Carlsson, Midthjell, and Grill 2004). In a recent Scandinavian study, smoking 20 or more cigarettes per day increased RR for type 2 diabetes (RR = 1.64) but appeared to reduce risk for type 1 diabetes (RR = 0.17) in adults (Carlsson, Midthjell, and Grill 2004).

In a study of a Pima Indian population, those who were exclusively breast-fed in the first two months of life had significantly lower rates of type 2 diabetes than those who were exclusively bottle-fed (OR = 0.41) (Carlsson, Midthjell, and Grill 2004). In a study of Native Canadians, breast-feeding for more than 12 months reduced risk of type 2 diabetes before 18 years of age to one-fifth of average risk (Young et al. 2002). In the recently published SEARCH for Diabetes in Youth Study, exposure to breast-feeding appeared to be protective against development of type 2 diabetes in African-American, Hispanic, and non-Hispanic white youth, with an OR adjusted for potential confounders of 0.43. When the BMI z score was added to the model, the OR was attenuated to 0.82. Longer duration of breast-feeding exposure appeared to provide greater protection, even accounting for current weight status (Mayer-Davis et al. 2008).

In data from the Nurses' Health Study (Hu et al. 2001), women with a BMI less than 25, a diet high in cereal fiber and polyunsaturated fat and low in *trans* fat and glycemic load, 30 minutes or more of moderate to vigorous physical activity a day, no current smoking, and average consumption of at least a half serving of alcohol per day had a RR of diabetes of 0.09, suggesting that the incidence of type 2 diabetes might nearly be eliminated in a culture or society where the adoption of healthy lifestyles was the norm.

Diabetes Complications

The prevalence of diabetes complications is quite high (*State of Diabetes Complications in America* 2007) (Table 10.1). Among people with diabetes, a variety of factors, such as smoking, obesity, and hypertension, interact to increase the risk of complications, including stroke and heart disease (Katon et al. 2004; Morse et al. 2006; Costa et al. 2004), as well as blindness, kidney damage, and lower-limb amputations. Working with their health care provider, patients with diabetes can reduce the risk for microvascular complications through improved glucose control (percentage point drop in A1c, e.g., 8.0% to 7.0%, decreases risk by 40%); BP control reduces risk of CVD by 33%–50% and microvascular complications by 33%; improved control of cholesterol or blood lipids reduces cardiovascular complications by 20% to 50%; and lowering BP can reduce the decline in kidney function when detected early by 30% to 70% (CDC 2008). Additionally,

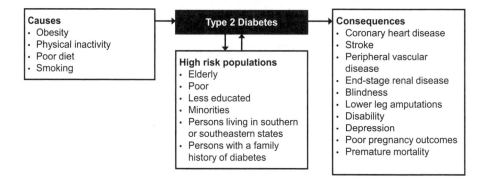

Figure 10.1. Type II diabetes: causes, consequences, and high-risk groups.

the higher risk for diabetes complications found in racial and ethnic minorities are accounted for by differences from the white, non-Hispanic population in such risk factors as smoking, socioeconomic status, income, education, and obesity (Lanting et al. 2005). The causes, consequences, and high-risk groups for type 2 diabetes are summarized in Figure 10.1

Population-Attributable Risk

Orchard, LaPorte, and Dorman (1992) have suggested that 70%–95% of type 1, immune-mediated diabetes may be attributed to environmental causes, including dietary practices and viral exposures. Between 20% and 90% of type 2 diabetes may be associated with obesity, although much of this may be attributable to abdominal adiposity (Kaye et al. 1991). In a nine-year follow-up of a national cohort of adults, the population-attributable risk for incidence of type 2 diabetes for weight increases of five kg or more was 27% (Ford, Williamson, and Liu 1997). In addition, approximately 24% of the incidence of type 2 diabetes may be attributable to a sedentary lifestyle (Manson et al. 1991a).

In data from the Framingham Heart Study, population-attributable risk associated with metabolic syndrome (including at least three of the following: abdominal adiposity, low HDL cholesterol, high triglycerides, hypertension, and IFG) for type 2 diabetes was 62% in men and 47% in women (Wilson et al. 2005). Population-attributable risk of gestational diabetes for development of diabetes in women is between 10% and 31% (Cheung and Byth 2003).

Prevention and Control

Prevention

Type 1 Diabetes

Attempts to prevent type 1 diabetes must first successfully identify those at risk for the disease. Large-scale studies have relied on the detection of islet cell autoantibodies in the relatives of individuals with type 1 diabetes, combined with subsequent assessment of insulin autoantibodies, first-phase insulin response to intravenous glucose, and oral glucose tolerance, excluding relatives with a known protective genetic allele (Will et al. 2001). Using such an approach in the Diabetes Prevention Trial (DPT)–Type 1 Study, investigators screening 100,000 relatives enrolled approximately 700 individuals with a reasonably high 5-year risk of developing type 1 diabetes (Tuomilehto et al. 2001). Only 10%–15% of the individuals with type 1 diabetes have a relative with the disease, but to identify the same size cohort from the general population would require screening one to two million people (Diabetes Prevention Program Research Group 2002).

Even with the DPT–1 Study's extraordinary effort to identify a large enough cohort of at-risk individuals, comparing outcomes for the two arms of the study (oral insulin and placebo) demonstrated no treatment benefit for the group taking oral insulin. A subgroup of the DPT–1 Study that had met a more stringent requirement for participation in the study (insulin autoantibody greater than 80 versus greater than 39 nU/ml) did appear to have had a successful outcome (i.e., potential delay in development of diabetes of four to five years). In another approach, the Trial to Reduce IDDM in the Genetically at Risk (TRIGR) Study Group is initiating a study to contrast the incidence of diabetes in infants weaned to an extensively hydrolyzed infant formula to infants weaned to conventional cow's milk-based formula (Ramachandran et al. 2006).

Lacking a relatively easy and economical means to identify those at risk for developing type 1 diabetes, combined with the lack of an established treatment or strategy that is both safe and effective for preventing type 1 diabetes, the translation of effective prevention strategies into clinical or community remains several years away.

Type 2 Diabetes

Unlike for type 1 diabetes, a clear path to the prevention or delayed onset of type 2 diabetes has been demonstrated in numerous large clinical trials published since 1997 (Diabetes Prevention Program Research Group 2002; Ramachandran et al. 2006; Tuomilehto et al. 2001; Chiasson et al. 2002; Buchanan et al. 2002; Pan et al. 1997; Gerstein et al. 2006; Torgerson et al. 2004). These studies clearly show that both lifestyle and pharmacological interventions prevent or delay the onset of type 2 diabetes in high-risk, prediabetic (IGT and/or IFG) populations. In these trials, the development of diabetes was reduced 25%–60% at follow-up, with the largest reductions accomplished most often through lifestyle interventions that supported weight loss and increased physical activity (Diabetes Prevention Program Research Group 2006).

In the Da Qing IGT and Diabetes Study in China, 110,000 people were screened for IGT and type 2 diabetes with 577 with IGT, then randomly assigned into four groups: control, diet only, exercise only, and diet plus exercise. At six-year follow-up, the diet, exercise, and diet-plus exercise intervention groups displayed 31%, 46%, and 42% reductions, respectively, in incidence of diabetes in comparison with the control (Pan et al. 1997). At 20-year follow-up, although intervention group subjects had 3.6 fewer years with diabetes and cumulative diabetes prevalence was 80% in intervention versus 93% in control subjects, there were no long-term differences between groups in first CV events, CV mortality, or all-cause mortality (Li et al. 2008).

The other most frequently cited, large prospective studies are the Finnish Diabetes Prevention Study (Tuomilehto et al. 2001) and the DPP (Diabetes Prevention Program Research Group 2002) conducted in the United States.

In the Finnish study, 522 overweight subjects with IGT were randomly assigned into a lifestyle intervention or control group. The treatment goal was to reduce weight by 5%, perform moderate-to-vigorous exercise at least 30 minutes a day, limit total and saturated fat, and increase consumption of fiber. The incidence of type 2 diabetes at follow-up was 11% in the intervention group and 23% in the control group, with the intervention group reducing their risk of diabetes by 58% after three years. The Finnish study recently reported extended median seven-year follow-up data conducted three years after the intervention was completed to assess the extent to which originally achieved lifestyle changes and risk reductions remained following discontinuation of active counseling (Lindsstrom et al. 2006). The absolute difference in diabetes risk between intervention and control remained at about 15%. Most who had maintained lifestyle goals at the conclusion of the intervention remained diabetes free at the extended follow-up.

The DPP in the United States randomly assigned 3,234 adults with IGT and a BMI greater than 24 kg/m^2 to placebo, metformin (850 mg twice daily), or a lifestyle modification program designed to achieve a 7% body weight loss and 150 minutes of physical activity per week (Diabetes Prevention Program Research Group 2002). The average follow-up was 2.8 years with respective incidence rates for diabetes in the placebo, metformin, and lifestyle groups of 11.0, 7.8, and 4.8 per 100 person-years. This represents a 58% and 31% risk reduction in the lifestyle and metformin groups compared with the placebo. The effect of the lifestyle intervention was associated with reduced risk for all age and racial/ethnic groups and in both sexes. The lifestyle intervention was especially effective in the older age group (60–85 years), while metformin was less effective than in younger adults (Diabetes Prevention Program Research Group 2006).

Large clinical drug trials have also been relatively efficacious in the prevention or delay of diabetes, although with the danger of side effects not present in lifestyle interventions (Diabetes Prevention Program Research Group 2002; Chiasson et al. 2002; Buchanan et al. 2002). The drugs used in pharmacological interventions, with the possible exception of generic metformin, are costly, have potentially dangerous side effects, are generally less effective than lifestyle interventions, and less likely than diet and physical activity to be of general benefit to the human body for diseases other than diabetes (Schulze and Hu 2005; Nathan et al. 2007).

A panel of experts was convened by the ADA in October 2006 for prediabetes (IFG and IGT). Based on their review of the evidence, a position statement was published (Tuomilehto and Wolf 1988) that recommends a program of lifestyle modification (i.e., 5%–10% weight loss and moderate-intensity physical activity of 30 minutes a day) for individuals with prediabetes. The use of metformin is recommended with or without lifestyle modification for those with IFG or IGT if they have any of the following characteristics: younger than 60 years old, BMI greater than or equal to 35 kg/m^2, family history of diabetes in first-degree relatives, elevated triglycerides, reduced HDL cholesterol, hypertension, or A1c greater than 6.0%. The panel felt that because of costs and potential side effects of other drugs, metformin was the only drug that should be considered for individuals with IFG/IGT.

Integrating two recently published statements from the ADA for nutrition (ADA 2007) and physical activity (Segal et al. 2006), it is recommended that lifestyle change programs to prevent type 2 diabetes include the following: moderate weight loss (7% of body weight), 150 minutes a week of moderate-to-vigorous physical activity, dietary strategies to reduce weight that includes reduced intake of fat and modest energy restriction, and consumption of 14 g fiber/1,000 kcal and foods containing whole grains (one-half of grain intake) daily.

Prevention of Type 2 Diabetes in Youth

Although multiple clinical trials have shown strong evidence that type 2 diabetes can be delayed or prevented by lifestyle modification or pharmacology in adults, there are no clinical trial data available on the prevention of type 2 diabetes in youth, largely because IGT and type 2 diabetes mellitus are much less common in children than in adults (Libman and Arslanian 2007).

Several investigations working in schools or with families have attempted to reduce or prevent the onset of obesity in high-risk youth, through physical activity and/or dietary interventions (Paradis et al. 2005; Carrell et al. 2005; Caballero et al. 2003; Teufel and Ritenbaugh 1998; Bishop et al. 2006; Trevino et al. 2004). The results of these studies have been mixed with most having little impact on obesity even when apparent lifestyle change was documented (Caballero et al. 2003; Campbell et al. 2004). In these studies, changes in glucose or insulin levels generally were not detected or were not measured (Libman and Arslanian 2007; Campbell et al. 2004).

Currently, the National Institute of Diabetes and Digestive and Kidney Diseases (NIDDK) and the ADA are sponsoring a collaborative research initiative called Studies to Treat or Prevent Pediatric Type 2 Diabetes (STOPP T2D) (USDHHS 2006). This collaboration, involving several major universities, launched the HEALTHY Study in the Fall of 2006 to determine if changes in school food services and physical education classes and other supportive activities in middle schools would lower risk factors for type 2 diabetes in youth. The intervention will last 2.5 years, with all students tested for diabetes risk factors (blood levels of glucose, insulin, and lipids) as well as measurement of fitness level, BP, height, weight, and waist circumference. Results of the HEALTHY Study are anticipated in 2009.

In practice, school-based interventions that target diabetes, cardiovascular, or obesity prevention have been quite similar in their general approach, putting strategies in place within the school environment designed to promote physical activity and healthy food choices. These interventions frequently target schools with student populations that are considered at high risk (i.e., American Indian, Latino, Asian, or African American student populations from predominantly low-income families and communities). Unfortunately, often intense academic expectations that society has placed upon the schools has limited the opportunity for school-based lifestyle interventions and greatly reduced the time devoted to physical education and activity during the school day, although there is no evidence that increased physical activity time in school diminishes academic achievement (Ahamed et al. 2007; Coe et al. 2006).

Secondary prevention of type 2 diabetes in youth necessarily includes the early detection of prediabetes followed by clinic- and family-based interventions that typically include nutrition education, physical activity, behavioral modification, and in some cases use of metformin (Goodman, Yoo, and Jack 2006). To date, family-based interventions have been limited in number, with small sample sizes, and conducted mostly with non-Hispanic ,white middle-class families rather than in populations where there is demonstrably greater need (Berry et al. 2004).

Barriers to Prevention

The approach taken in the large clinical trials (Tuomilehto et al. 2001; Chiasson et al. 2002; Pan et al. 1997) to prevent or delay diabetes onset were all resource-intense, conducted in clinical settings, and focused only on those at greatest risk of developing diabetes (Murphy, Chapel, and Clark 2004). The practicality and cost-effectiveness of a one-on-one approach such as that used in the DPP (Herman et al. 2003) is still an open question given the scope and complexity of both the diabetes and obesity epidemics, especially when it is those populations with the fewest resources and poorest access to care that most often have the greatest risk for developing diabetes.

Two recent studies on the cost-effectiveness of the DPP have come to different conclusions. Herman and colleagues (Herman et al. 2005) concluded that the lifestyle intervention, when implemented in routine clinical practice with impact projected across the life span, was cost-effective, but the metformin intervention was not cost-effective for those older than 65 years old. In contrast, Eddy, Schlessinger, and Kahn (2005) concluded that it was more cost-effective to delay intervention until onset of diabetes. The cost of the lifestyle intervention per QALY was estimated at $1,100 using a lifetime time horizon by Herman et al. (2005) and at $62,300 with a 30-year time horizon by Eddy, Schlessinger, and Kahn (2005). Eddy and colleagues emphasized the need for new methods to reduce cost of the lifestyle intervention to make it cost-effective.

One new approach with great potential is an adaptation of the DPP that shifts the core one-on-one curriculum to a group-based format offered in Indianapolis through the YMCA (Ackermann and Marrero 2007). Other changes for the YMCA adaptation included elimination of costly incentives, introduction of a formal exercise training partner system, and exercise components delivered by trained, local fitness club staff instead of specialized lifestyle coaches. The Group-Organized YMCA Diabetes Prevention Program (GO-YDPP) is currently being assessed through two National Institutes of Health (NIH) studies. Total cost in the first year was estimated at approximately $300 per participant compared with more than $1,400 for the original DPP (Herman et al. 2003; Ackermann and Marrero 2007).

In a recent review on the prevention of type 2 diabetes (Hussain et al. 2007), it was noted that roughly half of the risk for type 2 diabetes can be attributed to environmental exposure and that overweight is clearly the most critical risk factor and should be the primary target, especially in the young. The authors proposed, first, to target all people with IGT with increased physical activity and altered diet and, second, to introduce population-based measures that would encourage increased physical activity and decreased consumption of energy-dense foods in the community.

Upstream population-based measures, by definition, involve policy and environmental changes such as increased physical activity opportunities built into the school day and urban planning concepts such as "complete streets," which make possible and encourage alternative forms of transportation such as walking and biking. Although such upstream interventions have the greatest potential for ending the obesity and diabetes epidemics, rigorous scientific studies to demonstrate their worth are exceedingly difficult to conduct because the breadth, scale, and complexity of population-based interventions are not well-suited to assessment through the parameters of a clinical trial.

In summary, two basic approaches to primary prevention are appropriate, probably in combination. First, the upstream population approach seeks to alter or eliminate lifestyle and environmental characteristics that are known risk factors for diabetes from whole communities or populations. Strategies might include altering the food supply for whole populations and altering community attitudes and opportunities for exercise (Simmons et al. 1997). Second, the high-risk approach narrows the focus to particular individuals or groups with an especially high risk for developing diabetes (Zimmet 1988; Tuomilehto and Wolf 1988). A high-risk approach would target individuals with a family history of diabetes in combination with other metabolic and behavioral risk factors for the disease such as IGT.

Screening and Early Detection

Prediabetes

The benefits of primary prevention of diabetes are firmly established, because preventing or delaying the onset of diabetes appears to substantially reduce long-term complications of diabetes. Moreover, numerous randomized trials have shown effective strategies are available to prevent progression for prediabetic states to overt diabetes using lifestyle or pharmacological interventions. With a recent redefinition of prediabetes to include those whose blood glucose is 100–126 mg/dL, an estimated 57 million American adults are now classified as having prediabetes (CDC 2008).

Type 1 Diabetes

Population screening for type 1 diabetes is not recommended because of the infrequent occurrence of the disorder and the short time between the onset of hyperglycemia and the onset of symptoms in most patients (*Guide to Clinical Preventive Services* 2007).

Type 2 Diabetes

Mass, unselective population screening for type 2 diabetes is currently not recommended and is judged to not be cost-effective (U.S. Preventive Services Task Force 1996), even though the number of undiagnosed cases in the United States approaches six million (CDC 2008). Screening with a fasting plasma glucose test (no calorie consumption for eight hour before test) is recommended for defined high-risk groups such as Native Americans, Hispanics, African Americans, people with a strong family history of type 2 diabetes, women whose babies weighed more than nine pounds at birth, women with a morbid obstetric history, those with BMI greater than 30, or those with certain conditions including coronary heart disease, stroke, or transient ischemic attacks, peripheral vascular disease, hypertension, hypertriglyceridemia, or low HDL (ADA 2004). The sharp rise in the incidence of diabetes with increasing age has also lead the ADA to recommended screening every three years in all individuals 45 years and older (ADA 2004; Gilmer et al. 1997). It is important to recall that any patient presenting with symptoms suggestive of diabetes, such as polyuria, polydypsia, polyphagia, fatigue, blurry vision, or recurrent infections be evaluated for diabetes independent of screening criteria (O'Connor et al. 2006).

A fasting plasma glucose >126 mg/dL (7.0 mmol/L) confirmed on repeat testing a different day is considered diagnostic of diabetes. If an oral glucose tolerance test (OGTT) is used, the two hour glucose diagnostic level remains greater than 200 mg/dL (11.1 mmol/L). If the individual has consumed food or caloric beverages shortly before testing, a random plasma glucose test may be administered. A random plasma glucose greater than 200 mg/dL confirms the diagnosis in a patient with typical symptoms. A fasting plasma glucose level greater than 100 and less than 126 mg/dL indicates IFG and a two hour post glucose load plasma glucose between 140 and 200 mg/dL IGT (*Guide to Clinical Preventive Services* 2007).

Gestational Diabetes

Early diagnosis and aggressive treatment of GDM has been shown to reduce fetal morbidity and mortality. This has led to the recommendation that high-risk pregnant women be screened for gestational diabetes between the 24th and 28th weeks of pregnancy with a 50-g nonfasting one hour OGTT (Gregg et al. 2005). Women who are younger than 25 years old and of normal weight with no family history of diabetes and are not members of a high-risk ethnic group are excluded form screening due to low risk for gestational diabetes. When the screening test is positive (plasma glucose greater than or equal to 140 mg/dL at one hour), a three hour 100-g OGTT is subsequently administered. A diagnosis of gestational diabetes is confirmed when any two glucose values equal or exceed these limits: fasting, 105 mg/dL; one hour, 190 mg/dL; two hours, 165 mg/dL; three hours, 145 mg/dL (ADA 2003b).

Treatment, Rehabilitation, and Recovery

Diabetes mellitus is a chronic illness that requires lifelong care. Effective treatment is ideally provided by a health care team that includes a physician, a diabetes educator, a dietitian, and others. Yet, the majority of all diabetes care is necessarily self-care (Anderson 1991). Therefore, treatment should include not only initial evaluation, establishment of treatment goals, development of a management plan, cardiovascular risk factor reduction, and recognition of and care for complications, but also patient education in self-management and ongoing support. Standards of medical care as well as patient education criteria have been published by various entities (ADA 2008b; Funnell et al. 2007; Institute for Clinical Systems Improvement 2006; Pogach et al. 2004).

Type 1 Diabetes

The Diabetes Control and Complications Trial (DCCT), the longest prospective study for type 1 diabetes, showed that lowering blood glucose slows or prevents development of diabetes complications (ADA 2003c). The patient with type 1 diabetes requires exogenous insulin injections to survive; multiple daily, rapid- and long-acting insulin injections or use of an insulin infusion pump are often required. Diet is an essential factor in avoiding hyperglycemia and hypoglycemia (Galuk 1991). Nutritional and caloric intake must be synchronized with insulin action, with adjustments for varying levels of physical activity (ADA 2007). Current epidemiological evidence shows a substantial benefit from maintaining a physically active lifestyle and should be an important goal of treatment (Rachmeil, Buccino, and Daneman 2007; Guelfi, Jones, and Fournier 2007).

Type 2 Diabetes

The cornerstones of type 2 diabetes care are weight management, caloric restriction, and physical activity (Segal et al. 2006; ADA 2007; Institute for Clinical Systems Improvement 2006). However, 80%–90% of type 2 patients need pharmacotherapy to achieve recommended glucose. BP, LDL, cholesterol, nonuse of tobacco, and aspirin use goals may be as important or more important than glucose control in many adults with type 2 diabetes (Haire-Joshu, Glasgow, and Tibbs 1999; Ritz, Ogata, and Orth 2000; Eliasson

2003; Nobles-James, James, and Sowers 2004; Hansson et al. 1998; Harpaz et al. 1998; ADVANCE Collaborative Group 2008).

A wide range of pharmacological agents are available to help achieve glucose goals in type 2 diabetes (Karter et al. 2005, 2007). Initial treatment with metformin is often indicated. Metformin causes little hypoglycemia or weight gain, has favorable lipid effects, and has a proven safety record (Nathan et al. 2006). Metformin cannot be used in those with congestive heart failure or chronic kidney disease. Other agents including insulins, sulfonylureas, α-glucosidase inhibitors, thiazolidinediones, incretin agonists, DDP-4 inhibitors, or others may be added when indicated. Long-term safety of many of these medications has not been demonstrated. Thiazolidinediones, for example, increase congestive heart failure, fractures, eye problems, and rosiglitazone may increase rates of MIs (Nathan et al. 2008). The specifics of pharmacotherapy for diabetes are beyond the scope of this chapter but may be found in standard medial reference books or online (Grant et al. 2007).

Diabetes treatment requires the active involvement of the patients. Patient readiness to change is strongly predictive of improved diabetes care (Vallis et al. 2003; Jones et al. 2003; Nelson et al. 2007), and lower levels of health literacy are associated with poorer diabetes outcomes (Schillinger et al. 2002, 2006; Laramee, Morris, and Littenberg 2007). There is a body of well-conducted, positive research and descriptive literature on diabetes self-management (Haire-Joshu 1996; Clement 1995; Brown 1990; Anderson and Rubin 1996). Self-monitoring of blood glucose levels is useful in motivated insulin-treated patients and in patients prone to hypoglycemia without symptoms. In other patients, self-monitoring of blood glucose may be done less frequently but is useful as a feedback tool to patients and provides important information during acute illnesses (Burritt et al. 1991).

Continuing care is crucial in the management of diabetes, and frequent evaluation and adjustment in therapy may be required. Care can be effectively delivered through primary care, subspecialty care, or disease management models of care (Harris 1996; Wagner, Austin, and Von Korff et al. 1996; Wagner et al. 2001; Glasgow 2003). Essential components of diabetes management on a population basis include: identification of individuals or populations with diabetes, use of guidelines or performance standards to manage those identified, information systems to track and monitor interventions and patient- or population-based outcomes, and measurement and management of patient and population outcomes (Task Force on Community Preventive Services 2002).

As reviewed by the Task Force on Community Preventive Services, diabetes self-management education (DSME) teaches people to manage their own diabetes with the goal of optimizing metabolic control, prevention or early detection of acute and chronic complications, and optimizing quality of life at an acceptable cost both for the patient and the health care system (Task Force on Community Preventive Services 2002; Siminerio 2006; An Introduction to the Diabetes Initiative 2007; Fisher et al. 2007).

Examples of Public Health Interventions

The systems that impact diabetes in the United States are vast, especially if we consider the roles and responsibilities of government, communities, health care systems, insurers, employers, media, academia, foundations, persons with diabetes and their families, health professional organizations, and a myriad of other stakeholders. This broad perspective of public health has been well articulated in the Institute of Medicine's (IOM) *The Future of the Public's Health for the 21st Century* (IOM 2003). In this section, we will largely focus on diabetes within the governmental public health system. However, to be successful and to leverage limited resources, public-private partnerships are essential. Many of the government initiatives mentioned below are partnerships with the sectors discussed in *The Future of the Public's Health for the 21st Century*.

National Diabetes Prevention and Control Program

The Division of Diabetes Translation at the CDC supports an evolving and expanding National Diabetes Prevention and Control Program (NDPCP) with a mission to eliminate the preventable burden of diabetes through leadership, surveillance, research, programs, and policies that translate science into practice (Murphy et al. 2004; CDCf; Bowman et al. 2003). The NDPCP is guided by a multilevel ecologic framework constructed around the 10 Essential Public Health Services and a model of influence (Satterfield et al. 2004; CDCi; Safran, Mukhtar, and Murphy 2003). The framework is designed to stimulate and support broad-based partnerships to achieve population improvements.

A primary goal is to prevent diabetes and improve access to affordable, high-quality diabetes care and services recognizing (1) that moderate lifestyle modification (e.g., healthy eating, physical activity, and weight management), preventive care practices (e.g., influenza vaccinations, eye examinations, foot examinations, smoking cessation), and glucose, BP, and lipid control can delay or prevent diabetes and its complications; (2) many with prediabetes and diabetes are not achieving optimal care or are unaware they have the conditions; (3) the disproportionate burden for some racial, ethnic, and age groups; and (4) to reduce the impact of diabetes, efforts must focus on reshaping the health care system to deliver high-quality care and services, promote community programs to prevent diabetes and its complications, and create more formal linkages between health care systems and community programs (CDCf; Ockene et al. 2007).

The core NDPCP components are (1) defining the diabetes burden (public health surveillance), (2) conducting applied translational research, (3) strengthening state-based diabetes control programs, and (4) partnering on national diabetes efforts such as the National Diabetes Education Program (NDEP) (Narayan et al. 2000; CDCf; Association of State and Territorial Chronic Disease Directors 2005; NIH 2004). In 2007, the NDPCP received $63 million from Congress with almost $30 million distributed to 59 Diabetes Prevention and Control Programs (DPCPs) in all states, territories, and jurisdictions. Although some DPCPs receive additional state-level resources, most operate using the resources provided by the NDPCP.

Defining the Diabetes Burden

The Division of Diabetes Translation supports an NDSS that monitors the diabetes burden at the national and state levels (CDCb). The goals of the NDSS are to systematically collect, analyze, and interpret diabetes data; conduct studies to improve surveillance methods and better understand diabetes in specific populations or areas; and disseminate findings (Desai et al. 2003). To do this, multiple data sources are employed at the national and state level, including the NHANES, the NHIS, the National Hospital Discharge Survey, death certificates, and the Behavioral Risk Factor Surveillance System; hospital discharge data, U.S. Renal Data System, Medicare and Medicaid claims data, and managed care organization claims data (Desai et al. 2003; U.S. Renal Data System 2007; Hebert et al. 1999; McBean et al. 2004; Engelgau et al. 1998). Use of registries for surveillance is limited. New York City has recently created a citywide HbA1c registry (Steinbrook 2006). The various data sources have limitations including the validity and reliability of the data, the inability to distinguish between diabetes types, and monitoring mainly adults with diagnosed diabetes (Desai et al. 2003; Saydah et al. 2004b).

The NDSS is also involved in specific studies to improve diabetes surveillance. Examples include the Diabetes Primary Prevention Initiative (DPPI) for state-level diabetes prevention surveillance; the National Kidney Disease Initiative to monitor chronic kidney disease and its intermediate stages; the National Vision Health Initiative to track vision impairment and blindness; and the SEARCH for Diabetes in Youth Study to examine diabetes in youth (CDC 2006; Search for Diabetes in Youth 2007). Many other studies have been conducted or are underway to examine the burden of diabetes in managed care or in high-risk populations (CDC 2006; The TRIAD Study Group 2002).

As the NDSS expands, so does its reporting of the diabetes burden. The NDSS website provides information on diabetes morbidity and mortality, use of health care services, macrovascular and microvascular complications of diabetes, health status and disability, and other important diabetes indicators (CDCe). In addition, the NDSS communicates new findings through numerous publications and presentations and provides technical support such as the Diabetes Indicators and Data Sources Internet Tool (DIDIT), a web-based tool with in-depth descriptions of important diabetes indicators (CDCg; Mukhtar et al. 2005). Many states, territories, and jurisdictions also maintain diabetes surveillance websites with reports, publications, and fact sheets tailored to the needs of their state and local communities (CDCh).

Conducting Applied Translation Research

The goal of the NDPCP in conducting epidemiological and applied translational research is to accelerate the transfer of new scientific knowledge into clinical and public health practice. Translation research fills the niche between efficacy studies, such as randomized control trials, and the dissemination of these studies into the real-world environment or public health. The latter is concerned with sustainability, generalizability, and transferability to the majority of people and in diverse settings (Narayan et al. 2000). Significant contributions in this arena include the Translating of Research Into Action for Diabetes (TRIAD Study), the SEARCH for Diabetes in Youth Study, conducting systematic reviews for inclusion in *The Guide to Community Preventive Services*, and conducting numerous other studies examining the epidemiology and cost-effectiveness of diabetes and diabetes prevention interventions (The CDC Diabetes Cost-Effectiveness Group 2002; Mangione et al. 2006; Herman et al. 2005; SEARCH for Diabetes in Youth 2007; The TRIAD Study Group 2002; The Task Force on Community Preventive Services 2007; Ackermann et al. 2006; Hoerger et al. 2007; Zhang et al. 2003, 2005).

State-Based Diabetes Control Programs

The state DPCPs are an extension of the national program with the similar mission to eliminate the preventable burden of diabetes through providing leadership, conducting diabetes surveillance, developing novel approaches to address diabetes, and promoting and implementing evidenced-based programs (CDC 2003). In 2006, all 59 states, territories, and jurisdictions had DPCPs with CDC awards ranging from $58,000 to $1,200,000. The DPCPs are the link among national, state, and local efforts, often developing new approaches or tailoring existing programs to their local environments. Successful strategies are then fed back into the national program and to other DPCPs (Ottoson et al. 2007).

Most DPCPs facilitate and support statewide diabetes coalitions, councils, or committees. The coalitions are instrumental in statewide strategic planning to address diabetes at multiple levels (e.g., policy to patient care recommendations), in multiple settings (e.g., health care systems, work sites, schools), and in diverse populations (e.g., racial and ethnic groups, geographically defined groups, and age groups). DPCPs lead or support a wide array of diabetes programs, including surveillance. Many states host forums or conferences to educate health care providers about recommended diabetes care or strategies. DPCPs also partner with state professional chapters to support legislative efforts. As of December 2006, 46 states had laws requiring health insurance coverage include treatment for diabetes (CDCf).

DPCPs also participate in a variety of national projects. Since 1999, over 40 state DPCPs have participated in the Bureau for Primary Health Care's Health Disparities Collaborative (HDC), which is data-driven and uses the Chronic Care Model with Federally Qualified Health Centers to improve diabetes and prediabetes care (Landon et al. 2007; Health Disparities Collaborative 2007; Martin et al. 2007). The U.S.–Mexico Border Diabetes Prevention and Control Project began in 1999 and involves numerous academic, community, and public health partners in United States and Mexican border states, including the DPCPs of Arizona, California, New Mexico, and Texas (CDCf; Cohen and Ingram 2007; U.S.–Mexico Border Diabetes Prevention and Control Project 2007; Preventing Chronic Disease 2007). The goal of the Border project is to reduce the impact of diabetes among the predominantly Hispanic residents along the U.S.–Mexico border through a model of regional participation, shared leadership, and the development of acceptable and sustainable programs. In the wake of the DPP, in 2005, the NDPCP began the DPPI with California, Massachusetts, Michigan, Minnesota, and Washington. The purpose of the DPPI is to address diabetes prevention through enhanced strategic planning using systems thinking, surveillance, and promoting evidence-based programs through health care systems, work sites, community organizations, government programs, policy, and consumer awareness (CDC 2006). The DPPI Intervention focus area has compiled a tool kit of resources for public health professionals working with different constituents such as providers, policymakers, communities, insurers, and employers.

National Diabetes Partnerships and Programs

The NDPCP has several important national initiatives. The NDEP is a joint public education program of NIH and CDC (NDEP 2007). More than 200 organizations are partnering in developing and promoting resources, tools, and expertise to increase public awareness of the seriousness of diabetes and strategies for prevention of diabetes and its complications, promote healthy behaviors (diet and exercise), improve health care providers' diabetes knowledge, promote an integrated team approach to care, and promote health care policy that improves care quality and access. Current NDEP initiatives include *Control Your Diabetes for Life*; *Be Smart About Your Heart: Control the ABCs of Diabetes* and *Small Steps, Big Rewards, Prevent Type 2 Diabetes.* Target audiences include people with diabetes, health care providers, and employers. Additional communication activities are the Eagle's Books: Stories about Growing Strong and Preventing Diabetes, the Eagle's Nest website targeting school-age children, and the National Diabetes Translation Conference (DTC) for diabetes public health professionals to learn about the emerging science of diabetes and diabetes prevention and to learn from peers about the practical implementation programs.

The National Women's Health Initiative is a partnership with the ADA, the American Public Health Association, and the Association of State and Territorial Health Officials focusing on women's health and diabetes (CDCf). Other national initiatives include the National Vision Health Initiative, the National Kidney Disease Initiative, and the Native Diabetes Wellness Program (CDCf; CDC 2006).

Prevention Research Centers, Racial and Ethnic Approaches to Community Health, and Steps to a Healthier U.S.

The Prevention Research Centers (PRCs), the Racial and Ethnic Approaches to Community Health (REACH), and Steps to a Healthier U.S. are three CDC-sponsored initiatives that have a strong diabetes component. The 33 PRCs are an interdependent network of community, academic, and public health partners conducting prevention research and promoting the wide use of practices leading to good health (CDCj). They focus on community-based research, training, and the translation of research into practice. Currently, there are 40 REACH grantees throughout the United States, including 18 Centers of Excellence in the Elimination of Disparities and 22 Action Communities. The overarching goal for REACH is to eliminate racial and ethnic disparities in high-priority health areas including breast and cervical cancer, CVD, diabetes mellitus, hepatitis B, adult/older adult immunizations, tuberculosis, and infant mortality. Of the current grantees, 15 are addressing diabetes (CDCc). The REACH communities support community coalitions to develop, implement, and evaluate evidence-based community strategies for eliminating health disparities in diabetes and other diseases.

Steps to a Healthier U.S. is being implemented in 40 communities throughout the country with approximately $50 million (CDCd) working in partnership with their state and local health departments. The goal of Steps is to reduce the burden of obesity, diabetes, and asthma with an emphasis on addressing their common risk factors of physical inactivity, poor nutrition, and tobacco use. The ultimate goal is to slow the rising growth of overweight and obesity, reduce hospitalizations due to diabetes and asthma, and improve the health-related quality of life for community members (CDCi). All the objectives have a direct impact on persons with diabetes or at risk for diabetes.

Indian Health Service Division of Diabetes Treatment and Prevention

American Indians and Alaskan Natives are at dramatically increased risk for developing diabetes, exhibiting some of the highest and fastest growing diabetes rates in the United States. In 1979, the Indian Health Service (IHS) Diabetes Program was established. There are currently 19 model diabetes programs in the 12 IHS service areas supported by 12 area diabetes consultants; detailed diabetes, prediabetes, and metabolic clinical care guidelines; and strong clinical and community programs and assessment to track and improve diabetes awareness, care, and surveillance in the American Indian/Alaska Native population (IHS 2007).

In 1997, the Special Diabetes Program for Indians (SDPI) was implemented (IHS 2007). Funding began at $30 million per year and has steadily grown to $150 million per year since 2004. This influx of resources has allowed the SDPI to support tribes and tribal consortia, develop a community- and best practices–based approach to addressing diabetes, provide 399 noncompetitive and competitive diabetes program grants, and improve the diabetes data and evaluation infrastructure of the IHS. As a result, the SDPI has developed and implemented numerous innovative programs addressing primary, secondary, and tertiary prevention. Between 1997 and 2006, 67% of programs addressed primary prevention, 67% secondary prevention, and 32% tertiary prevention, with some focusing on multiple areas. The diabetes clinical infrastructure, nutrition education services, physical activity services, behavioral services, primary prevention and weight management programs for children, activities for obesity prevention, strategies for overweight children, and diabetes and prediabetes screening have all substantially increased (IHS 2007). Corresponding improvements in HbA1c levels and lipid levels are occurring (IHS 2007).

Diabetes Research and Training Centers

The Diabetes Research and Training Centers established by the NIH in 1977 develop and translate new behavioral and education programs for diabetes (The Diabetes Research and Training Center 2007). They conduct and support activities including health professional trainings, diabetes education programs, and community outreach. The Diabetes Research and Training Centers also provide tested evaluation and assessment instruments. Examples include Albert Einstein's multimodal weight control intervention involving an interactive computer system that can individually tailor the weight loss intervention, implementation of the Pathways Lifestyle Modification Program for African Americans by the University of Chicago, and the development of instructional materials and standardized instruments such as the Diabetes Care Profile by the University of Michigan.

Many other organizations also contribute greatly to the diabetes public health system. Professional organizations such as the ADA, the American Association of Diabetes Educators, the Society of Public Health Educators, the National Association of State and Territorial Chronic Disease Directors, and the National Association of City and County Health Officials collaborate on diabetes public health programs. Major health systems and insurers, such as the Center for Medicare and Medicaid Services, the Agency for Healthcare and Policy and Research, the Bureau of Primary Health Care, the Veterans Administration, and numerous community- and school-based organizations, are vital to supporting population-based approaches to improving diabetes care and reducing the diabetes burden throughout the United States.

Areas of Future Research and Demonstration

It is clear that in the face of the diabetes and obesity epidemics, primary prevention of diabetes through reduction in incidence and prevalence of obesity, increased levels of physical activity, healthier diet, and healthy body mass is a critical research priority, especially from the public health point of view. There is strong evidence that lifestyle interventions delay progression to diabetes in high-risk adults, but most high-risk subjects have not been exposed to these effective interventions (Tuomilehto et al. 2001; Diabetes Prevention Program Research Group 2006). Improving the knowledge base for customization of effective behavioral interventions to prevent diabetes, making a business case for the widespread dissemination of these strategies, and sustaining healthy lifestyle choices over long periods remain important research challenges.

For lifestyle interventions that prevent diabetes to be effectively adopted and widely disseminated, there are several research needs summarized by Samuel-Hodge et al. (Siminerio 2006) that must be addressed. Studies are needed to (1) determine the necessary intensity, frequency, and duration of physical activity; (2) better elucidate healthy/preventative dietary components and amounts; (3) investigate effectiveness of lifestyle interventions for obese adults with normal glucose tolerance or prediabetes; (4) examine potential effectiveness of lifestyle interventions that rely on "nonselective" community recruitment and conducted in diverse community settings (e.g., the YMCA adaptation of the DPP); (5) explore the role of physical activity independent of weight loss; (6) explore effectiveness of lifestyle weight loss interventions in combination with public health (physical and social environment) or pharmacological interventions; (7) determine effective lifestyle behavior change maintenance strategies; (8) investigate long-term outcomes of lifestyle interventions on diabetes complications; and (9) improve the quality of population-based lifestyle intervention study designs to include careful measurement of both processes and outcomes and the assessment of community and environmental indicators of risks and outcome (Siminerio 2006). Additional questions include: what is the most effective way to identify individuals at high risk for prediabetes, what changes in the health system and policy are needed to support and sustain lifestyle intervention, and what roles, responsibilities, and resources are most suitably placed in the hands of the physician, the health care system, or public health in a manner that will ensure effective collaboration (Wagner, Austin, and Von Korff et al. 1996; Wagner et al. 2001)?

Despite impressive improvement in diabetes care over the last decade, there is a persistent gap between recommended and actual levels of diabetes control. Factors that contribute to this gap in dissemination of effective interventions include lack of health insurance, low health literacy, patient noncompliance, failure of providers to intensify lifestyle or pharmacological therapy in a timely and persistent way until recommended goals of therapy are achieved, and inability to address external influences on outcomes within the patient's environment that are beyond the influence of the treatment setting. Future research is also needed on why women with diabetes appear to have even higher risk of stroke and other macrovascular events than men (Gregg et al. 2007; Chiasson et al. 2002). Evolving strategies for diabetes care that are promising include closed-loop insulin pumps, islet cell transplantation approaches, Roux-en-Y gastric bypass, which can now be done endoscopically using robotic equipment, and more effective use of electronic medical record systems to provide clinical decision support, customized patient interventions, and patient activation (Blonde and Parkin 2006; Wilke et al. 2007; Crosson et al. 2007).

As the science begins to determine effective prevention strategies for diabetes, models are also being developed to examine the cost utility of primary, secondary, and tertiary prevention based on QALYs (Herman et al. 2003; Eddy, Schlessinger, and Kahn 2005; CDC 2006; Vijgen et al. 2006). There are models that suggest cost-effectiveness of intensive therapy (i.e., the DCCT) (Herman et al. 2003; The Diabetes Control and Complications Trial Research Group 1996) is approximately $20,000 per QALY for type 1 diabetes and $16,000 for type 2 diabetes (Herman et al. 1997; Eastman et al. 1997), which is within the general range of intervention considered cost-effective in economic models. However, more detailed analyses of diabetes cost-effectiveness suggest that the cost of adding one QALY through intensive glucose control is approximately $41,000, dependent on age at diagnosis ranging from $9,614 for ages 25–34 years and $2.1 million for ages 85–94 years, whereas intensive efforts to control BP and lipids may actually provide cost savings to payers, especially with cheaper generic statins now available on the market (The CDC Diabetes Cost-Effectiveness Group 2002). These considerations underscore the importance of aggressive BP and LDL control in adults with type 2 diabetes.

There is also limited evidence suggesting the cost-effectiveness of behavioral interventions (i.e., diet plus exercise) for patients with type 2 diabetes (The Diabetes Control and Complications Trial Research Group 1996). A recent systematic review on studies on the cost-effectiveness of preventive interventions for type 2 diabetes found consistent evidence that strict BP control was more cost-effective than less strict control. Additionally, both primary and secondary prevention were highly cost-effective based on the limited number of studies available (Vijgen et al. 2006). Although there are good data from the DPP demonstrating the cost-effectiveness of lifestyle change (nutrition and physical activity) intervention for prediabetes, there remains a critical need for high-quality, clinical trial data targeting persons with diagnosed diabetes to provide information from which to model the cost utility of nutrition and physical activity interventions for that population (Dalziel and Segal 2007). Perhaps the strongest case can be made for primary prevention to lower incidence of type 2 diabetes through more physical activity, dietary change, combating obesity, and reducing rates of smoking.

There is a need for improved diabetes patient education models. Current information-based education models such as many sanctioned by the ADA are only marginally effective in improving glucose control. Models that use group approaches, problem-solving methods, and elicit powerful person stories appear promising (Task Force on Community Preventive Services 2002). However, much more research is needed to develop effective behavior change interventions that will lead to sustained adequate diabetes care in most patients.

Public health or population-based diabetes registries have been implemented in New York City and in many managed care plans or HMOs. In some of these clinical systems, there have been dramatic improvements in diabetes care since 1994. The use of electronic medical record system–derived registries that monitor not only A1c but also BP, LDL, and treatment patterns has revolutionized chronic disease surveillance and will likely lead to new approaches to diabetes management on a population basis in the near future.

Because of the increasing emphasis on primary care within the health care system; studies are needed that examine referral patterns between primary care and the diabetes specialty team to identify the essential "break points" where and when patients should move between them (Milstein et al. 2007; Codispoti et al. 2004). Team care models that include pharmacists and expanded role nurses and educators have shown promise as a way to improve care for diabetes and other chronic diseases. The cost-effectiveness of these models depends on a number of factors that are now being actively explored.

In the last two years, geneticists have successfully and consistently identified nearly a dozen genes that are associated with onset or progression of type 2 diabetes, obesity, and associated heart disease (Elbers et al. 2007; Frayling 2007). These and related research advances may soon make it possible to target screening and preventive strategies most effectively.

Factors related to the social and physical environment may influence onset and progression of type 2 diabetes (Deshpande et al. 2005). Obesity, sedentary behavior, and changing demographics of our society are driving a tidal wave of diabetes, and public health responses must address underlying issues in the social (stress, overwork, fragmented social systems) and physical (barriers to healthy eating and activity) environment. There is a great need for research on diabetes that is informed by the social and cultural context in which it occurs, including examination of family and friendship ties, community norms, the structure of community services, and health policy (Goodman, Yoo, and Jack 2006). Goodman and colleagues have reviewed community-based interventions for the primary prevention of diabetes and concluded that such prevention efforts need to focus more on the social, cultural, community, and environmental factors that contribute to health disparities than on behavioral modification strategies (Goodman, Yoo, and Jack 2006). Their recommended approach to a comprehensive community effort includes: (1) facilitating a meaningful and central role for the community, (2) giving primary attention to participatory processes before best practices, (3) emphasizing cultural relevance in intervention design sensitive to the cultural and racial or ethnic makeup of the community, and (4) incorporation of a social ecology approach that is holistic and addresses larger environmental influences and not individual behavior change alone. At the clinic level, their concerns are reflected in the Reach, Effectiveness, Adoption, Implementation, and Maintenance framework, proposed by Glasgow (2003) and emphasizes the importance of developing evidence-based interventions that balance effectiveness with generalizability (i.e., adoptability and effectiveness across many diverse settings).

Successful efforts to blunt the diabetes epidemic will require close collaboration among the medical, academic, and public health sectors of our society within a framework of strong government and community partnership. Upstream public policy interventions that involve government actions directed at entire populations or communities that alter tax structures, reimburse mechanisms for health promotion, and provide access to healthy dietary and physical activity opportunities within neighborhoods and communities are critical to any comprehensive strategy of diabetes treatment and prevention (Hussain et al. 2007; Cypress 2004; McKinlay and Marceau 2000). Such strategies are also among the most difficult to initiate and maintain for a period sufficient to adequately evaluate and justify the long-term commitment of public policy and resources necessary for change.

Resources

American Association of Diabetes Educators, 200 W. Madison, Suite 800, Chicago, IL 60606, tel.: (800) 338-3633; fax: (312) 424-2427; http://www.diabeteseducator.org

American Diabetes Association, ATTN: National Call Center, 1701 North Beauregard St., Alexandria, VA 22311, tel.: (800)-DIABETES (800-342-2383), http://www.diabetes.org

Diabetes Data and Trends, Centers for Disease Control and Prevention, National Diabetes Surveillance System, http://apps.nccd.cdc.gov/ddtstrs

Diabetes. Guide to Community Preventive Services website, Centers for Disease Control and Prevention, http://www.thecommunityguide.org/diabetes

Diabetes Prevention Program: Study Documents website, Diabetes Prevention Program Study Repository, DPP Coordinating Center, George Washington University Biostatistics Center, 6110 Executive Blvd., Suite 750, Rockville, MD 20852, http://www.bsc.gwu.edu/dpp/index.htmlvdoc

Diabetes Public Health Resource, National Center for Chronic Disease Prevention and Health Promotion, Centers for Disease Control and Prevention, 4770 Buford Highway NE, Mailstop K-10, Atlanta, GA 30341-3717, tel.: (770) 448-5000, fax: (770) 488-5966, CDC Diabetes Public Inquiries: 1-(800)-CDC-INFO, http://www.cdc.gov/diabetes

Juvenile Diabetes Research Foundation International, 120 Wall Street, 19th floor, New York, NY 10005-4001, tel.: (212) 479-7519, http://www.jdrf.org

National Diabetes Education Program, One Diabetes Way, Bethesda, MD 20814-9692, (301) 496-3583, e-mail: ndep@mail.nih.gov, http://www.ndep.nih.gov/index.htm

National Diabetes Information Clearinghouse, 1 Information Way, Bethesda, MD 20892-3560, tel.: 1-(800)-860-8747, fax: (703) 738-4929, e-mail: ndic@info.niddk.nih.gov, http://diabetes.niddk.nih.gov

Suggested Reading

Ackerman, R.T., and D.G. Marrero. Adapting the Diabetes Prevention Program Lifestyle Intervention for Delivery in the Community: The YMCA Model. *The Diabetes Educator* (2007):33:1:69. Available at http://tde.sagepub.com/cgi/content/abstract/33/1/69. Accessed September 5, 2008.

American Diabetes Association (ADA). Clinical Practice Recommendations 2008. *Diabetes Care* (2008):30(Suppl 1). Available at http://care.diabetesjournals.org/content/vol30/suppl_1/#top. Accessed September 5, 2008.

Centers for Disease Control and Prevention (CDC). *Take Charge of Your Diabetes* (3rd ed.) (2003). Atlanta, GA: U.S. Department of Health and Human Services. Available at http://www.cdc.gov/diabetes/pubs/tcyd. Accessed September 5, 2008.

Centers for Disease Control and Prevention (CDC). *Diabetes: Disabling Disease to Double by 2050: At-A-Glance 2007.* Available at http://www.cdc.gov/nccdphp/publications/aag/ddt.htm. Accessed September 5, 2008.

Centers for Disease Control and Prevention (CDC). *National Diabetes Fact Sheet.* General information and national estimates on diabetes in the United States (2007). Atlanta, GA: U.S. Department of Health and Human Services, Centers for Disease Control and Prevention. Available at http://www.cdc.gov/diabetes/pubs/factsheet07.htm. Accessed September 5, 2008.

Goodman, R.M., S. Yoo, and L.J. Jack. Applying Comprehensive Community-Based Approaches in Diabetes Prevention: Rationale, Principles, and Models. *J Public Health Management Practice* (2006):12(6):545–555.

Institute for Clinical Systems Improvement. *Management of Type 2 Diabetes Mellitus.* Released November 2006. Available at http://www.icsi.org/guidelines_and_more. Click on Other Health Care Conditions Guidelines. Accessed September 5, 2008.

Journal of Public Health Management and Practice, November 2003, Vol. 9 Supplement. Special issue featuring 12 articles from the Division of Diabetes Translation (DDT) at the Centers for Disease Control and Prevention on Public Health approaches to population-based diabetes prevention and control efforts.

SEARCH for Diabetes in Youth Fact Sheet. Available at http://www.cdc.gov/diabetes/pubs/pdf/search.pdf. Accessed September 5, 2008.

References

Ackermann, R.T., and D.G. Marrero. Adapting the Diabetes Prevention Program Lifestyle Intervention for Delivery in the Community: The YMCA Model. *Diabetes Educ* (2007):33(1):69, 74–75, 77–78.

Ackermann, R.T., D.G. Marrero, K.A. Hicks, et al. The Evaluation of Cost-Sharing to Finance a Diet and Physical Activity Intervention to Prevent Diabetes. *Diabetes Care* (2006):29:1237–1241.

Action to Control Cardiovascular Risk in Diabetes Study Group. Effects of Intensive Glucose Lowering in Type 2 Diabetes. *N Engl J Med* (2008):358(24):2545–2559.

Acton, K.J., N.R. Burrows, L.S. Geiss, and T. Thompson. Diabetes Prevalence among American Indians and Alaska Natives and the Overall Population—United States, 1994–2002. *MMWR* (2003):52:702–704.

Acton, K.J., N.R. Burrows, K. Moore, L. Querec, L.S. Geiss, and M.M. Engelgau. Trends in Diabetes Prevalence among American Indian and Alaska Native Children, Adolescents, and Young Adults. *Aust J Polit Hist* (2002):92(9):1485–1490.

ADVANCE Collaborative Group. Intensive Blood Glucose Control and Vascular Outcomes in Patients with Type 2 Diabetes. *N Engl J Med* (2008):358(24):2560–2572.

Ahamed, Y., H. Macdonald, K. Reed, P.J. Naylor, T. Liu-Ambrose, and H. McKay. School-Based Physical Activity Does Not Compromise Children's Academic Performance. *Med Sci Sports Exerc* (2007):39(2):371–376.

American Diabetes Association (ADA). Report of the Expert Committee on the Diagnosis and Classification of Diabetes Mellitus. *Diabetes Care* (2003a):26 (Suppl 1):S5–S20.

American Diabetes Association (ADA). Position Statement: Gestational Diabetes Mellitus. *Diabetes Care* (2003b):26(Suppl 1):S103–S105.

American Diabetes Association (ADA). Implications of the Diabetes Control and Complications Trial. *Diabetes Care* (2003c):26(Suppl 1):525–527.

American Diabetes Association (ADA). Position Statement: Screening for Type 2 Diabetes. *Diabetes Care* (2004):27(Suppl 1):S11–S14.

American Diabetes Association (ADA). Nutrition Recommendations and Interventions for Diabetes: A Position Statement of the American Diabetes Association. *Diabetes Care* (2007):30 (Suppl 1):S48–S65.

American Diabetes Association (ADA). Economic Costs of Diabetes in the U.S. in 2007. *Diabetes Care* (2008a):31(3):596–615.

American Diabetes Association (ADA). Position Statement: Standards of Medical Care in Diabetes—2008. *Diabetes Care* (2008b):31(Suppl 1):S12–S54.

An Introduction to the Diabetes Initiative and This Special Issue. *Diabetes Educ* (2007):33(Suppl 6): 123S–125S.

Anderson, B.J., and R.R. Rubin, editors. *Practical Psychology for Diabetes Clinicians: How to Deal with the Key Behavioral Issues Faced by Patients and Health Care Teams.* Alexandria, VA: American Diabetes Association (1996).

Anderson, R.J., K.E. Freedland, R.E. Clouse, and P.J. Lustman. The Prevalence of Comorbid Depression in Adults with Diabetes: A Meta-Analysis. *Diabetes Care* (2001):24:1069–1078.

Anderson, R.M. The Challenge of Translating Scientific Knowledge into Improved Diabetes Care in the 1990s. *Diabetes Care* (1991):14:418–421.

Association of State and Territorial Chronic Disease Directors. *The Primary Prevention of Diabetes: Recommendations from the Chronic Disease Directors' Project.* Atlanta, GA (2005).

Atkinson, M.A., and N.K. Maclaren. The Pathogenesis of Insulin-Dependent Diabetes. *N Engl J Med* (1994):331:1428–1436.

Baan, C., G. Bos, and M.A.M. van der Bruggen. *Modeling Chronic Diseases: The Diabetes Module: Justification of (New) Input Data.* RIVM Report 260801001/2005. Bilthoven, The Netherlands: Department for Prevention and Health Services Research (PZO) (2005).

Barr, E.L.M., P.Z. Zimmet, T.A. Welborn, et al. Risk of Cardiovascular and All-Cause Mortality in Individuals with Diabetes Mellitus, Impaired Fasting Glucose, and Impaired Glucose Tolerance. The Australian Diabetes, Obesity, and Lifestyle Study (AusDiab). *Circulation* published online June 18, 2007.

Berkman, N.D., D.A. DeWalt, M.P. Pignone, et al. *Literacy and Health Outcomes.* Evidence Report/Technology Assessment. Report No. 87. Rockville, MD: Agency for Healthcare Research and Quality (2004). Available at http://www.ncbi.nlm.nih.gov/books/bv.fcgi?rid=hstat1a. chapter.32213. Accessed September 24, 2007.

Berry, D., R. Sheehan, R. Heschel, K. Knafl, G. Melkus, and M. Grey. Family-Based Interventions for Childhood Obesity: A Review. *J Family Nurs* (2004):20:429–449.

Bishop, D.B., G.L. Taylor, R.A. Warren Mays, et al. American Indian Children Walking for Health: The Results of a Two-Year In-School Daily Walking Program. Presented at the CDC Diabetes and Obesity Conference, Denver, CO, May 2006.

Blonde, L., and C.G. Parkin. Internet Resources to Improve Health Care for Patients with Diabetes. *Endocr Pract* (2006):12(Suppl 1):131–137.

Bowman, B.A., E.W. Gregg, D.E. Williams, et al. Translating the Science of Primary, Secondary, and Tertiary Prevention to Inform the Public Health Response to Diabetes. *J Public Health Manage Pract* (2003):9:(Suppl 6):S8–S14.

Brancati, F.L., W.H. Kao, A.R. Folsom, R.L. Watson, and M. Szklo. Incident Type 2 Diabetes Mellitus in African American and White Adults: The Atherosclerosis Risk in Communities Study. *JAMA* (2000):283:2253–2259.

Brown, S.A. Studies of Educational Interventions and Outcomes in Diabetic Adults: A Meta-Analysis Revisited. *Patient Educ Couns* (1990):16:189–215.

Buchanan, T.A., A.H. Xiang, R.K. Peters, et al. Preservation of Pancreatic β-Cell Function and Prevention of Type 2 Diabetes by Pharmacological Treatment of Insulin Resistance in High-Risk Hispanic Women. *Diabetes* (2002):51:2796–2803.

Burke, J.P., K. Williams, S.P. Gaskill, et al. Rapid Rise in the Incidence of Type 2 Diabetes from 1987 to 1996: Results from the San Antonio Heart Study. *Arch Intern Med* (1999):159:1450–1456.

Burritt, M.F., E. Hanson, N.E. Munene, and B.R. Zimmerman. Portable Blood Glucose Meters: Teaching Patients How to Correctly Monitor Diabetes. *Postgrad Med* (1991):89:75–84.

Burrow, N.R., R. Valde, L.R. Geiss, M.M. Engelgau. Prevalence of Diabetes among Hispanics—Selected Areas, 1998–2002. *MMWR* (2004):53:941–944.

Caballero, B., T. Clay, S.M. Davis, et al. Pathways: A School-Based Randomized Controlled Trial for the Prevention of Obesity in American-Indian School Children. *Am J Clin Nutr* (2003):78:1030–1038.

Campbell, K., E. Waters, S. O'Meara, S. Kelly, and C. Summerbell. Interventions for Preventing Obesity in Children. *Cocharane Database Syst Rev* (2004):3.

Carlsson, S., N. Hammar, and V. Grill. Alcohol Consumption and Type 2 Diabetes Meta-Analysis of Epidemiological Studies Indicates a U-Shaped Relationship. (2005):48(6):1051–1054.

Carlsson, S., K. Midthjell, and V. Grill. Smoking is Associated with an Increased Risk of Type 2 Diabetes but a Decreased Risk of Autoimmune Diabetes in Adults: An 11-Year Follow-Up of Incidence of Diabetes in the Nord-Trondelag Study. *Diabetologia* (2004):47(11):1953–1956.

Carrell, A., A. Meinen, C. Garry, and R. Storandt. Effects of Nutrition Education and Exercise in Obese Children: The Ho-Chunk Youth Fitness Program. *Wisc Med J* (2005):104:(5):44–47.

CDC Diabetes Cost-Effectiveness Group. Cost-Effectiveness of Intensive Glycemic Control, Intensified Hypertension Control, and Serum Cholesterol Level Reduction for Type 2 Diabetes. *JAMA* (2002):287:2542–2551.

Centers for Disease Control and Prevention (CDC). Trends in the Prevalence and Incidence of Self-Reported Diabetes Mellitus—United States, 1980–1994. *MMWR* (1997):46:1027–1028.

Centers for Disease Control and Prevention (CDC). *Promising Practices in Chronic Disease Prevention and Control: A Public Health Framework for Action.* Atlanta, GA: U.S. Department of Health and Human Services (2003).

Centers for Disease Control and Prevention (CDC), Division of Diabetes Translation. *Diabetes Prevention and Control: Division of Diabetes Translation Program Review FY2006.*

Centers for Disease Control and Prevention (CDCa). *Behavioral Risk Factor Surveillance System (BRFSS)*. Available at http://www.cdc.gov/brfss. Accessed September 24, 2007.

Centers for Disease Control and Prevention (CDCb). *National Diabetes Surveillance System (NDSS)*. Available at http://www.cdc.gov/diabetes/statistics/index.htm. Accessed September 24, 2007.

Centers for Disease Control and Prevention (CDCc). *Racial and Ethnic Approaches to Community Health (REACH)*. Available at http://www.cdc.gov/reach. Accessed October 31, 2007.

Centers for Disease Control and Prevention (CDCd): *Steps to a Healthier U.S.* Available at: http://www.cdc.gov/steps. Accessed October 31, 2007.

Centers for Disease Control and Prevention (CDCe), Division of Diabetes Translation. *National Diabetes Surveillance System Data Reports*. Available at http://apps.nccd.cdc.gov/ddtstrs. Accessed October 31, 2007.

Centers for Disease Control and Prevention (CDCf), Division of Diabetes Translation. Available at http://www.cdc.gov/diabetes. Accessed October 31, 2007.

Centers for Disease Control and Prevention (CDCg), Division of Diabetes Translation. *Publications and Reports*. Available at http://www.cdc.gov/diabetes/pubs/index.htm. Accessed October 31, 2007.

Centers for Disease Control and Prevention (CDCh), Division of Diabetes Translation. *State Diabetes Prevention and Control Programs*. Available at http://www.cdc.gov/diabetes/states/index.htm. Accessed October 31, 2007.

Centers for Disease Control and Prevention (CDCi), Office of Public Health Practice. Available at http://www.cdc.gov/od/ocphp/nphpsp/EssentialPHServices.htm. Accessed October 31, 2007.

Centers for Disease Control and Prevention (CDCj), Prevention Research Centers. Available at http://www.cdc.gov/prc. Accessed October 31, 2007.

Centers for Disease Control and Prevention (CDC). *National Diabetes Fact Sheet: General Information and National Estimates on Diabetes in the United States, 2007*. Atlanta, GA: U.S. Department of Health and Human Services, Centers for Disease Control and Prevention (2008).

Chandalia, M., S.M. Grundy, B. Adams-Huet, and N. Abate. Ethnic Differences in the Frequency of ENPP1/PC1 121Q Genetic Variant in the Dallas Heart Study Cohort. *J Diabetes Complicat* (2007):21(3):143–148.

Cheung, N.W., and K. Byth. Population Health Significance of Gestational Diabetes. *Diabetes Care* (2003):26:2005–2009.

Chiasson, J.L., R.G. Josse, R. Gomis, M. Hanefetd, A. Karasik, and M. Laakso; The STOP-NIDDM Trial Research Group. Acarbose for Prevention of Type 2 Diabetes Mellitus: The STOP-NIDDM Randomized Trial. *Lancet* (2002):359:2072–2077.

Choi, H.K., W.C. Willett, M.J. Stampfer, E. Rimm, and F.B. Hu. Dairy Consumption and Risk of Type 2 Diabetes Mellitus in Men: A Prospective Study. *Arch Intern Med* (2005):165(9):997–1003.

Cleary, P.A., T.J. Orchard, S. Genuth, et al. DCCT/EDIC Research Group. The Effect of Intensive Glycemic Treatment on Coronary Artery Calcification in Type 1 Diabetic Participants of the Diabetes Control and Complications Trial/Epidemiology of Diabetes Interventions and Complications (DCCT/EDIC) Study. *Diabetes* (2006):55(12):3556–3565.

Clement, S. Diabetes Self-Management Education. *Diabetes Care* (1995):18:1204–1214.

Codispoti, C., M.R. Douglas, T. McCallister, and A. Zuniga. The Use of a Multidisciplinary Team Care Approach to Improve Glycemic Control and Quality of Life by the Prevention of Complications among Diabetic Patients. *J Okla State Med Assoc* (2004):97(5):201–204.

Coe, D.P., J.M. Pivarnik, C.J. Womack, M.J. Reeves, and R.M. Malina. Effect of Physical Education and Activity Levels on Academic Achievement in Children. *Med Sci Sports Exerc* (2006):38(8):151–159.

Cohen, S.J., and M. Ingram. Border Health Strategic Initiative: Overview and Introduction to a Community-Based Model for Diabetes Prevention and Control. *Prev Chronic Dis* (January, 2005) [serial online]. Available at http://www.cdc.gov/pcd/issue/2005/jan/04_0081.htm. Accessed October 2, 2007.

Costa, L.A., L.H. Canani, H.R. Lisboa, G.S. Tres, and J.L. Gross. Aggregation of Features of the Metabolic Syndrome is Associated with Increased Prevalence of Chronic Complications in Type 2 Diabetes. *Diabet Med* (2004):21(3):252–255.

Cowie, C.C., K.F. Rust, D.D. Byrd-Holt, et al. Prevalence of Diabetes and Impaired Fasting Glucose in Adults in the U.S. Population, National Health and Nutrition Examination Survey 1999–2002. *Diabetes Care* (2006):29:1263–1268.

Crosson, J.C., P.A. Ohman-Strickland, K.A. Hahn, et al. Electronic Medical Records and Diabetes Quality of Care: Results from a Sample of Family Medicine Practices. *Ann Fam Med* (2007):5(3):209–215.

Cypress, M. Looking Upstream. *Diabetes Spectr* (2004):17(4):249–253.

Dabelea, D., J.K. Snell-Bergeon, C.L. Hartsfield, et al. Increasing Prevalence of Gestational Diabetes Mellitus (GDM) Over Time and by Birth Cohort: Kaiser Permanente of Colorado GDM Screening Program. *Diabetes Care* (2005):28:579–584.

Dalziel, K., and L. Segal. Time to Give Nutrition Interventions a Higher Profile: Cost-Effectiveness of 10 Nutrition Interventions. *Health Promot Int* (2007):22(4):271–283.

DeFronzo, R.A. Pharmacologic Therapy for Type 2 Diabetes Mellitus. *Ann Intern Med* (1999): 131(4):281–303.

Desai, J., L. Geiss, Q. Mukhtar, et al. Public Health Surveillance of Diabetes in the United States. *J Public Health Manage Pract* (2003):Nov:(Suppl):S44-S51.

Deshpande, A.D., E.A. Baker, S.L. Lovegreen, and R.C. Brownson. Environmental Correlates of Physical Activity among Individuals with Diabetes in the Rural Midwest. *Diabetes Care* (2005):28(5):1012–1018.

Devlin, H.M., J. Desai, G.S. Holzmann, and D.T. Gilbertson. Trends and Disparities among Diabetes-Complicated Births in Minnesota, 1993–2003. *Aust J Polit Hist* (2008):98(1): 59–62.

Diabetes Control and Complications Trial Research Group. Lifetime Benefits and Costs of Intensive Therapy as Practiced in the Diabetes Control and Complications Trial. *JAMA* (1996):276:1409–1415.

Diabetes Prevention Program Research Group. Reduction in the Incidence of Type 2 Diabetes with Lifestyle Intervention or Metformin. *N Engl J Med* (2002):346:393–403.

Diabetes Prevention Program Research Group. The Influence of Age on the Effects of Lifestyle Modification and Metformin in Prevention of Diabetes. *J Gerontol Series A: Biol Sci and Med Sci* (2006):61:(40):1075–1081.

Diabetes Research and Training Center (DRTC) Program. Available at http://diabetes.niddk.nih. gov/dm/pubs/drtc/index.htm. Accessed October 31, 2007.

DIAMOND Project Group. Incidence and Trends of Childhood Type 1 Diabetes Worldwide 1990–1999. *Diabet Med* (2006):23:857–866.

Dluhy, R.G., and G.T. McMahon. Intensive Glycemic Control in the ACCORD and ADVANCE Trials. *N Engl J Med* (2008):358(24):2630–2633.

Dorman, J.S., B.J. McCarthy, L.A. O'Leary, and A.N. Koehler. Risk Factors for Insulin-Dependent Diabetes. In: Harris, M.I., C.C. Cowie, M.P. Stern, et al., editors, *Diabetes in America* (2nd ed.). Bethesda, MD: National Institutes of Health, National Institute of Diabetes and Digestive and Kidney Diseases (1995):165–177. NIH Publication 95-1468.

Eastman, R.C., M. Harris, S.A. Garfield, and J. Kotsanos. Model of Complications of NIDDM. II. Analysis of the Health Benefits and Cost-Effectiveness of Treating NIDDM with the Goal of Normoglycemia. *Diabetes Care* (1997):20(5):735–744.

Eddy, D.M., L. Schlessinger, and R. Kahn. Clinical Outcomes and Cost-Effectiveness of Strategies for Managing People at High Risk for Diabetes. *Ann Intern Med* (2005):143:251–264.

Egede, L.E. Diabetes, Major Depression, and Functional Disability among U.S. Adults. *Diabetes Care* (2004):27(2):421–428.

Eisenbarth, G.M. Type I Diabetes Mellitus. *N Engl J Med* (1986):314:1360–1368.

Elbers, C.C., N.C. Onland-Moret, L. Franke, et al. A Strategy to Search for Common Obesity and Type 2 Diabetes Genes. *Trends Endocrinol Metab* (2007):18(1):19–26.

Eliasson, B. Cigarette Smoking and Diabetes. *Prog Cardiovasc Dis* (2003):45(5):405–413.

Engelgau, M.M., L.S. Geiss, D.L. Manninen, et al. Use of Services by Diabetes Patients in Managed Care Organizations: Development of a Diabetes Surveillance System—CDC Diabetes in Managed Care Work Group. *Diabetes Care* (1998):21:2062–2068.

Engelgau, M.M., L.S. Geiss, J.B. Saadine, et al. The Evolving Diabetes Burden in the United States. *Ann Intern Med* (2004):140(11):945–951.

Everhart, J.E., D.J. Pertitt, P.H. Bennett, and W.C. Knowler. Duration of Obesity Increases the Incidence of NIDDM. *Diabetes* (1992):41:235–240.

Ferrara A. Increasing Prevalence of Gestational Diabetes Mellitus. *Diabetes Care* (2007):30(Suppl 2):S141–S146.

Fisher, E.B., C.A. Brownson, M.L. O'Toole, V.V. Anwuri, and G. Shetty. Perspectives on Self-Management from the Diabetes Initiative of the Robert Wood Johnson Foundation. *Diabetes Educ* (2007):33(6):216S–224S.

Ford, E.S., A.H. Mokdad, W.H. Giles, et al. Geographic Variation in the Prevalence of Obesity, Diabetes, and Obesity-Related Behaviors. *Obes Res* (2005):13:118–122.

Ford, E.S., D.F. Williamson, and S. Liu.Weight Change and Diabetes Incidence: Findings from a National Cohort of U.S. Adults. *Am J Epidemiol* (1997):14(3):214–222.

Fox, C.S., M.J. Pencina, J.B Meigs, et al. Trends in the Incidence of Type 2 Diabetes Mellitus from 1970s to the 1990s: The Framingham Heart Study. *Circulation* (2006):113:2914–2918.

Frayling, T.M. A New Ear in Finding Type 2 Diabetes Genes—The Usual Suspects. *Diabet Med* (2007):24(7):696–701.

Funnell, M.M., T.L. Brown, B.P. Childs, et al. National Standards for Diabetes Self-Management Education. *Diabetes Care* (2007):30(6):1630–1637.

Gale, E.A.M. The Rise of Childhood Type 1 Diabetes in the 20th Century. *Diabetes* (2002):51:3353–3361.

Galuk, D. Diabetes Mellitus Types I and II. *Adv Clin Care* (1991):March/April:5–7.

Geiss, L., M. Engelgau, L. Pogach, et al. A National Progress Report on Diabetes: Successes and Challenges. *Diabetes Technol Ther* (2005):7:198–203.

Geiss, L.S., W.H. Herman, and P.J. Smith. Mortality and Non-Insulin–Dependent Diabetes. In: Harris, M.I., C.C. Cowie, M.P. Stern, et al., editors, *Diabetes in America* (2nd ed.). Bethesda, MD: National Institutes of Health, National Institute of Diabetes and Digestive and Kidney Diseases (1995):233–257. NIH Publication 95-1468.

Geiss, L.S., L. Pan, B. Cadwell, E.W. Gregg, S.M. Benjamin, and M.M. Engelgan. Changes in Incidence of Diabetes in U.S. Adults, 1997–2003. *Am J Prev Med* (2006):30(5):371–377.

Gerstein, H.C. Cow's Milk Exposure and Type 1 Diabetes Mellitus: A Critical Overview of the Clinical Literature. *Diabetes Care* (1994):17:13–19.

Gerstein, H.C., S. Yusuf, J. Boxch, et al. DREAM (Diabetes Reduction Assessment with Ramipril and Rosiglitazone Medication) Trial Investigators: Effect of Rosiglitazone on the Frequency of Diabetes in Patients with Impaired Glucose Tolerance or Impaired Fasting Glucose: A Randomized Controlled Trial. *Lancet* (2006):368:1096–1105.

Getahun D., C. Nath, C.V. Ananth, et al. Gestational diabetes in the United States: temporal trends 1989 through 2004. *Am J Obstet Gynecol* (2008):198(5):525. e1–e5. Epub 2008 Feb 15.

Gilbertson, D.T., J. Liu, J.L. Xue, et al. Projecting the Number of Patients with End-Stage Renal Disease in the United States to the Year 2015. *J Am Soc Nephrol* (2005):16:3736–3741.

Gilmer, T.P., P.J. O'Connor, W.G. Manning, and W.A. Rush. The Cost to Health Plans of Poor Glycemic Control. *Diabetes Care* (1997):20(12):1847–1853.

Glasgow, R.E. Translating Research to Practice: Lessons Learned, Areas of Improvement, and Future Directions. *Diabetes Care* (2003):26(8):2451–2456.

Goodman, R.M., S.Yoo, and L.J. Jack. Applying Comprehensive Community-Based Approaches in Diabetes Prevention: Rationale, Principles, and Models. *J Public Health Manage Pract* (2006):12(6):545–555.

Grant, R.W., D.J. Wexler, A.J. Watson, et al. How Doctors Choose Medications to Treat Type 2 Diabetes: A National Survey of Specialists and Academic Generalists. *Diabetes Care* (2007):30:(6):1448–1453.

Gregg, E.W., B.L. Cadwell, Y.J. Cheng, et al. Trends in the Prevalence and Ratio of Diagnosed to Undiagnosed Diabetes According to Obesity Levels in the U.S. *Diabetes Care* (2004):27(12):2806–2810.

Gregg, E.W., Y.J. Cheng, B.L. Cadwell, et al. Secular Trends in Cardiovascular Disease Risk Factors According to Body Mass Index in U.S. Adults. *JAMA* (2005):293:1868–1874.

Gregg, E.W., Q. Gu, Y.J. Cheng, et al. Mortality Trends in Men and Women in Diabetes, 1971–2000. *Ann Intern Med* (2007):147(3):149–155.

Guelfi, K.J., T.W. Jones, and P.A. Fournier. New Insights into Managing the Risk of Hypoglycaemia Associated with Intermittent High-Intensity Exercise in Individuals with Type 1 Diabetes Mellitus: Implications for Existing Guidelines. *Sports Med* (2007):37(11):937–946.

Guide to Clinical Preventive Services, 2007. Recommendations of the U.S. Preventive Services Task Force. Rockville, MD: Agency for Healthcare Research and Quality (September 2007). AHRQ Publication 07-05100.

Haffner, S.M., M.P. Stern, H.P. Hazuda, B.D. Mitchell, and J.K. Patterson. Cardiovascular Risk Factors in Confirmed Prediabetic Individuals: Does the Clock for Coronary Heart Disease Start Ticking Before the Onset of Clinical Diabetes? *JAMA* (1990):263:2893–2898.

Haire-Joshu, D., editor. *Management of Diabetes Mellitus: Perspectives of Care across the Life Span* (2nd ed.). St. Louis, MO: Mosby (1996).

Haire-Joshu, D., R.E. Glasgow, and T.L. Tibbs. Smoking and Diabetes. *Diabetes Care* (1999):22(11):1887–1898.

Hansson, L., A. Zanchetti, S.G. Carruthers, et al. Effects of Intensive Blood-Pressure Lowering and Low-Dose Aspirin in Patients with Hypertension: Principal Results of the Hypertension Optimal Treatment (HOT) Randomized Trial. *Lancet* (1998):361:1755–1762.

Harding, A.H., N.E. Day, K.T. Khaw, et al. Dietary Fat and the Risk of Clinical Type 2 Diabetes. *Am J Epidemiol* (2004):159:73–82.

Harpaz, D., S. Gottlieb, E. Graff, et al. Effects of Aspirin Treatment on Survival in Non-Insulin–Dependent Diabetic Patients with Coronary Artery Disease. *Am J Med* (1998):105:494–499.

Harris, M.I. Undiagnosed NIDDM: Clinical and Public Health Issues. *Diabetes Care* (1993):16:642–652.

Harris, M.I. Medical Care for Patients with Diabetes: Epidemiologic Aspects. *Ann Intern Med* (1996):124(1 Pt 2):117–122.

Harris, M.I., R. Klein, C.C. Cowie, M. Rowland, and D. Byrd-Holt. Is the Risk of Diabetic Retinopathy Greater in Non-Hispanic Blacks and Mexican Americans than in Non-Hispanic Whites with Type 2 Diabetes? *Diabetes Care* (1998):21(8):1230–1235.

Harrison, T.A., L.A. Hindoff, H. Kim, et al. Family History of Diabetes as a Potential Public Health Tool. *Am J Prev Med* (2003):24(2):152–159.

Health Disparities Collaborative. Available at http://www.healthdisparities.net/hdc/html/home.aspx. Accessed October 31, 2007.

Hebert, P.L., L.S. Geiss, E.F. Tierney, et al. Identifying Persons with Diabetes Using Medicare Claims Data. *Am J Med Qual* (1999):14:(6):270–277.

Helmrich, S.P., D.R. Ragland, R.W. Leung, and R.S. Paffenbarger, Jr. Physical Activity and Reduced Occurence of Non-Insulin–Dependent Diabetes Mellitus. *N Engl J Med* (1991):325:147–152.

Herman, W.H., M. Brandle, P. Zhang, et al. Costs Associated with the Primary Prevention of Type 2 Diabetes Mellitus in the Diabetes Prevention Program. *Diabetes Care* (2003):26:36–47.

Herman, W.H., R.C. Eastman, T.J. Songer, and E.J. Dasbach. The Cost-Effectiveness of Intensive Therapy for Diabetes Mellitus. *Endocrinol Metab Clin North Am* (1997):26(3):679–695.

Herman, W.H., T.J. Hoerger, M. Brandle, et al., for the Diabetes Prevention Program Research Group. The Cost-Effectiveness of Lifestyle Modification or Metformin in Preventing Type 2 Diabetes in Adults with Impaired Glucose Tolerance. *Ann Intern Med* (2005):142:323–332.

Hoerger, T.J., K.A. Hicks, S.W. Sorensen, et al. The Cost-Effectiveness for Prediabetes among Overweight and Obese U.S. Adults. *Diabetes Care* (2007):30:2874–2879.

Hoerger, T.J., J.E. Segel, E.W. Gregg, and J.B. Saaddine. Is Glycemic Control Improving in U.S. Adults? *Diabetes Care* (2008):31(1):81–86.

Howard, A.A., J.H. Arnsten, and M.N. Gourevitch. Effect of Alcohol Consumption on Diabetes Mellitus: A Systematic Review. *Arch Intern Med* (2004):140:211–219.

Hu, F.B., J.E. Manson, M.J. Stampfer, et al. Diet, Lifestyle, and the Risk of Type 2 Diabetes Mellitus in Women. *N Engl J Med* (2001):345:790–797.

Hussain, A., B. Claussen, A. Ramachandran, and R. Williams. Prevention of Type 2 Diabetes: A Review. *Diabetes Res Clin Pract* (2007):76:317–326.

Imperatore, G., B.L. Cadwell, L. Geiss, et al. Thirty-Year Trends in Cardiovascular Risk Factor Levels among U.S. Adults with Diabetes: National Health and Nutrition Examination Surveys, 1971–2000. *Am J Epidemiol* (2004):160:531–539.

Indian Health Service (IHS). *Division of Diabetes Treatment and Prevention and the Special Diabetes Program for Indians (SDPI)*. Available at http://www.ihs.gov/medicalprograms/diabetes. Accessed October 31, 2007.

Institute for Clinical Systems Improvement. *Health Care Guideline: Management of Type 2 Diabetes Mellitus* (11th ed.). Bloomington, MN: Institute for Clinical Systems Improvement (November 2006). Available at www.icsi.org. Accessed on November 16, 2007.

Institute of Medicine (IOM). *The Future of the Public's Health in the 21st Century*. Washington, D.C.: National Academies Press (2003).

Jeon, C.Y., R.P. Loken, F.B. Hu, and R.M. van Dam. Physical Activity of Moderate Intensity and Risk of Type 2 Diabetes: A Systematic Review. *Diabetes Care* (2007):30(3):744–752.

Jiang, R., J. Ma, A. Ascherio, et al. Dietary Iron Intake and Blood Donations in Relation to Risk of Type 2 Diabetes in Men: A Prospective Cohort Study. *Am J Clin Nutr* (2004):79(1):70–75.

Jiang, R., J.E. Manson, M.J. Stampfer, et al. Nut and Peanut Butter Consumption and Risk of Type 2 Diabetes in Women. *JAMA* (2002):288:2554–2560.

Jones, H., L. Edwards, T.M. Vallis, et al. Diabetes Stages of Change (DiSC) Study. Changes in Diabetes Self-Care Behaviors Make a Difference in Glycemic Control: The Diabetes Stages of Change (DiSC) Study. *Diabetes Care* (2003):26(3):732–737.

Karter, A.J., H.H. Moffet, J. Liu, et al. Achieving Good Glycemic Control: Initiation of New Antihyperglycemic Therapies in Patients with Type 2 Diabetes from the Kaiser Permanente Northern California Diabetes Registry. *Am J Manag Care* (2005):11(4):262–270.

Karter, A.J., H.H. Moffet, J. Liu, et al. Glycemic Response to Newly Initiated Diabetes Therapies. *Am J Manag Care* (2007):13(11):598–606.

Katon, W.J., E.H.B. Lin, J. Russo, et al. Cardiac Risk Factors in Patients with Diabetes Mellitus and Major Depression. *J Gen Intern Med* (2004):19:1192–1199.

Kaye, S.A., A.R. Folsom, J.M. Sprafka, et al. Increased Incidence of Diabetes Mellitus in Relation to Abdominal Adiposity in Older Women. *J Clin Epidemiol* (1991):44:329–334.

Kenny, S.J., R.E. Aubert, and L.S. Geiss. Prevalence and Incidence of Non-Insulin–Dependent Diabetes. In: Harris, M.I., C.C. Cowie, M.P. Stern, et al., editors, *Diabetes in America* (2nd ed.). Bethesda, MD: National Institutes of Health, National Institute of Diabetes and Digestive and Kidney Diseases (1995):47–67. NIH Publication 95-1468.

Kerr, E.A., R.B. Gerzoff, S.L. Krein, et al. Diabetes Care Quality in the Veteran's Affairs Health Care System and Commercial Managed Care: The TRIAD Study. *Ann Intern Med* (2004):141:272–281.

Koopman, R.J., A.G. Mainous, V.A. Diaz, and M.E. Geesy. Change in Age at Diagnosis of Type 2 Diabetes Mellitus in the United States, 1988 to 2000. *Ann Fam Med* (2005):3(1):60–63.

Koppes, L.L., J.M. Dekker, H.F. Hendriks, et al. Moderate Alcohol Consumption Lowers the Risk of Type 2 Diabetes: A Meta-Analysis of Prospective Observational Studies. *Diabetes Care* (2005):23(3):719–725.

Krolewski, A.S., J.H. Warram, L.I. Rand, and C.R. Kahn. Epidemiologic Approach to the Etiology of Type I Diabetes Mellitus and Its Complications. *N Engl J Med* (1987):317:1390–1398.

Kurian, A.K., and K.M. Cardarelli. Racial and Ethnic Differences in Cardiovascular Disease Risk Factors: A Systematic Review. *Ethnic Dis* (2007):17:143–152.

Landon, B.E., L.S. Hicks, A.J. O'Malley, et al. Improving the Management of Chronic Disease at Community Health Centers. *N Engl J Med* (2007):356:921–934.

Lanting, L.C., I.M.A. Joung, J.P. Mackenbach, et al. Ethnic Differences in Mortality, End-Stage Complications, and Quality of Care among Diabetic Patients: A Review. *Diabetes Care* (2005):28(9):2280–2288.

Laramee, A.S., N. Morris, and B. Littenberg. Relationship of Literacy and Heart Failure in Adults with Diabetes. *BMC Health Serv Res* (2007):7:98.

Lee, D.H., A.R. Folsom, and D.R. Jacobs, Jr. Dietary Iron Intake and Type 2 Diabetes Incidence in Postmenopausal Women: The Iowa Women's Health Study. *Diabetologia* (2004):47(2): 185–194.

Leibson, C.L., P.C. O'Brien, E. Atkinson, et al. Relative Contributions of Incidence and Survival to Increasing Prevalence of Adult-Onset Diabetes Mellitus: A Population-Based Study. *Am J Epidemiol* (1997):146:12–22.

Leslie, D.G. and R.B. Elliott. Early Environmental Events as a Cause of IDDM: Evidence and Implications. *Diabetes* (1994):43:843–850.

Li, G., P. Shang, J. Wang, et al. The Long-Term Effect of Lifestyle Interventions to Prevent Diabetes in the China Da Qing Diabetes Prevention Study: A 20-Year Follow-Up Study. *Lancet* (2008):371(9626):1731–1733.

Liao, Y., P. Tucker, C.A. Okoro, et al. REACH 2010 Surveillance for Health Status in Minority Communities—United States, 2001–2002. *MMWR CDC Surveill Summ* (2004):53 (SS-6):1–35.

Libman, I.M., and S.A. Arslanian. Prevention and Treatment of Type 2 Diabetes in Youth. *Horm Res* (2007):67:22–34.

Lindsstrom, J., P. Llanne-Parikka, M. Peltonen, et al., on behalf of the Finnish Diabetes Prevention Study Group. Sustained Reduction in the Incidence of Type 2 Diabetes by Lifestyle Intervention: Follow-Up of the Finnish Diabetes Prevention Study. *Lancet* (2006):368: 1673–1679.

Liu, S., H.K. Choi, E. Ford, et al. A Prospective Study of Dairy Intake and the Risk of Type 2 Diabetes in Women. *Diabetes Care* (2006):29(7):1579–1584.

Lopez-Ridaura, R., W.C. Willett, E.B. Rimm, et al. Magnesium Intake and Risk of Type 2 Diabetes in Men and Women. *Diabetes Care* (2004):27(1)134–140.

Lovejoy, J.C. The Impact of Nuts in Diabetes and Diabetes Risk. *Curr Diab Rep* (2005):5: 379–384.

Mangione, C.M., R.B. Gerzoff, D.F. Williamson, et al. The Association between Quality of Care and the Intensity of Diabetes Disease Management Programs. *Ann Intern Med* (2006):145: 107–116.

Manson, J.E., D.M. Nathan, A.S. Krolewski, et al. A Prospective Study of Exercise and Incidence of Diabetes among U.S. Male Physicians. *JAMA* (1991a):268:63–67.

Manson, J.E., E.B. Rimm, M.J. Stampfer, et al. Physical Activity and Incidence of Non-Insulin–Dependent Diabetes in Women. *Lancet* (1991b):338:774–778.

Martin, J.A., B.E. Hamilton, P.D. Sutton, et al. Births: Final Data for 2004. *Natl Vital Stat Rep* (2006):55(1):1–104.

Martin, M., B. Larsen, L. Shea, et al. State Diabetes Prevention and Control Program Participation in the Health Disparities Collaborative: Evaluating the First 5 Years. *Prev Chronic Dis* [serial online January 2007]. Available at http://www.cdc.gov/pcd/issues/2007/jan/06_0027.htm. Accessed October 12, 2007.

Mayer-Davis, E.J., D. Dabelea, A.P. Lamichhane, et al. Breast-Feeding and Type 2 Diabetes in the Youth of Three Ethnic Groups: The Search for Diabetes in Youth Case-Control Study. *Diabetes Care* (2008):31:470–475.

McBean, A.M., S. Li, D.T. Gilbertson, and A.J. Collins. Differences in Diabetes Prevalence, Incidence, and Mortality among the Elderly of Four Racial/Ethnic Groups: Whites, Blacks, Hispanics, and Asians. *Diabetes Care* (2004):27:2317–2324.

McEwen, L.N., C. Kim, M. Haan, et al., and The TRIAD Study Group. Diabetes Reporting as a Cause of Death: Results from Translating Research into Action for Diabetes (TRIAD). *Diabetes Care* (2006):29(2):247–253.

McEwen, L.N., C. Kim, A.J. Karter, et al. Risk Factors for Mortality among Patients with Diabetes: The Translating Research into Action for Diabetes (TRIAD) Study. *Diabetes Care* (2007):30(7):1736–1741.

McKinlay, J., and L. Marceau. U.S. Public Health and the 21st Century: Diabetes Mellitus. *Lancet* (2000):356:757–761.

McNeely, M.J., and E.J. Boyko. Type 2 Diabetes Prevalence in Asian Americans. *Diabetes Care* (2004):27(1):66–69.

Milstein, B., A. Jones, J.B. Homer, et al. Charting Plausible Futures for Diabetes Prevalence in the United States: A Role for System Dynamics Simulation Modeling. *Prev Chron Dis* [serial online July 2007]. Available at http://www.cdc.gov/pcd/issues/2007/jul/06_0070.htm.

Minino, A.M., M.P. Heron, S.L. Murphy, and K.D. Kochanek. *Deaths: Final Data for 2004.* National Vital Statistics Reports; Vol. 55, No. 19. Hyattsville, MD: National Center for Health Statistics (2007).

Mokdad, A.H., E.S. Ford, B.A. Bowman, et al. Diabetes Trends in the U.S.: 1990–1998. *Diabetes Care* (2000):23(9):1278–1283.

Montonen, J., P. Knekt, R. Järvinen, et al. Whole-Grain and Fiber Intake and the Incidence of Type 2 Diabetes. *Am J Clin Nutr* (2003):77(3):622–629.

Morse, S.A., P.S. Ciechanowski, W.J. Katon, and I.B. Hirsch. Isn't This Just Bedtime Snacking? The Potential Adverse Effects of Night-Eating Symptoms on Treatment Adherence and Outcomes in Patients with Diabetes. *Diabetes Care* (2006):29(8)1800–1804.

Mukhtar, Q., E.R. Brody, P. Mehta, et al. An Innovative Approach to Enhancing the Surveillance Capacity of State-Based Diabetes Prevention and Control Programs: The Diabetes Indicators and Data Sources Internet Tool (DIDIT). *Prev Chronic Dis* [serial online July 2005]. Available at http://www.cdc.gov/pcd/issues/2005/jul/04_0126.htm or http://www.cdc.gov/diabetes/statistics/didit/index.htm. Accessed October 31, 2007.

Murphy, D., T. Chapel, and C. Clark. Moving Diabetes Care from Science to Practice: The Evolution of the National Diabetes Prevention and Control Program. *Ann Intern Med* (2004):140(11):978–984.

Nakanishi, N., K. Nakamura, Y. Matsuo, et al. Cigarette Smoking and Risk for Impaired Fasting Glucose and Type 2 Diabetes in Middle-Aged Japanese Men. *Ann Intern Med* (2000):133:183–191.

Narayan, K.M.V., J.P. Boyle, L.S. Geiss, et al. Impact of Recent Increase in Incidence on Future Diabetes Burden: U.S., 2005–2050. *Diabetes Care* (2006):29(9):2114–2116.

Narayan, K.M.V., J.P. Boyle, T.J. Thompson, et al. Lifetime Risk for Diabetes Mellitus in the United States. *JAMA* (2003):290(14):1884–1890.

Narayan, K.M.V., J.P. Boyle, T.J. Thompson, et al. Effect of BMI on Lifetime Risk for Diabetes in the U.S. *Diabetes Care* (2007):30(6):1562–1566.

Narayan, K.M.V., E.W. Gregg, M.M. Engelgau, et al. Translation Research for Chronic Disease: The Case of Diabetes. *Diabetes Care* (2000):23:1794–1798.

Nathan, D.M., J.B. Buse, M.B. Davidson, et al. Management of Hyperglycemia in Type 2 Diabetes: A Consensus Algorithm for the Initiation and Adjustment of Therapy: A Consensus Statement from the American Diabetes Association and the European Association for the Study of Diabetes. *Diabetes Care* (2006):29(8):1963–1972.

Nathan, D.M., J.B. Buse, M.B. Davidson, et al. Management of Hyperglycemia in Type 2 Diabetes: A Consensus Algorithm for the Initiation and Adjustment of Therapy: Update Regarding Thiazolidinediones: A Consensus Statement from the American Diabetes Association and the European Association for the Study of Diabetes. *Diabetes Care* (2008):31(1):173–175.

Nathan, D.M., M.B. Davidson, R.A. DeFronzo, et al. Impaired Fasting Glucose and Impaired Glucose Tolerance: Implications for Care. *Diabetes Care* (2007):30(3):753–759.

National Center for Health Statistics (NCHS). *Health, United States, 2007. With Chartbook on Trends in the Health of Americans.* Washington, D.C.: U.S. Government Printing Office (2007). Library of Congress No. 76-641496.

National Diabetes Education Program. Available at http://www.nih.ndep.gov. Accessed October 31, 2007.

National Institutes of Health (NIH). *From Clinical Trials to Community: The Science of Translating Diabetes and Obesity Research.* Bethesda, MD: National Institutes of Health (December 2004). NIH Publication 04-5540.

Nelson, K.M., L. McFarland, and G. Reiber. Factors Influencing Disease Self-Management among Veterans with Diabetes and Poor Glycemic Control. *J Gen Intern Med* (2007):22(4):442–447.

Nobles-James, C., E.A. James, and J.R. Sowers. Prevention of Cardiovascular Complications of Diabetes Mellitus by Aspirin. *Cardiovasc Drug Rev* (2004):22(3):215–226.

Norris, J., K. Barriga, G. Klingensmith, et al. Timing of Initial Cereal Exposure in Infancy and Risk of Islet Autoimmunity. *JAMA* (2003):290(13):1713–1719.

O'Connor, P.J., E. Gregg, W. Rush, et al. Diabetes: How Are We Diagnosing and Initially Managing It? *Ann Fam Med* (2006):4(1):15–22.

Ockene, J.K., E.A. Edgerton, S.M. Teutsch, et al. Integrating Evidence-Based Clinical and Community Strategies to Improve Health. *Am J Prev Med* (2007):32:244–252.

Ogden, C.L., M.D. Carroll, L.R. Curtin, et al. Prevalence of Overweight and Obesity in the United States, 1999–2004. *JAMA* (2006):295:1549–1555.

Ogden, C.L., C.D. Fryar, M.D. Carroll, and K.M. Flegal. Mean Body Weight, Height, and Body Mass Index, United States 1960–2002. *Adv Data* (2004):October 27(347):1–17.

Onkamo, P., S. Vaananen, M. Karvonen, and J. Tuomilehto. Worldwide Increase in Incidence of Type 1 Diabetes—The Analysis of the Data on Published Incidence Trends. *Diabetologia* (1999):42:1395–1403.

Orchard, T.J., R.E. LaPorte, and J.S. Dorman. Diabetes. In: Last, J.M., and R.B. Wallace, editors, *Maxcy-Rosenau-Last Textbook of Public Health and Preventive Medicine* (13th ed.). Norwalk, CT: Appelton and Lange (1992):873–883.

Ottoson, J., M. Rivera, A. DeGroff, et al. On the Road to the National Objectives: A Case Study of Diabetes Prevention and Control Programs. *J Public Health Managet Pract* (2007):13:287–295.

Pan, X.R., G.W. Li , Y.H. Hu, et al. Effects of Diet and Exercise in Preventing NIDDM in People with Impaired Glucose Tolerance: The Da Qing IGT and Diabetes Study. *Diabetes Care* (1997):20(4):537–544.

Paradis, G., L. Levesque, A.C. Macaulay, et al. Impact of a Diabetes Prevention Program on Body Size, Physical Activity, and Diet among Kanien'keha:ka (Mohawk) Children Age 6–11 Years Old: Eight-Year Results from the Kahnawake Schools Diabetes Prevention Project. *Pediatrics* (2005):115:333–339.

Paterson, A.D., B.N. Rutledge, P.A. Cleary, et al. Diabetes Control and Complications Trial/Epidemiology of Diabetes Interventions and Complications Research Group. The Effect of Intensive Diabetes Treatment on Resting Heart Rate in Type 1 Diabetes: The Diabetes Control and Complications Trial/Epidemiology of Diabetes Interventions and Complications Study. *Diabetes Care* (2007):30(8):2107–2112.

Pavkov, M.E., R.L. Hanson, W.C. Knowler, et al. Changing Patterns of Type 2 Diabetes Incidence among Pima Indians. *Diabetes Care* (2007):30(7):1758–1763.

Peng, H., and W. Hagopian. Environmental Factors in the Development of Type 1 Diabetes. *Rev Endocr Metab Disord* (2006):7(3):149–162.

Pereira, M.A., E.D. Parker, and A.R. Folsom. Coffee Consumption and Risk of Type 2 Diabetes Mellitus: An 11-Year Prospective Study of 28,812 Postmenopausal Women. *Arch Intern Med* (2006):166(12):1311–1316.

Perry, I.J., S.G. Wannamethee, M.K. Walker, et al. Prospective Study of Risk Factors for Development of Non-Insulin Dependent Diabetes in Middle-Aged British Men. *BMJ* (1995):310: 560–564.

Pettitt, D.J., P.H. Bennett, W.C. Knowler, et al. Breastfeeding and Incidence of Non-Insulin–Dependent Diabetes Mellitus in Pima Indians. *Lancet* (1997):350(9072):166–168.

Pogach, L.M., S.A. Brietzke, C.L. Cowan, Jr., et al. VA/DoD Diabetes Guidelines Development Group. Development of Evidence-Based Clinical Practice Guidelines for Diabetes: The Department of Veterans Affairs/Department of Defense Guidelines Initiative. *Diabetes Care* (2004):27(Suppl 2):B82–B89.

Preventing Chronic Disease. Special Focus on the Border Health Strategic Initiative (*Border Health ¡SI!*). Available at http://www.cdc.gov/pcd/issues/2005/jan/toc.htm. Accessed October 31, 2007.

Rachmeil, M., J. Buccino, and D. Daneman. Exercise and Type 1 Diabetes Mellitus in Youth: Review and Recommendations. *Pediatr Endocrinol Rev* (2007):5(2):656–665.

Rajpathak, S., J. Ma, J. Manson, et al. Iron Intake and the Risk of Type 2 Diabetes in Women: A Prospective Cohort Study. *Diabetes Care* (2006):29(6):1370–1376.

Ramachandran, A., C. Snehalatha, S. Mary, et al. Indian Diabetes Prevention Programme (IDPP): The Indian Diabetes Prevention Programme Shows That Lifestyle Modification and Metformin Prevent Type 2 Diabetes in Asian Indian Subjects with Impaired Glucose Tolerance (IDPP-1). *Diabetologia* (2006):49(2):289–297.

Rewers, M., and R.F. Hamman. Risk Factors for Non-Insulin–Dependent Diabetes. In: Harris, M.I., C.C. Cowie, M.P. Stern, et al., editors, *Diabetes in America* (2nd ed.). Bethesda, MD: National Institutes of Health, National Institute of Diabetes and Digestive and Kidney Diseases (1995):179–220. NIH Publication 95-1468.

Rimm, E.B., J. Chan, M.J. Stampfer, et al. Prospective Study of Cigarette Smoking, Alcohol Use, and the Risk of Diabetes in Men. *BMJ* (1995):310(6979):555–559.

Rimm, E.B., J.E. Manson, M.J. Stampfer, et al. Cigarette Smoking and the Risk of Diabetes in Women. *Aust J Polit Hist* (1993):83:211–214.

Ritz, E., H. Ogata, and S.R. Orth. Smoking: A Factor Promoting Onset and Progression of Diabetic Nephropathy. *Diabetes Metab* (2000):(26 Suppl 4):54–63.

Robbins, J.M., V. Vaccarino, H. Zhang, and S.V. Kasl. Socioeconomic Status and Type 2 Diabetes in African American and Non-Hispanic White Women and Men: Evidence from the Third National Health and Nutrition Examination Survey. *Aust J Polit Hist* (2001):91:76–83.

Robbins, J.M., V. Vaccarino, H. Zhang, and S.V. Kasl. Socioeconomic Status and Diagnosed Diabetes Incidence. *Diabetes Res Clin Pract* (2005):68:230–236.

Ryerson, B., E.F. Tierney, T.J. Thompson, et al. Excess Physical Limitations among Adults with Diabetes in the U.S. Population, 1997–1999. *Diabetes Care* (2003):26(1):2006–2010.

Saaddine, J.B., B. Cadwell, E.W. Gregg, et al. Improvements in Diabetes Processes of Care and Intermediate Outcomes: United States, 1988–2002. *Ann Intern Med* (2006):144:465–474.

Safran, M.A., Q. Mukhtar, and D.L. Murphy. Implementing Program Evaluation and Accountability for Population Health: Progress of a National Diabetes Control Effort. *J Public Health Manag Pract* (2003):9:58–65.

Satterfield, D.W., D. Murphy, J.D. Essien, et al. Using the Essential Public Health Services as Strategic Leverage to Strengthen the Public Response to Diabetes. *Public Health Rep* (2004):119: 311–321.

Saydah, S.H., J. Fradkin, and C.C. Cowie. Poor Control of Risk Factors for Vascular Disease among Persons with Previously Diagnosed Diabetes. *JAMA* (2004a):291:335–342.

Saydah, S.H., L.S. Geiss, E. Tierney, et al. Review of the Performance of Methods to Identify Diabetes Cases among Vital Statistics, Administrative, and Survey Data. *Ann Epidemiol* (2004b):14:507–516.

Schillinger, D., L.R. Barton, A.J. Karter, et al. Does Literacy Mediate the Relationship between Education and Health Outcomes? A Study of a Low-Income Population with Diabetes. *Public Health Rep* (2006):121(3):245–254.

Schillinger, D., K. Grumbach, J. Piette, et al. Association of Health Literacy with Diabetes Outcomes. *JAMA* (2002):288(4):475–482.

Schulz, L.O., P.H. Bennett, E. Ravussin, et al. Effects of Traditional and Western Environments on Prevalence of Type 2 Diabetes in Pima Indians in Mexico and the U.S. *Diabetes Care* (2006):29(8):1866–1871.

Schulze, M.B., and F.B. Hu. Primary Prevention of Diabetes: What Can Be Done and How Much Can be Prevented? *Annu Rev Public Health* (2005):26:445–467.

Schulze, M.B., J.E. Manson, W.C. Willet, and F.B. Hu. Processed Meat Intake and Incidence of Type 2 Diabetes in Younger and Middle-Aged Women. *Diabetologia* (2003):46(11):1465–1473.

Schulze, M.B., M. Schulz, C. Heidemann, et al. Fiber and Magnesium Intake and Incidence of Type 2 Diabetes: A Prospective Study and Meta-Analysis. *Arch Intern Med* (2007):167(9):956–965.

SEARCH for Diabetes in Youth. Available at http://www.searchfordiabetes.org. Accessed October 31, 2007.

SEARCH for Diabetes in Youth Study Group. The Burden of Diabetes Mellitus among US Youth: Prevalence Estimates from the SEARCH for Diabetes in Youth Study. *Pediatrics* (2006):118:1510–1518.

Segal, R.J., G.P. Kenny, D.H. Wasserman, et al. Consensus Statement: Physical Activity/Exercise and Type 2 Diabetes: A Consensus Statement from the American Diabetes Association. *Diabetes Care* (2006):29(6):1433–1438.

Selvin, E., J. Coresh, and F.L. Brancati. The Burden and Treatment of Diabetes in Elderly Individuals in the U.S. *Diabetes Care* (2006):29(11):2415–2419.

Siminerio, L.M. Implementing Diabetes Self-Management Training Programs: Breaking Through the Barriers in Primary Care. *Endocr Pract* (2006):12(Suppl 1):124–130.

Simmons, D., K. O'Dea, B. Swinburn, and J. Voyle. Community-Based Approaches for the Primary Prevention of Non-Insulin–Dependent Diabetes Mellitus. *Diabet Med* (1997):14(7):519–526.

Soltesz, G., C.C. Patterson, and G. Dahlquist. Worldwide Childhood Type 1 Diabetes—What Can We Learn from Epidemiology? *Pediatr Diabetes* (2007):8(Suppl 6):6–14.

Song, Y., J.E. Manson, J.E. Buring, and S. Liu. A Prospective Study of Red Meat Consumption and Type 2 Diabetes in Middle-Aged and Elderly Women: The Women's Health Study. *Diabetes Care* (2004):27(9):2108–2115.

State of Diabetes Complications in America. A Comprehensive Report Issued by the American Association of Clinical Endocrinologists, in Partnership with Amputee Coalition of America Mended Hearts National Federation of the Blind National Kidney Foundation (April 2007). Available at http://harrisschool.uchicago.edu/News/press-releases/media/Diabetes%20Complications%20Report_FINAL.PDF.

Steinbrook, R. Facing the Diabetes Epidemic—Mandatory Reporting of Glycosylated Hemoglobin Values in New York City. *N Engl J Med* (2006):354(6):545–548.

Steyn, N.P., J. Mann, P.H. Bennett, et al. Diet, Nutrition, and the Prevention of Type 2 Diabetes. *Public Health Nutr* (2004):7(14):147–165.

Task Force on Community Preventive Services. Recommendations for Healthcare System and Self-Management Education Interventions to Reduce Morbidity and Mortality from Diabetes. *Am J Prev Med* (2002):22(4 Suppl):10–14.

Task Force on Community Preventive Services. *The Guide to Community Preventive Services.* Available at http://www.thecommunityguide.org/diabetes/default.htm. Accessed October 31, 2007.

Teufel, N.I., and C.K. Ritenbaugh. Development of a Primary Prevention Program: Insight Gained in the Zuni Diabetes Prevention Program. *Clin Pediatr (Phila)* (1998):37:131–141.

Thorpe, L.E., D. Berger, J.A. Ellis, et al. Trends and Racial/Ethnic Disparities in Gestational Diabetes among Pregnant Women in New York City, 1990–2001. *Aust J Polit Hist* (2005):95:1536–1539.

Torgerson, J.S., J. Hauptman, M.N. Boldrin, and L. Sjostrom. Xenical in the Prevention of Diabetes in Obese Subjects (XENDOS) Study: A Randomized Study of Orlistat as an Adjunct to Lifestyle Changes for the Prevention of Type 2 Diabetes in Obese Patients. *Diabetes Care* (2004):27:151–161.

Trevino, R.P., Z. Yin, A. Hernandez, et al. Bienestar School-Based Diabetes Mellitus Prevention Program on Fasting Capillary Glucose Levels: A Randomized Controlled Trial. *Arch Pediatr Adolesc Med* (2004):158:911–917.

TRIAD Study Group. The Translating Research Into Action for Diabetes (TRIAD) Study: A Multicenter Study of Diabetes in Managed Care. *Diabetes Care* (2002):25:386–389.

Tuomilehto, J., J. Lindstrom, J.G. Eriksson, et al. the Finnish Diabetes Prevention Study Group. Prevention of Type 2 Diabetes Mellitus by Changes in Lifestyle among Subjects with Impaired Glucose Tolerance. *N Engl J Med* (2001):344:1343–1350.

Tuomilehto, J., and E. Wolf. The Challenge in the Future: Primary Prevention of Diabetes Mellitus. In: Larkins, R., P. Zimmet, and D. Chisholm, editors, *Prevention of Diabetes and Its Complications: International Conference Proceedings* (1988):993–999. Abstract 800.

Unwin, N., J. Shaw, P. Zimmet, and K.G.M.M. Alberti. Impaired Glucose Tolerance and Impaired Fasting Glycaemia: The Current Status on Definition and Intervention. *Diabet Med* (2002):19:708–723.

U.S. Department of Health and Human Services (USDHHS). *New Study Seeks to Lower Diabetes Risk in Youth.* Bethesda, MD: NIH News: National Institutes of Health (August 28, 2006). Press release.

U.S. Mexico Border Diabetes Prevention and Control Project: Phase 1 Report. Available at http://www.fep.paho.org/english/publicaciones/Diabetes/Diabetes%20first%20report%20of%20Results.pdf. Accessed October 31, 2007.

U.S. Preventive Services Task Force. *Guide to Clinical Preventive Services* (2nd ed.). Washington, D.C.: U.S. Department of Health and Human Services (1996).

U.S. Renal Data System. *USRDS 2007 Annual Data Report: Atlas of End-Stage Renal Disease in the United States* (2007). Bethesda, MD: National Institutes of Health, National Institute of Diabetes and Digestive and Kidney Diseases. Available at http://www.usrds.org/adr.htm. Accessed September 24, 2007.

U.S. Renal Data System. Available at http://www.usrds.org. Accessed October 31, 2007.

Vaccaro, O., L.E. Eberly, J.D. Neaton, et al., for the Multiple Risk Factor Intervention Trial (MRFIT) Research Group. Impact of Diabetes and Previous Myocardial Infarction on Long-Term Survival. *Arch Intern Med* (2004):164:1438–1443.

Valdez, R., P.W. Yoon, T. Liu, and M.J. Khoury. Family History and Prevalence of Diabetes in the U.S. Population: 6-Year Results from the National Health and Nutrition Examination Survey (NHANES 1999–2004). *Diabetes Care* (2007):30:2515–2522 [published online July 18, 2007].

Vallis, M., L. Ruggiero, G. Greene, et al. Stages of Change for Healthy Eating in Diabetes: Relation to Demographic, Eating-Related, Health Care Utilization, and Psychosocial Factors. *Diabetes Care* (2003):26(5):1468–1474.

van Dam, R.M., and F.B. Hu. Coffee Consumption and Risk of Type 2 Diabetes: A Systematic Review. *JAMA* (2005):294(1):97–104.

van Dam, R.M., W.C. Willett, J.E. Manson, and F.B. Hu. Coffee, Caffeine, and Risk of Type 2 Diabetes: A Prospective Cohort Study in Younger and Middle-Aged U.S. Women. *Diabetes Care* (2006):29(2):398–403.

van Dam, R.M., W.C. Willet, E.B. Rimm, et al. Dietary Fat and Meat Intake in Relation to Risk of Type 2 Diabetes in Men. *Diabetes Care* (2002):25:417–424.

Vijgen, S.M., M. Hoogendoorn, C.A. Baan, et al. Cost Effectiveness of Preventive Interventions in Type 2 Diabetes Mellitus: A Systematic Literature Review. *Pharmacoeconomics* (2006):24(5):425–441.

Wagner, E.H., B.T. Austin, and M. Von Korff. Organizing Care for Patients with Chronic Illness. *Milbank Q* (1996):74:511–544.

Wagner, E.H., R.E. Glasgow, C. Davis, et al. Quality Improvement in Chronic Illness Care: A Collaborative Approach. *Joint Comm J Qual Improv* (2001):27:63–80.

Wannamethee, S.G., A.G. Shaper, and I.J. Perry. Smoking as a Modifiable Risk Factor for Type 2 Diabetes in Middle-Aged Men. *Diabetes Care* (2001):24:1590–1595.

Wilke, R.A., R.L. Berg, P. Peissig, et al. Use of an Electronic Medical Record for the Identification of Research Subjects with Diabetes Mellitus. *Clin Med Res* (2007):5(1):1–7.

Will, J.C., D.A. Galuska, E.S. Ford, et al. Cigarette Smoking and Diabetes Mellitus: Evidence of a Positive Association with a Large Prospective Cohort Study. International *J Epidemiology* (2001):30:540–546.

Williams, D.E., B.L. Cadwell, Y.J. Cheng, et al. Prevalence of Impaired Fasting Glucose and Its Relationship with Cardiovascular Disease Risk Factors in U.S. Adolescents, 1999–2000. *Pediatrics* (2005):116(5):1122–1126.

Wilson, P.W., R.B. D'Agostino, H. Parise, et al. Metabolic syndrome as a precursor of cardiovascular disease and type 2 diabetes mellitus. *Circulation* (2005):112(20):3066-3072. Epub 2005 Nov 7.

Writing Group for the SEARCH for Diabetes in Youth Study Group. Incidence of Diabetes in Youth in the United States. *JAMA* (2007):297(24):2716–2724.

Young, T.K., P.J. Martens, S.P. Taback, et al. Type 2 Diabetes Mellitus in Children: Prenatal and Early Infancy Risk Factors among Native Canadians. *Arch Pediatr Adolesc Med* (2002):156:651–655.

Zhang, C., C.G. Solomon, J.E Manson, and F.B. Hu. A Prospective Study of Pregravid Physical Activity and Sedentary Behaviors in Relation to the Risk for Gestational Diabetes Mellitus. *Arch Intern Med* (2006):166(5):543–548.

Zhang, P., M.M. Engelgau, R. Valdez, et al. Costs of Screening for Prediabetes among U.S. Adults: A Comparison of Different Screening Strategies. *Diabetes Care* (2003):26(9):2536–2542.

Zhang, P., M.M. Engelgau, R. Valdez, et al. Efficient Cutoff Points for Three Screening Tests for Detecting Undiagnosed Diabetes and Prediabetes: An Economic Analysis. *Diabetes Care* (2005):28:1321–1325.

Ziegler, A., S. Schmid, D. Huber, et al. Early Infant Feeding and Risk of Developing Type 1 Diabetes-Associated Autoantibodies. *JAMA* (2003):290(13):1721–1727.

Zimmet, P.Z. Primary Prevention of Diabetes Mellitus. *Diabetes Care* (1988):11:258–262.

CHAPTER 11

HIGH BLOOD PRESSURE (ICD-10 I10-I15)

Leonelo E. Bautista, M.D., Dr.P.H.

Introduction

Arterial blood pressure is the force that the circulating blood exerts on the walls of the larger, low-resistance arteries of the vascular system. The level of blood pressure cannot be perceived, and therefore, high blood pressure (also called hypertension) is asymptomatic. However, high blood pressure has a large impact on morbidity and mortality in almost all populations due to its high prevalence and strong association with the incidence of cardiovascular and renal disease (Figure 11.1). Fortunately, hypertension is fairly easy to diagnose, and blood pressure control results in significant health benefits.

The precise blood pressure levels defining high blood pressure are those above which blood pressure-lowering interventions have been shown to reduce the risk of stroke and coronary heart disease (Zanchetti et al. 1993). Accordingly, the definition of high blood pressure has changed over time as new knowledge about the consequences of hypertension and the benefits of blood pressure lowering accumulated. Although arbitrary, the definition of hypertension is very useful for clinicians making treatment decisions, as well as for epidemiological surveillance.

Owing to the natural variability in blood pressure, the diagnosis of hypertension is based on the average of at least two blood pressure measurements taken on at least two sequential clinic visits, following standard measurement guidelines (Pickering et al. 2005). Current guidelines for blood pressure staging (Table 11.1) include normal blood pressure (systolic blood pressure [SBP] <120 mmHg and diastolic blood pressure [DBP] <80 mmHg), prehypertension (SBP 120–139 mmHg and/or DBP 80–89 mmHg), stage 1 hypertension (SBP 140–159 mmHg and/or DBP 90–99 mmHg), and stage 2 hypertension (SBP ≥160 mmHg and/or DBP ≥100 mmHg) (Chobanian et al. 2003). During the last 30 years, individuals ≥18 years old who are not acutely ill and have SBP ≥140 mmHg and/or DBP ≥90 mmHg have been diagnosed as hypertensive because they have an important increase in cardiovascular risk and they benefit from additional examinations or blood pressure–lowering interventions (Moser et al. 1977). The term "prehypertension" has been recently introduced to emphasize the need for preventive interventions, because individuals with blood pressures in the prehypertensive range have been found to be 3–7 times more likely to become hypertensive and 2 times more likely to develop cardiovascular diseases (Vasan et al. 2001a, 2001b) and can benefit from nonpharmacological

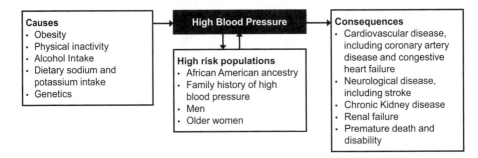

Figure 11.1. High blood pressure: causes, consequences, and high-risk groups.

interventions aimed to reduce blood pressure (He et al. 2000; Sacks et al. 2001; Whelton et al. 2002b).

Pathophysiology

Mean arterial pressure is the product of cardiac output, the volume of blood pumped by the heart by unit of time, and systemic vascular resistance, the force that small peripheral arteries oppose to the circulation of the blood. The mechanisms that cause essential hypertension are not completely understood. However, it is well recognized that the kidney, the sympathetic nervous system, and the renin–angiotensin system play central roles in blood pressure regulation. Under normal conditions, the human body maintains a precise balance between the intake and output of fluids and electrolytes. If this balance is compromised, the volume of body fluids could expand or contract to a point where the circulatory system would fail. The long-term regulation of body fluids volume depends greatly on the ability of the kidneys to excrete and reabsorb sodium chloride. When the extracellular concentration of sodium increases, the blood volume increases, leading to an increase in cardiac output and blood pressure. In response to the increase in blood pressure, the kidney increases sodium excretion, leading to lower blood volume, reduced cardiac output, and normal blood pressure. Conversely, when blood pressure falls below normal, the kidney retains water and sodium as a way to increase blood volume and cardiac output and reestablish normal blood pressure.

All forms of essential hypertension are characterized by impaired pressure natriuresis, i.e., higher levels of blood pressure are required to stimulate the kidney to excrete sodium as a way to maintain normal body fluid volumes. Impaired pressure natriuresis could be caused by intrarenal or extrarenal factors. A reduced glomerular filtration rate and/or an increased tubular reabsorption of sodium are intrarenal mechanisms that may lead to hypertension. When the intrinsic balance between glomerular filtration rate and tubular reabsorption is altered, blood pressure increases as a way to increase natriuresis and preserve normal body fluid volume.

Increased activity of the sympathetic nervous system is an extrarenal mechanism often associated with the pathogenesis of hypertension. In fact, increased sympathetic activity has been proposed as a mechanism for obesity and stress-related hypertension. Activation of the sympathetic nervous system can cause short-term increases in blood

Table 11.1. Blood Pressure Staging Guidelines of the Joint National Committee on Detection, Evaluation and Treatment of High Blood Pressure

Stage	JNC IV (1988)[a]	JNC V (1993)	JNC VI (1997)[b]	JNC VII (2003)
Optimal				
SBP			<120	
DBP			<80	
Normal				
SBP		<130	<130	<120
DBP	<85	<85	<85	<80
High normal				
SBP		130–139	130–139	
DBP	85–89	85–89	85–89	
Prehypertension				
SBP				120–139
DBP				80–89
Hypertension				
Stage 1 (mild)				
SBP		140–159	140–159	140–159
DBP	90–104	90–99	90–99	90–99
Stage 2 (moderate)				
SBP		160–179	160–179	≥160
DBP	105–114	100–109	100–109	≥100
Stage 3 (severe)				
SBP		180–209	≥180	
DBP	≥115	110–119	≥110	
Stage 4 (very severe)				
SBP		≥210		
DBP		≥120		

[a]Patients with DBP <90 mmHg and SBP 140–159 or SBP ≥160 mmHg were classified as "borderline systolic hypertension" and "isolated systolic hypertension," respectively. Patients with elevated DBP and SBP were classified by their DBP level.

[b]Concords with the 1999 World Health Organization/International Society of Hypertension Guidelines (Black 1999) and the 2007 European Society of Hypertension/European Society of Cardiology Guidelines (Mancia et al. 2007).

References: JNC IV: JNC 1988; JNC V: Gifford et al. 1993; JNC VI: Sheps et al. 1997; JNC VII: Chobanian et al. 2003.

pressure by increasing heart rate, heart contractility, and cardiac output and by increasing vasoconstriction and systemic vascular resistance. More importantly, activation of renal sympathetic activity increases sodium retention, impairs pressure natriuresis, and could cause essential hypertension.

Disorders that induce arterial vasoconstriction or sodium retention can also play a role in the pathogenesis of hypertension. For example, an increased activity of the renin–angiotensin system results in high levels of angiotensin II, a powerful vasoconstrictor that helps to maintain blood pressure in situations such as low blood volume or low cardiac contractility. High levels of angiotensin II increase vasoconstriction and systemic vascular resistance and also impair pressure natriuresis. Thus, high angiotensin II could lead to chronic hypertension because higher levels of blood pressure are needed to preserve normal sodium excretion and body fluid volume. Finally, vasodilating (e.g., nitric oxide) and vasoconstricting (e.g., endothelin-1) factors produced by the vascular endothelium in response to mechanical and biochemical agonists participate in blood pressure control, but their role on the pathogenesis of hypertension has yet to be fully elucidated.

Significance

High blood pressure (hypertension) imposes an extraordinary health burden in almost all populations. According to a worldwide study, high blood pressure is the second largest contributor to the burden of disease in both developed countries and developing countries with low mortality and the fifth largest contributor in developing countries with high mortality (World Health Organization 2002). About 7.1 million (13%) of all annual deaths in the world are caused by high blood pressure. The lost disability adjusted life years (DALYs) attributed to high blood pressure (64 million, 4.4% of the total) is considerably larger than that lost to smoking (59 million) and alcohol (58 million). In the United States, the age-adjusted death rate from hypertension increased 25.2% from 1994 to 2004, and the estimated total cost of hypertension in 2007 was $66.4 billion (Rosamond et al. 2007).

The effect of blood pressure on cardiovascular mortality has been recently estimated in a meta-analysis of cohort studies including more than 1 million adults (Lewington et al. 2002). In this study, an increase of 20 mmHg in SBP increased the coronary heart disease death rate by 50% in 80- to 89-year-olds, 70% in 70- to 79-year-olds, 90% in 60- to 69-year-olds, and 100% in 50- to 59- and 40- to 49-year-olds. Corresponding changes for an increase of 10 mmHg in DBP were 40%, 60, 80%, 90%, and 110%, respectively. For the same age groups and SBP difference, the risk of stroke mortality increased by 50%, 100%, 130%, 160%, and 180%, respectively. Corresponding changes associated with DBP were 60%, 110%, 150%, 190%, and 190%, respectively. These results show that the relative effect of high blood pressure on cardiovascular mortality is higher in younger subjects. However, because cardiovascular disease mortality increases with age, the absolute differences in mortality are larger in older groups. The relative increase in mortality associated with an absolute difference in blood pressure was the same at all levels of blood pressure down to at least 115 mmHg of SBP and 75 mmHg of DBP.

Table 11.2 displays the relative risk and population attributable risk for various diseases associated with hypertension. Among middle-class white persons who participated in the Framingham study, those with high blood pressure were about two times more likely to develop coronary heart disease (Kannel 1996). However, in a more recent cohort study including a large sample of African Americans, high blood pressure was a stronger predictor of coronary heart disease in African American women than in other race–sex groups, with a relative risk of 4.8, as compared with 2.0 in African American men, 2.1 in white women, and 1.6 in white men (Jones et al. 2002). Limited data from cohort studies (D'Agostino et al. 2001; Otiniano et al. 2005; Wei et al. 1996) suggest that high blood pressure doubles the risk of coronary heart in Hispanics (pooled relative risk 1.9), but no sex-specific estimates have been reported in this ethnic group.

High blood pressure is the strongest independent risk factor for stroke. Estimates of the relative risk of stroke associated with high blood pressure have been remarkably consistent in different cohort studies (Li et al. 2005; Ohira et al. 2006; Qureshi et al. 2002). In these cohorts, the incidence of stroke was on average 2.2 times higher in hypertensive as compared with normotensive subjects. The relative effect of high blood pressure on stroke does not seem to depend on race or sex (Kittner et al. 1990; Lawes et al. 2004; MacMahon et al. 1990). High blood pressure is also a major risk factor for the development of congestive heart failure. Hypertensive subjects are 1.8 times more likely to develop congestive heart failure than normotensive subjects (Levy et al. 1996; McNeill et al. 2006; Williams et al. 2002). Although the increase in risk is similar in men and women (Kannel, Ho, and Thom 1994; McNeill et al. 2006), it is currently uncertain whether the effect of high blood pressure on the risk of congestive heart failure depends on race.

High blood pressure can also lead to the development of chronic kidney disease, a progressive loss of renal function, and to end-stage renal disease (ESRD), an advanced stage of chronic kidney disease requiring dialysis or renal transplant as a form of renal replacement therapy (Levey et al. 2003). The average relative risk from two prospective cohort studies (Fox et al. 2004; Kurella, Lo, and Chertow 2005) of high blood pressure and risk of chronic kidney disease (glomerular filtration rate <60 mL/min per 1.73 m^2 was 1.72 (95% confidence interval 1.48–2.01). ESRD incidence also increases progressively with higher levels of blood pressure. Pooled estimates from three large cohort studies show that the relative risk of ESRD associated with high normal blood pressure, stage 1, 2, and 3 hypertension as compared with optimal blood pressure (JNC VI categories, Table 11.1) (Sheps et al. 1997) were 1.5, 2.0, 2.8, 4.8, and 7.0 (Haroun et al. 2003; Hsu et al. 2005; Klag et al. 1997). The strength of the association between blood pressure and chronic kidney disease is similar in men and women (Haroun et al. 2003) as well as in African Americans and whites (Klag et al. 1997).

A considerable fraction of all new cases of cardiovascular disease in the United States is attributable to high blood pressure. About 16% of all cases of coronary heart disease in men and almost 40% in women are associated with high blood pressure (Table 11.2). It is unknown whether a similar sex disparity also occurs in Hispanics. The larger absolute impact of high blood pressure among women is due to both a larger relative risk and higher prevalence of high blood pressure in women than in men. About a quarter of all cases or coronary heart disease in white women are associated with high blood pressure, compared with almost 60% in African American women. Approximately 25% of all strokes, 20% of all cases of congestive heart failure, and 18% of all cases of chronic kidney disease are attributable to high blood pressure. Overall, about one out of every four cases of cardiovascular diseases in the United States could be theoretically prevented by eliminating high blood pressure.

The population attributable risks presented in Table 11.2 likely underestimate the impact of elevated high blood pressure, since they do not take into account the fact that

Table 11.2. Relative Risk and Population Attributable Risk for Diseases Associated with Hypertension in Men (M) and Women (W) by Race/Ethnicity: United States, 1999–2003

Disease	Relative Risk[a]	Population Attributable Risk (%)[b]							
		White		African American		Hispanic		All	
		M	W	M	W	M	W	M	W
Coronary heart disease[c]	2.2	15.5	25.8	25.5	59.8	18.5	20.3	16.2	38.6
Stroke	2.2	26.9	27.5	29.1	32.0	18.5	20.3	26.0	27.2
Congestive heart failure	1.8	19.7	20.2	21.5	23.9	13.2	14.5	18.9	19.9
Chronic kidney disease	1.7	17.7	18.1	19.3	21.5	11.7	12.9	17.0	17.9

[a]Relative risks were calculated by the author by pooling the estimates from the references cited in the text.
[b]Population attributable risks were calculated by the author using Levin's formula (Szklo and Nieto 2007). Population attributable risks for coronary heart disease were calculated using the sex–race-specific relative risks reported in the text. Estimates of the prevalence of hypertension used in the calculation of the population attributable risk come from NHANES (1999–2003)
[c]Pooled relative risks of coronary heart disease for men and women are 1.66 and 3.02, respectively.

the risk of developing cardiovascular disease increases with blood pressure even with blood pressure levels "within the normal range." Indeed, individuals with SBP of 130–139 mmHg and DBP of 85–89 mmHg are 2.5 and 1.6 times more likely to develop cardiovascular disease, respectively, than those with SBP of <120 mmHg and DBP of <80 mmHg (Vasan et al. 2001a). In the Atherosclerosis Risk in Communities (ARIC) study, the risk of ischemic stroke increased about 50% for each increase of 19 mmHg in SBP (Ohira et al. 2006). Also, in the Framingham study, an increase of 20 mmHg in SBP or 10 mmHg in DBP was associated with corresponding increases of 56% and 24%, respectively, in the incidence of congestive heart failure (Haider et al. 2003). Finally, an increase of 16 mmHg in SBP or 10 mmHg in DBP resulted in a similar increase of 76% in the risk of ESRD (Klag et al. 1996).

The effect of high blood pressure on cardiovascular complications varies by race/ethnic group, age, and the type of blood pressure measured. In middle-aged Europeans and Americans, coronary heart disease is the main complication of high blood pressure, whereas stroke is more important among Asians and older individuals (Staessen et al. 2003). African Americans tend to have higher prevalence of high blood pressure and higher rates of high blood pressure–related complications than other racial groups. The relative effect of blood pressure is larger in younger persons, but the absolute effect is larger in older individuals. Moreover, different blood pressure measures have different impacts on disease incidence. In persons younger than 50 years, DBP is the strongest predictor of coronary heart diseases. From age 50–59 years, SBP, DBP, and their difference (pulse pressure) are equally predictive of coronary heart disease. From 60 years old and on, pulse pressure becomes a better predictor than SBP, and higher levels of DBP are associated with lower risk of coronary heart disease (Franklin et al. 2001). Moreover, SBP seems to be a better predictor of stroke incidence than DBP and pulse pressure (Bowman et al. 2006; Inoue et al. 2006; Kannel et al. 1981; Nielsen et al. 1997; Psaty et al. 2001). SBP and pulse pressure also confer a greater risk of congestive heart disease than DBP (Chae et al. 1999; Haider et al. 2003; Vaccarino, Holford, and Krumholz 2000). Although all blood pressure measurements are directly associated with increased risk of chronic kidney disease, results from a large observational study and from several clinical trials suggest that SBP is a stronger predictor of chronic kidney disease than DBP and pulse pressure (Klag et al. 1996; Mentari and Rahman 2004).

Descriptive Epidemiology

High-Risk Populations

Average blood pressure increases with age in most populations, except those isolated and with low sodium intake (Bazzano, He, and Whelton 2007; Whelton 1994; Wolf-Maier et al. 2003). Age- and sex-related changes in blood pressure are illustrated here using data from the National Health and Nutrition Examination Survey in the United States (NHANES 1999–2004; NCHS 1996, 2006).

SBP increases with age in both men and women, from about 110 mmHg in women age 20 years to about 160 mmHg in women age 80 years and from about 120 mmHg in men age 20 years to about 150 mmHg in men age 80 years. As a consequence, SBP is higher in young men than in young women but becomes higher in women than in men around age 50 (Figure 11.2). Sex- and age-specific average SBP tends to be higher among African Americans than in other racial/ethnic groups.

Average DBP increases with age until about 50 years old and remains constant or decreases thereafter (Figure 11.3). Among whites and Hispanics, DBP peaks and then levels off around age 40 years in men and age 50 years in women. Corresponding changes occur around age 50 and 60 years among African Americans. DBP is slightly and consistently higher among men than in women of the same age and race/ethnicity. Age-related changes in blood pressure are mostly explained by the loss of elasticity of the aorta and other large arteries (arterial stiffness) that occurs normally with aging.

Estimates of the prevalence of high blood pressure come mostly from epidemiological studies where cases are defined using the average of multiple measures of blood pressure taken in a single evaluation, instead of multiple sequential clinic visits. However, most prospective studies linking blood pressure and cardiovascular risk have relied on this epidemiological definition of high blood pressure (Kannel, Gordon, and Schwartz 1971; MacMahon et al. 1990).

High blood pressure is common in almost all populations. Just like the average blood pressure, high blood pressure prevalence depends strongly on age, sex, and race/ethnicity.

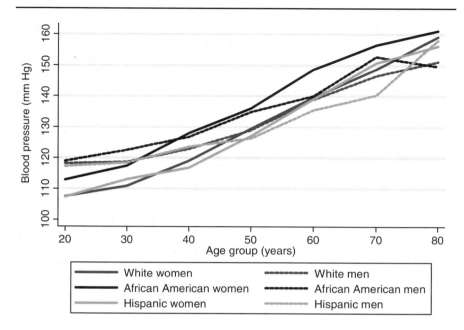

Figure 11.2. Average SBP by age, sex, and race (NHANES 1999–2004).

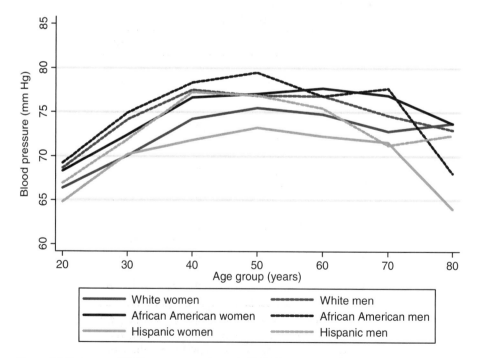

Figure 11.3. Average DBP by age, sex, and race (NHANES 1999–2004).

A recent meta-analysis of population-based cross-sectional studies suggests that about a quarter of the adult world population in 2000 had high blood pressure (Kearney et al. 2005), but data from most countries were not available. Estimates of the prevalence of high blood pressure in the United States based on data from NHANES 1999–2004 are presented in Table 11.3. The overall prevalence of high blood pressure in U.S. adults ($\geq$20 years old) is 31.4% but ranges from about 5% in 20- to 29-year-olds to over 75% in those 80- to 89-years-old. Similar to the pattern observed for average SBP, the prevalence of high blood pressure is higher in young men than in young women, but higher in older women than in older men (Table 11.3, Figure 11.4). This pattern is consistent in all race/ethnicity groups, but the age at which high blood pressure prevalence becomes higher in women than in men is about 30 years in African Americans and 50 years in other race/ethnicity groups.

Data on the incidence of high blood pressure are limited because they require active follow-up of populations with frequent blood pressure measurements for long periods. The risk of developing high blood pressure has been estimated among Framingham Heart Study participants who had remained free of the condition at age 55 or 65 years (Vasan et al. 2002). About 90% of all participants developed high blood pressure during a follow-up period corresponding to their median residual lifetime expectancy (20 years for 65-year-olds and 25 years for 55-year-olds) (Vasan et al. 2002).

In addition to age, the incidence of high blood pressure depends greatly on starting blood pressure values. Individuals with SBP <140 mmHg and DBP 85–89 mmHg are 2–3 times more likely to develop high blood pressure than those with similar SBP and

Table 11.3. Prevalence of Hypertension (%) by Sex and Age in the United States (NHANES 1999–2004)

Age	Women	Men	All
20–29	2.0	7.4	4.9
30–39	8.2	14.5	11.5
40–49	24.0	26.7	25.3
50–59	42.8	41.3	42.5
60–69	61.3	59.4	60.4
70–79	77.2	63.9	71.5
80–89	82.6	66.7	76.8
All	32.7	30.2	31.4

Note: Hypertension was defined as SBP $\geq$140 mmHg or DBP $\geq$90 mmHg or self-reported history of a diagnosis of hypertension plus current use of antihypertensive medication. Pregnant women were excluded.

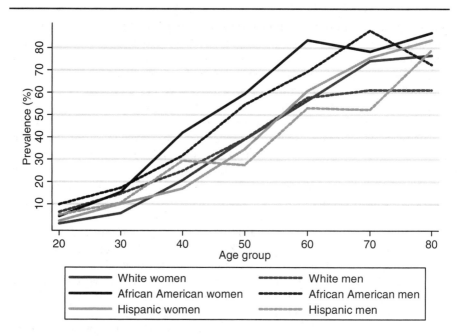

Figure 11.4. Prevalence of hypertension by age, sex, and race (NHANES 1999–2004).

DBP<85 mmHg (Leitschuh et al. 1991). Among Framingham Heart Study participants with optimum, normal, or high normal blood pressure according to JNC VI (Table 11.1) (Sheps et al. 1997), the 4-year risk of high blood pressure was 5.1%, 18.1%, and 39.4% in individuals 35–64 years old and 18.5%, 29.0%, and 52.5% in individuals 65–94 years old, respectively (Vasan et al. 2001b). Race/ethnicity also has a large impact in high blood pressure incidence. In the ARIC cohort (n=15,972), the 6-year risks of high blood pressure in men and women were 27% and 30% among African Americans and 17% and 16% among whites, respectively (Fuchs, et al. 2001).

Geographic Trends

Since the rates of high blood pressure are higher among African Americans, the prevalence of high blood pressure is higher in states and communities with a higher proportion of African Americans, such as the south and southeastern United States. On the other hand, in a group of six European countries, age-specific prevalence of high blood pressure was considerably higher than those in the United States and Canada (Wolf-Maier et al. 2003).

Time Trends

Overall, the age-adjusted average SBP and DBP in the U.S. population 18–74 years old decreased from 131 to 119 mmHg and from 83 to 73 mmHg, respectively, from 1971 to 1991 (Burt et al. 1995). Correspondingly, the age-adjusted prevalence of high blood pressure declined from 36.3% to 20.4%. This decline in the prevalence of high blood pressure was observed across all age, sex, and racial/ethnic groups, with the exception of African American men aged 50 years and older, who experienced a small increase (Burt et al. 1995). During this period, the distribution of both SBP and DBP in the whole U.S. population shifted downward, suggesting population-wide behavioral and environmental influences on blood pressure and not only a reduction in average blood pressure due to treatment of hypertensive people had shaped the distribution of blood pressure values (Goff et al. 2001). Moreover, there is evidence that the age-related increase in both SBP and DBP is smaller in more recent birth cohorts than in earlier birth cohorts (Goff et al. 2001).

The downward trend in the prevalence of high blood pressure has reversed during the last two decades. In fact, from 1988–1991 to 1999–2000, the age-adjusted prevalence of high blood pressure in the United States increased almost 4 percentage points, from 25.0% to 28.7% (Hajjar and Kotchen 2003). Larger increases occurred among persons ≥60 years old (7.5%) and in women (5.6% compared with 2.2% in men), particularly those of African American race/ethnicity (7.2%). An increase in the average body mass index (BMI=weight in kilograms/[height in meters]^2) observed during the same period was responsible for more than 50% of the increase in the prevalence of high blood pressure, independently of age, sex, and race/ethnicity (Hajjar and Kotchen 2003). Comparable estimates obtained from the last waves of NHANES suggest that the prevalence of high blood pressure has not changed recently: 30.5% in 1999–2000, 30.0% in 2001–2002, and 32.2% in 2003–2004 (p=.27).

Causes

Various genetic and environmental factors promote the development and persistence of high blood pressure (Figure 11.1). Nonmodifiable risk factors for elevated blood pressure include age, sex, and genetic susceptibility. Known modifiable risk factors include dietary intake of sodium, potassium, and alcohol, as well as physical activity and obesity. Other potential risk factors have been identified, but it is still uncertain whether they have an independent effect on blood pressure levels. These include low birth weight; socioeconomic status; insulin resistance; dietary fat, protein, calcium, and fiber intake; mild chronic inflammation; and psychological and emotional stress.

Genetic Factors

Blood pressure level aggregates in families, partly as a result of shared genetic predisposition. In fact, about 40% of the variability in blood pressure is explained by genetic factors (Harrap et al. 2000), and the risk of developing high blood pressure in persons younger than 50 years doubles for each first-degree relative with a history of high blood pressure (Hopkins and Hunt 2003). However, identifying genetic causes has been particularly difficult due to the etiologic heterogeneity of high blood pressure. Blood pressure is regulated by several mechanisms involving multiple nonallelic genes with small additive effects. The altered mechanism can not be identified in 90% of the cases because high blood pressure looks the same in all individuals. This compromises our ability to identify gene variants (alleles) or combinations of variants (haplotypes) associated with the development of high blood pressure.

Obesity

Excessive accumulation of body fat commonly leads to higher blood pressure. This effect could be mediated by overactivation of the sympathetic nervous system and the renin–angiotensin system and by alterations in endothelial and renal function. The prevalence of high blood pressure in U.S. adults (NHANES 1999–2004) increases progressively with BMI, from 18.0% in those with normal BMI (<25 kg/m^2) to 30.8% in those with overweight (BMI ≥25 kg/m^2 and <30 kg/m^2) and 42.0% in those with obesity (BMI ≥30 kg/m^2). Combining data from two large cohort studies, Field et al. (2001) showed that the risk of high blood pressure increases 2.1, 2.7, 2.4, and 3.9 times in overweight women, obese women, overweight men, and obese men, respectively, as compared with those with normal BMI. About 30% of all new cases of hypertension in men and women in the U.S. population could be attributable to overweight, while 36% of the cases in women and 45% of the cases in men could be attributed to obesity. Overall, about 50% of all new cases of high blood pressure are attributable to overweight and obesity combined (Table 11.4). Multiple randomized controlled trials (RCTs) of nonpharmacological weight reduction interventions have corroborated the effect of obesity on blood pressure (see below) (Neter et al. 2003).

Salt Intake

A high dietary intake of salt (sodium chloride) is associated with the development of high blood pressure. Over prolonged periods, a high intake of salt compromises the kidney's capacity to excrete sodium, leading to a persistent increase in blood volume and blood pressure. INTERSALT, a standardized epidemiological study of more than 10,000 persons from 32 countries, showed that an increase of 100 mmol/day of urinary sodium (an additional intake of ~5 g of salt) increased SBP by 3–6 mmHg and DBP by 0–3 mmHg

Table 11.4. Relative Risk and Population Attributable Risk for Risk Factors for Hypertension: United States, 1999–2003

Risk Factor	Relative Risk[a]	Population Attributable risk (%)
Overweight and obesity	2.5	49.5
Salt intake (>4.6 g/day)	1.5[b]	30.4
Alcohol intake in men[c]	1.2	15.5
Alcohol intake in women[c]	1.5	5.0
Low physical activity[d]	1.7	16.6

[a]Relative risks were calculated by pooling the estimates mentioned in the text and prevalence of risk factors came from NHANES 1999–2004.
[b]This is a conservative estimate base on the report of Khaw et al. (2004).
[c]Exposure corresponds to ≥1 drink/day in men and ≥4 drinks/day in women.
[d]Exposure corresponds to <3 hours/week of moderate or vigorous physical activity.

(Stamler 1997). In a more recent study of more than 23,000 individuals, SBP and DBPs were 7.2 and 3.0 mmHg higher, respectively, in those with a daily salt intake ≥12.6 g/day as compared with ≤4.6 g/day (Khaw et al. 2004). Accordingly, the risk of having a SBP ≥ 160 mmHg was about 2.5 times higher in those in the highest as compared with the lowest salt intake group. In fact, the population attributable risk of high blood pressure for a salt intake of >4.6 g/day is about 30% in the United States (Table 11.4). The relationship between salt intake and blood pressure has been confirmed in multiple RCTs of sodium intake reduction (Cutler, Follmann, and Allender 1997; He and MacGregor 2004; Sacks et al. 2001).

Potassium Intake

Increased dietary intake of potassium has been associated with lower blood pressure (Dyer et al. 1994). Administration of dietary potassium increases renal sodium and chloride excretion, reduces blood volume, and decreases blood pressure (Gallen et al. 1998). In INTERSALT, an increase of 30 mmol/day in urinary potassium excretion was associated with an independently significant reduction of 2.0 mmHg in SBP and 1.1 mmHg in DBP (Dyer et al. 1994). However, large epidemiological studies using dietary records have failed to show an independent association between potassium intake and self-reported incidence of high blood pressure (Ascherio et al. 1992, 1996). This is probably explained by inaccuracy in the measurement of dietary potassium intake. On the contrary, randomized clinical trials have confirmed that potassium supplementation is associated with significant reductions in SBP and DBP (Whelton et al. 1997).

Alcohol Intake

There is ample evidence linking alcohol intake (ethanol) and high blood pressure. Although the biological mechanisms of the long-term effect of alcohol intake on blood pressure are unclear, the hypertensive effect of alcohol has been shown in observational studies (Fuchs et al. 2001; Marmot et al. 1994) as well as randomized clinical trials of reduction (Xin et al. 2001) and increase (McFadden et al. 2005) in alcohol intake. In the INTERSALT study, men who drank 3–5 drinks/day had a 2.7-mmHg higher SBP and 1.6-mmHg higher DBP than nondrinkers, independently of other factors (Marmot, et al. 1994). In the ARIC study, participants who drank ≥3 drinks/day were 1.2 to 2.3 times more likely to develop high blood pressure after 6 years of follow-up (Fuchs et al. 2001). Also, a low to moderate alcohol intake (up to 3 drinks/day) was associated with higher incidence of high blood pressure or increased blood pressure in African Americans, but not in whites, suggesting higher alcohol sensitivity among African Americans. Interestingly, in two large cohort studies, Sesso et al. (2008) found that women who consumed from 1 drink/month to 1 drink/day were about 10% less likely, those who drank 2–3 drinks/day were as likely, and those who drank ≥4 drinks/day were 53% more likely to develop high blood pressure than never drinkers. In contrast, light-to-moderate alcohol intake did not change the risk of high blood pressure in men, but consumption of ≥1 drink/day increased the risk by at least 20%. These levels of alcohol intake correspond to a population attributable risk of 5.0% in women and 15.5% in men. A lower blood pressure following a reduction in alcohol intake has been demonstrated in randomized clinical trials (Xin et al. 2001).

Physical Activity

An inverse relationship has been observed between leisure time physical activity and blood pressure. Reduced stroke volume, systemic arterial resistance, sympathetic activity, urinary sodium retention, and insulin resistance may explain how long-term physical activity lowers blood pressure. In a cohort study of more than 8,000 men, Hu et al. (2004) found that those who reported moderate or high level of physical activity were on average about 40% less likely to develop high blood pressure after 11 years of follow-up. Some (Hu et al. 2004; Katzmarzyk et al. 2000; Levenstein, Smith, and Kaplan 2001) but not all (Folsom et al. 1990; Haapanen et al. 1997; Pereira et al. 1999) cohort studies have shown a lower risk of high blood pressure among physically active women. Similarly, no beneficial effects of physical activity on blood pressure were observed in African Americans from the ARIC and the CARDIA cohorts (Dyer et al. 1999; Pereira et al. 1999). These inconsistencies may be due to lack of accuracy in the measurement of physical activity in women and African Americans. Although two meta-analyses of randomized clinical trials have shown that aerobic physical training was associated with reductions in SBP and DBP (Fagard 2001; Whelton et al. 2002b), the evidence from randomized clinical trials in women and African Americans is inconclusive. If the effect of physical activity observed in white men also applies to women and individuals of other races, low physical activity carries a population attributable risk for high blood pressure of about 17% (Table 11.4).

Prevention and Control Measures

Prevention of high blood pressure can and should be implemented at the individual and at the population level. At the individual level, primary prevention is aimed at persons at high risk, with the goal of limiting the risk of becoming hypertensive, while secondary prevention is aimed at hypertensive and prehypertensive subjects, with the goal of avoiding the cardiovascular, neurological, renal, and ocular complications of high blood pressure. The strategy of population prevention is aimed at a collection of individuals, with the goal of shifting the whole blood pressure distribution to lower values (Whelton et al. 2002a). A change in the average blood pressure in the population would likely be small but should result in a large reduction in the incidence of hypertension-related complications and mortality (Stamler 1991).

Prevention at the Individual Level

Screening and Early Detection

Screening for high blood pressure has a substantial net benefit because blood pressure can be reliably and safely measured and treating hypertensive patients significantly reduces their risk of cardiovascular morbidity and mortality. In adults, blood pressure should be measured at every routine clinic visit, then remeasured in 2 years in those with normal blood pressure and in 1 year in those with prehypertension (Calonge et al. 2007; Chobanian et al. 2003). In addition to blood pressure measurement, screening for high blood pressure should be aimed to identify high-risk patients, i.e., those with a family history of hypertension, African American ancestry, overweight or obesity, a sedentary lifestyle, and a high alcohol intake (Whelton et al. 2002a). High salt and low potassium intake are also risk factors for high blood pressure, but they are difficult to identify in the context of a regular clinic visit. Although high blood pressure is easily diagnosed, data from NHANES 1999–2004 show that only 76% of all hypertensive persons are aware of their condition (Ong et al. 2007). Awareness of high blood pressure did not change significantly between 1988 and 2000 (Hajjar and Kotchen 2003), but there is evidence of a significant increase in awareness from 1999–2000 (68%) to 2003–2004 (76%) (Ong et al. 2007).

Primary Prevention: Lifestyle Modifications (Nonpharmacological Interventions)

Primary prevention of high blood pressure resides in the detection and management of modifiable risk factors through lifestyle changes. The efficacy of lifestyle changes in decreasing blood pressure and reducing the incidence of high blood pressure has been shown in randomized clinical trials. JNC VII recommended the use of lifestyle modifications in prehypertensive and hypertensive subjects and also encouraged their use in persons with normal blood pressure (Chobanian et al. 2003). Lifestyle modifications known to effectively reduce blood pressure are discussed below.

Weight Reduction

In a meta-analysis of 25 randomized clinical trials of weight control through increased physical activity and/or decreased energy intake, body weight reduction of 1 kg was associated with a decrease of approximately 1 mmHg in both SBP and DBP (Table 11.5) (Neter et al. 2003). Similar to other interventions, the beneficial effect of weight loss tended to be larger in hypertensive patients. In the Trials of Hypertension Prevention (TOHP), 181 men and women with high normal blood pressure were randomly assigned to an 18-month lifestyle modification intervention aimed at either weight loss or dietary sodium reduction or to a usual care control group (He et al. 2000). By the end of the intervention, there was a net intervention-to-control difference of −3.5 kg in body weight, −5.8 mmHg in SBP, and −3.2 mmHg in DBP. After 7 years of follow-up, body weight was similar in both treatment groups, but the incidence of high blood pressure was still 77% lower in the weight loss intervention group. Randomized clinical trials also suggest that patients require less intensive antihypertensive drug therapy if they follow a weight-reducing diet (Mulrow et al. 2000). The American Heart Association (AHA) recommends maintaining a BMI <25 kg/m^2 (Appel et al. 2006).

Salt Intake Reduction

Numerous randomized clinical trials support a blood pressure-lowering effect of reduced salt intake. In a meta-analysis of 40 trials, an average urinary sodium decrease of 77 mmol/day (about 4.5 g salt/day) resulted in a reduction of 2.5 and 2.0 mmHg in DBP and SBP, respectively (Table 11.5) (Geleijnse, Kok, and Grobbee 2003). Blood pressure reduction was at least twice as large in hypertensive as in normotensive subjects (SBP −5.24 versus −1.26 mmHg; DBP: −3.69 versus −1.14 mmHg). In TOHP, a difference of 33.3 mmol/day in urinary sodium excretion between intervention and control groups by the end of the intervention resulted in significant reductions of 3.3 mmHg in SBP and 1.7 mmHg in DBP (He et al. 2000). After 7 years of follow-up, urinary sodium excretion was similar but incidence of high blood pressure was still 35% lower in the sodium reduction arm.

Table 11.5. Effects of Lifestyle Interventions to Reduce Blood Pressure, Quantified in RCTs[a]

Intervention	Change	Reduction in Blood Pressure (mmHg)		Recommended Level
		SBP	DBP	
Weight loss	−1 kg	1.0	1.0	18.5–24.9 kg/m²
Reduce Na intake	−77 mmol/day urinary sodium	2.0	2.5	100 mmol/day (5.7 g salt/day)
Increase potassium intake	75 mmol/day (supplement)	3.1	2.0	120 mmol/day (4.7 g/day, diet)
Moderation in alcohol intake	−25%	3.0	2.0	≤2 drinks/d in men ≤1 drink/day in women
Aerobic physical activity	≥3 sessions/week, 30–60 minutes	3.5	2.5	30 min/day, most days of the week
DASH diet	Diet rich in fruits, vegetables, and low-fat dairy products and low in saturated and total fat	5.5	3.0	Regularly

[a]See references in text.

A lower need of antihypertensive medication in patients following a low-salt diet has also been demonstrated in RCTs (Whelton et al. 1998). The AHA currently recommends a maximum salt intake of 5.7 g/day (100 mmol/day of sodium) (Lichtenstein et al. 2006).

Dietary Potassium Increase

A consistently inverse relationship between increased potassium intake and blood pressure has been demonstrated in meta-analyses of RCTs (Table 11.5) (Geleijnse, Kok, and Grobbee 2003; Whelton et al. 1997). In one of these meta-analyses, potassium supplementation (median 75 mmol/d) reduced SBP and DBP by 3.1 and 2.0 mmHg, respectively (Whelton et al. 1997). The average effect size was larger in hypertensive subjects and in African Americans. Similar results were obtained in a meta-analysis of trials in normotensive persons (Geleijnse, Kok, and Grobbee 2003). Moreover, the effect of potassium supplementation on blood pressure is larger in the context of a concurrent high intake of sodium, and vice versa (Morris et al. 1999). Based on findings from randomized clinical trials, the AHA sets the recommended potassium intake level as 120 mmol/d

(4.7 g/d) in healthy individuals (Appel et al. 2006). Importantly, this level of potassium intake can and should be achieved through consumption of fruits, vegetables, and nuts in the diet, instead of diet pill supplements.

Moderation of Alcohol Intake

A dose-dependent association between alcohol intake and risk of high blood pressure has been documented in observational and experimental studies. A recent meta-analysis showed that an average reduction of about 25% in alcohol intake lowers SBP and DBP by 3.3 and 2.0 mmHg, respectively (Table 11.5) (Xin et al. 2001). Although the effect was similar in normotensive and hypertensive subjects, the effect of the intervention was larger in those with higher baseline blood pressure. Alcohol intake should be limited to 2 drinks/day in most men and 1 drink/day in women and lighter-weight persons (1 drink equals 12 ounces of regular beer, 5 ounces of wine, or 1.5 ounces of 80-proof distilled spirits) (Appel et al. 2006).

Physical Activity

Regular physical activity lowers blood pressure and prevents the development of high blood pressure. Two meta-analyses of randomized clinical trials have shown that aerobic physical training is associated with reductions in SBP and DBP of about 3.5 and 2.5 mmHg, respectively (Table 11.5) (Fagard 2001; Whelton, et al. 2002b). The effect of physical activity on blood pressure seems to be slightly greater in hypertensive subjects, independent of baseline body weight and weight loss. Unfortunately, there is currently inconclusive evidence on the effect of physical activity among women and African Americans. On the other hand, the influence of resistance training, such as weight lifting, on blood pressure is currently uncertain. JNC VII recommends at least 30 min/day of aerobic physical activity of moderate intensity, such as quick walking, most days of the week (Chobanian et al. 2003).

Change in Dietary Pattern

A considerable proportion of the between population variability in blood pressure could be explained not by differences in single nutrients but by large variations in dietary patterns. The effect of three dietary patterns on blood pressure was evaluated in the Dietary Approaches to Stop Hypertension (DASH) Trial, a controlled dietary intervention study (Appel et al. 1997; Sacks et al. 2001). The DASH Trial included 133 hypertensive and 326 normotensive adults who received carefully controlled diets for 11 weeks. One group received a control diet low in fruits, vegetables, and dairy products, with a fat content typical of the average diet in the United States; the second group received a diet rich in fruits and vegetables; and the third group received the DASH diet, i.e., a combination diet rich in fruits, vegetables, and low-fat dairy products and with reduced saturated and total fat. The DASH diet significantly reduced SBP and DBP by 5.5 and 3.0 mmHg more, respectively, than the control diet (Table 11.5). The effect of the DASH diet was significantly larger among participants with high blood pressure (reductions of 11.4 and 5.5 mmHg in SBP and DBP, respectively) and among African Americans as compared with whites (6.9 versus 3.3 mmHg in SBP and 3.7 versus 2.4 mmHg in DBP, respectively) (Appel et al. 1997; Svetkey et al. 1999). Importantly, the effect of the DASH diet was evident within the first 2 weeks of the trial. The DASH diet is currently recommended by the AHA and by JNC VII as a way to prevent and treat high blood pressure (Appel et al. 2006; Chobanian et al. 2003).

Secondary Prevention: Pharmacological Treatment

Secondary prevention is aimed at avoiding the complications of high blood pressure. Interventions for secondary prevention are indicated in prehypertensive and hypertensive individuals. Blood pressure–lowering lifestyle modifications were recommended by JNC VII (Table 11.6) (Chobanian et al. 2003) for all prehypertensive persons and are justifiable on the following grounds. First, prehypertensive individuals are several times more likely than normotensive individuals to become hypertensive within a few years (Vasan et al. 2001b; Winegarden 2005) and about 1.5 to 2.5 times more likely to develop cardiovascular disease (Hsia et al. 2007; Vasan et al. 2001a). Second, prehypertension is highly prevalent. About a quarter of the U.S. population is prehypertensive, 20% of women and 31% of men (NHANES 1999–2004). Third, randomized clinical trials have documented that changes in lifestyle significantly reduce blood pressure in normotensive persons. In fact, the DASH study gave support to the JNC VII's recommendation for proactive management of prehypertension. There are, at present, no intervention studies with cardiovascular end-points to support antihypertensive drug therapy in prehypertensive subjects. In contrast to the JNC VII guidelines, the guidelines from the European Society of Cardiology and the European Society of Hypertension call for initiation of lifestyle modification in prehypertensive persons only if they have 1–2 additional cardiovascular risk factors (Mancia et al. 2007).

Table 11.6. Management of High Blood Pressure According to JNC VII

Blood Pressure Stage	SBP (mmHg)		DBP (mmHg)	Starting Treatment
Normal	<120	and	<80	Encourage lifestyle modifications
Prehypertension	120–139	or	80–89	Lifestyle modifications
Stage 1 hypertension	140–159	or	90–99	Lifestyle modifications + one drug
Stage 2 hypertension	≥160	or	≥100	Lifestyle modifications + two drugs

Note: All patients with blood pressure ≥120/80 mmHg and a compelling indication (heart failure, postmyocardial infarction, high risk of coronary heart disease, diabetes, chronic kidney disease, or recurrent stroke) should receive drugs for the compelling indication independently of their blood pressure level. In these cases, the antihypertensive drug selected will depend on the compelling indication (Chobanian et al. 2003).

In a departure from previous guidelines, JNC VII called for pharmacological treatment of all patients with high blood pressure (≥140/90 mmHg) without consideration of other risk factors (Chobanian et al. 2003). In contrast, JNC VI recommended immediate drug therapy in patients without other risk factors only if they had a blood pressure ≥160/100 mmHg (stage 2 and 3 hypertension). Similarly, the current guidelines from the European Societies of Hypertension and Cardiology (Mancia et al. 2007) recommend immediate drug treatment in patients without other cardiovascular risk factors only if blood pressure is ≥180/110 mmHg. The treatment goal for individuals with high blood pressure and no other compelling conditions is to reduce SBP and DBP to <140 mmHg and <90 mmHg, respectively, but the primary focus should be on SBP (Chobanian et al. 2003; Mancia et al. 2007). A treatment goal of SBP <130 mmHg and of DBP <80 mmHg has been proposed in most guidelines for patients with diabetes mellitus, chronic kidney disease, and ischemic heart disease (Chobanian et al. 2003; Mancia et al. 2007; Rosendorff et al. 2007). This goal is mostly based on the higher risk of cardiovascular disease observed in cohort studies in patients with these diseases (Cushman 2007).

In most patients with uncomplicated high blood pressure, JNC VII recommends a thiazide diuretic as preferred initial drug (Chobanian et al. 2003). The benefits of thiazide diuretics in preventing cardiovascular complications, as compared with placebo or other active drugs, have been clearly demonstrated in randomized clinical trials, and thiazide diuretics are less expensive than other antihypertensive drugs (Psaty et al. 2003). Other drugs with demonstrated cardiovascular benefits and recommended by JNC VII are long-acting calcium channel blockers, angiotensin-converting enzyme inhibitors, angiotensin type I receptor blockers, and β-blockers. However, a recent meta-analysis suggests that β-blockers are no better at preventing heart attacks and are less effective at preventing stroke than other antihypertensive drugs (Lindholm, Carlberg, and Samuelsson 2005), a finding that has led to calls for a change of the endorsement of β-blockers as a first-line drug for the treatment of uncomplicated high blood pressure (Beevers 2005; Cushman 2007).

There is irrefutable evidence that treatment of hypertensive patients with commonly used drugs greatly reduces the risk of cardiovascular events and that the reduction in risk is proportional to the reduction in blood pressure (Psaty et al. 2003; Turnbull 2003). In randomized clinical trials, antihypertensive drugs have been associated with an average reduction of 19% to 38% in the risk of stroke, about 20% in the risk of coronary heart disease, 16% to 49% in the risk of congestive heart failure, and about 10% in the risk of overall mortality (Table 11.7) (Lindholm, Carlberg, and Samuelsson 2005; Psaty et al. 2003; Turnbull 2003). Importantly, β-blockers and Ang II type I receptor blockers do not seem to prevent heart attacks or to reduce mortality, and calcium antagonists may increase the risk of congestive heart failure, although the increase was not statistically significant (Table 11.7). In addition, reducing SBP by 12 mmHg over 10 years results in preventing one death for every 25, 20, and 10 treated patients with stage 1, 2, and 3 hypertension (JNC VI) without additional risk factors, respectively. The number of patients needed to treat decreases to 10, 9, and 8 in patients with similar blood pressure and target organ damage, cardiovascular disease, or diabetes (Ogden et al. 2000).

In spite of the proven benefit of blood pressure lowering, current rates of high blood pressure treatment and control are well below the U.S. *2010 Healthy People* goal of 50%. Currently, 61.1% of the hypertensive men and 67.9% of the hypertensive women are receiving pharmacological treatment (NHANES 1999–2004), but only 38% of all hypertensive people have their blood pressure controlled (<140/90 mmHg), 36% of women

Table 11.7. Effects of Pharmacological Interventions to Reduced Blood Pressure, Ascertained in Randomized Placebo-Controlled Trials

Intervention	% Reduction in Risk of Outcome					
	Stroke	CHD	CHF	CV Events	CV Deaths	Total Mortality
Diuretics (Psaty et al. 2003)	29	21	49	24	19	10
β-Blockers (Lindholm, Carlberg, and Samuaelsson 2005)	19	7[a]	–	–	–	5[a]
Angiotensin converting enzyme inhibitors (Turnbull 2003)	28	20	18	22	20	12
Calcium antagonists (Turnbull 2003)	38	22	21[a]	18	22	11
Angiotensin II type I receptor blockers (Turnbull 2003)	21	4[a]	16	10	4[a]	6[a]

[a]Not statistically significant.

Note: CHD = coronary heart disease; CHF = congestive heart failure; CV = cardiovascular.

and 39% of men. Blood pressure control is considerably more likely in persons who are receiving antihypertensive drugs (57%) (Ong et al. 2007), but still far from ideal. In a multivariate analysis, the probability of being treated increased significantly with age, in men (5%; p=.04), in African Americans (11%; p=.03), and in 2003–2004 as compared to 1999–2000 (13%; p=.03). Also, the probability of having blood pressure controlled increased progressively with age, but the rate of increase decreased after age 70 years. Sex was not associated with blood pressure control, but Hispanics were 16% less likely to be have their blood pressure controlled (p=.04) and the blood pressure control rate increased 28% from 1999–2000 to 2003–2004 (p=.004). These results are consistent with those from Ong et al. (2007).

Failure by patients to use medications as prescribed is a major contributor to poor blood pressure control. Studies based on pharmacy claims databases have shown that

32% to 53% of newly treated hypertensive patients stop using their medication by the end of the first year of treatment (Bourgault et al. 2005; Perreault et al. 2005). In a study based on NHANES data, stopping treatment (nonpersistence) was 12 times higher in patients younger than 30 years than in those ≥50 years old ($p<.001$), 31% higher in men than in women ($p=.01$), and 43% higher in Hispanics, as compared with other racial groups ($p=.03$) (Bautista 2008). Moreover, nonpersistence rates were almost twice as high in patients with low income ($p<.001$) and those without insurance ($p<.001$), and 10 times as high in patients who did not visit their doctor during the last year ($p<.001$).

Prevention at the Population Level

Primary prevention at the population level complements the detection and treatment of high blood pressure at the individual level. The aim of public health interventions is to lower the average blood pressure in the whole population. Even modest decreases in the average blood pressure can delay the onset of high blood pressure and substantially reduce hypertension-related morbidity and mortality. Using data from observational studies and clinical trials, Cook et al. have shown that a reduction of 2 mmHg in the average DBP in the U.S. population would result in a 17% decrease in the prevalence of high blood pressure, a 6% lower risk of coronary heart disease, and a 15% lower risk of stroke (Cook et al. 1995). Because the number of persons with normal blood pressure is considerably larger than the number of hypertensive persons, a greater number of prevented cases should occur in the first group. Therefore, from a public health point of view, it is useful to focus efforts toward the lowering of blood pressure not only in hypertensive and prehypertensive people, but also in individuals with blood pressure within the "normal range" (MacMahon 2000; van den Hoogen et al. 2000).

Lifestyle modifications recommended for primary prevention in individuals are also recommended as interventions to reduce blood pressure in the general population (Whelton et al. 2002a). During the last few decades, community-based programs have been effective means to raise awareness, increase knowledge, and promote lifestyle changes to improve blood pressure control (Kotchen 2007). Community-based demonstration projects funded by the National Heart, Lung, and Blood Institute (NHLBI) in the 1970s and early 1980s tested different educational strategies and showed significant but inconsistent reductions in average blood pressure (Welch and Hill 2002). In 1972, the NHLBI established the National High Blood Pressure Education Program as a cooperative effort to translate research into practice. This program has developed and promulgated several guidelines for the evaluation and management of high blood pressure. Although there has been no empiric evaluation of the National Program, since its inception, there has been a large increase in public and professional knowledge on high blood pressure.

A framework for prevention of high blood pressure was set by the U.S. Department of Health and Human Services (USDHHS 2008) as part of *Healthy People 2010*. Two main blood pressure–related goals were to reduce the prevalence of high blood pressure to 16% and to increase the proportion of adults with controlled hypertension to 50% by 2010. It is now obvious that these goals will not be achievable by that time. More prevention efforts are clearly needed. Improved access to care, additional education of health care professionals and the general public, promoting adherence to drug treatment, providing support for those attempting to change their lifestyle, and reducing the burden and obstacles associated with those changes are essential for making progress in the prevention of high blood pressure.

Resources

American Heart Association, http://www.americanheart.org/presenter.jhtml?identifier=1200000.
American Society of Hypertension, http://www.ash-us.org.
Centers for Disease Control, High Blood Pressure Program, http://www.cdc.gov/bloodpressure/index.htm.
National Heart, Lung, and Blood Institute, http://www.nhlbi.nih.gov.
British Hypertension Society, http://www.bhsoc.org/default.stm.

Suggested Reading

Chobanian, A.V., G.L. Bakris, H.R. Black, et al. Seventh Report of the Joint National Committee on Prevention, Detection, Evaluation, and Treatment of High Blood Pressure. *Hypertension* (2003):42:1206–1252.
Cushman, W.C. JNC-7 Guidelines: Are They Still Relevant? *Curr. Hypertens Rep.* (2007):9:380–386.
Hajjar, I., and T.A. Kotchen. Trends in Prevalence, Awareness, Treatment, and Control of Hypertension in the United States, 1988–2000. *JAMA* (2003):290:199–206.
Kearney, P.M., M. Whelton, K. Reynolds, P. Muntner, P.K. Whelton, and J. He. Global Burden of Hypertension: Analysis of Worldwide Data. *Lancet* (2005):365:217–223.
Lewington, S., R. Clarke, N. Qizilbash, R. Peto, R. Collins, and the Prospective Studies Collaboration. Age-Specific Relevance of Usual Blood Pressure to Vascular Mortality: A Meta-analysis of Individual Data for One Million Adults in 61 Prospective Studies. *Lancet* (2002):360:1903–1913.
Ong, K.L., B.M. Cheung, Y.B. Man, C.P. Lau, and K.S. Lam. Prevalence, Awareness, Treatment, and Control of Hypertension among United States Adults 1999–2004. *Hypertension* (2007):49:69–75.
Staessen, J.A., J. Wang, G. Bianchi, and W.H. Birkenhager. Essential Hypertension. *Lancet* (2003):361:1629–1641.
Whelton, P.K., J. He, L.J. Appel, et al. Primary Prevention of Hypertension: Clinical and Public Health Advisory from The National High Blood Pressure Education Program. *JAMA* (2002):288:1882–1888.

References

Appel, L.J., T.J. Moore, E. Obarzanek, et al. A Clinical Trial of the Effects of Dietary Patterns on Blood Pressure. DASH Collaborative Research Group. *N Engl J Med* (1997):336:1117–1124.
Appel, L.J., M.W. Brands, S.R. Daniels, et al. Dietary Approaches to Prevent and Treat Hypertension: A Scientific Statement from the American Heart Association. *Hypertension* (2006):47:296–308.
Ascherio, A., E.B. Rimm, E.L. Giovannucci, et al. A Prospective Study of Nutritional Factors and Hypertension among US Men. *Circulation* (1992):86:1475–1484.
Ascherio, A., C. Hennekens, W.C. Willett, et al. Prospective Study of Nutritional Factors, Blood Pressure, and Hypertension among US Women. *Hypertension* (1996):27:1065–1072.
Bautista, L.E. Predictors of Persistence with Antihypertensive Therapy: Results from the NHANES. *Am J Hypertens* (2008):21:183–188.
Bazzano, L.A., J. He, and P. Whelton. Blood Pressure in Westernized and Isolated Populations. In: Lip, G. Y. H. and J. E. Hall, editors, *Comprehensive Hypertension*. Philadelphia, PA: Mosby Elsevier (2007):21–30.

Beevers, D.G. The End of Beta Blockers for Uncomplicated Hypertension? *Lancet* (2005):366:1510–1512.

Black, H.R. The Paradigm has Shifted, to Systolic Blood Pressure. *Hypertension* (1999):34:386–387.

Bourgault, C., M. Senecal, M. Brisson, M.A. Marentette, and J.P. Gregoire. Persistence and Discontinuation Patterns of Antihypertensive Therapy among Newly Treated Patients: A Population-Based Study. *J Hum Hypertens* (2005):19:607–613.

Bowman, T.S., J.M. Graziano, C.S. Kase, H.D. Sesso, and T. Kurth. Blood Pressure Measures and Risk of Total, Ischemic, and Hemorrhagic Stroke in Men. *Neurology* (2006):67:820–823.

Burt, V.L., J.A. Cutler, M. Higgins, et al. Trends in the Prevalence, Awareness, Treatment, and Control of Hypertension in the Adult US Population. Data from the Health Examination Surveys, 1960 to 1991. *Hypertension* (1995):26:60–69.

Chae, C.U., M.A. Pfeffer, R.J. Glynn, G.F. Mitchell, J.O. Taylor, and C.H. Hennekens. Increased Pulse Pressure and Risk of Heart Failure in the Elderly. *JAMA* (1999):281:634–639.

Chobanian, A.V., G.L. Bakris, H.R. Black, et al. Seventh Report of the Joint National Committee on Prevention, Detection, Evaluation, and Treatment of High Blood Pressure. *Hypertension* (2003):42:1206–1252.

Cook, N.R., J. Cohen, P.R. Herbert, J.O. Taylor, and C.H. Hennekens. Implications of Small Reductions in Diastolic Blood Pressure for Primary Prevention. *Arch Intern Med* (1995):155:701–709.

Cushman, W.C. JNC-7 Guidelines: Are They Still Relevant? *Curr Hypertens Rep* (2007):9:380–386.

Cutler, J.A., D. Follmann, and P.S. Allender. Randomized Trials of Sodium Reduction: An Overview. *Am J Clin Nutr* (1997):65:643S–651S.

D'Agostino, R.B., Sr., S. Grundy, L.M. Sullivan, P. Wilson, and the CHD Risk Prediction Group. Validation of the Framingham Coronary Heart Disease Prediction Scores: Results of a Multiple Ethnic Groups Investigation. *JAMA* (2001):286:180–187.

Dyer, A.R., P. Elliot, M. Shipley, R. Stamler, and J. Stamler. Body Mass Index and Associations of Sodium and Potassium with Blood Pressure in INTERSALT. *Hypertension* (1994):23:729–736.

Dyer, A.R., K. Liu, M. Walsh, C. Kiefe, D.R. Jacobs, Jr., and D.E. Bild. Ten-Year Incidence of Elevated Blood Pressure and Its Predictors: The CARDIA Study. Coronary Artery Risk Development in (Young) Adults. *J Hum Hypertens* (1999):13:13–21.

Fagard, R.H. Exercise Characteristics and the Blood Pressure Response to Dynamic Physical Training. *Med Sci Sports Exerc* (2001):33:S484–S492.

Field, A.E., E.H. Coakley, A. Must, et al. Impact of Overweight on the Risk of Developing Common Chronic Diseases During a 10-Year Period. *Arch Intern Med* (2001):161:1581–1586.

Folsom, A.R., R.J. Prineas, S.A. Kaye, and R.G. Munger. Incidence of Hypertension and Stroke in Relation to Body Fat Distribution and Other Risk Factors in Older Women. *Stroke* (1990):21:701–706.

Fox, C.S., M.G. Larson, E.P. Leip, B. Culleton, P.W. Wilson, and D. Levy. Predictors of New-Onset Kidney Disease in a Community-Based Population. *JAMA* (2004):291:844–850.

Franklin, S.S., M.G. Larson, S.A. Khan, et al. Does the Relation of Blood Pressure to Coronary Heart Disease Risk Change with Aging? The Framingham Heart Study. *Circulation* (2001):103:1245–1249.

Fuchs, F.D., L.E. Chambless, P.K. Whelton, F.J. Nieto, and G. Heiss. Alcohol Consumption and the Incidence of Hypertension: The Atherosclerosis Risk in Communities Study. *Hypertension* (2001):37:1242–1250.

Gallen, I.W., R.M. Rosa, D.Y. Esparaz, et al. On the Mechanism of the Effects of Potassium Restriction on Blood Pressure and Renal Sodium Retention. *Am J Kidney Dis* (1998):31:19–27.

Geleijnse, J.M., F.J. Kok, and D.E. Grobbee. Blood Pressure Response to Changes in Sodium and Potassium Intake: A Metaregression Analysis of Randomised Trials. *J Hum Hypertens* (2003):17:471–480.

Goff, D.C., G. Howard, G.B. Russell, and D.R. Labarthe. Birth Cohort Evidence of Population Influences on Blood Pressure in the United States, 1887–1994. *Ann Epidemiol* (2001):11: 271–279.

Guidelines Sub-Committee of WHO/ISH Mild Hypertension Liaison Committee. Summary of 1993 WHO/ISH Guidelines for the Management of Mild Hypertension: Memorandum from a WHO/ISH Meeting. Guidelines Sub-Committee of WHO/ISH Mild Hypertension Liaison Committee. *Clin Exp Pharmacol Physiol* (1993):20:801–808.

Haapanen, N., S. Milunpalo, I. Vuori, P. Oja, and M. Pasanen. Association of Leisure Time Physical Activity with the Risk of Coronary Heart Disease, Hypertension and Diabetes in Middle-Aged Men and Women. *Int J Epidemiol* (1997):26:739–747.

Haider, A.W., M.G. Larson, S.S. Franklin, and D. Levy. Systolic Blood Pressure, Diastolic Blood Pressure, and Pulse Pressure as Predictors of Risk for Congestive Heart Failure in the Framingham Heart Study. *Ann Intern Med* (2003):138:10–16.

Hajjar, I., and T.A. Kotchen. Trends in Prevalence, Awareness, Treatment, and Control of Hypertension in the United States, 1988–2000. *JAMA* (2003):290:199–206.

Haroun, M.K., B.G. Jaar, S.C. Hoffman, G.W. Comstock, M.J. Klag, and J. Coresh. Risk Factors for Chronic Kidney Disease: A Prospective Study of 23,534 Men and Women in Washington County, Maryland. *J Am Soc Nephrol* (2003):14:2934–2941.

Harrap, S.B., M. Stebbing, J.L. Hopper, H.N. Hoang, and G.G. Giles. Familial Patterns of Co-variation for Cardiovascular Risk Factors in Adults: The Victorian Family Heart Study. *Am J Epidemiol* (2000):152:704–715.

He, F.J., and G.A. MacGregor. Effect of Longer-Term Modest Salt Reduction on Blood Pressure. *Cochrane Database Syst Rev* (2004):CD004937.

He, J., P.K. Whelton, L.J. Appel, J. Charleston, and M.J. Klag. Long-Term Effects of Weight Loss and Dietary Sodium Reduction on Incidence of Hypertension. *Hypertension* (2000):35:544–549.

Hopkins, P.N., and S.C. Hunt. Genetics of Hypertension. *Genet Med* (2003):5:413–429.

Hsia, J., K.L. Margolis, C.B. Eaton, et al. Prehypertension and Cardiovascular Disease Risk in the Women's Health Initiative. *Circulation* (2007):115:855–860.

Hsu, C.Y., C.E. McCulloch, J. Darbinian, A.S. Go, and C. Iribarren. Elevated Blood Pressure and Risk of End-Stage Renal Disease in Subjects Without Baseline Kidney Disease. *Arch Intern Med* (2005):165:923–928.

Hu, G., N.C. Barengo, J. Tuomilehto, T.A. Lakka, A. Nissinen, P. Jousilahti. Relationship of Physical Activity and Body Mass Index to the Risk of Hypertension: A Prospective Study in Finland. *Hypertension* (2004):43:25–30.

Inoue, R., T. Ohkubo, M. Kikuya, et al. Predicting Stroke Using 4 Ambulatory Blood Pressure Monitoring-Derived Blood Pressure Indices: The Ohasama Study. *Hypertension* (2006):48:877–882.

Joint National Committee on Detection, Evaluation, and Treatment of High Blood Pressure. Report of the Joint National Committee on Detection, Evaluation, and Treatment of High Blood Pressure. A Cooperative Study. *JAMA* (1977):237:255–261.

Joint National Committee on Detection, Evaluation, and Treatment of High Blood Pressure. The Fifth Report of the Joint National Committee on Detection, Evaluation, and Treatment of High Blood Pressure (JNC V). *Arch Intern Med* (1993):154–183.

Joint National Committee on Detection, Evaluation, and Treatment of High Blood Pressure. The 1988 report of the Joint National Committee on Detection, Evaluation, and Treatment of High Blood Pressure. *Arch Intern Med* (1988):148(5):1023–1038.

Joint National Committee on Prevention, Detection, Evaluation, and Treatment of High Blood Pressure. *The Sixth Report of the Joint National Committee on Prevention, Detection, Evaluation, and Treatment of High Blood Pressure*. Bethesda, MD. National Institutes of Health (1997).

Jones, D.W., L.E. Chambless, A.R. Folsom, et al. Risk Factors for Coronary Heart Disease in African Americans: The Atherosclerosis Risk in Communities Study, 1987–1997. *Arch Intern Med* (2002):162:2565–2571.

Kannel, W.B. Blood Pressure as a Cardiovascular Risk Factor: Prevention and Treatment. *JAMA* (1996):275:1571–1576.

Kannel, W.B., T. Gordon, and M.J. Schwartz. Systolic Versus Diastolic Blood Pressure and Risk of Coronary Heart Disease. The Framingham study. *Am J Cardiol* (1971):27:335–346.

Kannel, W.B., K. Ho, and T. Thom. Changing Epidemiological Features of Cardiac Failure. *Br Heart J* (1994):72:S3–S9.

Kannel, W.B., P.A. Wolf, D.L. McGee, T.R. Dawber, P. McNamara, and W.P. Castelli. Systolic Blood Pressure, Arterial Rigidity, and Risk of Stroke. The Framingham Study. *JAMA* (1981):245:1225–1229.

Katzmarzyk, P.T., T. Rankinen, L. Perusse, R.M. Malina, and C. Brouchard. 7-Year Stability of Blood Pressure in the Canadian population. *Prev Med* (2000):31:403–409.

Kearney, P.M., M. Whelton, K. Reynolds, P. Muntner, P.K. Whelton, and J. He. Global Burden of Hypertension: Analysis of Worldwide Data. *Lancet* (2005):365:217–223.

Khaw, K.-T., S. Bingham, A. Welch, et al. Blood Pressure and Urinary Sodium in Men and Women: The Norfolk Cohort of the European Prospective Investigation into Cancer (EPIC-Norfolk). *Am J Clin Nutr* (2004):80:1397–1403.

Kittner, S.J., L.R. White, K.G. Losonczy, P.A. Wolf, and J.R. Hebel. Black–White Differences in Stroke Incidence in a National Sample. The Contribution of Hypertension and Diabetes Mellitus. *JAMA* (1990):264:1267–1270.

Klag, M.J., P.K. Whelton, B.L. Randall, et al. Blood Pressure and End-Stage Renal Disease in Men. *N Engl J Med* (1996):334:13–18.

Klag, M.J., P.K. Whelton, B.L. Randall, J.D. Neaton, F.L. Brancati, and J. Stamler. End-Stage Renal Disease in African-American and White Men. 16-Year MRFIT Findings. *JAMA* (1997):277:1293–1298.

Kotchen, T.A. Hypertension Control: Trends, Approaches, and Goals. *Hypertension* (2007):49:19–20.

Kurella, M., J.C. Lo, and G.M. Chertow. Metabolic Syndrome and the Risk for Chronic Kidney Disease among Nondiabetic Adults. *J Am Soc Nephrol* (2005):16:2134–2140.

Lawes, C.M., D.A. Bennett, V.L. Feigin, and A. Rodgers. Blood Pressure and Stroke: An Overview of Published Reviews. *Stroke* (2004):35:1024.

Leitschuh, M., L.A. Cupples, W. Kannel, D. Gagnon, and A. Chobanian. High-Normal Blood Pressure Progression to Hypertension in the Framingham Heart Study. *Hypertension* (1991):17:22–27.

Levenstein, S., M.W. Smith, and G.A. Kaplan. Psychosocial Predictors of Hypertension in Men and Women. *Arch Intern Med* (2001):161:1341–1346.

Levey, A.S., J. Coresh, E. Balk, et al. National Kidney Foundation Practice Guidelines for Chronic Kidney Disease: Evaluation, Classification, and Stratification. *Ann Intern Med* (2003):139:137–147.

Levy, D., M.G. Larson, R.S. Vasan, W.B. Kannel, and K.K. Ho. The Progression from Hypertension to Congestive Heart Failure. *JAMA* (1996):275:1557–1562.

Lewington, S., R. Clarke, N. Qizilbash, R. Peto, R. Collins, and the Prospective Studies Collaboration. Age-Specific Relevance of Usual Blood Pressure to Vascular Mortality: A Meta-Analysis of Individual Data for One Million Adults in 61 Prospective Studies. *Lancet* (2002):360:1903–1913.

Li, C., G. Engstrom, B. Hedblad, G. Berglund, and L. Janzon. Blood Pressure Control and Risk of Stroke: A Population-Based Prospective Cohort Study. *Stroke* (2005):36:725–730.

Lichtenstein, A.H., L.J. Appel, M. Brands, et al. Diet and Lifestyle Recommendations Revision 2006: A Scientific Statement from the American Heart Association Nutrition Committee. *Circulation* (2006):114:82–96.

Lindholm, L.H., B. Carlberg, and O. Samuelsson. Should Beta Blockers Remain First Choice in the Treatment of Primary Hypertension? A Meta-Analysis. *Lancet* (2005):366:1545–1553.

MacMahon, S. Blood Pressure and the Risk of Cardiovascular Disease. *N Engl J Med* (2000):342:50–52.

MacMahon, S., R. Peto, J. Cutler, et al. Blood Pressure, Stroke, and Coronary Heart Disease. Part 1, Prolonged Differences in Blood Pressure: Prospective Observational Studies Corrected for the Regression Dilution Bias. *Lancet* (1990):335:765–774.

Mancia, G., G. Backer, A. Dominiczak, et al. 2007 Guidelines for the Management of Arterial Hypertension: The Task Force for the Management of Arterial Hypertension of the European Society of Hypertension (ESH) and of the European Society of Cardiology (ESC). *J Hypertens* (2007):25:1105–1187.

Marmot, M.G., P. Elliot, M.J. Shipley, et al. Alcohol and Blood Pressure: The INTERSALT Study. *BMJ* (1994):308:1263–1267.

McFadden, C.B., C.M. Brensinger, J.A. Berlin, and R.R. Townsend. Systematic Review of the Effect of Daily Alcohol Intake on Blood Pressure. *Am J Hypertens* (2005):18:276–286.

McNeill, A.M., R. Katz, C.J. Girman, et al. Metabolic Syndrome and Cardiovascular Disease in Older People: The Cardiovascular Health Study. *J Am Geriatr Soc* (2006):54:1317–1324.

Mentari, E., and M. Rahman. Blood Pressure and Progression of Chronic Kidney Disease: Importance of Systolic, Diastolic, or Diurnal Variation. *Curr Hypertens Rep* (2004):6:400–404.

Morris, R.C., Jr., A. Sebastian, A. Forman, M. Tanaka, and O. Schmidlin. Normotensive Salt Sensitivity: Effects of Race and Dietary Potassium. *Hypertension* (1999):33:18–23.

Mulrow, C.D., E. Chiquette, L. Angel, et al. Dieting to Reduce Body Weight for Controlling Hypertension in Adults. *Cochrane Database Syst Rev* (2000):CD000484.

National Center for Health Statistics (NCHS), Centers for Disease Control and Prevention. *Analytic and Reporting Guidelines. The National Health and Nutrition Examination Survey (NHANES). National Center for Health Statistics Centers for Disease Control and Prevention* (2006). Available at http://www.cdc.gov/nchs/about/major/nhanes/nhanes2003-2004/analytical_guidelines.htm. Accessed April 16, 2008.

National Center for Health Statistics (NCHS), Centers for Disease Control and Prevention. *Analytic and Reporting Guidelines: The Third National Health and Nutrition Examination Survey, NHANES III (1988–94). National Center for Health Statistics, Centers for Disease Control and Prevention* (1996). Available at http://www.cdc.gov/nchs/about/major/nhanes/nhanes2003-2004/analytical_guidelines.htm. Accessed April 16, 2008.

Neter, J.E., B.E. Stam, F.J. Kok, D.E. Grobbee, and J.M. Geleijnse. Influence of Weight Reduction on Blood Pressure: A Meta-Analysis of Randomized Controlled Trials. *Hypertension* (2003):42:878–884.

Nielsen, W.B., E. Lindenstrom, J. Vestbo, and G.B. Jensen. Is Diastolic Hypertension an Independent Risk Factor for Stroke in the Presence of Normal Systolic Blood Pressure in the Middle-Aged and Elderly? *Am J Hypertens* (1997):10:634–639.

Ogden, L.G., J. He, E. Lydick, and P.K. Whelton. Long-Term Absolute Benefit of Lowering Blood Pressure in Hypertensive Patients According to the JNC VI Risk Stratification. *Hypertension* (2000):35:539–543.

Ohira, T., E. Shahar, L.E. Chambless, W.D. Rosamond, T.H. Mosley, Jr., and A.R. Folsom. Risk Factors for Ischemic Stroke Subtypes: The Atherosclerosis Risk in Communities Study. *Stroke* (2006):37:2493–2498.

Ong, K.L., B.M. Cheung, Y.B. Man, C.P. Lau, and K.S. Lam. Prevalence, Awareness, Treatment, and Control of Hypertension among United States Adults 1999–2004. *Hypertension* (2007):49:69–75.

Otiniano, M.E., X.L. Du, M.R. Maldonado, L. Ray, and K. Markides. Effect of Metabolic Syndrome on Heart Attack and Mortality in Mexican-American Elderly Persons: Findings of 7-Year Follow-up from the Hispanic Established Population for the Epidemiological Study of the Elderly. *J Gerontol A Biol Sci Med Sci* (2005):60:466–470.

Pereira, M.A., A.R. Folsom, P.G. McGovern, et al. Physical Activity and Incident Hypertension in Black and White Adults: The Atherosclerosis Risk in Communities Study. *Prev Med* (1999):28:304–312.

Perreault, S., D. Lamarre, L. Blais, et al. Persistence with Treatment in Newly Treated Middle-Aged Patients with Essential Hypertension. *Ann Pharmacother* (2005):39:1401–1408.

Pickering, T.G., J.E. Hall, L.J. Appel, et al. Recommendations for Blood Pressure Measurement in Humans and Experimental Animals: Part 1: Blood Pressure Measurement in Humans: A Statement for Professionals from the Subcommittee of Professional and Public Education of the American Heart Association Council on High Blood Pressure Research. *Circulation* (2005):111: 697–716.

Psaty, B.M., C.D. Furberg, L.H. Culler, et al. Association Between Blood Pressure Level and the Risk of Myocardial Infarction, Stroke, and Total Mortality: The Cardiovascular Health Study. *Arch Intern Med* (2001):161:1183–1192.

Psaty, B.M., T. Lumley, C.D. Furberg, et al. Health Outcomes Associated with Various Antihypertensive Therapies Used as First-Line Agents: A Network Meta-Analysis. *JAMA* (2003):289:2534–2544.

Qureshi, A.I., M.F.K. Suri, Y. Mohammad, L.R. Guterman, and L.N. Hopkins. Isolated and Borderline Isolated Systolic Hypertension Relative to Long-Term Risk and Type of Stroke: A 20-Year Follow-up of the National Health and Nutrition Survey. *Stroke* (2002):33:2781–2788.

Rosamond, W., K. Flegal, G. Friday, et al. Heart Disease and Stroke Statistics—2007 Update: A Report from the American Heart Association Statistics Committee and Stroke Statistics Subcommittee. *Circulation* (2007):115:e69–e171.

Rosendorff, C., H.R. Black, C.P. Cannon, et al. Treatment of Hypertension in the Prevention and Management of Ischemic Heart Disease: A Scientific Statement from the American Heart Association Council for High Blood Pressure Research and the Councils on Clinical Cardiology and Epidemiology and Prevention. *Circulation* (2007):115:2761–2788.

Sacks, F.M., L.P. Svetkey, W.M. Vollmer, et al. Effects on Blood Pressure of Reduced Dietary Sodium and the Dietary Approaches to Stop Hypertension (DASH) Diet. DASH-Sodium Collaborative Research Group. *N Engl J Med* (2001):344:3–10.

Sesso, H.D., N.R. Cook, J.E. Buring, J.E. Manson, and J.M. Graziano. Alcohol Consumption and the Risk of Hypertension in Women and Men. *Hypertension* (2008):51:1080–1087.

Staessen, J.A., J. Wang, G. Bianchi, and W.H. Birkenhager. Essential Hypertension. *Lancet* (2003):361:1629–1641.

Stamler, J. The INTERSALT Study: Background, Methods, Findings, and Implications. *Am J Clin Nutr* (1997):65:626S–642S.

Stamler, R. Implications of the INTERSALT Study. *Hypertension* (1991):17:I16–I20.

Svetkey, L.P., D. Simons-Morton, W.M. Vollmer, et al. Effects of Dietary Patterns on Blood Pressure: Subgroup Analysis of the Dietary Approaches to Stop Hypertension (DASH) Randomized Clinical Trial. *Arch Intern Med* (1999):159:285–293.

Szklo, M., and F.J. Nieto. *Epidemiology: Beyond the Basics*. Sudbury, MA: Jones and Barlett Publishers (2007):85–88.

Turnbull, F. Effects of Different Blood-Pressure–Lowering Regimens on Major Cardiovascular Events: Results of Prospectively-Designed Overviews of Randomised Trials. *Lancet* (2003):362:1527–1535.

U.S. Department of Health and Human Services (USDHHS). *Healthy People 2010* (2008). Available at http://www.healthypeople.gov/. Accessed on April 16, 2008.

U.S. Preventive Services Task Force. Screening for High Blood Pressure: U.S. Preventive Services Task Force Reaffirmation Recommendation Statement. *Ann Intern Med* (2007):147:783–786.

Vaccarino, V., T.R. Holford, and H.M. Krumholz. Pulse Pressure and Risk for Myocardial Infarction and Heart Failure in the Elderly. *J Am Coll Cardiol* (2000):36:130–138.

van den Hoogen, P.C., E.J. Feskens, N.J. Nagelkerke, A. Menotti, A. Nissinen, and D. Kromhout. The Relation Between Blood Pressure and Mortality Due to Coronary Heart Disease among Men in Different Parts of the World. Seven Countries Study Research Group. *N Engl J Med* (2000):342:1–8.

Vasan, R.S., M.G. Larson, E.P. Leip, et al. Impact of High-Normal Blood Pressure on the Risk of Cardiovascular Disease. *N Engl J Med* (2001a):345:1291–1297.

Vasan, R.S., M.G. Larson, E.P. Leip, W.B. Kannel, and D. Levy. Assessment of Frequency of Progression to Hypertension in Non-Hypertensive Participants in the Framingham Heart Study: A Cohort Study. *Lancet* (2001b):358:1682–1686.

Vasan, R.S., A. Beiser, S. Seshadri, et al. Residual Lifetime Risk for Developing Hypertension in Middle-Aged Women and Men: The Framingham Heart Study. *JAMA* (2002):287:1003–1010.

Wei, M., B.D. Mitchell, S.M. Haffner, and M.P. Stem. Effects of Cigarette Smoking, Diabetes, High Cholesterol, and Hypertension on All-Cause Mortality and Cardiovascular Disease Mortality in Mexican Americans. The San Antonio Heart Study. *Am J Epidemiol* (1996):144:1058–1065.

Welch, V.L., and M.N. Hill. Effective Strategies for Blood Pressure Control. *Cardiol Clin* (2002): 20:321–333, vii.

Whelton, P.K. Epidemiology of Hypertension. *Lancet* (1994):344:101–106.

Whelton, P.K., J. He, J.A. Cutler, et al. Effects of Oral Potassium on Blood Pressure. Meta-Analysis of Randomized Controlled Clinical Trials. *JAMA* (1997):277:1624–1632.

Whelton, P.K., L.J. Appel, M.A. Espeland, et al. Sodium Reduction and Weight Loss in the Treatment of Hypertension in Older Persons: A Randomized Controlled Trial of Nonpharmacologic Interventions in the Elderly (TONE). TONE Collaborative Research Group. *JAMA* (1998):279:839–846.

Whelton, P.K., J. He, L.J. Appel, et al. Primary Prevention of Hypertension: Clinical and Public Health Advisory from The National High Blood Pressure Education Program. *JAMA* (2002a):288:1882–1888.

Whelton, S.P., A. Chin, X. Xin, and J. He. Effect of Aerobic Exercise on Blood Pressure: A Meta-Analysis of Randomized, Controlled Trials. *Ann Intern Med* (2002b):136:493–503.

Williams, S.A., S.V. Kasl, A. Heiat, J.L. Abramson, H.M. Krumholz, and V. Vaccarino. Depression and Risk of Heart Failure among the Elderly: A Prospective Community-Based Study. *Psychosom Med* (2002):64:6–12.

Winegarden, C.R. From "Prehypertension" to Hypertension? Additional Evidence. *Ann Epidemiol* (2005):15:720–725.

Wolf-Maier, K., R.S. Cooper, J.R. Banegas, et al. Hypertension Prevalence and Blood Pressure Levels in 6 European Countries, Canada, and the United States. *JAMA* (2003):289:2363–2369.

World Health Organization (WHO). The World Health Report 2002. *Reducing Risks, Promoting Healthy Life.* Geneva, Switzerland: World Health Organization (2002).

Xin, X., J. He, M.G. Frontini, L.G. Ogden, O.I. Motsamai, and P.K. Whelton. Effects of Alcohol Reduction on Blood Pressure: A Meta-Analysis of Randomized Controlled Trials. *Hypertension* (2001):38:1112–1117.

CHAPTER 12

HIGH BLOOD CHOLESTEROL (ICD-10 E78.0–E78.5)

Heather M. Johnson, M.D. and Patrick E. McBride, M.D., M.P.H.

Introduction

Multiple longitudinal studies demonstrate that elevated serum cholesterol is a major risk factor for atherosclerosis and coronary heart disease (CHD) (Figure 12.1). Cardiovascular disease remains the number one cause of death in the United States for men and women (Kannel et al. 1971; NCEP 1990, 2002). High blood cholesterol or hypercholesterolemia is defined as a total serum cholesterol of ≥240 mg/dL. The relationship between total serum cholesterol and the risk of CHD is continuous and graded (Stamler 1986) and even borderline elevations are associated with an increased risk of atherosclerosis and CHD (Kannel et al. 1971; NCEP 1990, 2002).

Significance

A large percentage of Americans are at risk for CHD due to hypercholesterolemia. According to the 2001–2004 Third National Health and Nutrition Examination Survey (NHANES), 16.5% of the U.S. population ages 20–74 years have high serum cholesterol, and the mean U.S. total cholesterol is 202 mg/dL (National Center for Health Statistics 2006). The public health burden from hypercholesterolemia results from the health and economic consequences of CHD, as well as other atherosclerotic diseases. High blood cholesterol is thought to account for 20–30% of CHD in the United States (NCEP 2002). In addition, considerable health care resources are required for the screening and treatment of persons with hypercholesterolemia.

Pathophysiology and Genetics

Cholesterol is insoluble in water and is therefore transported in the blood in complex particles called lipoproteins, which are a combination of the cholesterol lipid and apoproteins. The apoproteins on the surface act as ligands for receptors on cells in the body and make lipoproteins water soluble by creating a hydrophilic composition of the surface layer of the particle (Stone 2005). There are four major classes of lipoprotein particles.

- Low-density lipoprotein (LDL) carries most of the cholesterol ester and is pivotal to atherosclerotic development
- Very low-density lipoprotein (VLDL) is composed mainly of triglycerides
- Intermediate density lipoprotein (IDL) transports both cholesterol and triglycerides

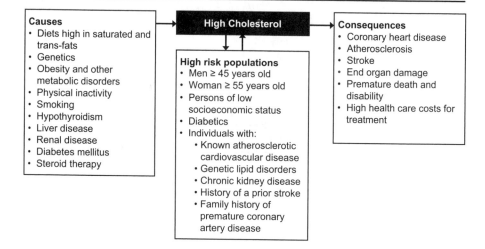

Figure 12.1. High cholesterol: causes, consequences, and high-risk groups.

- High-density lipoprotein (HDL) transports cholesterol to be removed from the body via a process called "reverse cholesterol transport" (Fuster et al. 2005). There is an inverse relationship between HDL cholesterol and CHD risk (NCEP 2002).

Cholesterol is necessary for the human body to function normally. However, when there is an excess of cholesterol, it accumulates in the arterial walls, initiating atherosclerosis development (Ross 1999). This can progress to plaque development and arterial thrombosis, resulting in a vascular event (Fuster et al. 2005). Fatty streaks are the earliest atherosclerotic lesions and are the result of the accumulation of lipoproteins and lipid-laden macrophages (Fuster et al. 2005). These lesions are flat or only slightly elevated and do not significantly narrow the involved artery (Fuster et al. 2005). It has been known for several decades that fatty streaks begin in early childhood and that the extent of fatty streaks in early life is directly related to levels of serum cholesterol and other risk factors (Berenson 1987; Strong et al. 1999; Newman et al. 1986). Fatty streaks progress into intermediate lesions that contain numerous lipid particles and disrupt smooth muscle cells (Fuster et al. 2005).

Fibrous plaques (atheromas) are advanced, raised lesions resulting from the accumulation of lipid deposition, macrophages, smooth muscle cells, and the proliferation of connective tissue in the arterial wall (Fuster et al. 2005; Stary et al. 1995). Cholesterol is incorporated into atherosclerotic lesions and becomes a component of plaques via complex interactions with the vessel endothelium and macrophages. These lesions generally appear in the second decade of life and are associated with serum lipoprotein concentrations (McGill et al. 1997; Solberg and Strong 1983; Stary et al. 1995).

Fibrous plaques progress in complexity and can become calcified, hemorrhage, and/or ulcerate (Stary et al. 1995). Platelet aggregation and thrombus (clot) formation can occur and become incorporated into these complicated plaques. Ultimately, thrombus formation and rupture of the plaque can result in infarction and organ damage (Fuster et al. 2005; Stary et al. 1995). Atherosclerotic lesions do not need to be stenotic to be prone to rupture; in fact, the vast majority of sudden cardiac events occur in atherosclerotic lesions that occupy less than 80% of the lumen of coronary arteries (Falk et al. 1995). Physical stress and inflammatory cascades along the thin fibrous cap of the plaque can cause rupture and precipitate an acute myocardial infarction or other vascular event (Fuster et al. 2005). These partially occluding lesions are also more likely to respond to lipid-lowering therapy that may delay and possibly reverse atherosclerotic development (Stoll and Bendszus 2006).

Damage to the endothelial lining of arteries and lipid infiltration initiates an inflammatory response that is involved in the genesis of atherosclerosis (Stoll and Bendszus 2006). The lipids contained in atherosclerotic lesions are thought to be primarily derived from oxidized LDL particles, although other lipoproteins are also atherogenic (Stoll and Bendszus 2006; Ross 1999). LDL cholesterol is delivered to cells, primarily in the liver, by a process involving the attachment of circulating LDL cholesterol to LDL receptors, which are located on the surface of the cell. The cholesterol is used by the cell for the synthesis of plasma membranes, bile acids, and steroid hormones or is stored by the cell (Stone 2005). When LDL receptor function is diminished in response to regulatory signals (such as a high saturated fat diet) or as a result of genetic defects, LDL is cleared by other mechanisms, including macrophage foam cells, which can promote atherogenesis (Stone 2005).

Epidemiologic studies have demonstrated that elevated triglyceride levels are associated with increased CHD events in both women and men (Sarwar et al. 2007). In addition, the rate of CHD risk may increase faster in women as triglyceride levels increase (LaRosa 1997). The mechanism of how increased triglycerides correlate with CHD events is unclear, although triglyceride-rich remnants are atherogenic, and high triglyceride levels are associated with other metabolic changes (Nordestgaard et al. 2007) Animal and human studies have demonstrated that elevated triglyceride and lipid levels after eating may cause foam cell formation (Bansal et al. 2007). Recent clinical trials reported that nonfasting triglyceride levels predict CHD events in both men and women, and may be a stronger independent predictor of CHD in women than fasting triglyceride levels (Nordestgaard et al. 2007; Bansal et al. 2007).

Genetic factors play an important role in determining cholesterol levels (Garg and Simha 2007). Familial hypercholesterolemia (FH) is an autosomal dominant genetic disorder marked by impaired LDL clearance, leading to greatly elevated LDL cholesterol levels (Stone 2005; McCrindle et al. 2007). Internationally, it affects approximately 10 million people (Marks et al. 2003). About 1 in every 500 persons is heterozygous for FH; the number of LDL receptors is reduced by about half in these persons, resulting in LDL cholesterol levels that are approximately twice normal. Homozygous FH occurs with a frequency of 1 per million people and results in LDL cholesterol levels that are 5 times the normal rate (Garg and Simha 2007). In these persons, advanced atherosclerosis before age 20 and premature CHD events are common (Stone 2005; Garg and Simha 2007).

Many other genetically determined abnormalities involving cholesterol metabolism have been described; the most common of these is familial-combined hyperlipidemia or combined dyslipidemia (Stone 2005). Persons with this disorder have multiple abnormalities of lipoproteins, including high LDL, high triglycerides, and low HDL (Stone 2005; Garg and Simha 2007). Low HDL (hypoalphalipoproteinemia), high lipoprotein (a), and other genetic lipid disorders are commonly noted in persons with premature CHD (Genest et al. 1992; Garg and Simha 2007).

Descriptive Epidemiology

High-Risk Populations

The populations bearing the highest risk for this condition are those with known athero-sclerotic cardiovascular disease, especially those with a prior cardiovascular or peripheral vascular event. In addition, the proportion at risk of high blood cholesterol increases with age, specifically in men ≥45 years old and women ≥55 years old (NCEP 2002). Those with diabetes mellitus, a genetic lipid disorder, chronic kidney disease, prior stroke, or a family history of premature coronary artery disease are also considered high-risk groups (NCEP 2002) (Figure 12.1).

In the United States, according to the 2006 NHANES report, Hispanic males have slightly higher rates of high blood cholesterol (17.0%) compared to Hispanic females (12.8%), white males (16.5%), and white females (16.7%) (National Center for Health Statistics 2006). Epidemiologic and early genomic research has begun to demonstrate that African ancestry is associated with slightly decreased total cholesterol, LDL cholesterol, and triglycerides compared to European ancestry (Reiner et al. 2007; LaRosa and Brown 2005).

Geographic Distribution

There have been multiple longitudinal studies evaluating the global burden of CHD and its associated risk factors. The MONICA (Multinational MONItoring of trends and de-terminants in CArdiovascular disease) Study was a 10-year longitudinal study that ended in the mid-1990s and incorporated 21 countries (WHO MONICA 1988). The study demonstrated that Beijing, China, had the lowest prevalence of hypercholesterolemia for both men and women, whereas Ticino, Switzerland, and Novi Sa, Yugoslavia, had the highest prevalence of hypercholesterolemia for men and for women, respectively (To-lonen et al. 2005; Petersen et al. 2005). More recent data has demonstrated that among European countries, Eastern Europe has the highest serum cholesterol levels (McKay et al. 2004).

The Seven Countries Study, a 25-year longitudinal study comparing populations, found a correlation between the proportion of men with serum cholesterol of more than 250 mg/dL and CHD mortality rate for the country (Worth et al. 1975) The Ni-Hon-San Study was a migration study evaluating three cohorts of Japanese men living in southern Japan, Hawaii, and San Francisco, CA. Both CHD incidence and serum cholesterol levels were higher in those who reside in San Francisco than in Hawaii, and higher in Hawaii residents than in Japan residents, which suggests a cultural contribution to increased risk of CHD (Worth et al. 1975; NCEP 1990). In addition, a study conducted in Spain has demonstrated increased serum cholesterol levels in children correlating with westerniza-tion of dietary habits (Couch et al. 2000).

Time Trends

In general, the average serum total cholesterol and prevalence of high blood cholesterol has steadily decreased in the United States since 1960, and has continued to decline re-cently in both men and women (Figure 12.2) (National Center for Health Statistics 2006;

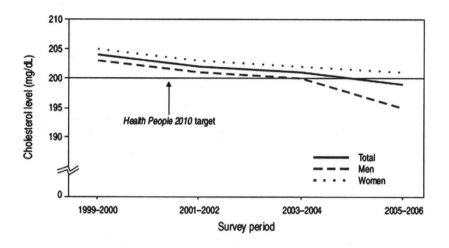

Figure 12.2. Mean cholesterol levels (mg/dL) by gender in the United States, 1999–2006.

QuickStats MMWR 2005). Between the 1960–1962 and the 2001–2004 surveys, the age-adjusted mean serum cholesterol values decreased from 220 to 201 mg/dL for men and from 224 to 201 mg/dL for women (National Center for Health Statistics 2006). This population decline in serum cholesterol levels is estimated to have contributed significantly to the decline in CHD in the United States in the past 40 years (Goldman et al. 2001; Ford et al. 2007). The mean cholesterol level has continued to decline since 2000, meeting the 2010 Objective for the Nation by 2005 (see Figure 12.2).

Causes

Modifiable Risk Factors

The most important modifiable risk factor for high blood cholesterol is dietary fat intake, specifically dietary saturated and trans fats (Figure 12.1). Recent National Institutes of Health guidelines have emphasized that there is a dose–response relationship between saturated fat intake and LDL cholesterol levels (NCEP 2002). The Seven Countries Study demonstrated that populations whose diets are substantially lower in saturated and trans fat also have decreased mean cholesterol levels and lower cardiovascular disease mortality (Kromhout et al. 1995; Menotti et al. 1999). This idea is supported by migration studies such as the Ni-Hon-San Study (Worth et al. 1975). In addition, a population's rate of CHD is related to the population intake of saturated fat (NCEP 2002). Most of the fat in human diets is in the form of fatty acids, with "medium chain" fatty acids (chain lengths of 12, 14, 16, or 18 carbons) being the most common.

These fatty acids are divided into three groups: saturated (completely saturated with hydrogen with no double bonds), monounsaturated (one double bond), and polyunsaturated (two or more double bonds). Intake of saturated fatty acids raises total serum cholesterol levels and LDL cholesterol levels by decreasing the activity of LDL receptors (Grundy and Denke 1990; Hu and Willett 2002). A high intake of dietary cholesterol also raises LDL cholesterol levels (NCEP 2002). Reviews on the association of dietary intake of cholesterol with the risk of CHD conclude that dietary cholesterol is atherogenic in humans (Stone 1996; Hu and Willett 2002). Therefore, current guidelines for cholesterol reduction focus primarily on the amount of saturated fats and dietary cholesterol in the diet.

Polyunsaturated fatty acids are of two types, omega-6 and omega-3, named based on the location of the double bond. Omega-6 polyunsaturated fatty acids are common in plant oils (corn, safflower, soybean, sunflower oils). Clinical and animal studies provide evidence that when substituted for saturated fatty acids in the diet, omega-6 polyunsaturated fatty acids result in lowering of total and LDL cholesterol, but also usually some lowering of HDL cholesterol (Hu and Willett 2002; Stone 1996). Omega-3 polyunsaturated fatty acids are common in marine fish and some plant oils. These fatty acids help to lower LDL cholesterol and triglyceride levels, in addition to decreasing coronary events (Stone 1996; Hu and Willett 2002).

Monounsaturated fatty acids are especially abundant in olive oil and canola oil (Grundy and Denke 1990; Hu and Willett 2002). Clinical studies indicate that substitution of monounsaturated for saturated fatty acids reduces serum total and LDL cholesterol without significantly reducing HDL cholesterol (Hu and Willett 2002).

Recently, there has been more evidence on the harm caused by trans fatty acids (or "trans-fats"), which get their name from the arrangement of the carbon molecules around the double bond. Trans fatty acids both raise LDL cholesterol levels and lower HDL cholesterol levels. In addition, trans fats in the diet raise triglycerides, lipoprotein (a) levels, and the total cholesterol/HDL ratio (Hu and Willett 2002; NCEP 2002).

Obesity and other metabolic disorders are associated with an increase in LDL cholesterol levels, a decrease in HDL cholesterol levels, and an increase in the fasting triglyceride levels (Baumgartner et al. 1987; Lichtenstein et al. 2006). Body mass index is positively correlated with total cholesterol levels (Lichtenstein et al. 2006; Higgins et al. 1988). Physical inactivity and smoking are associated with lower levels of HDL cholesterol and increased risk of CHD (Haskell et al. 1980; Criqui 1980; Stoll and Bendszus 2006; Pearson et al. 2003). Although alcohol use is associated with higher levels of HDL cholesterol, it is not recommended as a means for raising HDL cholesterol due to other potentially negative effects of alcohol and the risk of abuse (Stone 1996). Hypothyroidism, liver disease, renal disease, diabetes mellitus, and other metabolic disorders may also significantly affect cholesterol levels in humans (Garg and Simha 2007) (Figure 12.1).

Socioeconomic status has also been shown to affect the cholesterol profile. According to a 1999–2002 NHANES cross-sectional survey, HDL cholesterol positively correlates with income and education level after controlling for lifestyle, environmental, and genetic risk factors (Muennig et al. 2007).

Prevention and Control

Prevention

Although diet is the cornerstone for cholesterol management, CHD risk reduction by the use of cholesterol-lowering medications is strongly supported by many randomized clinical trials (Holme 1990; McCrindle et al. 2007; NCEP 2002). Both primary and secondary prevention trials demonstrate that cholesterol treatment is safe and reduces cardiovascular events and total mortality for men, women, and elderly patients (Sacks et al. 1996; Frick et al. 1987; Shepherd et al. 1995; Kane et al. 1990; Salonen et al. 1995; Scandinavian Simvastatin Survival Study 1994; Furberg et al. 1994). The benefits of cholesterol treatment have the greatest impact on high-risk patients, especially those with known CHD or multiple cardiovascular risk factors, by stabilizing atherosclerotic plaques (Scandinavian Simvastatin Survival Study 1994; Furberg et al. 1994; Sacks et al. 1996). The results of randomized trials using cholesterol-lowering medications have been extensively reviewed (McCrindle et al. 2007; NCEP 2002; Baigent et al. 2005; O'Regan et al. 2008; Bucher et al. 1999; Law et al. 2003).

The National Cholesterol Education Program (NCEP) was launched in 1987 to develop national health policy and specific recommendations to reduce the risk of CHD by lowering cholesterol levels in the United States. The NCEP guidelines, *The Expert Panel on the Detection, Evaluation and Treatment of High Blood Cholesterol in Adults*, include population and individual clinical approaches to cholesterol screening, diagnosis, and management with the goal of CHD risk reduction (NCEP 1990, 2002; NHLBI Public Health Service 1995). The NCEP recently published the full guidelines in 2002 (NCEP 2002) and updated guidelines in 2004 (Grundy et al. 2004). The NCEP *Adult Treatment Panel III* (ATP III) summarizes both the clinical and population approaches (NCEP 2002). The NCEP ATP III cholesterol guidelines are the standard for most health organizations.

The population strategy focuses on widespread lifestyle changes with the goal of substantially reducing the CHD burden. The clinical approach addresses the needs of persons with cholesterol abnormalities, CHD risk factors, or preexisting CHD who have a significantly increased risk for future CHD events and would benefit most from cholesterol reduction. The obesity epidemic may negatively affect recent population cholesterol reductions and should be a focus of population approaches. Despite the apparent differences in the two strategies for cholesterol reduction, they should not be viewed as mutually exclusive. In fact, universal screening of adults is a part of both the population and clinical approaches (NCEP 1990, 2002).

Screening

The focus of the population approach by the NCEP is to lower the risk of CHD events in the United States through cholesterol screening and treatment, nutritional changes, weight management, and increasing physical activity. The NCEP's ATP III guidelines recommended that a full serum lipid panel—including total cholesterol, HDL cholesterol, triglyceride level, and LDL cholesterol—be measured in all adults 20 years of age and older, at least once every 5 years in the fasting state. If the patient is not fasting, the total cholesterol and HDL cholesterol may be obtained.

A key objective of the national campaign, *Healthy People 2010*, is to increase the number of adults ≥20 years old who have been screened in the preceding 5 years for high blood cholesterol to 80% (MMWR 2005). The Behavior Risk Factor Surveillance System demonstrated that in 2005, 73% of the population surveyed had their cholesterol checked in the preceding 5 years (Chowdhury et al. 2005). However, by ethnicity, Hispanics and Asian/Pacific Islanders have had much lower screening rates, at 65.5% and 69.6%, respectively (MMWR 2005). The Population Panel recommended that public screening be used to supplement screening in the health care setting only under conditions that ensure adherence to high quality standards (NCEP 1990; NHLBI Public Health Service

1995). These standards include assuring the performance and standardization of choles-terol analyzers, providing appropriate training and supervision of staff, and providing reli-able information to the individual screened about cholesterol levels and dietary practices to lower cholesterol.

An individual's baseline total cholesterol level can vary by 5 mg/dL and HDL cho-lesterol by 1.5 mg/dL on a daily basis (Pereira et al. 2004). In addition, lipid profiles can fluctuate widely secondary to acute or chronic infection, stress, hormones, seasonal variation, and in the setting an acute myocardial infarction (Pereira et al. 2004; Ro-senson 1993; Cooper et al. 1992). The total cholesterol and HDL levels may decrease precipitously in the initial 12–24 hours after the onset of symptoms and may not return to baseline until after 2 or 3 months of the initial event. The classification of total cho-lesterol into three groups—desirable, borderline high, and high—and the recommended follow-up and referral pattern are shown in Table 12.1. It should be emphasized that public screening is not a substitute for health care and should not be used for monitoring the cholesterol levels of individuals under treatment.

Treatment

Population-Based Treatment Guidelines

Community education for lifestyle modification, including physical activity, dietary rec-ommendations, and weight management, is a cornerstone of the Population Approach for cholesterol management. Weight reduction has been shown to decrease LDL cholesterol and regular physical activity of moderate intensity should be performed most days of the week (NCEP 2002; Lichtenstein et al. 2006). *Dietary Guidelines for Americans* is a publi-cation by the Department of Health and Human Services and the United States Depart-ment of Agriculture that is updated every 5 years with the goal of decreasing the risk of CHD and other chronic diseases. The NCEP recommends incorporating these guidelines along with other key lifestyle modifications for healthy people older than 2 years. This

Table 12.1. National Cholesterol Education Program (NCEP) Categories of Total Cholesterol and the Referral Recommendations for Public Screenings

Category (level)	Referral Recommendation
Desirable (total cholesterol <200 mg/dL)	Repeat blood cholesterol measurement within 5 years
Borderline-high (total cholesterol 200–239 mg/dL)	Refer to physician if patient has a history of CHD or if two or more CHD risk factors are detected by interview. Otherwise, repeat cholesterol measurement within 1 year
High (total cholesterol ≥240 mg/dL)	Refer patient to physician for follow-up lipoprotein analysis

CHD, Coronary heart disease.

recommendation is summarized in Table 12.2. If an individual has a cholesterol disorder, has had a CHD event, or is at moderate to high risk for CHD, stricter dietary guidelines are recommended under the individualized clinical approach discussed below.

Patient-Based Treatment Guidelines

A full lipoprotein analysis should be performed if: a person's total cholesterol is >200 mg/dL or the HDL cholesterol is <40 mg/dL, there is known atherosclerotic disease, a family history of premature CHD, or there are multiple CHD risk factors (NCEP 2002). Secondary causes of dyslipidemia, including diabetes, hypothyroidism, chronic renal or liver disease, and steroid therapy, should be investigated (NCEP 2002).

The ATP III guidelines focus on intensive LDL cholesterol lowering as the primary target of therapy for primary and secondary CHD prevention. The NCEP classifies CHD risk into three categories and has specific LDL cholesterol goals for each (Table 12.3). The first category includes individuals with established CHD or the presence of CHD risk equivalents. "CHD risk equivalents" may include peripheral arterial disease, abdominal aortic aneurysm, carotid artery disease, and diabetes mellitus. This category has a >20% risk of having a CHD event according to the Framingham 10-year CHD Risk Score

Table 12.2. NCEP: Role of Physician and Other Health Care Professionals in Implementing Population and Clinical Approaches to Lifestyle Modification (Principles) and Cholesterol

	Population Approach	**Clinical Approach**
Principles	Promote change in lifestyle habits by serving as a role model to patients Provide general advice and access to credible sources of information regarding healthy lifestyle habits	Promote targeted changes in individual lifestyle to produce significant reductions in an individual patient's risk Initiate outcome measurements that will be tracked during scheduled follow-up visit Physicians, dietitians, and other relevant health professionals should go beyond monitoring adherence to actively helping individuals overcome barriers and promote new behaviors
Cholesterol	Ensure that all adults age 20 years and older have their blood cholesterol measured and their results explained in keeping with ATP III guidelines. Ensure that children and first-degree relatives of adults in whom a genetic lipoprotein disorder is suspected undergo cholesterol screening	Follow ATP III guidelines for detection, evaluation, and treatment of persons with lipid disorders

Table 12.3. NCEP Categories of CHD and Associated Target LDL Cholesterol Goals

Category	Risk of a CHD Event	LDL Cholesterol Goal
Established CHD or CHD risk equivalents	>20%	<100 mg/dL (<70mg/dL in setting of acute coronary syndrome or presence of other major risk factors)
Multiple (2) risk factors	10–20%	<130 mg/dL (<100 mg/dL if baseline is <130 mg/dL or risk factors poorly controlled)
One or less risk factors	<10%	<160 mg/dL

(NCEP 2002). The target LDL cholesterol level for this group should be <100 mg/dL. However, in the setting of an acute coronary syndrome (heart attack), or for those with CHD and other major risk factors (e.g., smoking, metabolic syndrome), recent updates recommend an LDL cholesterol goal of <70 mg/dL (Grundy et al. 2004).

The second risk category includes individuals with multiple (2) risk factors and has a Framingham risk score of 10–20%. According to the NCEP ATP III guidelines, the LDL cholesterol goal is <130 mg/dL. However, recent clinical trials suggests an LDL goal of <100 mg/dL if the patient's baseline LDL cholesterol is <130 mg/dL with the risk factors, or if the risk factors are poorly controlled (Grundy et al. 2004). The final group includes individuals with zero or one risk factor. The Framingham risk score is <10% and the goal LDL cholesterol is <160 mg/dL for this group (NCEP 2002).

Non-HDL cholesterol is the difference between the total cholesterol and HDL cholesterol. It incorporates atherogenic particles including IDL, VLDL, LDL, and lipoprotein (a), and is itself a predictor of CVD events and mortality (Cui et al. 2001). In the setting of high triglycerides, the LDL cholesterol level is inaccurate. The ATP III panel recommends using non-HDL cholesterol as a secondary target in the presence of hypertriglyceridemia. The goal non-HDL level should be 30 mg/dL higher than the target LDL concentration (NCEP 2002).

The classification of patients and therapy is based on the level of LDL cholesterol calculated from lipoprotein analysis, the lipid disorder identified, and the presence of CHD risk factors. The initial step in the clinical approach of the 2002 NCEP ATP III guidelines is to achieve the LDL cholesterol using a "multifactorial lifestyle approach" entitled Therapeutic Lifestyle Changes (TLC) (NCEP 2002). The four main areas of focus are weight reduction, physical activity, decreased intake of saturated fats and cholesterol, and therapeutic dietary options for decreasing LDL cholesterol levels (NCEP 2002). The TLC dietary recommendations are summarized in Table 12.2. The ATP III TLC diet incorporates the necessary dietary requirements as outlined in the *Dietary Guidelines for Americans* (US DHHS 2005).

If, after 6 weeks of increasing physical activity and decreasing saturated fat intake, the target LDL is not achieved, the incorporation of plant stanols and sterols and increased soluble fiber is recommended. Plant stanols and sterols are present in some margarines available in community grocery stores. They may lower LDL cholesterol by up to 15% (Lichtenstein et al. 2006). Increased soluble fiber may be achieved by increasing intake of fruits, vegetables, and some cereal grains and legumes. It is not known whether the reduction of serum cholesterol by increasing dietary fiber is due to a concomitant reduction of dietary fat or to an intrinsic cholesterol-lowering property of soluble fiber (Ripsin 1992).

If, after 3 months of the ATP III TLC approach, the target cholesterol reduction is not achieved, initiation of medications may be considered. However, diet and lifestyle reinforcement should continue indefinitely, regardless of medication use. The detailed algorithm is provided in the full guidelines (NCEP 2002).

If medications are necessary, there are four categories that may be used alone or in combination to help optimize cholesterol levels: statins, bile acid sequestrants, niacin (nicotinic acid), and fibrates.

Statins are the most efficacious in lowering LDL cholesterol levels for both men and women. Numerous clinical trials demonstrate their role in decreasing major adverse vascular events and mortality, specifically in high-risk populations (Pasternak et al. 2002; NCEP 2002; Grundy et al. 2004; Baigent et al. 2005; O'Regan et al. 2008; Bucher et al. 1999; Law et al. 2003). Cholesterol absorption inhibitors, such as ezetimibe and bile acid sequestrants decrease LDL cholesterol by reducing absorption of cholesterol in the intestines and assisting with elimination of cholesterol through the gastrointestinal system. Niacin (vitamin B_3) can decrease LDL cholesterol and triglyceride levels, in addition to raising HDL cholesterol. Fibrates assist with lowering triglyceride levels and raising HDL cholesterol (NCEP 2002). An individualized approach is essential for choosing the appropriate pharmacotherapy. Patients who are high risk, or are not responding to cholesterol treatment appropriately, may need referral to a lipid specialist.

Antioxidants

In the past, in vitro studies demonstrated that antioxidant supplementation decreased LDL oxidation (Martin and Frei 1997; Lynch et al. 1996; Jialal and Fuller 1993). Based on these findings, it was suggested that antioxidant supplementation with vitamin A, C, E, beta carotene, and/or selenium may alter lipid metabolism, decrease atherogenesis, and ultimately decrease cardiovascular morbidity and mortality. However, prospective clinical trials have demonstrated that antioxidant vitamin supplementation does not significantly decrease the atherosclerotic burden, nor does it prevent primary or secondary CHD events (Waters et al. 2002; Lee et al. 2005; Lee 1999). In fact, vitamins A, C, and E, and beta carotene supplementation may increase cardiovascular events and overall mortality in both men and women, and may increase the risk of lung cancer, specifically in smokers (Omenn et al. 1996; Waters et al. 2002; Lichtenstein et al. 2006). Antioxidant supplementation is not recommended for lipid therapy or for the prevention of atherosclerosis or cardiovascular events. If antioxidants are important for lipid metabolism, the source should be from fruits and vegetables.

Hormone Replacement Therapy

Hormone replacement therapy (HRT), which includes estrogen with or without progesterone, is not recommended for the treatment or prevention of lipid disorders. Women's

Health Initiative (WHI) was a randomized, primary-prevention trial of estrogen plus progesterone in 16,608 postmenopausal women ages 50–79 years. Based on this landmark study, HRT did not provide protection from cardiovascular events but suggested a possible increased risk, and was statistically significant for an increased risk of stroke (Manson et al. 2003; Rossouw et al. 2007). The Women's Angiographic Vitamin and Estrogen trial (mean age = 65 years) did not demonstrate improvement in atherosclerotic burden by coronary angiography with HRT (Waters et al. 2002). In 2005, the United States Preventive Services Task Force concluded that "the harmful effects of combined estrogen and progestin are likely to exceed the chronic disease prevention benefits in most women" (USPSTF 2005). A recent clinical trial published in 2007 from the WHI demonstrated that HRT may decrease calcified atherosclerotic burden when initiated in early menopause, in a younger population (Manson et al. 2007). However, it will be prudent to conduct additional clinical trials before recommending HRT to specific populations.

Guidelines for Children and Adolescents

Guideline development for children and adolescents was based on several major factors. First, studies indicate that the process of atherosclerosis begins in childhood and that its progression is related to elevated levels of blood cholesterol (Strong et al. 1999; Berenson 1987; NCEP 1990; McCrindle et al. 2007; Newman et al. 1986). Second, cholesterol levels in children "track" over time and adolescents with high cholesterol levels are more likely to have high levels as adults (Freedman et al. 1985; McCrindle et al. 2007). Third, high blood cholesterol aggregates in families as a result of shared environments and genetic factors, and children and adolescents with elevated total or LDL cholesterol frequently come from families with a high incidence of CHD (Lauer et al. 1988; McCrindle et al. 2007). Finally, U.S. children and adolescents have higher blood cholesterol levels and higher intakes of saturated fatty acids and cholesterol than their counterparts in many other countries (McCrindle et al. 2007). Therefore, the American Heart Association's guidelines, "Drug Therapy of High-Risk Lipid Abnormalities in Children and Adolescents," recommends both a population and individualized approach that includes selective screening of children and adolescents (McCrindle et al. 2007).

As with adults, the *population approach* is intended to reduce the average levels of blood cholesterol of children and adolescents through population-wide changes in eating patterns of children over the age of 2 years. The diet is the same as recommended for adults, focusing on fruits and vegetables, whole grains, low-fat dairy products, and lean meat (Gidding et al. 2005). Infants and children up to the age of 2 years have a fast growth rate and require a diet with a higher percentage of calories from fat; the recommendations are not intended for this age range. Toddlers 2 and 3 years of age may safely make the transition to the recommended eating pattern as they begin to eat with the family.

The *individualized approach* is designed to identify and treat children who are at greatest risk of having high blood cholesterol levels as adults and an increased risk of CHD. To accomplish this, selective screening of children and adolescents who have a family history of premature cardiovascular, peripheral vascular or cerebrovascular disease, or at least one parent with high blood cholesterol is recommended. In addition, children and adolescents who have comorbidities such as hypertension, diabetes mellitus, nephrotic syndrome, systemic lupus erythematous, or who are obese are also considered high risk and should be screened. This screening should be conducted in the context of regular and continuing health care, and evaluation for the metabolic syndrome should be included (McCrindle et al. 2007).

The screening protocol varies according to the reason for screening. For young people screened because of hypercholesterolemia in a parent, the initial test should be total cholesterol. Advanced lipoprotein analysis should be performed if there is a family history of premature cardiovascular disease, complex cholesterol disorder, or if the child has other cardiovascular risk factors because of the high proportion of lipoprotein abnormalities in these children (McCrindle et al. 2007).

As with adults, at least 6 months of lifestyle modifications, including increasing physical activity and dietary therapy with the TLC diet, is recommended before initiating medication. Medication therapy should only be considered for children more than 10 to 12 years old if the target LDL cholesterol of <130 mg/dL is not achieved with lifestyle changes alone (McCrindle et al. 2007). Randomized clinical trials of lipid-lowering medications have been performed in children and adolescents and data regarding the safety and efficacy of statin therapy in children and adolescents continue to emerge (Wiegman et al. 2004; McCrindle et al. 2007). If statin therapy is initiated, it is recommended that the lowest dose be initiated with appropriate education, clinical laboratory monitoring, and continued lifestyle modifications (McCrindle et al. 2007).

Examples of Public Health Interventions

National institutions and organizations, including the National Cholesterol Education Panel, the Centers for Disease Control, and the American Heart Association, have focused on public education, screening, and intervention for cholesterol and CHD risk reduction. Sources for educational material and presentations for public education are available at their websites. Efforts continually need to be focused on improving awareness and control of high cholesterol in the community for overall population health. *The American Heart Association Guide for Improving Cardiovascular Health at the Community Level* addresses strategies to increase physical activity and access to healthy foods at places of employment, schools, grocery stores, and restaurants (Pearson et al. 2003).

The National Heart, Lung, and Blood Institute has funded local community intervention projects to address cardiovascular disease risk factors, including high blood cholesterol, to decrease cardiovascular disease rates. Examples of large community-based intervention projects include the Stanford Five City Project, the Pawtucket Heart Health Program, and the Minnesota Heart Health Program.

The Stanford Five City Project began in 1978 and incorporated multiple community interventions, including a media advocacy program, to disseminate information and promote behavioral change (Fortmann et al. 1995). The Pawtucket Heart Health Program was a hospital-based community project from 1980 to 1991, that used community volunteers to develop and sustain cardiovascular risk reduction programs (Carleton et al. 1995). The Minnesota Heart Health Program also began in 1980 and incorporated extensive community organization efforts, school programs, and environmental change programs (Luepker et al. 1994). Although the results are mixed about the effectiveness of these programs, all the projects demonstrated the importance of integrating efforts at the community, state, and national levels to help encourage, and sustain behavioral change for population cardiovascular risk reduction.

Areas of Future Research and Demonstration

Although clinical trials of cholesterol-lowering medications have shown that the risk of CHD is lowered by cholesterol reduction, the estimated public health benefit in terms of total event and mortality reduction appears to vary substantially by age, cholesterol level, and presence of other CHD risk factors (Stone 2005; Grundy et al. 2004). Secondary prevention trials have included women and the elderly and have documented benefits for these patients with cholesterol therapy (Grundy et al. 2004; NCEP 2002). Further information is needed on the benefits of cholesterol reduction as primary prevention among the young adult population related to mortality and long-term outcomes, including the progression of atherosclerosis.

The "optimal" diet in terms of dietary fat and carbohydrate composition to attain the optimal weight and for prevention of CHD continues to evolve. The goal is continued lowering of LDL cholesterol and VLDL cholesterol with proper nutrition requirements. Data are emerging about functional foods, such as flavonoids, that may benefit lipid panels.

Cholesterol disorders with heterogeneous lipoproteins need careful evaluation for absolute risk prediction and to improve treatment of these disorders. Emerging risk factors, such as lipoprotein (a), need to be further investigated regarding their roles in atherogenesis and future implications for possible screening and therapy. Genetic testing and gene therapy will be important areas of research to develop enhanced screening and treatment strategies for high-risk individuals.

Studies on motivating behavior change, both for population and individual levels, are key to further reducing CHD. Much is known about preventing disease and managing risk factors; yet, the United States has not met its goal for screening, awareness, and treatment of cholesterol disorders. Methods to support improved adherence to lifestyle changes and medical guidelines are sorely needed. Health care systems must be reorganized to ensure the delivery of proven preventive strategies and medical therapies. Efforts to control the obesity epidemic could have significant impact on blood cholesterol levels and comorbid conditions related to cardiovascular disease. Population health efforts focusing on policy and prevention, such as efforts to reduce the intake of trans fats, could have far-reaching implications on public health.

Resources

Websites

American Heart Association—Clinical Guidelines (www.americanheart.org)
National Heart, Lung, and Blood Institute—National Cholesterol Education Program (www.nhlbi. nih.gov/about/ncep/index.htm)
National Lipid Association (http://www.lipid.org)
U.S. Department of Health and Human Services, Healthy People 2010 and 2020 Campaigns (http://www.healthypeople.gov)
U.S. Department of Agriculture, Center for Nutrition Policy and Promotion—Dietary Guidelines (http://www.cnpp.usda.gov/Dietaryguidelines.htm)

Suggested Reading

Denke, M.A. Cholesterol-Lowering Diets: A Review of the Evidence. *Arch Intern Med* (1995):155:17–26.

Miller, M., and R. Vogel. *The Practice of Coronary Disease Prevention.* Baltimore, MD: William and Wilkins (1996).

National Institutes of Health. *Report of the Expert Panel on Blood Cholesterol Levels in Children and Adolescents.* Washington, D.C.: Dept of Health and Human Services, Public Health Service; November 1990. NIH publication 91-2732.

National Institutes of Health. *Report of the Expert Panel on Population Strategies for Blood Cholesterol Reduction.* Washington, D.C.: Dept of Health and Human Services, Public Health Service. NIH publication 90-3046.

Report of the Expert Panel on Detection, Evaluation, and Treatment, of High Blood Cholesterol in Adults. National Cholesterol Education Program: Third report of the Expert Panel on Detection, Evaluation, and Treatment of High Blood Cholesterol in Adults (Adult Treatment Panel III). *Circulation* (2002):106:3143–3421.

Grundy, S.M., J.I. Cleeman, C.N. Bairey Merz, et al. Implications of Recent Clinical Trials for the National Cholesterol Education Program Adult Treatment Panel III Guidelines. *Circulation* 2004:110:227–239.

Stone, N.J., C.B. Blum, and E. Winslow. *Management of Lipids in Clinical Practice.* Caddo, OK: Professional Communications Inc (2005).

References

Baigent, C., A. Keech, P.M. Kearney, et al. Cholesterol Treatment Trialists' (CTT) Collaborators. Efficacy and Safety of Cholesterol-Lowering Treatment: Prospective Meta-Analysis of Data from 90,056 Participants in 14 Randomised Trials of Statins. *Lancet* (2005):366:1267–1278.

Bansal, S., J.E. Buring, N. Rifai, et al. Fasting Compared with Nonfasting Triglycerides and Risk of Cardiovascular Events in Women. *JAMA* (2007):298:309–316.

Baumgartner, R.N., A.F. Roche, W.C. Chumlea, R.M. Siervogel, and C.J. Glueck. Fatness and Fat Patterns: Associations with Plasma Lipids and Blood Pressures in Adults, 18 to 57 Years of Age. *Am J Epidemiol* (1987):126:614–628.

Berenson, G.S., S.R. Srinivasan, D.S. Freedman, B. Radhakrishnamurthy, and E.R. Dalferes, Jr. Atherosclerosis and Its Evolution in Childhood. *Am J Med Sci* (1987):294:429–440.

Bucher, H.C., L.E. Griffith, and G.H. Guyatt. Systematic Review on the Risk and Benefit of Different Cholesterol-Lowering Interventions. *Arterioscler Thromb Vasc Biol* (1999):19:187–195.

Carleton, R.A., T.M. Lasater, A.R. Assaf, H.A. Feldman, S. McKinlay, and the Pawtucket Heart Health Program Writing Group. The Pawtucket Heart Health Program: Community Changes in Cardiovascular Risk Factors and Projected Disease Risk. *Am J Public Health* (1995):85: 777–785.

Chowdhury, P., L. Balluz, W. Murphy, et al. Surveillance of Certain Health Behaviors among States and Selected Local Areas—United States, 2005. *MMWR* (2005):56:1–160.

Cooper, G.R., G.L. Myers, S.J. Smith, and R.C. Schlant. Blood Lipid Measurements. Variations and Practical Utility. *JAMA* (1992):267:1652–1260.

Couch, S.C., A.T. Cross, K. Kida, et al. Rapid Westernization of Children's Blood Cholesterol in 3 Countries: Evidence for Nutrient–Gene Interactions? *Am J Clin Nutr* (2000):72:1266S–1274S.

Criqui, M.H., R.B. Wallace, G. Heiss, et al. Cigarette Smoking and Plasma High-Density Lipoprotein Cholesterol. The Lipid Research Clinics Program Prevalence Study. *Circulation* (1980):62:IV70–IV76.

Cui, Y., R.S. Blumenthal, J.A. Flaws, et al. Non-High-Density Lipoprotein Cholesterol Level as a Predictor of Cardiovascular Disease Mortality. *Arch Intern Med* (2001):161:1413–1419.

Dept. of Health and Human Services, United States Dept. of Agriculture, United States Dietary Guidelines Advisory Committee. Dietary guidelines for Americans, 2005. Washington, D.C.: G.P.O. (2005):ix, 71 pp.

Falk, E., P.K. Shah, and V. Fuster. Coronary Plaque Disruption. *Circulation* (1995):92:657–671.

Ford, E.S., U.A. Ajani, J.B. Croft, et al. Explaining the Decrease in U.S. Deaths from Coronary Disease, 1980–2000. *N Engl J Med.* (2007):356:2388–2398.

Fortmann, S.P., J.A. Flora, M.A. Winkleby, C. Schooler, C.B. Taylor, and J.W. Farquhar. Community Intervention Trials: Reflections on the Stanford Five-City Project Experience. *Am J Epidemiol* (1995):142:576–586.

Freedman, D.S., C.L. Shear, S.R. Srinivasan, L.S. Webber, and G.S. Berenson. Tracking of Serum Lipids and Lipoproteins in Children over an 8-Year Period: The Bogalusa Heart Study. *Prev Med* (1985):14:203–216.

Frick, M.H., O. Elo, K. Haapa, et al. Helsinki Heart Study: Primary-Prevention Trial with Gemfibrozil in Middle-Aged Men with Dyslipidemia. Safety of Treatment, Changes in Risk Factors, and Incidence of Coronary Heart Disease. *N Engl J Med* (1987):317:1237–1245.

Furberg, C.D., H.P Adams, Jr., W.B. Applegate, et al. Effect of Lovastatin on Early Carotid Atherosclerosis and Cardiovascular Events. Asymptomatic Carotid Artery Progression Study (ACAPS) Research Group. *Circulation* (1994):90:1679–1687.

Fuster, V., P.R. Moreno, Z.A. Fayad, R. Corti, J.J. Badimon. Atherothrombosis and High-Risk Plaque: Part I. Evolving Concepts. *J Am Coll Cardiol* (2005):46:937–954.

Garg, A., and V. Simha. Update on Dyslipidemia. *J Clin Endocrinol Metab* (2007):92:1581–1589.

Genest, J., Jr., J.R. McNamara, J.M. Ordovas, et al. Lipoprotein Cholesterol, Apolipoprotein A-I and B and Lipoprotein (a) Abnormalities in Men with Premature Coronary Artery Disease. *J Am Coll Cardiol* (1992):19:792–802.

Gidding, S.S., B.A. Dennison, L.L. Birch, et al. Dietary Recommendations for Children and Adolescents: A Guide for Practitioners: Consensus Statement from the American Heart Association. *Circulation* (2005):112:2061–2075.

Goldman, L., K.A. Phillips, P. Coxson, et al. The Effect of Risk Factor Reductions between 1981 and 1990 on Coronary Heart Disease Incidence, Prevalence, Mortality and Cost. *J Am Coll Cardiol* (2001):38:1012–1017.

Grundy, S.M., and M.A. Denke. Dietary Influences on Serum Lipids and Lipoproteins. *J Lipid Res* (1990):31:1149–1172.

Grundy, S.M., J.I. Cleeman, C.N. Merz, et al. Implications of Recent Clinical Trials for the National Cholesterol Education Program Adult Treatment Panel III guidelines. *Circulation* (2004):110:227–239.

Haskell, W.L., H.L. Taylor, P.D. Wood, H. Schrott, and G. Heiss. Strenuous Physical Activity, Treadmill Exercise Test Performance and Plasma High-Density Lipoprotein Cholesterol. The Lipid Research Clinics Program Prevalence Study. *Circulation* (1980):62:IV53–IV61.

Higgins, M., W. Kannel, R. Garrison, J. Pinsky, and J. Stokes, 3rd. Hazards of Obesity—The Framingham Experience. *Acta Med Scand Suppl* (1988):723:23–36.

Holme, I. An analysis of Randomized Trials Evaluating the Effect of Cholesterol Reduction on Total Mortality and Coronary Heart Disease Incidence. *Circulation* (1990):82:1916–1924.

Hu, F.B., and W.C. Willett. Optimal Diets for Prevention of Coronary Heart Disease. *JAMA* (2002):288:2569–2578.

Jialal, I., and C.J. Fuller. Oxidized LDL and Antioxidants. *Clin Cardiol* (1993):16:I6–I9.

Kane, J.P., M.J. Malloy, T.A. Ports, N.R. Phillips, J.C. Diehl, and R.J. Havel. Regression of Coronary Atherosclerosis during Treatment of Familial Hypercholesterolemia with Combined Drug Regimens. *JAMA* (1990):264:3007–3012.

Kannel, W.B., W.P. Castelli, T. Gordon, and P.M. McNamara. Serum Cholesterol, Lipoproteins, and the Risk of Coronary Heart Disease. The Framingham study. *Ann Intern Med* (1971):74:1–12.

Kromhout, D., A. Menotti, B. Bloemberg, et al. Dietary Saturated and Trans Fatty Acids and Cholesterol and 25-Year Mortality from Coronary Heart Disease: The Seven Countries Study. *Prev Med* (1995):24:308–315.

LaRosa, J.C. Triglycerides and Coronary Risk in Women and the Elderly. *Arch Intern Med* (1997): 157:961–968.

LaRosa, J.C., and C.D. Brown. Cardiovascular Risk Factors in Minorities. *Am J Med* (2005):118: 1314–1322.

Lauer, R.M., J. Lee, and W.R. Clarke. Factors Affecting the Relationship between Childhood and Adult Cholesterol Levels: The Muscatine Study. *Pediatrics* (1988):82:309–318.

Law, M.R., N.J. Wald, and A.R. Rudnicka, Quantifying Effect of Statins on Low Density Lipoprotein Cholesterol, Ischaemic Heart Disease, and Stroke: Systematic Review and Meta-Analysis. *BMJ* (2003):326:1423.

Lee, I.M., N.R. Cook, J.M. Graziano, et al. Vitamin E in the Primary Prevention of Cardiovascular Disease and Cancer: The Women's Health Study: A Randomized Controlled Trial. *JAMA* (2005):294:56–65.

Lee, I.M. Beta-Carotene Supplementation and Incidence of Cancer and Cardiovascular Disease: The Women's Health Study. *J Natl Cancer Inst* (1999):91:2102–2106.

Lichtenstein, A.H., L.J. Appel, M. Brands, et al. Diet and Lifestyle Recommendations Revision 2006: A Scientific Statement from the American Heart Association Nutrition Committee. *Circulation* (2006):114:82–96.

Luepker, R.V., D.M. Murray, D.R. Jacobs, Jr., et al. Community Education for Cardiovascular Disease Prevention: Risk Factor Changes in the Minnesota Heart Health Program. *Am J Public Health* (1994): 84:1383–1393.

Lynch, S.M., J.M. Gaziano, and B. Frei. Ascorbic Acid and Atherosclerotic Cardiovascular Disease. *Subcell Biochem* (1996):25:331–367.

Manson, J.E., J. Hsia, K.C. Johnson, et al. Estrogen Plus Progestin and the Risk of Coronary Heart Disease. *N Engl J Med* (2003):349:523–534.

Manson, J.E., M.A. Allison, J.E. Rossouw, et al. Estrogen Therapy and Coronary-Artery Calcification. *N Engl J Med* (2007):356:2591–2602.

Marks, D., M. Thorogood, H.A. Neil, and S.E. Humphries. A Review on the Diagnosis, Natural History, and Treatment of Familial Hypercholesterolaemia. *Atherosclerosis* (2003):168: 1–14.

Martin, A., and B. Frei. Both Intracellular and Extracellular Vitamin C Inhibit Atherogenic Modification of LDL by Human Vascular Endothelial Cells. *Arterioscler Thromb Vasc Biol* (1997):17:1583–1590.

McCrindle, B.W., E.M. Urbina, B.A. Dennison, et al. Drug Therapy of High-Risk Lipid Abnormalities in Children and Adolescents: A Scientific Statement from the American Heart Association: Atherosclerosis, Hypertension, and Obesity in Youth Committee, Council of Cardiovascular Disease in the Young, with the Council on Cardiovascular Nursing. *Circulation* (2007):115:1948–1967.

McGill, H.C., Jr., C.A. McMahan, G.T. Malcom, M.C. Oalmann, and J.P. Strong. Effects of Serum Lipoproteins and Smoking on Atherosclerosis in Young Men and Women. The PDAY Research Group. Pathobiological Determinants of Atherosclerosis in Youth. *Arterioscler Thromb Vasc Biol* (1997):17:95–106.

McKay, J., and G.A. Mensah. World Health Organization. The Atlas of Heart Disease and Stroke. Geneva: World Health Organization (2004) 112 pp.

Menotti, A., D. Kromhout, H. Blackburn, F. Fidanza, R. Buzina, and A. Nissinen. Food Intake Patterns and 25-Year Mortality from Coronary Heart Disease: Cross-Cultural Correlations in the Seven Countries Study. The Seven Countries Study Research Group. *Eur J Epidemiol* (1999):15:507–515.

Muennig, P., N. Sohler, and B. Mahato. Socioeconomic Status as an Independent Predictor of Physiological Biomarkers of Cardiovascular Disease: Evidence from NHANES. *Prev Med* (2007):45:35–40.

National Center for Health Statistics (U.S.). Chartbook on Trends in the Health of Americans. Hyattsville, MD: U.S. Dept. of Health and Human Services, Centers for Disease Control and Prevention, National Center for Health Statistics; Washington, D.C. (2006): DHHS publication; no. (PHS) 2007–1560, vi, 153 pp.

National Cholesterol Education Program (U.S.). Expert Panel on Population Strategies for Blood Cholesterol Reduction. *Report of the Expert Panel on Population Strategies for Blood Cholesterol Reduction.* Washington, D.C.: The Program (1990): ix, 139 pp.

National Heart Lung and Blood Institute. *Recommendations Regarding Public Screening for Measuring Blood Cholesterol.* Washington, D.C.: U.S. Dept. of Health and Human Services, Public Health Service (1995).

Newman, W.P., 3rd, D.S. Freedman, A.W. Voors, et al. Relation of Serum Lipoprotein Levels and Systolic Blood Pressure to Early Atherosclerosis. The Bogalusa Heart Study. *N Engl J Med* (1986):314:138–44.

Nordestgaard, B.G., M. Benn, P. Schnohr, and A. Tybjaerg-Hansen. Nonfasting Triglycerides and Risk of Myocardial Infarction, Ischemic Heart Disease, and Death in Men and Women. *JAMA* (2007):298:299–308.

Omenn, G.S., G.E. Goodman, M.D. Thornquist, et al. Effects of a Combination of Beta Carotene and Vitamin A on Lung Cancer and Cardiovascular Disease. *N Engl J Med* (1996):334:1150–1155.

O'Regan, C., P. Wu, P. Arora, D. Perri, and E.J. Mills. Statin Therapy in Stroke Prevention: A Meta-Analysis Involving 121,000 Patients. *Am J Med* (2008):121:24–33.

Pasternak, R.C., S.C. Smith, C.N. Bairey-Merz, et al. ACC/AHA/NHLBI Clinical Advisory on the Use and Safety of Statins. *J Am Coll Cardiol* (2002):40:567–572.

Pearson, T.A., T.L. Bazzarre, S.R. Daniels, et al. American Heart Association Guide for Improving Cardiovascular Health at the Community Level: A Statement for Public Health Practitioners, Healthcare Providers, and Health Policy Makers from the American Heart Association Expert Panel on Population and Prevention Science. *Circulation* (2003):107:645–651.

Pereira, M.A., R.M. Weggemans, D.R. Jacobs, Jr., et al. Within-Person Variation in Serum Lipids: Implications for Clinical Trials. *Int J Epidemiol* (2004):33:534–541.

Petersen, S., V. Peto, M. Rayner, J. Leal, R. Luengo-Fernandez, and A. Gray. *European Cardiovascular Disease Statistics.* London: British Heart Foundation (2005).

QuickStats: Trends in Mean Total Cholesterol among Adults Aged 20–74 Years, by Age Group—United States, 1960–1962 to 1999–2002. *Morb Mortal Wkly Rep* (2005):54:1288.

Reiner, A.P., C.S. Carlson, E. Ziv, C. Iribarren, C.E. Jaquish, and D.A. Nickerson. Genetic Ancestry, Population Sub-Structure, and Cardiovascular Disease-Related Traits among African-American Participants in the CARDIA Study. *Hum Genet* (2007):121:565–575.

Ripsin, C.M., J.M. Keenan, D.R. Jacobs, Jr., et al. Oat Products and Lipid Lowering. A Meta-Analysis. *JAMA* (1992):267:3317–3325.

Rosenson, R.S. Myocardial Injury: The Acute Phase Response and Lipoprotein Metabolism. *J Am Coll Cardiol* (1993):22:933–940.

Ross, R. Atherosclerosis—An Inflammatory Disease. *N Engl J Med* (1999):340:115–1126.

Rossouw, J.E., R.L. Prentice, J.E. Manson, et al. Postmenopausal Hormone Therapy and Risk of Cardiovascular Disease by Age and Years Since Menopause. *JAMA* (2007):297:1465–1477.

Sacks, F.M., M.A. Pfeffer, L.A. Moye, et al. The Effect of Pravastatin on Coronary Events after Myocardial Infarction in Patients with Average Cholesterol Levels. Cholesterol and Recurrent Events Trial Investigators. *N Engl J Med* (1996):335:1001–1009.

Salonen, R., K. Nyyssonen, E. Porkkala, et al. Kuopio Atherosclerosis Prevention Study (KAPS). A Population-Based Primary Preventive Trial of the Effect of LDL Lowering on Atherosclerotic Progression in Carotid and Femoral Arteries. *Circulation* (1995):92:1758–1764.

Sarwar, N., J. Danesh, G. Eiriksdottir, et al. Triglycerides and the Risk of Coronary Heart Disease: 10,158 Incident Cases among 262,525 Participants in 29 Western Prospective Studies. *Circulation* (2007):115:450–458.

Scandinavian Simvastatin Survival Study (4S). Randomised Trial of Cholesterol Lowering in 4444 Patients with Coronary Heart Disease: The Scandinavian Simvastatin Survival Study (4S). *Lancet* (1994):344:1383–1389.

Shepherd, J., S.M. Cobbe, I. Ford, et al. Prevention of Coronary Heart Disease with Pravastatin in Men with Hypercholesterolemia. West of Scotland Coronary Prevention Study Group. *N Engl J Med* (1995):333:1301–1307.

Solberg, L.A., and J.P. Strong. Risk Factors and Atherosclerotic Lesions. A Review of Autopsy Studies. *Arteriosclerosis* (1983):3:187–198.

Stamler J., D. Wentworth, and J.D. Neaton. Is Relationship between Serum Cholesterol and Risk of Premature Death from Coronary Heart Disease Continuous and Graded? Findings in 356,222 Primary Screenees of the Multiple Risk Factor Intervention Trial (MRFIT). *JAMA* (1986):256:2823–2828.

Stary, H.C., A.B. Chandler, R.E. Dinsmore, et al. A Definition of Advanced Types of Atherosclerotic Lesions and a Histological Classification of Atherosclerosis. A Report from the Committee on Vascular Lesions of the Council on Arteriosclerosis, American Heart Association. *Circulation* (1995):92:1355–1374.

Stoll, G., and M. Bendszus. Inflammation and Atherosclerosis: Novel Insights into Plaque Formation and Destabilization. *Stroke* (2006):37:1923–1932.

Stone, N.J. Fish Consumption, Fish Oil, Lipids, and Coronary Heart Disease. *Circulation* (1996):94:2337–2340.

Stone, N.J., and C.B. Blum. *Management of Lipids in Clinical Practice.* Caddo, OK: Professional Communications (2005).

Strong, J.P., G.T. Malcom, C.A. McMahan, et al. Prevalence and Extent of Atherosclerosis in Adolescents and Young Adults: Implications for Prevention from the Pathobiological Determinants of Atherosclerosis in Youth Study. *JAMA* (1999):281:727–735.

The World Health Organization MONICA Project (Monitoring Trends and Determinants in Cardiovascular Disease): A Major International Collaboration. WHO MONICA Project Principal Investigators. *J Clin Epidemiol* (1988):41:105–114.

Third Report of the National Cholesterol Education Program (NCEP) Expert Panel on Detection, Evaluation, and Treatment of High Blood Cholesterol in Adults (Adult Treatment Panel III) final report. *Circulation* (2002):106:3143–3421.

Tolonen, H., U. Keil, M. Ferrario, A. Evans, and WHO MONICA Project. Prevalence, Awareness and Treatment of Hypercholesterolaemia in 32 Populations: Results from the WHO MONICA Project. *Int J Epidemiol* (2005):34:181–192.

Trends in Cholesterol Screening and Awareness of High Blood Cholesterol—United States, 1991–2003. *Morb Mortal Wkly Rep* (2005):54:865–870.

U.S. Preventive Services Task Force (USPSTF) Hormone Therapy for the Prevention of Chronic Conditions in Postmenopausal Women: Recommendations from the U.S. Preventive Services Task Force. *Ann Intern Med* (2005):142:855–860.

Waters, D.D., E.L. Alderman, J. Hsia, et al. Effects of Hormone Replacement Therapy and Antioxidant Vitamin Supplements on Coronary Atherosclerosis in Postmenopausal Women: A Randomized Controlled Trial. *JAMA* (2002):288:2432–2440.

Wiegman, A., B.A. Hutten, E. de Groot, et al. Efficacy and Safety of Statin Therapy in Children with Familial Hypercholesterolemia: A Randomized Controlled Trial. *JAMA* (2004):292: 331–337.

Worth, R.M., H. Kato, G.G. Rhoads, K. Kagan, and S.L. Syme. Epidemiologic Studies of Coronary Heart Disease and Stroke in Japanese Men Living in Japan, Hawaii and California: Mortality. *Am J Epidemiol* (1975):102:481–490.

CHAPTER 13

CARDIOVASCULAR DISEASE (ICD-10 I20–I25, I50, I60–I69, I73)

Craig J. Newschaffer, Ph.D., Longjian Liu, M.D., Ph.D., M.Sc., and Alan Sim, M.S.

Introduction

Cardiovascular disease (CVD) refers to a wide variety of heart and blood vessel diseases, including coronary heart disease (CHD), stroke, and peripheral artery disease (PAD). In the United States today, CVD is of paramount public health importance because of its widespread nature and the potential for intervention. An estimated 80 million Americans have one or more type of CVD (Lloyd-Jones et al. 2009), and CVD is the leading cause of death and disability in the United States. More than 864,000 Americans died of CVD in 2005, accounting for just over 35% of all U.S. deaths in that year (Lloyd-Jones et al. 2009). Poor diet, lack of physical activity, and smoking are the leading causes of CVD, leading to high rates of CVD among the poor, less educated, and minorities (see Figure 13.1).

This is despite the fact that CVD death rates have declined precipitously over the last decade, falling more than 26% from 1995 to 2005 (Lloyd-Jones et al. 2009). This decline has been driven by continuing reductions in mortality from both coronary heart disease

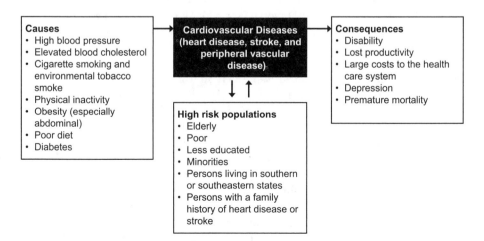

Figure 13.1. CVD: causes, consequences, and high-risk groups.

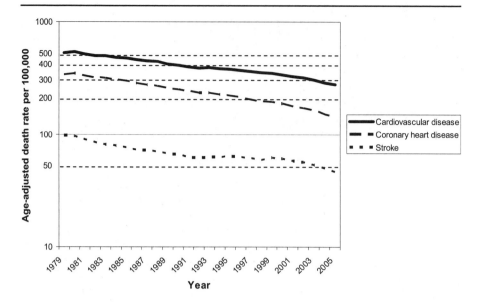

Figure 13.2. Trends in age-adjusted CVD mortality by year (1979–2005). *Note:* From CDC (2009b, 2009c).

and stroke (Figure 13.2). CVD remains a major public health challenge with heart disease still the first, and cerebrovascular disease is still the third, leading overall causes of death in the United States (Kung et al. 2008).

Significance

Death rates for CVD vary markedly by age, race, and sex (Lloyd-Jones et al. 2009). Although mortality from CVD is greater among older adults, more than 154,000 Americans younger than 65 years died from CVD in 2005 (Lloyd-Jones et al. 2009). Also, despite the fact that the age-adjusted CVD mortality rate for U.S. men in 2005 was 45% higher than for women, CVD remains the leading cause of death in U.S. women. In fact, in 2005, more women (454,600) than men (409,867) in the United States died from CVD. In that year, the age-adjusted mortality rates were 438 per 100,000 for African American men, 325 for white men, 319 for African American women, and 230 for white women (Lloyd-Jones et al. 2009). Hispanic and Asian Americans appear to be at lower risk of heart disease and stroke mortality than whites. However, CVD-related diseases remain the leading contributors to mortality for these racial and ethnic groups (CDC 1994).

Yet, mortality alone captures only a portion of the health burden imposed by CVD. CVD was a primary diagnosis for approximately 6.2 million inpatient hospital discharges, 6.6 million outpatient visits, and almost 4.4 million emergency department encounters in 2006 (DeFrances 2008; Lloyd-Jones et al. 2009) and is a leading cause of disability as an estimated 5 million American adults self-reported heart trouble, stroke or high blood pressure as the main reason for their disability in 2005 (CDC 2009a). The estimated direct and indirect costs of CVD in 2009 will reach $475 billion, according to the American Heart Association (AHA) (Lloyd-Jones et al. 2009).

CVD mortality rates remain higher in the United States than in many other industrialized nations; however, reflective of the worldwide spread of CVD, the United States ranked 165th out of 192 nations in 2004 age-adjusted CVD mortality data in the WHO Global Burden of Disease database (WHO 2008). While CVD mortality is expected to continue to decline in the developed world, in the developing world projections suggest that heart disease mortality will increase 120% for women and 137% for men from 1990 to 2020 with a tripling of both heart disease and stroke mortality expected in Latin America, the Middle East and sub-Saharan Africa (Leeder et al. 2004).

Pathophysiology

Atherosclerosis, the underlying disease process of the major forms of CVD, is a slowly progressive condition in which the inner layers of the artery walls become thick, irregular, and rigid. The process is complex, with contributing factors including deposition of fat and cholesterol, inflammation, migration and proliferation of smooth muscle cells, formation of raised fibrous lesions, and calcification. With the progression of atherosclerosis, the arteries narrow, the blood flow is decreased, and there is greater likelihood that the built-up material, or plaque, will disrupt, creating a traveling blood clot (or embolism) (See also Chapter 12, High Blood Cholesterol).

CVD usually manifests clinically in middle age or later—the lifetime risk for incident CVD for 40-year-old men is about 66% and just over 50% for like-aged women (Lloyd-Jones et al. 2009). However, atherosclerosis typically initiates in childhood and there is growing speculation that fetal factors may also be etiologically significant. Atherosclerosis is associated with several modifiable risk factors including those well known as risk factors for CVD: high blood cholesterol, high blood pressure, cigarette smoking, physical inactivity, diabetes, and obesity (Labarthe et al. 1991). The advent of noninvasive means of evaluating atherosclerosis has fostered the epidemiologic study of asymptomatic CVD. Control of modifiable risk factors, at both the population and individual levels, remains the key to primary and secondary prevention of CVD.

Coronary heart disease (CHD), congestive heart failure (CHF), stroke, and PAD share, but are not influenced equally by, many of the same CVD risk factors. CHD is rarely found in populations without elevated cholesterol. In contrast, stroke is a disease most strongly associated with high blood pressure with less contribution coming from cholesterol and other risk factors. Diabetes and smoking are most strongly associated with PAD. This chapter provides a more detailed discussion of each of these four major types of CVD.

CORONARY HEART DISEASE
(ICD-10 I20–I25)

Significance

CHD is the single largest killer of American men and women today, accounting for nearly 452,000 deaths in 2004. CHD represents over half (52%) of the CVD deaths and over one fifth (21%) of all-cause mortality. Each year there are more than 1.2 million new or recurrent heart attacks, with an estimated additional 175,000 silent first heart attacks occurring each year (Rosamond et al. 2007). The AHA estimates that among adults 20 years and older, over 15 million Americans alive today have a history of CHD (Lloyd-Jones et al. 2009). About two million hospital admissions each year involve diagnoses of CHD, and the costs associated with medical care, lost earnings, and lost productivity due to CHD were estimated at $151.6 billion for 2004 (Rosamond et al. 2007).

Pathophysiology

CHD, also called ischemic heart disease or coronary artery disease, is a term used to identify several disorders that reduce the blood supply to the heart muscle. This impairment of circulation to the heart is most frequently the result of narrowing of the coronary arteries by atherosclerosis. The onset, and much of the progression, of atherosclerosis is subclinical (i.e., without symptoms), with the most common emergent clinical manifestations of coronary atherosclerosis being angina pectoris (chest pain), myocardial infarction (MI, heart attack), and sudden death. Historically, CHD epidemiology has been dependent on studies of these clinical manifestations as endpoints. However, the incorporation of new technologies into epidemiologic investigations, such as the B-mode ultrasound of the carotid arteries used in the Atherosclerosis Risk in Communities (ARIC) studies, is allowing for new insights about risk factors for early-stage CHD. Those implicated through these studies thus far include: traditional CHD risk factors, genetic changes at the cellular level, circulating markers of inflammation, infectious agents, micronutrients, and hemostatic factors (de Andrade et al. 1995; Folsom 1993, 1994; Ma et al. 1995; Nieto et al. 1996).

Descriptive Epidemiology

High-Risk Populations

Throughout life, men have much higher CHD mortality rates than women. Overall, the age-adjusted death rate for CHD in the United States is more than twice as high for men as it is for women. The incidence of CHD in women lags behind men by 10 years for total CHD and by 20 years for more serious clinical events such as MI and sudden death. However, in women, CHD is still the single greatest mortality risk, with the age-adjusted mortality rate three times greater than that for breast cancer (Anderson et al. 1997).

CHD risk increases with age independent of known CHD risk factors. Approximately 55% of all heart attacks occur in people aged 65 or older and 85% of the people who die of heart attacks are older than 65 years (Rosamond et al. 2007). CHD is the leading cause of death for men and women over 65 years of age and the second leading cause of disability in older men and women (Corti et al. 1996). For men, major increases in CHD begin in the 35- to 44-year age group, while for women, the marked increase is delayed until after menopause. CHD incident rates in women after menopause are two to three times those of women the same age before menopause. Subclinical CHD is more prevalent in older than in younger individuals and has been shown to be associated with the same risk factors linked to clinical disease at younger ages, thereby suggesting that risk factor modification in older individuals may still be a very cost-effective public health strategy (Corti et al. 1996).

For men and women combined, age-adjusted CHD death rates are higher among African Americans than whites until advanced age, at which point they are higher among whites. African American men experience a slightly higher death rate from CHD than white men. In 2005, the overall age-adjusted CHD death rate was 144.4 per 100,000 population, with death rates of 187.7 for white men and 213.3 per 100,000 for African American men. More strikingly, the rate for white women was 111.7, while for African American women, it was 140.9 per 100,000. It is the difference in female death rates that accounts for the bulk of the discrepancy in CHD mortality between African Americans and whites (CDC 2009b).

Although national data on CHD mortality among Americans of Hispanic origin are limited, existing data suggest that age-adjusted death rates in 2003 for CHD were 130.0 per 100,000 for Hispanics or Latinos, 114.1 per 100,000 for American Indians or Alaska Natives, and 92.8 for Asians or Pacific Islanders (Rosamond et al. 2007).

A family history of premature CHD increases the risk of CHD. The clustering of CHD in families is not fully understood but is believed to be a combination of genetics and higher levels of risk factors within these families (e.g., similar dietary patterns).

CHD incidence and mortality rates are higher among people of lower socioeconomic status than among those in the middle or upper classes (Jenkins 1988). The greatest declines in CHD mortality over time among white men and women in the United States have been among those with the highest levels of income and education and among workers in white-collar jobs (Wing et al. 1988, 1992). Not surprisingly, the gradient of CHD mortality associated with socioeconomic status is similar to the gradient of risk factors; for example, cigarette smoking, obesity, and high blood pressure are more common among people with lower income and education levels (Jenkins 1988). In addition, neighborhood socioeconomic status effects may persist above those related to differing distributions of individual-level risk factors. In general, living in deprived neighborhoods is associated with increased risk of CHD and increased levels of risk factors. However, complex interaction between individual- and neighborhood-level socioeconomic status on CHD risk factors in African American men have been observed. For example, one analysis of African American men living in Jackson, Mississippi found that lower individual SES was associated with increased serum cholesterol in higher-SES neighborhoods and decreased serum cholesterol in lower-SES neighborhoods (Diez-Roux et al. 1997).

Geographic Distribution

In the United States, age-adjusted CHD death rates show striking variation by geographic region. In 1998, the age-adjusted death rates (adjusted to the U.S. 2000 population) in the United States varied from a high of 440.6 per 100,000 in New York to a low of 208.1 per 100,000 in New Mexico (CDC 2000). The CHD death rate for the United States is approximately midway between those of other industrialized countries. A World Health Organization study of CHD deaths rates from 1985 showed extremely high rates in the United Kingdom, Ireland, and some of the Nordic and eastern European countries. Low rates were noted in certain southern European countries and Asia, France, and Japan. In the countries studied, the highest CHD death rate observed was as much as 10 times the lowest rate (Uemura 1988).

Time Trends

CHD has been the leading cause of death in the United States for most of this century, with death rates from CHD peaking in 1963. Since 1968, the decline in CHD mortality has been consistent and nearly uniform across race and sex groups, but is steeper in younger than in older age groups (Higgins et al. 1988). From 1980 to 2000, the age-adjusted death rate of CHD fell from 542.9 to 266.8 deaths per 100,000 population among men aged 25 to 84 years and from 263.3 to 134.4 deaths per 100,000 population among women aged 25 to 84 years. In 1980, a total of 462,984 deaths among people in this age group were recorded as due to CHD. By 2000, that had dropped to 337,658 recorded CHD deaths. Had the age-specific death rates from 1980 remained in 2000, an additional 341,745 deaths from CHD would have occurred (Ford et al. 2007). Declines in age-adjusted mortality since 1999 have been comparable across race/sex subgroups (CDC 2009b) (see Figure 13.3). Factors responsible for the decline in CHD mortality are not fully understood, but changes in lifestyle, reductions in risk factor prevalence, and improvements in medical care and treatment of CHD are thought to have contributed (Goldman et al. 1988). A recent study by Ford and colleagues indicates that approximately 47% of the decline in the CHD death rate from 1980 to 2000 was attributed to evidence-based medical treatments, including secondary preventive therapies after MI or revascularization (11%), initial treatment for acute MI or unstable angina (10%), treatments for heart failure (9%), revascularization for chronic angina (5%), and other therapies (12%). Approximately 44% was attributed to changes in major risk factors, including reductions in total cholesterol (24%), systolic blood pressure (20%), smoking prevalence (12%), and physical inactivity (5%), although these reductions were partially offset by increases in the Body Mass Index (BMI) and the prevalence of diabetes, which accounted for an increased number of CHD deaths (8% and 10%, respectively) (Ford et al. 2007).

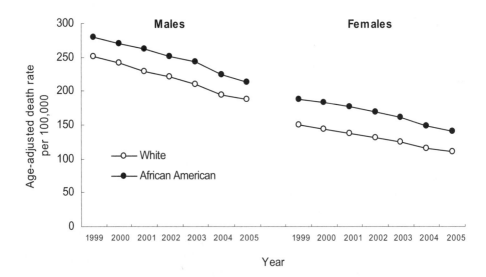

Figure 13.3. Age-adjusted death rates for coronary heart disease by sex and race in the United States from 1999 to 2005. *Rates are age adjusted to 2000 standard. *Note:* From CDC (2009b).

Causes

Coronary risk factors can be classified as either modifiable or nonmodifiable. Among modifiable risk factors, the major independent risk factors for CHD are high blood pressure, elevated blood cholesterol, cigarette smoking, physical inactivity, abdominal obesity, low daily fruit and vegetable consumption and diabetes. Other modifiable risk factors include elevated blood C-reactive protein (CRP), fibrinogen, homocysteine, and environmental tobacco smoke. Alcohol overconsumption and stress may also contribute to CHD risk. Nonmodifiable risk factors are discussed under the previous heading of high-risk groups. Note, however, that not all high-risk groups are defined by nonmodifiable factors. Improved socioeconomic status, for example, while not typically a direct goal of medical or public health intervention, certainly is a legitimate objective for social and economic policy.

Modifiable Risk Factors

High blood pressure, or hypertension (see Chapter 11), is a strong independent risk factor for morbidity and mortality from CHD (Hennekens 1988). People with elevated blood pressure are 2 to 4 times as susceptible to CHD as are people with normal blood pressure (Table 13.1) (Jenkins 1988). However, it is important to note that risk of CHD generally increases as levels of systolic or diastolic blood pressure rise whether or not one is looking at a population group above or below a particular hypertension cutpoint. Therefore, blood pressure reduction by individuals labeled "normotensive" by conventional definitions can also be beneficial. Studies suggest that a prolonged reduction of only 5 to 6 mmHg in diastolic blood pressure results in a 20% to 25% reduction in CHD (MacMahon 1996). Although drug therapy to reduce high blood pressure has resulted in lower overall rates of CVD deaths, major studies of drug treatment for high blood pressure have failed to demonstrate a reduction in CHD deaths, possibly as a result of the untoward effects of antihypertensive therapy on other risk factors (Collins 1990).

Tobacco use (see Chapter 5) is a major cause of CHD among both men and women. Smokers have twice the risk of heart attack as nonsmokers. Smoking is also the major risk factor for sudden death from heart attack, with smokers having 2 to 4 times the risk of nonsmokers. The risk increases with the number of cigarettes smoked (U.S. Department of Health and Human Services 1983).

Following the first Surgeon General's Report on smoking in 1964, cigarette smoking declined sharply for men and at a slower pace for women (NCHS 2009) (see Figure 13.4). Overall, cigarette smokers are 2–4 times more likely to develop CHD than nonsmokers. Cigarette smokers have CHD death rates 70% higher than those of nonsmokers, with heavy smokers (i.e., those who smoke two or more packs per day) dying from CHD at a rate 2–3 times that of nonsmokers. Studies have shown, however, that people who stop smoking experience a rapid and substantial reduction in CHD mortality. For people who have smoked a pack or less per day, within 10 years of quitting, death rates from CHD drop to the level of people who have never smoked (USDHHS 1983).

In addition, a number of studies suggest that exposure to environmental tobacco smoke (also called passive smoking or secondhand smoke) increases the risk of CHD (Glantz et al. 1991; Steenland et al. 1992). For example, follow-up of a very large group of never-smoking U.S. women showed that those with regular exposure to passive smoke at home or at work had a 90% increased risk of developing CHD compared with those

Table 13.1. Modifiable Risk Factors for Coronary Heart Disease, United States

Magnitude	Risk Factor	Best Estimate (%) of PAR (Range)
Strong (relative risk >4)	None	–
Moderate (relative risk 2–4)	High blood pressure (≥140/90 mmHg)	25 (20–29)
	Cigarette smoking	22 (17–25)
	Elevated cholesterol (≥200 mg/dL)	43 (39–47)
	Diabetes (fasting glucose ≥140 mg/dL)	8 (1–15)
Weak (relative risk <2)	Obesity[a]	17 (7–32)
	Physical inactivity	35 (23–46)
	Environmental tobacco smoke exposure	18 (8–23)
	Elevated plasma C-reactive protein (>3.0 mg/L)	19 (11–25)
	Elevated fibrinogen (>3.74 g/L)	21 (17–25)
	Elevated plasma homocysteine (>15 μmol/L) 5 (2–9)	5 (2–9)
Possible	Psychological factors	–
	Alcohol use[b]	–
	Elevated plasma homocysteine	–
	Infectious agents	–

[a]Based on BMI >27.8 kg/m^2 for men and >27.3 kg/m^2 for women.
[b]Moderate to heavy alcohol use may increase risk, whereas light use may reduce risk.
Note: Data from Anonymous (1988), Abbott et al. (1987), Danesh et al. (1998, (2004), Fibrinogen Studies Collaboration (2005), He et al. (1996), Hennekens et al. (1988), Howard et al. (1998), Kawachi et al. (1997), Kovar et al. (1987), Lam et al. (2000), Nygard et al. (1995), Powell et al. (1994), Ridker et al. (2006), Stamler et al. (1986), Stampfer et al. (1992), Thom et al. (2006), and U.S. Department of Health and Human Services (1991).

unexposed (Kawachi 1997). An estimated 35,052 nonsmokers die from CHD each year as a result of exposure to environmental tobacco smoke (Thom et al. 2006). The association between environmental tobacco smoke exposure and CHD mortality is elevating the importance of this critical public health issue to new heights. Cholesterol (see Chapter 12) is the blood lipid most strongly associated with CHD. The risk of CHD increases steadily as blood cholesterol levels in a population increase. Studies have shown that a 10% decrease in total cholesterol levels may result in an estimated 30% reduction in incidence of CHD (CDC 2000). For people with cholesterol levels in the 250- to 300-mg/dL range, each 1% reduction in cholesterol level results in about a 2% reduction in CHD morbidity and mortality (Sempos et al. 1989).

Cholesterol is transported in the blood by low-density lipoproteins (LDL), very-low density lipoproteins (VLDL), and high-density lipoproteins (HDL) (NHLBI 2002). High levels of LDL are a leading factor in the progression of atherosclerosis and in the subsequent development of CHD (Blackburn 1992; NHLBI 2002). The VLDLs, which are composed primarily of triglyceride, comprise 10% to 15% of the total serum cholesterol. Evidence supporting the association between elevated blood triglyceride and CHD has been mounting in recent years (Hokanson 1996).

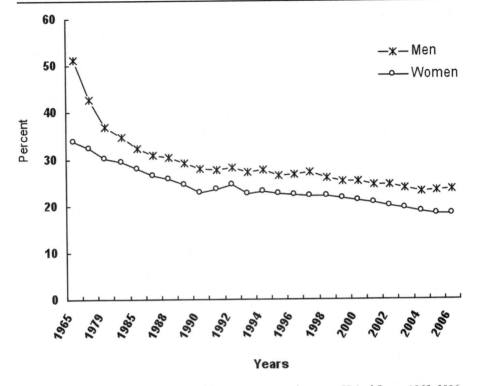

Figure 13.4. Prevalence of cigarette smoking among men and women: United States, 1965–2006. *Note:* From National Center for Health Statistics (2009).

The level of HDL is inversely related to CHD; the lower the level of HDL, the higher the risk of CHD, particularly at levels below 35 mg/dL (NHLBI 2002; Rifkind 1990). HDL level correlates inversely with LDL size and triglyceride level, and this coupled with the complex metabolic interrelationships of these particles makes it more difficult to separate the independent contributions of various lipids to CHD. It is quite possible that all play a role; one hypothesis is that LDL may be more important in early-stage athero-genesis, while low HDL and triglycerides elevation develops closer to the clinical onset of CHD (Sharrett et al. 1994).

CRP is an inflammatory biomarker that is strongly associated with CHD, inflammation, and the metabolic syndrome. Although CRP, synthesized primarily in the liver, was discovered in 1930 (Ridker et al. 2006), this protein has received substantial attention in recent years as a promising biological predictor of atherosclerotic disease (Pearson 2003). An evolving body of work suggests that even small increases in CRP within the normal range are predictive of future vascular events in apparently healthy, asymptomatic individuals (Hackam et al. 2003). Danesh et al. (2000, 2004) recently reported a meta-analysis of 14 prospective long-term studies of CRP and the risk of nonfatal MI or death from CHD. The analysis comprised 2,557 cases with a mean age at entry of 58 years and a mean follow-up eight years. The combined adjusted risk ratio was 1.9 (95% confidence interval [CI] 1.5–2.3) for the development of CHD among individuals in the top third of baseline

CRP concentrations compared with those in the bottom third. A number of prospective studies have demonstrated that CRP also predicts recurrent events and increased mortality in patients with acute coronary syndromes, chronic stable angina, ischemic stroke and peripheral vascular disease (Hackam et al. 2003).

Fibrinogen is a circulating glycoprotein that acts at the final step in the coagulation response to vascular and tissue injury. Epidemiological data support an independent association between elevated levels of fibrinogen and CHD (Fibrinogen Studies Collaboration 2005; Lam et al. 2000). Two meta-analyses involving 18 and 22 prospective, long-term studies demonstrated strong, statistically significant risk for individuals in the upper third of baseline fibrinogen concentration compared with those in the lower third (relative risk 1.8, 95% CI 1.6–2.0) (Danesh et al. 1998; Fibrinogen Studies Collaboration 2005; Hackam et al. 2003; Maresca et al.1999).

Another plasma constituent, homocysteine, is receiving increased attention as a potentially modifiable risk factor for acute CHD events. Plasma homocysteine levels have been found to be positively associated with risk of CHD events (Nygard et al. 1997; Stampfer et al. 1992). A recent review conducted by Humphrey and colleagues (2008) searching MEDLINE (between 1966 and March 2006) identified 26 articles of good or fair quality. The results indicated that most studies found elevations of 20% to 50% in CHD risk for each increase of five mol/L in homocysteine level. A meta-analysis yielded a combined risk ratio for coronary events of 1.18 (95% CI 1.10–1.26) for each increase of five mol/L in homocysteine level. The association between homocysteine and CHD was similar when analyzed by sex, length of follow-up, outcome, study quality, and study design (Humphrey et al. 2008).

Although the underlying mechanisms linking diabetes (see Chapter 10) and CHD are still not well understood, diabetes mellitus is generally considered a major CHD risk factor. CHD is the most common cause of morbidity and mortality among people with diabetes, and individuals with diabetes experience CHD at rates two to four times greater than those without the disease (National Research Council 1989). Data from national studies showed a disproportionately high prevalence of diabetes in African Americans (11.7%) when compared with whites (4.8%). The 2003 overall death rate per 100,000 population from diabetes was 25.2. Death rates were 26.8 for white men, 50.5 for African American men, 20.0 for white women and 47.3 for African American women. At least 65% of people with diabetes die of some form of heart or blood vessel disease (Thom et al. 2006).

Obesity has widely been defined using BMI (weight [kg]/height [m^2]). A BMI of 25 and higher indicates overweight, and 30 or higher indicates obesity in adults (Thom et al. 2006). Obesity and overweight have significant associations with increases in blood pressure, serum total cholesterol and glucose, and with decreases in serum HDL levels. In addition, obesity has been well-documented as an independent risk factor for CVD and diabetes (see Chapter 9).

Recent studies suggest that the distribution of fat deposits on the body may also affect CHD risk. Upper body or abdominal fat ("central obesity" "apple shape") appears to increase risk more than lower body fat (pear shape). Men and women in the upper quintile of subscapular skin fold as well as men with a waist-to-hip ratio greater than 1.0 and women with a ratio greater than 0.8 experience increased CHD risk (Barrett-Connor et al. 1985; Freedman et al. 1995; USPSTF 1989). The tendency toward abdominal disposition of body fat seems to increase CHD risk across all levels of BMI (Prineas et al. 1993).

Physical inactivity (see Chapter 7) is increasingly recognized as a major risk factor for CHD. About 60% of U.S. adults do not engage in the recommended amount of regular leisure-time physical activity (defined as light-moderate activity for ≥30 minutes, ≥5 times per week or vigorous activity for ≥20 minutes, ≥3 times per week) (Thom et al. 2006). Physical activity decreases body weight, decreases blood pressure, and improves insulin sensitivity (USDHHS 1996). Mounting evidence suggests that small amounts of physical activity can also have a significant impact on heart disease mortality (Blair et al. 1989; Hakim et al. 1998). The greatest benefits appear to occur with the move from a completely sedentary lifestyle to very modest levels of activity.

Moderate to heavy alcohol consumption is known to raise blood pressure levels and to increase CHD mortality. However, in most studies, including several recent investigations (Hanna et al. 1997; Keil et al. 1997; Wannamethee et al. 1997), light regular drinking (two or fewer drinks per day) has been associated with modest reductions in CHD risk. The principal pathway for this protection appears to be through increased HDL-cholesterol (Criqui 1996). The relationship to other risk factors and the social consequences of alcohol use, however, preclude any public health recommendation for alcohol use (see Chapter 8).

Psychological factors and stress also have been studied in relation to the development of CHD (Greenwood et al. 1996; Williams 1987). Perhaps the most widely studied is the Type A behavior pattern, characterized by excessive competitiveness, hostility, impatience, fast speech, and quick motor movements (McQueen et al. 1982). Considerable attention has been devoted to the exploration of specific psychological factors, including anger, job stress, anxiety, and social support. Causal connections between these specific psychological risk factors and CHD have yet to be clearly established, but evidence supporting a causal role for anger, both as an event trigger and a long-term risk factor, and social support, particularly important in extending survival among those with disease, is mounting (Greenwood et al. 1996; Kawachi et al. 1996).

Lastly, risk factors for heart disease tend to cluster; that is, individuals with CHD are likely to have more than one risk factor. The greater the level of any single risk factor, the greater the chance of developing CHD. Moreover, the likelihood of developing CHD increases markedly when risk factors manifest simultaneously. There is at least an additive contribution to CHD risk for the major risk factors of high blood pressure, high LDL-cholesterol and fibrinogen, as evident in the findings of the Prospective Cardiovascular Munster (PROCAM) study (Figure 13.5) (Anonymous 1991; Abbott et al. 1987; CDC 1989; Heinrich et al. 1994; Kovar et al. 1987; Powell et al. 1994; Stamler et al. 1986).

Population-Attributable Risk

CHD is a multifactorial disease, and precisely quantifying the contribution of each risk factor to overall heart disease is difficult. We can, however, roughly gauge the importance of risk factors by estimating population-attributable risk (PAR), which is the percentage of CHD that could be prevented by eliminating a particular risk factor in the population. There are several things that need to be remembered when considering PARs, the two most important being that (1) when there are many factors contributing to a disease, as is the case with CHD, these percentages will sum to more than 100% and (2) when risk factors are continuous, like blood pressure or cholesterol level, the PAR estimated depends greatly on the cutpoint chosen to designate who is at high risk. Table 13.1 shows

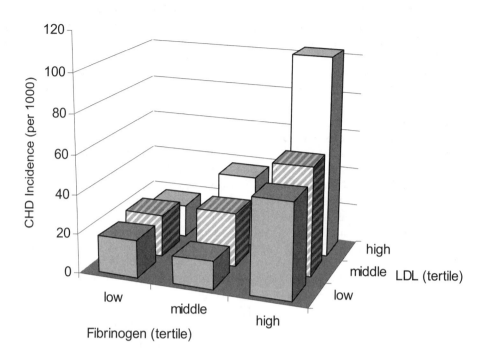

Figure 13.5. CHD incidence rates (per 1,000) in a 6-year follow-up, the PROCAM study. Heinrich, J. et al. Fibrinogen and Factor VII in the Prediction of Coronary Risk. Results from the PROCAM Study in Healthy Men. *Arterioscler Thromb* (1994):14:54–59. Reprinted with Permission. ©1994, American Heart Association, Inc.

the proportion of CHD mortality that can be attributed to the risk factors discussed above.

Prevention and Control Measures

Prevention

Because of the multiple risk factors involved in coronary heart disease, modest changes in one or more risk factors can have a large public health impact. Primary prevention of CHD involves controlling the major preventable risk factors: hypertension, high blood cholesterol, tobacco use, diet and physical inactivity (see Chapters 11, 12, 5, 6 and 7, respectively). Other effective methods of prevention include diabetes control, weight management, and limitations in alcohol consumption (see Chapters 10, 9 and 8, respectively).

The multifactorial nature of CHD etiology calls for multiple intervention strategies. In addition to the early detection and control of risk factors in adults, prevention approaches may include early and systematic health education regarding the importance of lifestyle behaviors in young people, such as avoiding tobacco, eating a healthy diet, and performing adequate physical activity. Other prevention interventions can include policy-related or environmental changes such as improved food choices in schools, improved food labeling in grocery stores, elimination of cigarette vending machines, and provision of smoke-free environments. (The multifaceted approach to risk reduction is discussed in Chapter 3 on intervention strategies.)

When considering prevention strategies, it is also important to recognize that CHD is affected by the social and economic characteristics of a community, including levels of income and education and occupations. Positive changes in public health are, therefore, often the result of general social and economic development policies, rather than public health policies per se (Wing et al. 1988).

Screening

The principal methods of early detection for CHD include screening for high blood pressure and elevated serum cholesterol, and assessing behavioral factors such as tobacco use, dietary fat intake, and physical activity level.

Screening electrocardiograms are not recommended for the general population but may be appropriate for individuals at increased risk of CHD. This group includes men older than 40 years with two or more CHD risk factors, high-risk sedentary men planning to begin an exercise program, and people who would endanger the safety of others if they were to experience sudden cardiac events (USPSTF 1989).

Treatment

Advances in the treatment of CHD have contributed substantially to major reductions in mortality over the past four decades. Treatment for CHD is tailored to each patient, depending on the cause and severity of the coronary artery disease. Treatment options mainly comprise: (1) healthy lifestyle programs, (2) medications, (3) surgical and other invasive procedures, and (4) gene therapy. Of them, adopting a healthy lifestyle is one of the best treatments for CHD. Either by itself or in combination with medical treatment, a healthy lifestyle can prevent or attenuate the disease progress.

When medications and lifestyle adjustments cannot relieve the chest pain symptomatic of CHD, surgery may be necessary to restore adequate function to the heart. Patients may benefit from one or more of these surgical treatment options. (a) Catheter-assisted procedures: a thin, flexible tube (catheter) is inserted into the patient's artery, usually in the leg, and then is threaded through the arteries to the heart. (b) Coronary angioplasty and stents: angioplasty opens blocked coronary arteries to allow blood to flow more freely to the heart. When the catheter tip reaches a blocked artery, a small balloon expands in the artery to push open the blood vessel. (c) Radiation brachytherapy: in cases where coronary artery blockage reoccurs, the patient may benefit from brachytherapy. In this procedure, the coronary artery segment is reopened during angioplasty and exposed to radiation. (d) Atherectomy: a catheter is inserted into the blocked artery and one of several types of small devices removes plaque build-up. (e) Coronary artery bypass surgery: Bypass surgery, also called coronary artery bypass grafting, creates a detour around a blocked coronary artery with a new blood vessel, or graft.

Gene therapy is another one of the newest potential treatment modalities, but its effectiveness is still under investigation. Gene therapists are attempting to introduce into the heart a gene that codes for a blood vessel growth factor, to stimulate and repair adequate blood growth (Goldstein et al. 2006; Mayo Foundation for Medical Education and Research

2009). Finally, cardiac rehabilitation—prevention of CHD complications through diet, exercise, weight control, and smoking cessation—has reduced mortality and improved functional capacity and quality of life among patients with clinical CHD (Oldridge et al. 1988).

Examples of Evidence-Based Interventions

Two major primary prevention strategies have been used in attempts to reduce cardiovascular mortality rates: the high-risk and the community-based (or population-based) approaches. The high-risk approach aims to identify high-risk individuals through population screening and to refer them for treatment. The Oslo Heart Study (Hjermann et al. 1981), the Multiple Risk Factor Intervention Trial (Anonymous 1982), the European Collaborative Trial of Multifactorial Prevention of Coronary Heart Disease (Levy 1985), and the Lipid Research Clinics Coronary Primary Prevention Trial (Anonymous 1984) are examples of this approach.

Community-based interventions are a cornerstone of the public health approach to CHD prevention. They are defined as programs that attempt to modify the prevalence of one or more CHD risk factors (i.e., hypertension, smoking, hyperlipidemia, physical inactivity, unhealthy diet), CHD mortality, or both within a specifically identified, circumscribed community. Community-based interventions have typically used education or environmental change to promote and facilitate changes in the lifestyles and other behaviors of a population (Papadakis et al. 2008).

The oldest community-based CVD prevention program is the North Karelia (Finland) Project, which began in 1972 and provided a broad range of risk factor interventions. Those targeted at individuals and groups included smoking cessation programs, nutrition education aimed at housewives, and the use of natural helper networks. At the community level, interventions were directed at the media and at food producers and distributors. Physicians and community nurses played a key role in providing both clinical services and health education. Combined, these efforts resulted in reduced heart disease morbidity and mortality in North Karelia (Puska et al. 1989).

Subsequently, the National Heart Lung and Blood Institute (NHLBI) funded four sites for major research and demonstration field trials: the Stanford (California) Three Community Study, the Stanford Five-City Project, the Minnesota Heart Health Program, and the Pawtucket (Rhode Island) Heart Health Program. The Three Community Study, funded in 1971, investigated the influence of a large-scale media intervention on health behavior. Evaluation showed the use of media to be effective and the addition of face-to-face intervention even more powerful in producing behavior changes (Farquhar et al. 1977; Flora et al. 1989).

In the Five-City Project, funded from 1978 through 1992, two treatment and two control cities were compared for changes in knowledge and changes in risk factors. The 5-year intervention was based on social learning theory, a communication-behavior change model, community organization principles, and social marketing methods. The treatment cities received 26 hours of exposure to general education and specific risk factor campaigns, resulting in increased knowledge and a reduction of CHD risk factors (Farquhar et al. 1990).

In 1980, the Minnesota Heart Health Program was initiated by the University of Minnesota. The program combined community organization, CVD risk factor screening and counseling, smoking cessation contests, physical activity promotion, mass media campaigns, and other interventions to reduce heart disease risk factors in three communities in Minnesota and North Dakota (Mittelmark et al. 1986).

The Pawtucket Heart Health Program, funded for 11 years beginning in 1980, was based on community psychology principles. A cornerstone of this program's approach was the use of volunteers. The intervention strategy involved mobilizing the community and involving them in all aspects of the program (Lasater et al. 1984; Lefebvre et al. 1990).

Largely because of a strong favorable but unanticipated secular trend in CHD risk factors in control communities, these interventions tended to have less power to demonstrate overall effectiveness at the community level than originally anticipated. However, within each intervention program individual components frequently were shown to be successful in analyses of intermediate or process measures and in analyses of principal endpoints that were limited to subpopulations most likely to be exposed to the component (e.g., school children participating in school-based components of community interventions) (Schooler et al. 1997). A recent review of 21 published major community-based CVD intervention programs worldwide, showed positive impact on CHD risk factors within a distinct population. More recent community-based CHD prevention programs have focused on discrete populations including the socioeconomically deprived, ethnic minorities, and rural communities (Papadakis et al. 2008).

From the Stanford projects, the utility of channel-specific interventions (e.g., worksite exercise challenges) to maximize reach and change behavior became evident (Anonymous 1994). In addition, interventionists learned that they needed to work within the formal political and institutional structure and the informal opinion leadership network. In some instances, community members need to be mobilized to modify the formal rules and regulations of a community to implement and maintain changes in risk factors (Fortmann et al. 1995). In Minnesota, it was apparent that changes in different outcomes (e.g., knowledge, behavior changes) necessitated different targeted strategies. For example, awareness was most influenced by general community events (fun walks, health fairs, etc.) for older persons and women. Similar to the experience of the Stanford study, specific settings such as work sites yielded better behavior change results than general community settings (Anonymous 1994). The most cost-effective efforts were those done in existing community channels (schools, work sites, etc.) where participants spend considerable time. The need to institutionalize these competitions and programs with limited resources and staff time from service providers was an ongoing issue (Anonymous 1994). Finally, Pawtucket investigators found it useful and important not only to establish formal, continuing relationships with community organizations already providing CVD risk reduction services but also to establish and maintain positive working relationships with community organizations that did not ordinarily view themselves as having a role in CVD risk reductions (e.g., places of worship). Leaders in these sites needed to buy in and be actively involved in planning and implementation for greatest participation to be realized (Anonymous 1994).

Since the NHLBI demonstrations, smaller-scale efforts have been undertaken at other sites. One is the New York State Healthy Heart Program, an effort based on community wide strategies for influencing risk behaviors developed and tested in the major NHLBI studies. The challenge has been to apply these strategies on a limited budget for hard-to-affect populations. The eight programs in high-risk communities are sponsored and coordinated by the New York State Department of Health through its Mary Lasker Heart and Hypertension Institute (New York State Healthy Heart Program 1992).

Also employing some of the methods and lessons learned from the early NHLBI projects, the Centers for Disease Control and Prevention (CDC) joined with states and other agencies to fund other community-based intervention programs, including the South Carolina Cardiovascular Disease Prevention Project (South Carolina Department of Health and Environmental Control 1991), the Bootheel Heart Health Project (Brownson et al. 1996), the Bemidji (Minnesota) Cardiovascular Disease Prevention Project, a collaborative project with the Indian Health Service (Indian Health Service 1992), and several projects using their Planned Approach to Community Health (Krueter 1992).

A recent report by Chen et al. described two successful community-based CVD intervention programs in China—the Capital Steel and Iron Company cardiovascular intervention program (CSICIP) and the Beijing Fangshan cardiovascular prevention program (BFCP). The two programs each included >110,000 participants. The CSICIP, a work site–based intervention, began with a cardiovascular health survey covering 60,000 employees in 1974, and grew to 110,000 persons by 1995. The program targeted altering diet (particularly reducing salt and fat intake), keeping alcohol consumption to modest levels, and quitting smoking, together with a strategy of controlling high risks such as hypertension. The BFCP was a comprehensive prevention trial in Fangshan rural area during the period of 1991–1999. BFCP covered a total of 120,000 residents in five rural communities, including three serving as intervention communities with a total of 66,000 residents and two as control communities with a total of 54,000 residents. In the CSICIP, significant reductions in blood pressure occurred in both intervention and control sites, with greater reductions at the intervention site. In addition, intervention sites experienced a marked additional reduction in salt intake and better overall control of hypertension. In the BFCP, blood pressure fell in all communities to a more modest degree than that in the CSICIP. In the intervention communities of BFCP, participants had greater blood pressure declines and higher smoking cessation rates, and also kept alcohol consumption to more modest levels than those in the control communities (Chen et al. 2008).

In sum, there were numerous insights gained learned from these pioneering community CVD prevention interventions, relating to the following: using of mass media effectively, building on existing settings/institutions, creating strategies for making a healthy heart lifestyle "doable"; developing approaches to support environmental as well as legislative and policy changes; and establishing and maintaining community coalitions. One of the most important common threads in the truly exemplary prevention and control programs was their reliance on multiple channels and multiple levels. This strategy appears to be critical in effecting lasting change. A model exemplifying this approach is the Multilevel Approach to Community Health (MATCH) model (CDC 1998). Under the model, the four specific channels suggested are work sites, schools, health care, and community sites. Interventions can be directed to the individual, organizational, or policy level in any of these sites. Table 13.2 gives an example of an organizational-level MATCH intervention in the "school" channel. Other multilevel models that appear to be successful include the Spectrum of Prevention, used successfully in California for their tobacco control program, and the social ecology approach being used in other countries, such as Australia.

Public health leaders are now approaching consensus on high yield strategies to help change social/community norms regarding other critical CHD risk factors, including physical activity and nutrition. As these strategies are tested and refined, various experts are recommending that they be implemented through the population-based approach like MATCH (Association of State and Territorial Chronic Disease Program Directors 1997;

Table 13.2. Example of an Organizational-Level MATCH Intervention in the "School" Channel: Organizational Change for School Lunch Modifications for Cardiovascular Health

Intervention objectives	*Policy:* Adopt "Go for Health" program, establish and distribute policy supporting lower fat and sodium diets for children authorizing changes in school food service menus, food purchasing, and food preparation practices.
	Practice: Implement low-salt and low-fat school lunches through the modification of recipes and food preparation practices.
Targets of intervention	*Policymakers:* School superintendent, food service director, school principals.
	Staff: School food service workers, cafeteria managers.
Intervention approaches:	*Policy:* Consulting to policymakers.
	Practice: Training of staff.

Simons-Morton, D.G., et al. Influencing Personal and Environmental Conditions for Community Health: A Multilevel Intervention Model. *Fam Community Health* (1988):11:25–35. Used with permission.

King et al. 1995; Sallis et al. 2002; Schmid et al. 1995; Simons-Morton et al. 1988). However, to date, large variability has also been noted in the success of population-level CHD prevention trials. Developing an in-depth understanding of best practice derived from experiences to date with community-based intervention trials is essential for the design of future population-level cardiovascular prevention interventions. The burgeoning epidemics of chronic disease will necessitate the application of population health interventions to effectively address a multiplicity of issues, disease states, and management challenges. It is also important that these interventions be delivered appropriately (Papadakis et al. 2008).

Areas of Future Research

Epidemiologic research on CHD will likely focus on emerging, yet not completely understood, modifiable factors, like plasma CRP, fibrinogen, homocysteine, as well as known, but complex, risk factors like serum cholesterol. Studies focusing on subclinical endpoints will be important in revealing undiscovered risk factors potentially significant in primary prevention. For example, further exploration of the importance of infection and inflammation in increasing the risk of atherosclerosis may prove fruitful. Population-based studies devising novel means of using information on known risk factors may also be crucial to advancing secondary prevention strategies.

There is also growing interest and recognition of the importance of conducting more research and demonstration efforts involving policy and environmental approaches to reduce CHD risk factors. Partnerships with nontraditional partners will be essential for success. Population-based prevention research should focus on CHD research in special populations such as women, children, older adults, and racial and ethnic minorities, addressing the applicability of current knowledge to these populations and designing population-specific interventions, like the recent proposed Multiethnic Study of Atherosclerosis (MESA) (Bild et al. 2002) and The Hispanic Community Health Study/Study of

Latinos (HCHS/SOL) (Anonymous 2007). The MESA is designed to study the prevalence, correlation, and progression of subclinical CVD in multiple ethnicities (white, African American, Hispanic and Chinese) (Bild et al. 2002). The HCHS/SOL is a multicenter epidemiologic study in Hispanic/Latino populations to determine the role of acculturation in the prevalence and development of disease and to identify risk factors playing a protective or harmful role in Hispanics/Latinos (Anonymous 2007). Finally, despite the huge potential for public health benefits, CHD control efforts have been modest at many state and local health department levels. Both levels need to have an infusion of resources and expertise to build capacity and expand activities in CHD control.

CEREBROVASCULAR DISEASE (ICD-10 I60-I69)

Significance

Cerebrovascular disease, also referred to as stroke, is the third leading cause of death in the United States, accounting for 137,119 deaths in 2006. It represents over one fifth of all CVD deaths and approximately 6% of all cause mortality; the age-adjusted death rate due to stroke for 2006 was 43.6 per 100,000 (Heron et al. 2009). Stroke mortality rates are down 29.7% over the decade between 1995 and 2005 (Lloyd-Jones et al. 2009). Despite this steady decline (Kung et al. 2008), stroke remains a major cause of morbidity, with an estimated 795,000 Americans suffering new or recurrent strokes each year (Lloyd-Jones et al. 2009). Slightly over three quarters of such incident cases represent new strokes, while under a quarter represent recurrent cases. The impact of stroke is substantial with over 6 million American survivors, many of whom endure short- and long-term disabilities (Lloyd-Jones et al. 2009). Stroke-associated societal costs, including direct costs associated with medical care and indirect costs due to lost productivity, are estimated at $68.9 billion in 2009 (Lloyd-Jones et al. 2009). Racial disparities in the incidence of stroke, particularly among African Americans, and observed regional differences in stroke continue to be explored. Stroke is also observed in children. In 1999, the overall incidence rate for stroke for children less than 15 years of age was 6.4 per 100,000 (Lloyd-Jones et al. 2009).

Pathophysiology

Stroke occurs when an artery in the brain is either ruptured or clogged by a blood clot resulting in an interruption or a severe restriction of blood supply used to provide oxygen and nutrients to brain tissue. Two major types of stroke include ischemic and hemorrhagic. Ischemic strokes account for approximately 87% of all strokes and are caused by blockage due to a blood clot (thrombus), a wandering clot (embolus) or narrowing of the artery due to atherosclerotic plaque (Lloyd-Jones et al. 2009). The major form of ischemic stroke, cerebral thrombosis, is caused when a blood clot forms and blocks blood flow in the cerebral artery. This is generally the result of atherosclerosis in the cerebral vessels. Cerebral embolism occurs when a clot breaks loose from another part of the body, often the heart, and lodges in a cerebral artery. Transient ischemic attacks (TIA) or "ministrokes" exhibit symptoms similar to ischemic strokes but are "transient" in nature with a thrombus or embolus quickly dislodging, allowing restored blood flow. Typically, a TIA does not result in lasting neurological impairment or deficits. However, TIAs are important in predicting future strokes, with about half of strokes following a TIA event occurring within a year (AHA 2003).

The other type of stroke, hemorrhagic, is caused by intracerebral or subarachnoid hemorrhaging. The rupturing of blood vessels due to head injury or a burst aneurysm can lead to bleeding into brain tissue (intracerebral hemorrhage) or into the space between the brain and the skull (subarachnoid hemorrhage) (AHA 2003). The severity of hemorrhagic stroke is dependent on the location and amount of bleeding. Although subarachnoid hemorrhaging is life-threatening with mortality averaging 40% within the first month of bleeding, those who survive the initial stroke and following critical period often make remarkable recoveries. Hemorrhagic strokes account for 13% of all strokes (Lloyd-Jones et al. 2009).

Descriptive Epidemiology

Age is a strong risk factor for stroke. After age 55 years, the rate of stroke incidence doubles in each successive decade. Stroke mortality also increases sharply with age. In 2005, the stroke death rate ranged from 33 per 100,000 in those aged 55 to 64 years to 1,142 per 100,000 in people aged 85 years and older (Lloyd-Jones et al. 2009).

Men generally have higher mortality rates than women between the ages of 35 to 85 years. Women, however, represent approximately 60% of all strokes each year and generally surpass male incidence of stroke after age 85 years. The Framingham Heart Study examined sex differences in stroke incidence and estimated lifetime risk as one in five for women and one in six for men (Petrea et al. 2009). The increased lifetime risk for women can be explained in large part due to the longer life expectancy of women. Study researchers found women to be significantly older (75.1 years) than men (71.1 years) at first-ever stroke event (Petrea et al. 2009).

Distinct differences in stroke prevalence, incidence, and mortality rates exist among racial groups. According to the 2005 BRFSS, prevalence rates are distributed as follows: 2.3% for whites, 4.0% for African Americans, 1.6% for Asian/Pacific Islanders, 2.6% for Hispanics, 6% for American Indian/Alaska Natives, and 4.6% for multiracial individuals. In the Atherosclerosis Risk in Communities (ARIC) cohort study, for people aged 42 to 84 years, from 1987 to 2001, African American men had nearly double the age-adjusted incidence rates for stroke than white men (6.6 vs. 3.6 per 1,000 person-years, respectively) (NHLBI 2006). Similarly, African American women had greater than two times the age-adjusted incidence rates for stroke than white women (4.9 vs. 2.3 per 1,000 person years, respectively). Age-adjusted mortality rates for African Americans in 2005 were similarly greater than whites (65.2 vs. 44.7 per 100,000) (Lloyd-Jones et al. 2009).

Results from the Brain Attack Surveillance in Corpus Christi (BASIC) study suggest that Mexican Americans have twofold higher cumulative incidence for stroke (first-ever, recurrent, and TIA) compared with non-Hispanic whites in younger populations (aged 42–59 years) (Morgenstern et al. 2004). For older populations, this difference was not observed (Morgenstern et al. 2004). Despite the higher prevalence and incidence rates of stroke for Hispanics compared with non-Hispanic whites in younger populations,

Hispanic stroke survivors tend to live longer as evidenced by an approximately 15% to 20% decrease in mortality compared with non-Hispanic whites in 2005 (Kung et al. 2008; Lloyd-Jones et al. 2009). However, caution should be taken when interpreting Hispanic mortality rates due to potential reporting inconsistencies on death certificates and surveys.

Risk of stroke is greatly increased among people who have previously had a stroke or a TIA. Approximately one-third to one-half of people who have had one or more TIA will later have a stroke (Lloyd-Jones et al. 2009; Kleindorfer et al. 2005). Risk of TIA increases with age and occurs more often in men. After TIA, the 90 day risk of stroke ranges from 9% to 17% (Lloyd-Jones et al. 2009). People who have had TIAs are nearly 10 times more likely to have a stroke than are people of the same age and sex who have not had a TIA. However, only about 15% of all strokes are preceded by TIAs (Lloyd-Jones et al. 2009).

The risk for stroke is higher for people with a family history of stroke. Positive paternal family history is associated with a doubling of stroke risk, while maternal family history increases stroke risk about 40%. The effect of family history appears to be about the same in African Americans and whites (Kim et al. 2004). Current smoking combined with family history may place an individual at even greater risk (OR 6.4, 95% CI 3.1–13.2) compared with nonsmokers with no family history of stroke (Woo et al. 2009).

The "stroke belt" is represented by a group of states clustered in the Southeast with some of the highest stroke rates in the country: Alabama, Arkansas, Georgia, Louisiana, Mississippi, North Carolina, South Carolina, and Tennessee (Figure 13.6). In 2005, age-adjusted stroke mortality ranged from a high of 60 per 100,000 in Alabama to a low of 31.1 per 100,000 in New York (Howard et al. 2006). Estimates of 10-year stroke risk by region and race show differences in regional risk due to mean age-, race-, and sex-adjusted stroke risk varying slightly by region (10.7% in stroke belt vs. 10.1% elsewhere). Racial differences in 10-year stroke risk are evident (11.3% for African Americans vs. 9.7% for whites) with primary differences observed in hypertension, systolic blood pressure, diabetes and smoking (Cushman et al. 2008). Countries with the highest rate of stroke in 2005 were the Russian Federation, Romania, and China (rural areas). Those with very low rates were Canada, Australia, France, and Switzerland (Lloyd-Jones et al. 2009). In developed

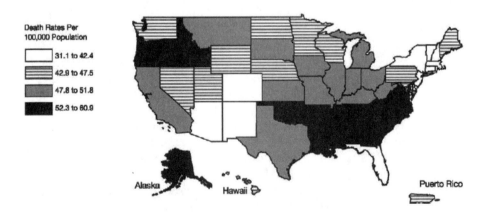

Figure 13.6. Stroke age-adjusted death rates per 100,000 population by state, United States, 2005. Lloyd-Jones, D. et al. Heart Disease and Stroke Statistics—2009 Update: A Report from the American Heart Association Statistics Committee and Stroke Statistics Subcommittee. *Circulation.* (2009):119:480–486. Reprinted with Permission. © 2009, American Heart Association, Inc.

countries, incidence of stroke is declining due to efforts to lower blood pressure and reduce smoking (CDC 2007). Stroke rates remain high in areas where the population is aging.

Stroke mortality rates have been declining steadily since the 1950s. Between 1979 and 1995, mortality rates declined approximately 20%, declining another 25% from 1999 to 2005, five years ahead of the AHA 2010 goal to reduce stroke mortality. The trend has been uniformly downward for both sexes and all race groups. The marked decline is attributed to a number of factors including (1) decrease in mean blood pressure levels, (2) improved diagnosis and prevention of stroke and CVD, (3) reduction in smoking, and (4) improved treatment and control of primary risk factors such as hypertension (CDC 1999, 2007). Despite success in combating stroke to date, public health experts continue to monitor mortality rates in light of the increasing rate of diabetes, hypertension, and other risk factors.

Causes

The major modifiable risk factors for stroke include hypertension, nonvalvular atrial fibrillation (AF), diabetes, cigarette smoking, physical inactivity, obesity, and dyslipidemia. Hypertension, physical inactivity, diabetes, and AF contribute the highest PAR percentages in those aged 80–89 years (See Table 13.3). Since most of the risk factors are also associated with atherosclerotic cerebrovascular disease, treatment, management and primary and secondary prevention of stroke remain targeted at reduction of these factors. Some studies also show possible increased risk associated with race and genetic factors including increased risk for stroke in identical twins where one has suffered a stroke.

Modifiable Risk Factors

Hypertension remains the single most significant modifiable and treatable risk factor for stroke and has been shown to increase stroke risk for persons with blood pressures as low

Table 13.3. Modifiable Risk Factors for Stroke

Relative Magnitude Risk	Risk Factor	Estimated PAR (%)
Strong		
4	Hypertension (age 50 years)	40
4	Atrial fibrillation (age 50–59 years)	1.5
Moderate		
1.8	Cigarette smoking	12–18
1.8–6	Diabetes	5–27
2.0	Dyslipidemia (high total cholesterol)	15
1.75–2.37	Obesity	12–20
Possible		
2.7	Physical inactivity	30
1.5–2.5	Dyslipidemia (low HDL-cholesterol)	10
1.4	Postmenopausal Hormone Therapy	7

Note: Data from Sacco et al. (2006).

as 110/75, well within the normal range (Lewington et al. 2002). The risk increases with increasing blood pressure, both systolic and diastolic. In a meta-analysis by Collins et al. (1990) of randomized trials with antihypertensive drugs, mostly diuretics and beta-blockers, a reduction of as little as five to six mmHg (average 5.8 mmHg) was associated with approximately 35% to 40% reduction in stroke incidence (Collins et al. 1990). Li et al. (2005) confirmed that even individuals with blood pressures below 140/90 had an increased risk of stroke. Because of the recognized significant role of hypertension in stroke, the AHA and American Stroke Association (AHA/ASA) issued guidelines in 2006 with recommendations for antihypertensive treatment for all patients with ischemic stroke and TIA. While strict values are not defined, most practitioners direct therapy with goals guided by the Joint National Committee's (JNC) definition of prehypertension as 120–139/80–89 mmHg and have goals for diabetics of maintaining blood pressure less than 130/80, with caution in lowering the blood pressure in the elderly.

Nonvalvular atrial fibrillation (AF) is associated with worse outcomes such as fatality (two times more likely) or more severe disability (with 30-day mortality of 25% vs. 14% in AF vs. non-AF strokes, respectively), lower functional status, and greater rates of recurrences of stroke (Lin et al. 1996). In addition, the risk of stroke due to AF increases with age from 1.5% in those aged 50–59 years to 23.5% in those aged 80–89 (Lloyd-Jones et al. 2009). Because of the severity of outcomes, unless there is a strong contraindication to anticoagulation, long-term therapy with warfarin anticoagulation is warranted for primary and secondary prevention.

Diabetes is also an independent risk factor for stroke. Uncontrolled diabetes leads to arterial damage as well as increased risk for dyslipidemia, atherosclerosis, and hypertension—all which confer high risk for stroke. The occurrence of stroke is two to five times higher among people with diabetes than among those without it. Stroke risk is highest in black diabetics aged 35 to 54 years, while white diabetics are at highest risk from 45 to 64 years of age (Lloyd-Jones et al. 2009). A few studies (and subsequently the AHA/ASA 2006 guidelines) have suggested intensive therapy and aggressive glycemic control to a hemoglobin A1c <7% are associated with a decrease in microvascular and cardiovascular complications; however, these studies are limited on macrovascular complications and the risks of hypoglycemic complications in elderly patients seem to outweigh the benefits of tight control.

Several studies have shown the association of cigarette smoking with an increased risk of stroke. The Framingham Heart Study in 1988 assessed cigarette smoking as a risk factor for stroke and found that the risk increase is dose-dependent. Cigarette smoking has been shown to be strongly associated with carotid stenosis as well (Wilson et al. 1997). Haheim et al (1996) confirmed that daily cigarette smoking increases the risk of fatal stroke up to 3.5 times in men aged 40–49 years and furthermore found that combined cigarette and pipe or cigar smoking conferred an even higher risk than cigarettes alone (Haheim et al. 1996). Smoking cessation, but not necessarily reduction, resulted in decreased risk and incidence of strokes and sustained ex-smokers' risk for stroke was not significantly different from never-smokers' risk (Bjartveit et al. 2009). Smoking has also been identified as a risk factor for aneurysm formation, rupture of which results in hemorrhagic stroke.

Physical activity level is inversely proportional to stroke risk. Several studies including the Physicians' Health Study (Lee et al. 1999), the EPIC-Norfolk study (Myint et al. 2006), the Nurses' Health Study (Hu et al. 2000), and the Northern Manhattan Stroke Study (Sacco et al. 1998) support this relationship. A meta-analysis of 31 studies showed not only a reduced risk but also protective effects of moderate and high levels of physical activity on strokes, both ischemic and hemorrhagic (Wendel-Vos et al. 2004).

Although there are limited data that support weight reduction directly reducing the risk of recurrent stroke, the AHA/ASA 2006 guidelines recommend that persons with ischemic stroke and TIA be considered for weight reduction based on data from the Nurses' Health Study which found an increased risk of ischemic (but not hemorrhagic) stroke with increased BMI. The risk increases with increasing BMI. Weight reduction also indirectly affects stroke incidence reduction through its effects on other modifiable risks such as hypertension, diabetes, dyslipidemia, and physical inactivity.

While epidemiological data has been conflicting concerning the direct association of cholesterol levels with ischemic and hemorrhagic strokes, a meta-analysis of lipid-lowering therapy with statins found that treatment decreases the risk of nonhemorrhagic stroke (Hankey 2008).

Several trials including the Women's Estrogen for Stroke Trial (WEST) and the landmark Women's Health Initiative (WHI) trial showed an increased rate of fatal stroke and increased risk of ischemic stroke up to 55%, respectively, with unopposed estrogen therapy. Furthermore, data suggested the use of estrogen and progestin also increased the risk of stroke in postmenopausal women (Hendrix et al. 2006; Rossouw et al. 2002; Viscoli et al. 2001; Wassertheil-Smoller et al. 2003).

Population-Attributable Risk

As shown in Table 13.3, an estimated 20%–40% (varies by age group) of stroke deaths are attributed to elevated blood pressure with the greatest PAR percentage demonstrated in the 50-year-old age group. Smoking PAR varies from 12 to 18% with risk differences varied by age and sex (Goldstein et al. 2006). It is important to note that modifiable risk factors often interact or are accompanied by nonmodifiable risk factors (e.g., age, sex, genetic factors). Such individuals are at greater risk and benefit from targeted prevention screenings and treatment of modifiable risk factors. Although the PAR for diabetes, ranging from 5% to 27%, is less than that observed for hypertension, the increasing prevalence and incidence of diabetes suggests the rise of future comorbid cases. Effective lifestyle modifications and interventions will be necessary to combat the growing obesity epidemic and the associated sedentary lifestyle (12%–20% and 30% PAR, respectively) (Goldstein et al. 2006).

Prevention and Control

As described earlier, there are a number of primary risk factors associated with first and recurrent stroke. Risk assessment tools, such as the Framingham Stroke Profile, can be used to identify and classify individuals based on risk score (see Table 13.4) (Goldstein et al. 2006). Regardless of whether a formal risk assessment tool is used, the evidence is clear that primary prevention of stroke is most effective when controlling hypertension. Studies have shown that reducing blood pressure, whether through diet and exercise or through antihypertensive medication, significantly decreases risk of stroke. Other established, modifiable risk factors to target include cigarette smoking, diabetes, and dyslipidemia (elevated cholesterol, LDL, and/or triglycerides). Nonmodifiable risk factors that should factor in the planning and implementation of appropriate therapeutic interventions include age, family history, and other genetic factors. Due to the broad scope of factors that

Table 13.4. Modified Framingham Stroke Risk Profile

					Points						
	0	+1	+2	+3	+4	+5	+6	+7	+8	+9	+10
Men											
Age (years)	54–56	57–59	60–62	63–65	66–68	69–72	73–75	76–78	79–81	82–84	85
Untreated systolic blood pressure (mmhg)	97–105	106–115	116–125	126–135	136–145	146–155	156–165	166–175	176–185	186–195	196–205
Treated systolic blood pressure (mmhg)	97–105	106–112	113–117	118–123	124–129	130–135	136–142	143–150	151–161	162–176	177–205
History of diabetes	No		Yes								
Cigarette smoking	No			Yes							
Cardiovascular disease	No				Yes						
Atrial fibrillation	No				Yes						
Left ventricular hypertrophy on electrocardiogram	No					Yes					
Women											
Age (years)	54–56	57–59	60–62	63–64	65–67	68–70	71–73	74–76	77–78	79–81	82–84
Untreated systolic blood pressure (mmhg)		95–106	107–118	119–130	131–143	144–155	156–167	168–180	181–192	193–204	205–216
Treated systolic blood pressure (mmhg)		95–106	107–113	114–119	120–125	126–131	132–139	140–148	149–160	161–204	205–216
History of diabetes	No			Yes							
Cigarette smoking	No			Yes							
Cardiovascular disease	No		Yes								
Atrial fibrillation	No						Yes				
Left ventricular hypertrophy on electrocardiogram	No				Yes						

Note: Data from Sacco et al. (2006).

directly and indirectly impact the risk of stroke to both the individual and population, the CDC published "A Public Health Action Plan to Prevent Heart Disease and Stroke" as a means to assist in the Healthy People 2010 goal of "improving cardiovascular health through the prevention, detection, and treatment of risk factors" (AHA 2008).

Screening

Survivors of stroke or TIA are at increased risk for another stroke. All survivors should be monitored for hypertension on a routine basis. In addition to routine monitoring, anti-hypertensive treatment is recommended for prevention of recurrent stroke and other vascular events (Sacco et al. 2006). This is recommended regardless of whether an individual has a history of hypertension. Treatment is also associated with a benefit of approximately 10/5 mmHg average reduction in blood pressure (Sacco et al. 2006). For survivors with diabetes, particular attention is placed in controlling blood pressure, lipids, glucose, and hemoglobin A1c ($\leq$7%). Stroke survivors with comorbid coronary artery disease or elevated cholesterol levels are similarly monitored to ensure proper lipid management following lifestyle modifications, dietary guidelines, and treatment recommendations (Sacco et al. 2006). Statin agents, in particular, are recommended in lowering cholesterol to reduce the risk of vascular events. Further research is needed to determine its efficacy in preventing recurrent stroke or TIA events. Other factors associated with increased risk of CVD and stroke such as smoking, weight gain (obesity), and excessive alcohol consumption should also be avoided.

Treatment

Long-term effects of stroke can be devastating; therefore initial assessment and proper management are crucial to minimizing complications and preventing recurrence. Some common medical complications of stroke include heart attack, heart failure, difficulty swallowing, aspiration pneumonia, deep vein thrombosis/pulmonary embolism, and residual paralysis. It is important to acknowledge the severity of complications as approximately half of deaths after strokes are due to medical complications.

Acutely, goals of assessment and management include attempts at determining the etiology of the stroke and minimizing brain injury through interventions ranging from thrombolytic therapy to cautious lowering of blood pressure with medications to surgical procedures (Adams et al. 2007). Because even the acute management of stroke depends on the type of stroke, (i.e., ischemic vs. hemorrhagic), standard of care includes prompt brain imaging either by computerized axial tomography (CAT) scanning or magnetic resonance imaging (MRI). Ultrasound imaging of the carotid arteries, now standard of care for assessment of causes of stroke, can reveal blockages that can be opened with surgery or less invasive methods (Adams et al. 2007).

The National Institutes of Health (NIH) developed a scale known as the NIH Stroke Scale (NIHSS) to help diagnose stroke based on the person's level of consciousness, eye muscle and visual impairments, facial muscle deficits, extremity muscle deficits, sensory deficits, and language and speech deficits. There are 11 criteria resulting in a total possible score ranging from 0 to 42. The NIHSS is one of the most widely used and validated scales. Adams et al. (1999) found that the baseline NIHSS score strongly predicted ischemic stroke outcome at seven days and three months. Previously, Goldstein et al.

(1997) confirmed the reliability of the NIHSS score for nonneurologists as well as neurologists. The landmark trial of thrombolytic therapy tissue plasminogen activator (t-PA) conducted by the National Institute of Neurological Disorders and Stroke Recombinant t-PA Stroke Study Group found that sufferers of ischemic stroke treated with t-PA within three hours after the onset of symptoms were at least 30% more likely than patients given placebo to have minimal or no disability at three months and one year (Anonymous 1995). Long-term goals include minimizing the physical manifestations of neurological deficits through physical therapy, speech and swallowing therapy, and occupational therapy, and minimizing the risk of recurrence of stroke, including antiplatelet or anticoagulation therapy as necessary and strict control or modification of risk factors such as diabetes, dyslipidemia, hypertension, arrhythmias, and smoking cessation. As mentioned, equally important to the individual's recovery and long-term prognosis is the addressing and prevention of the common medical complications.

Examples of Evidence-Based Interventions

In 2004, USDHHS funded the Stroke Belt Elimination Initiative (SBEI) to promote prevention and control of hypertension and stroke. SBEI is part of the larger Closing the Health Gap Initiative with the mission of reducing racial and ethnic disparities in health care. SBEI funds programs targeting the seven southeastern states in the "stroke belt" with the highest stroke death rates. SBEI is community-focused with four key public health interventions to develop and implement: (1) a community-wide awareness and education campaign, (2) a communications network to inform the public of free blood pressure screening activities, (3) a health professional component that emphasizes improvement of blood pressure control among persons with hypertension, and (4) a component for health systems and health plans that emphasizes improvement of blood pressure control rates for persons with hypertension.

The Well-Integrated Screening and Evaluation for Women Across the Nation (WISEWOMAN) project targets low-income and uninsured women (http://www.cdc.gov/WISEWOMAN/). This initiative is coordinated by the CDC and offers cholesterol and hypertension screening, lifestyle interventions, and other services to enable women to address and reduce risk factors for heart disease and stroke. Health care providers and health departments partner with the state to provide such services to participants.

Areas of Future Research

Despite decreasing stroke incidence during the second half of the twentieth century, stroke continues to be a major cause of death and disability worldwide. There has been increasing recognition that early risk factor detection and lifestyle modification can prevent and/or reduce stroke disease burden. Future research to detect surrogate and other potentially modifiable risk factors, including elevated cholesterol and body weight, is being defined. Further refinement is needed to promote specific interventions to high risk populations (using risk assessment and other diagnostic tools). Guidelines are needed to tailor interventions to a variety of subpopulations. Creative methods to encourage lifestyle interventions such as diet, occupational and leisure physical activity along with appropriate treatment to reduce first and/or recurrent stroke and TIA is desired to combat the multifactoral nature of the disease. National initiatives partnered with community-based research will provide individual and population level support to ensure patients are properly screened, treated, and monitored for primary risk factors. As the world's population ages, development of effective methods of primary and secondary prevention of stroke will be crucial to reduce long-term disability and disease burden.

HEART FAILURE (ICD-10 I50.0)

Significance

Heart failure (HF) represents a new epidemic of CVD, affecting nearly 5 million people in the United States. Every year, approximately 300,000 people die as a result of HF, and 550,000 new cases are diagnosed. In contrast to other CVDs, the prevalence, incidence, and mortality from HF are increasing, and prognosis remains poor (Hunt et al. 2005). HF results in high hospitalization rates and mortality; up to 40% of patients die within one year of first hospitalization, making the survival rate bleaker than that for nearly all cancers. In addition to the cost in human suffering, care for patients with HF places a large economic strain on the health care system, including the Medicare program. In the United States, in 2005, for example, there were about 1,079,000 hospital admissions with a principal diagnosis of HF, accounting for $28 billion in health care costs (Hunt et al. 2005).

Pathophysiology

Heart failure (HF) is a multisystem disorder characterized by abnormalities of cardiac function, skeletal muscle, and renal function, stimulation of the sympathetic nervous system, and a complex pattern of neurohormonal change that impairs the ability of either ventricle to fill with or eject blood (Jackson et al. 2000; Mann 1999). The cardinal manifestations of HF are dyspnea and fatigue, which may limit exercise tolerance, and fluid retention, which may lead to pulmonary and peripheral edema. Both abnormalities can impair the functional capacity and quality of life of affected individuals, but they may not necessarily dominate the clinical picture at the same time (Hunt et al. 2005). Over the past decades, three clinical pathophysiological models (hypotheses) for HF have been suggested: (1) the cardiorenal model, in which HF is reviewed as a problem of excessive salt and water retention that is caused by abnormalities of renal blood flow; (2) the cardiocirculatory, or hemodynamic, model, in which HF is thought to arise largely as a result of abnormalities in the pumping capacity of the heart and excessive peripheral vasoconstriction; and (3) the neurohormonal model, in which HF progresses as a result of the overexpression of biologically active molecules that are capable of exerting toxic effects on the heart and circulation (Batlle et al. 2007; Mann et al. 2005).

In terms of left ventricular dysfunction (LVD), there are two mechanisms of reduced cardiac output: systolic dysfunction and diastolic dysfunction. Systolic dysfunction refers to impaired ventricular contraction. It is defined by a left-ventricular ejection fraction of less than 50%. The most common causes of systolic dysfunction are ischemic heart disease, idiopathic dilated cardiomyopathy, hypertension, and valvular heart disease. Diastolic dysfunction (defined as left ventricular ejection fraction ≥50%) results from impaired myocardial relaxation, with increased stiffness in the ventricular wall and reduced left ventricular compliance, leading to impairment of diastolic ventricular filling. Diastolic dysfunction can occur in many of the same conditions that lead to systolic dysfunction. The most common causes of diastolic dysfunction are hypertension, ischemic heart disease, hypertrophic cardiomyopathy, and restrictive cardiomyopathy (Figueroa et al. 2006).

Descriptive Epidemiology

High-Risk Groups

Heart failure disproportionately affects the older population. The incidence of HF approaches 10 per 1,000 population after age 65 years, and approximately 80% of patients hospitalized with HF are more than 65 years old (Hunt et al. 2005). People with coronary artery disease, hypertension, and diabetes are at particular risk of developing HF. About seven of ten people with HF had high blood pressure before being diagnosed. About 22% of men and 46% of women will develop HF within six years of having a heart attack (Thom et al. 2006). African Americans with HF are an average of 10 years younger than whites, have more hospital admissions and readmissions, and suffer a different spectrum of disease that predispose them to HF. Specifically, African Americans have a higher incidence of hypertension, left ventricular hypertrophy and diabetes (Yancy 2001; Young 2004). The annual rates per 1,000 population of new and recurrent HF events for white men are 21.5 for ages 65–74 years, 43.3 for ages 75–84 years, and 73.1 for age 85 years and older. For white women in the same age groups the rates are 11.2, 26.3 and 64.9, respectively. For African American men, the rates are 21.1, 52.0 and 66.7 years, and for African American women, the rates are 18.9, 33.5 and 48.4 years, respectively (Thom et al. 2006). Data from the NHANES 1999–2000 indicates that the overall prevalence of HF is about the same for white and African American groups (2%), but among those 60 years and older, it is higher in African Americans than whites, 9% vs 6%, respectively (Hunt et al. 2005). African Americans also have higher mortality rates from HF than whites. In the United States, the 2003 death rates for HF were 20.5 for white men, 23.4 for African American men, 18.4 for white women and 20.4 per 100,000 for African American women (Thom et al. 2006).

Geographic Distribution

Age-adjusted mortality rates for heart failure among all ages vary substantially among the states in the United States. For example, in 1995, the age-adjusted rates ranged from 3.4 (New Hampshire) to 29.7 (Mississippi) per 100,000 population for all ages. For persons aged 65 years or more, the five highest age-adjusted mortality rates in 1995 were 255.6 (Alabama), 247.6 (Mississippi), 226.0 (Arkansas), 196.6 (Kentucky), and 181.5 (Oklahoma) per 100,000 population, and the five lowest age-adjusted mortality rates were 30.7 (New Hampshire), 32.4 (Rhode Island), 33.0 (Iowa), 34.5 (Florida), and 46.9 (Hawaii) per 100,000 population (CDC 1998).

Time Trends

Most current information on the epidemiology of heart failure is derived from three major epidemiologic studies in the United States published since 1993 (CDC 1998; Gillum 1993; Kannel 2000). There have been several consistent findings, including a sharp increase in prevalence with age and strong male preponderance. The prevalence of HF has increased in the United States since 1980 in both sexes (Kannel 2000). From 1990 to 1999, the annual number of hospitalizations has increased from approximately 810,000 to over one million for HF as a primary diagnosis and from 2.4 to 3.6 million for HF as a primary or secondary diagnosis (Haldeman et al. 1999; Hunt et al. 2005). The aging of the post-World War II "baby boom" generation is likely to swell the number of patients with HF further (Young 2004). Data from the National Hospital Discharge Surveys between 1980 and 2006 indicated that age-adjusted HF hospitalization rates in patients aged 65 and older significantly increased from 1980 to 2006, with an estimated annual percentage increase rate of 1.20% (95% CI 0.76%–3.17%) in men and of 1.55% (95% CI 0.42%–3.51%) in women. Poisson regression models indicate that the relative risk of being hospitalized due to HF in subjects living in the last five year period (2002–2006) was 1.37 times higher (95% CI 1.31–1.42) than those living in the early years of 1980 to 1984. Subjects aged 85 years or older had four times higher risk of being hospitalized due to HF as compared with those aged 65–74 years (Libbey et al. 2005). Crude death rates for HF increased during 1980–1988 for persons aged 65 years or older and declined slightly from 1989 to 1990. For persons aged 65 or older, age-adjusted death rates for HF increased during 1980–1988 for both white and African American men and women; however, death rates were higher among African Americans and men (CDC 1998).

Causes

Modifiable Risk Factors

The most common causes of heart failure are coronary artery disease, hypertension, diabetes, heart rhythm disorders (arrhythmias), congenital heart disease, and heart muscle disease (cardiomyopathy). Other risk factors associated with these diseases in general also contribute to HF by putting extra stress on the heart, including high cholesterol, cigarette smoking, alcohol abuse, and a family history of HF or other CVDs. The odds of developing HF are especially high in people who have more than one of these risk factors. For example, a study of the predictors of HF among women with coronary heart disease (CHD) found that CHD patients with diabetes had the highest risk of developing HF. Among diabetic participants with no additional risk factors, the annual incidence of HF was 3.0% compared with 8.2% among diabetics with at least three additional risk factors. Diabetics with fasting glucose greater than 300 mg/dL had a threefold adjusted risk of developing HF, compared with diabetics with controlled fasting blood sugar levels (Bibbins-Domingo et al. 2004; Liu et al. 2009; Thom et al. 2006).

Population-Attributable Risk

Data from the Framingham Heart Study indicate that hypertension is one of the major predisposing risk factors for the development of HF in the general population. In terms of PAR, hypertension accounts for 39% of HF events in men and 59% in women. MI, despite only a 3%-10% prevalence in the population, accounts for 34% of HF in men and 13% in women. Prevalence of diabetes in the Framingham cohort study was 8% in men and 5% in women. Diabetes accounted for 6% of HF in men and 12% in women (Kannel 2000).

Prevention and Control

Early identification of heart failure risk factors and appropriate prevention and treatment will have the greatest impact in reducing progression of the disease. Earlier guidelines for HF health care emphasized the functional status and appropriate treatment of HF patients. According to the New York Heart Association (NYHA) Functional Classification, HF is classified into four classes that range from patients with asymptomatic LVD (Class I) to those with severe symptoms at rest or with minimal exertion (Class IV) (Table 13.5). This classification helps clinicians assess the severity of a patient's symptoms, guides the choice of therapy, and helps with subjective documentation of response or lack of response to therapy (Caboral et al. 2003). In 2001, to further emphasize prevention of HF, the American College of Cardiology (ACC) and the AHA created a new conceptual framework to help health professionals understand the continuum of disease progression in HF (Hunt et al. 2005). Rather than replacing the NYHA classification, the framework defines disease progression in four stages: A, B, C, and D, beginning with patients who have risk factors for developing HF all the way to patients with end-stage disease (Hunt et al. 2005; Rasmusson et al. 2007). Figure 13.7 shows the stages in the development of heart failure and recommendations for preventing and treating HF by stages (Hunt et al. 2005).

Stage A: Patients in Stage A do not have any diagnosed structural heart disease but have risk factors that can lead to HF. At this stage, patient education is key, given that lifestyle modifications that reduce the risk of developing CVD include maintaining an appropriate diet, regular exercise, maintaining a normal body weight, smoking cessation, and limiting alcohol consumption (Rasmusson et al. 2007; Thom et al. 2006).

Stage B: Like patients in Stage A, HF patients at Stage B are asymptomatic, but have either structural heart disease or evidence of LVD. Treatments for Stage B are added to all those mentioned for Stage A, in an attempt to prevent the development of overt, symptomatic HF. Medications are requested for patients when appropriate (Rasmusson et al. 2007; Thom et al. 2006).

Stage C: Patients in Stage C have structural heart disease and current or previous symptoms of HF, such as reduced activity tolerance, dyspnea, and fluid retention. Rec-

Table 13.5. Heart Failure Classification

Level	Description	Simple Description
I	Cardiac disease without resulting limitations of physical activity.	Asymptomatic.
II	Slight limitation of physical activity—comfortable at rest, but ordinary physical activity results in fatigue, dyspnea, or anginal pain.	Symptomatic with moderate exertion.
III	Marked limitation in physical activity—comfortable at rest, but less than ordinary physical activity causes fatigue, dyspnea, or anginal pain.	Symptomatic with minimal exertion.
IV	Inability to carry on any physical activity without discomfort of symptoms at rest.	Symptomatic at rest.

Note: Data from Hunt et al. (2005) and Chavey et al. (2001).

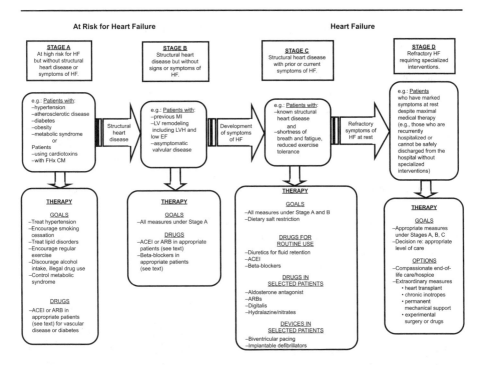

Figure 13.7. Stages in the development of heart failure with recommended therapy by stage. ACEI, angiotensin converting enzyme inhibitor; ARB, angiotensin receptor blocker; HF, heart failure. Hunt, S.A., et al. ACC/AHA 2005 Guideline Update for the Diagnosis and Management of Chronic Heart Failure in the Adult. *Circulation*. (2005):112:e154–e235. Reprinted with Permission. © 2005, American Heart Association, Inc.

ommended therapies for patients with Stage C are the same as those for patients with Stages A and B. But because these patients are symptomatic, most patients receive medications (such as a diuretic and digoxin along with angiotensin-converting enzyme (ACE) inhibitors, angiotensin receptor blockers, and beta-blockers). Other important measures include sodium restriction, administration of the influenza and pneumococcal vaccine, and physical activity except for patients in an acute decompensated state (Caboral et al. 2003; Hunt et al. 2005; Rasmusson et al. 2007; Thom et al. 2006).

Stage D: Stage D is reserved for HF patients with end-stage HF. These patients are markedly symptomatic, despite maximal tolerated therapy. In addition to the care outlined for patients in Stages A to C, these patients usually require specialized interventions to control and manage their HF such as mechanical assist devices (biventricular pacemaker or left ventricular assist device) (Caboral et al. 2003; Hunt et al. 2005; Rasmusson et al. 2007; Thom et al. 2006).

Because of the clear-cut relationship between preventable difficulties such as coronary heart disease and the tremendous burdens of HF medications, comorbidity, and mortality (e.g., Stages C and D), a great deal of attention should be focused on preventing the development of ventricular dysfunction in the first place. Clearly, early identification and prevention of patients at risk for HF (Stages A and B) are critical to control HF.

Examples of Evidence-Based Interventions

Since the overwhelming majority of heart failure cases are traced to three preventable and treatable conditions (hypertension, coronary artery disease, and diabetes), prevention and treatment of these conditions and risk factors is the focus of efforts to reduce incidence of HF (Baker 2002). For example, several studies have shown that treating elevated blood pressure can dramatically decrease the risk of developing HF (Baker 2002; Dahlof et al. 1991; Kostis et al. 1997). Results from the Swedish Trial in Old Patients with Hypertension indicated that treatment of hypertension reduced the risk of developing HF from 4.8% to 2.3%, a 52% relative reduction in those who received active treatment as compared with the placebo (Dahlof et al. 1991). Among patients with diabetes, controlling hypertension and hyperglycemia is also critical for preventing HF. In the United Kingdom Prospective Diabetes Study Group (UKPDS), for example, effective blood pressure control reduced the relative risk of developing HF by a dramatic 56%, as compared with those who received less effective blood pressure control (UKPDS 1998).

Areas of Future Research

Over the last decade, although there have been many studies on the etiology of heart failure and advances in the care of patients with heart failure, the causes remain poorly understood and the prognosis remains poor. Further research should include (1) identifying HF risk factors to develop more effective methods of primary prevention, (2) continued studies of secondary prevention of HF to reduce the mortality of HF and to improve quality of life for HF patients, and (3) community based studies, along with regional, national, and international cooperative studies to identify specific prevention and treatment strategies for HF among different populations.

PERIPHERAL ARTERIAL DISEASE (ICD-10 I73.9)

Significance

Peripheral arterial disease is a condition involving atherosclerosis of the lower extremities that is common in older populations. In epidemiologic studies PAD is typically confirmed with the ankle-brachial index (ABI)—a ratio of Doppler-recorded systolic blood pressure in the upper compared with the lower extremities. An ABI below 0.90 is the conventional cutpoint for PAD case confirmation.

PAD causes functional morbidity and increases the risk for other CVD morbidity and mortality. PAD is associated with intermittent claudication, a classic presentation that involves calf pain and other symptoms. However, intermittent claudication is now believed to be present in only approximately 10% of the estimated eight million U.S. adults with PAD (Lloyd-Jones et al. 2009). Large numbers of individuals with PAD report different constellations of leg symptoms and a substantial subgroup (estimated at 40%) presents without pain (Lloyd-Jones et al. 2009). However, when present, the pain of PAD is strongly associated with diminished functional status and quality of life. Individuals with asymptomatic PAD have also been found to be at significant risk for decline in lower limb functioning (McDermott 2006). PAD is the leading cause of lower limb amputation in the United States and accounted for $3.9 billion worth of health care expenses by the Medicare program in 2001, most of it going toward inpatient hospital stays (Hirsch et al. 2008). Annual Medicare spending for PAD is comparable with annual spending for CHF and cerebrovascular disease.

The major public health burden of peripheral arterial disease stems from its strong association with CVD mortality—individuals with PAD are over three times more likely to experience CVD death than like-aged non-PAD patients (Heald et al. 2006). This excess risk of CVD mortality in PAD patients is independent of the effects of other CVD risk factors (McDermott 2006) and represents a very large attributable mortality risk since baseline CVD death rates are high in the older age-groups most affected by PAD. The five year all-cause mortality rate in PAD patients is higher than that among those with either breast cancer or Hodgkin's disease (Criqui 2001). Finally, in addition to the morbidity associated with lower limb function and the mortality burden, there is a growing body of evidence linking PAD with cognitive decline (Rafnsson et al. 2009).

Pathophysiology

Peripheral arterial disease is caused by atherosclerosis of the arteries—consequently its pathophysiology is not unique from that of other atherosclerosis-related CVDs. The presence of PAD is, therefore, a strong indication that there are also atherosclerotic manifestations in other vascular territories—particularly the heart or brain. Confirmed coronary atherosclerosis is found in very large proportions of patients diagnosed with PAD and also in patients with borderline ABI values (McDermott 2006). PAD appears to be more frequently associated with disease at multiple vascular territories than either coronary artery disease or cerebrovascular disease (Steg et al. 2007) and, moreover, the coronary atherosclerosis present in patients with concomitant PAD tends to be more severe than that found in patients with coronary disease alone (Brevetti et al. 2009).

Descriptive Epidemiology

Prevalence of ankle-brachial index defined peripheral arterial disease in individuals 40 years of age or above was estimated at 4.3%, according to NHANES 2000 data (Selvin et al. 2004). Prevalence is strongly associated with age, even within older age groups (Ostchega et al. 2007) and approximately doubles with each successive decade after age forty (Allison et al. 2007). The prevalence estimates for the U.S. population aged 65 or more years range from 12% to 20% (Lloyd-Jones et al. 2009). Strong sex differences in PAD prevalence have not been consistently documented. PAD prevalence in African Americans 50 years or older is at least twofold higher than in non-Hispanic whites (Allison et al. 2007). Prevalence in Hispanic Americans is similar to, or perhaps modestly higher, than that for non-Hispanic whites (Allison et al. 2007; Criqui et al. 2005). Prevalence of PAD may be underestimated because individuals with PAD who have undergone revascularization procedures may have normal ABIs and because up to 25% of individuals with ABIs in the 0.90 to 0.99 range, above the conventional cutpoint for defining PAD, may actually have disease (Allison et al. 2007).

Causes

Individuals with diabetes, hypertension, and renal disease have higher prevalences of PAD. Based on NHANES 2000 data for individuals over age 40 years, prevalence of PAD was over 10% among those with diabetes and nearly 7% in those with hypertension (Selvin et al. 2004). Patients with renal insufficiency also appear to have at least double the PAD prevalence of those with normal kidney function (Selvin et al. 2004) and prospective data from the ARIC cohort suggest that individuals with chronic kidney disease had a 1.5 fold higher risk for developing incident PAD than do those with normal kidney function (Wattanakit et al. 2007).

In addition to age and the high-risk groups noted above, the constellation of risk factors for PAD is similar to those for other CVD. Smoking appears to have a particularly strong effect. A cohort study of PAD incidence suggested a 2.55 increased PAD risk associated with current smoking (Newman et al. 1993), and case-control studies estimating current smoking RRs yield even higher estimates (Cole et al. 1993). The prevalence ratio of PAD in current compared with never smokers is nearly seven (Selvin et al. 2004). In a study of individuals with diabetes, and therefore already at high risk for PAD, active smoking was still associated with a doubling of PAD incidence (Wattanakit et al. 2005). Hypertension and dyslipidemia RRs are more modest than those for smoking or diabetes (Criqui 2001; Selvin et al. 2004). A recent, large, cross-sectional study of PAD patients in France suggested that isolated systolic hypertension occurred more commonly among patients with PAD than CAD or CVD—a finding worthy of follow-up in epidemiologic studies (Safar et al. 2009).

Two less-traditional PAD risk factors worth considering as research moves forward are inflammatory biomarkers and genetics. Prospective studies of large cohorts have suggested that CRP, as well as certain other circulating markers of inflammation, are significant predictors of symptomatic PAD incidence (Pradhan et al. 2008; Ridker et al. et al. 2001). In large cross-sectional studies, CRP levels were significantly different in those with and without prevalent PAD (Selvin et al. 2004). Inflammatory biomarkers also have been significantly associated with all-cause mortality risk through two years of follow-up in a small cohort of PAD patients (Vidula et al. 2008). While not directly modifiable risk factors, CRP and other inflammatory factors may ultimately prove useful as component biomarkers in the assessment of subclinical PAD, PAD severity, or treatment responsiveness.

As with other CVDs, genetic susceptibility likely plays a role in PAD etiology but the mechanisms are complex involving multiple genes and gene–environment interactions. The limited number of family studies of PAD completed to date do support a role for heritable genetics in PAD etiology—but the degree of genetic influence is difficult to quantify and gene-finding and candidate gene studies have not yielded putative PAD risk genes (Knowles et al. 2007). Larger candidate gene studies are now underway with researchers also now contemplating the optimal strategies needed to mount large genome-wide association studies that could potentially reveal common genetic variants associated with PAD.

Prevention and Control

Strategies for primary prevention of peripheral arterial disease do not differ from those for any atherosclerotic chronic disease and will not be discussed here in detail. With respect to treatment, the foundational intervention for the management of symptomatic PAD is exercise. Exercise is hypothesized to improve PAD symptoms via adaptive responses of the muscle or increasing collateral blood flow in the affected limbs (Carman et al. 2006). Higher levels of physical activity have been associated with increased survival among PAD patients (Garg et al. 2006). Smoking cessation is also advised for the improvement of leg pain symptoms of PAD (Hankey et al. 2006). More recently, options for pharmacological therapy of symptomatic PAD have become available including statins and cilostazol (Garg et al. 2006; Hankey et al. 2006). The 2005 treatment guidelines for PAD are available through the AHRQ National Guideline Clearinghouse at http://www.guideline.gov/summary/summary.aspx?doc_id=8503&nbr=4740.

In instances where limb pain is severely disabling or the limb is threatened because of ulceration or gangrene, endovascular surgical procedures, such as angioplasty with and without stents and arterial bypass surgery, are recommended; however, it has been argued that the evidence supporting efficacy of such procedures for PAD is much weaker than that for coronary artery disease (Cao et al. 2009). Despite this, endovascular procedures for PAD are one of the fastest growing surgical procedures in the United States (Almahameed et al. 2006).

By far, the single biggest issue related to PAD prevention and control, from a public health perspective, is secondary prevention. Given the high risk of mortality from CVD-related events among PAD patients, individuals diagnosed with PAD are obvious candidates for interventions designed to reduce coronary heart disease and stroke risks. The pursuit of appropriate atherothrombotic risk factor reduction is a cornerstone of PAD treatment guidelines. Smoking cessation, blood pressure control, and cholesterol lowering have been linked with decreased CVD mortality while blood glucose control and weight loss have been connected with other benefits. Antiplatelet therapy, including aspirin, has been demonstrated in multiple studies to prevent progression of atherosclerosis in PAD patients, and in some studies to prevent CVD mortality. PAD researchers have advocated the use of more formal clinical staging approaches for PAD patients to guide intensity of intervention (Haugen et al. 2007). However, at the same time, studies have shown that physician awareness of the strong link between PAD and future cardiovascular events is low (Gornik et al. 2006). Also well documented is the fact that PAD patients are less likely to receive CVD risk reduction pharmacotherapy than patients with atherosclerotic disease in other vascular beds (Bennett et al. 2009; Cacoub et al. 2009). This suggests diagnosed PAD patients are not receiving potentially effective interventions as often as indicated. The REACH Registry, an international, prospective, observational registry of more than 68,000 patients with coronary artery disease, cerebrovascular disease or PAD, recently reported that PAD patients had significantly fewer CVD risk factors under control than did the patients in either of the other two diagnostic groups (Cacoub et al. 2009). Moreover, as mentioned earlier, a large proportion of PAD is currently undiagnosed, implying a pressing need to improve disease detection. The ABI measure, while inexpensive and noninvasive, unfortunately has not been found sufficiently sensitive to be used as a population-based screening tool (Hankey et al. 2006) and secondary prevention in asymptomatic PAD patients is largely still a function of direct recognition of adverse CVD risk factor profiles. Consequently the vigilant monitoring of and intervention on classic CVD risk factors remains the most promising path for secondary prevention of PAD moving forward.

Resources

American Heart Association, http://www.americanheart.org/presenter.jhtml?identifier=1200000.
American Stroke Association, http://www.strokeassociation.org/presenter.jhtml?identifier=1200037.
Centers for Disease Control, Division for Heart Disease and Stroke Prevention, http://www.cdc.gov/DHDSP.
National Heart Lung and Blood Institute, http://www.nhlbi.nih.gov.
National Institute of Neurological Disorders and Stroke, http://www.ninds.nih.gov.
National Center for Health Statistics Fast Stats, http://www.cdc.gov/nchs/fastats/heart.htm and http://www.cdc.gov/nchs/fastats/stroke.htm.
WHO MONICA Project, http://www.ktl.fi/monica.
Framingham Heart Study, http://www.framinghamheartstudy.org.
American College of Cardiology, http://www.acc.org.
Heart Failure Society of America, http://www.hfsa.org.
National Heart Failure Quality Improvement Project, http://www.nationalheartfailure.org.
Heart Failure Online, http://www.heartfailure.org.

Suggested Reading

Ammar, K.A., S.J. Jacobsen, D.W. Mahoney, et al. Prevalence and Prognostic Significance of Heart Failure Stages: Application of the American College of Cardiology/American Heart Association Heart Failure Staging Criteria in the Community. *Circulation* (2007):115:1653–1670.
Centers for Disease Control and Prevention (CDC). Update to: A Public Health Action Plan to Prevent Heart Disease and Stroke (2008).
Lloyd-Jones, D., R. Adams, M. Carnethon, et al. Heart Disease and Stroke Statistics—2009 Update: A Report from the American Heart Association Statistics Committee and Stroke Statistics Subcommittee. *Circulation* (2009):119:480–486.
McDermott, M.M. The Magnitude of the problem of Peripheral Arterial Disease: Epidemiology and Clinical Significance. *Cleve Clin J Med* (2006):73(Suppl 4): S2–S7.
McMurray, J.J., and S. Stewart. Epidemiology, Aetiology, and Prognosis of Heart Failure. *Heart.* (2000):83:596–602.
O'Donnell, C.J., and R. Elosua. Cardiovascular Risk Factors. Insights from Framingham Heart Study. *Rev Esp Cardiol* (2008):61:299–310.
Ostchega, Y., R. Paulose-Ram, C.F. Dillon, Q. Gu, and J.P. Hughes. Prevalence of Peripheral Arterial Disease and Risk Factors in Persons aged 60 and Older: Data from the National Health and Nutrition Examination Survey 1999–2004. *J Am Geriatr Soc* (2007):55:583–589.
Papadakis, S., and I. Moroz. Population-Level Interventions for Coronary Heart Disease Prevention: What Have We Learned Since the North Karelia Project? *Curr Opin Cardiol* (2008):23: 452–461.

References

Anonymous. *Hispanic Community Health Study/Study of Latinos.* University of North Carolina: Chapel Hill, NC. Available at: http://www.cscc.unc.edu/hchs. Accessed October 24, 2007.

Anonymous. Tissue Plasminogen Activator for Acute Ischemic Stroke. The National Institute of Neurological Disorders and Stroke Rt-PA Stroke Study Group. *N Engl J Med* (1995):333: 1581–1587.

Anonymous. Moving on: International Perspectives on Promoting Physical Activity. In: Killoran, A.J., P. Fentem, and C. Caspersen, editors, *Health Education Authority*. London, UK (1994).

Anonymous. National Education Programs Working Group Report on the Management of Patients with Hypertension and High Blood Cholesterol. *Ann Intern Med* (1991):114:224–237.

Anonymous. The Lipid Research Clinics Coronary Primary Prevention Trial Results. I. Reduction in Incidence of Coronary Heart Disease. *JAMA* (1984):251:351–364.

Anonymous. Multiple Risk Factor Intervention Trial. Risk Factor Changes and Mortality Results. Multiple Risk Factor Intervention Trial Research Group. *JAMA* (1982):248:1465–1477.

Abbott, R.D., R.P. Donahue, S.W. MacMahon, D.M. Reed, and K. Yano. Diabetes and the Risk of Stroke. The Honolulu Heart Program. *JAMA* (1987):257:949–952.

Adams, H.P., Jr., P.H. Davis, E.C. Leira, et al. Baseline NIH Stroke Scale Score Strongly Predicts Outcome After Stroke: A Report of the Trial of Org 10172 in Acute Stroke Treatment (TOAST). *Neurology* (1999):53:126–131.

Adams, H.P., Jr., G. del Zoppo, M.J. Alberts, et al. Guidelines for the Early Management of Adults with Ischemic Stroke. A Guideline from the American Heart Association/American Stroke Association Stroke Council, Clinical Cardiology Council, Cardiovascular Radiology and Intervention Council, and the Atherosclerotic Peripheral Vascular Disease and Quality of Care Outcomes in Research Interdisciplinary Working Groups. *Circulation* (2007):115: e478–e534.

Allison, M.A., E. Ho, J.O. Denenberg, et al. Ethnic-Specific Prevalence of Peripheral Arterial Disease in the United States. *Am J Prev Med* (2007):32:328–333.

Almahameed, A., and D.L. Bhatt. Contemporary Management of Peripheral Arterial Disease: III. Endovascular and Surgical Management. *Cleve Clin J Med* (2006):73(4 Suppl):S45–S51.

American Heart Association. *Update to a Public Health Action Plan to Prevent Heart Disease and Stroke*. Atlanta, GA: Centers for Disease Control and Prevention (2008).

American Heart Association. Heart Disease and Stroke Statistics—2003 Update. American Heart Association, Dallas, Texas (2003).

Anderson, R.N., K.D. Kockanck, and S.L. Murphey. Report of final mortality statistics, 1995. *Mon Vital Stat Rep* (1997):45:1–40.

Association of State and Territorial Chronic Disease Program Directors. Physical Activity Issue Paper. (1997).

Baker, D.W. Prevention of Heart Failure. *J Card Fail* (2002):8:333–346.

Barrett-Connor, E., and T. Orchard. Diabetes and Heart Disease. In: National Diabetes Data Group, editor, *Diabetes in America: Diabetes Data Compiled 1984*. U.S. Department of Health and Human Services, Public Health Service, National Institutes of Health, National Institute of Arthritis, Diabetes, and Digestive and Kidney Diseases: Bethesda, MD (1985):XVI-1–XVI-41.

Batlle, M., F. Perez-Villa, E. Garcia-Pras, et al. Down-Regulation of Matrix Metalloproteinase-9 (MMP-9) Expression in the Myocardium of Congestive Heart Failure Patients. *Transplant Proc* (2007):39:2344–2346.

Bennett, P.C., S. Silverman, and P. Gill. Hypertension and Peripheral Arterial Disease. *J Hum Hypertens* (2009):23:213–215.

Bibbins-Domingo, K., F. Lin, E. Vittinghoff, et al. Predictors of Heart Failure Among Women with Coronary Disease. *Circulation* (2004):110:1424–1430.

Bild, D.E., D.A. Bluemke, G.L. Burke, et al. Multi-Ethnic Study of Atherosclerosis: Objectives and Design. *Am J Epidemiol* (2002):156:871–881.

Bjartveit, K., and A. Tverdal. Health Consequences of Sustained Smoking Cessation. *Tob Control* (2009):18:197–205.

Blackburn, H. Ancel Keys Lecture. The Three Beauties. Bench, Clinical, and Population Research. *Circulation* (1992):86:1323–1331.

Blair, S.N., H.W. Kohl, III, R.S. Paffenbarger, Jr., D.G. Clark, K.H. Cooper, and L.W. Gibbons. Physical Fitness and All-Cause Mortality. A Prospective Study of Healthy Men and Women. *JAMA* (1989):262:2395–2401.

Brevetti, G., G. Sirico, G. Giugliano, et al. Prevalence of Hypoechoic Carotid Plaques in Coronary Artery Disease: Relationship with Coexistent Peripheral Arterial Disease and Leukocyte Number. *Vasc Med* (2009):14:13–19.

Briefel, R.R., and C.L. Johnson. Secular Trends in Dietary Intake in the United States. *Annu Rev Nutr* (2004):24:401–431.

Brownson, R.C., C.A. Smith, M. Pratt, et al. Preventing Cardiovascular Disease Through Community-Based Risk Reduction: The Bootheel Heart Health Project. *Am J Public Health* (1996):86:206–213.

Caboral, M., and J. Mitchell. New Guidelines for Heart Failure Focus on Prevention. *Nurse Pract* (2003):28:13, 16, 22–23; quiz 24–25.

Cacoub, P.P., M.T. Abola, I. Baumgartner, et al. Cardiovascular Risk Factor Control and Outcomes in Peripheral Artery Disease Patients in the Reduction of Atherothrombosis for Continued Health (REACH) Registry. *Atherosclerosis* (2009):204:e86–e92.

Cao, P., and P. De Rango. Endovascular Treatment of Peripheral Artery Disease (PAD): So Old Yet So Far from Evidence. *Eur J Vasc Endovasc Surg* (2009):37:501–503.

Carman, T.L., and B.B. Fernandez, Jr. Contemporary Management of Peripheral Arterial Disease: II. Improving Walking Distance and Quality of Life. *Cleve Clin J Med* (2006):73(4 Suppl): S38–S44.

Centers for Disease Control and Prevention (CDC). Prevalence and Most Common Causes of Disability Among Adults—United States, 2005. *MMWR* (2009):58:421–426.

Centers for Disease Control and Prevention (CDCa). Wonder System Compressed Mortality Files, 1999–2005. Accessed July, 2009.

Centers for Disease Control and Prevention (CDCb). Wonder System Compressed Mortality Files, 1979–1998. Accessed July, 2009.

Centers for Disease Control and Prevention (CDC). Prevalence of stroke—United States, 2005. *MMWR* (2007):56:469–474.

Centers for Disease Control and Prevention (CDC). State-Specific Cholesterol Screening Trends— United States, 1991–1999. *MMWR* (2000):49:750–755.

Centers for Disease Control and Prevention (CDC). Decline in Deaths from Heart Disease and Stroke—United States, 1900–1999. *MMWR* (1999):48:649–656.

Centers for Disease Control and Prevention (CDC). Changes in Mortality from Heart Failure— United States, 1980–1995. *MMWR* (1998):47:633–637.

Centers for Disease Control and Prevention (CDC). *Chronic Disease in Minority Populations.* Atlanta, GA: U.S. Department of Health and Human Services, Public Health Service, Centers for Disease Control and Prevention (1994).

Centers for Disease Control and Prevention (CDC). Chronic Disease Reports: Coronary Heart Disease Mortality—United States, 1986. *MMWR* (1989):38:285–288.

Chavey, W.E., 2nd, C.S. Blaum, B.E. Bleske, R.V. Harrison, S. Kesterson, and J.M. Nicklas. Guideline for the Management of Heart Failure Caused by Systolic Dysfunction: Part I. Guideline Development, Etiology, and Diagnosis. *Am Fam Physician* (2001):64:769–774.

Chen, J., X. Wu, and D. Gu. Hypertension and Cardiovascular Diseases Intervention in the Capital Steel and Iron Company and Beijing Fangshan Community. *Obes Rev* (2008):9(1 Suppl):142–145.

Cole, C.W., G.B. Hill, E. Farzad, et al. Cigarette Smoking and Peripheral Arterial Occlusive Disease. *Surgery* (1993):114:753–756; discussion 756–757.

Collins, R., R. Peto, S. MacMahon, et al. Blood Pressure, Stroke, and Coronary Heart Disease. Part 2, Short-Term Reductions in Blood Pressure: Overview of Randomised Drug Trials in their Epidemiological Context. *Lancet* (1990):335:827–838.

Corti, M.C., J.M. Guralnik, and C. Bilato. Coronary Heart Disease Risk Factors in Older Persons. *Aging (Milano)* (1996):8(2):75–89.

Criqui, M.H. Peripheral Arterial Disease—Epidemiological Aspects. *Vasc Med* (2001):6:3–7.

Criqui, M.H. Alcohol and Coronary Heart Disease: Consistent Relationship and Public Health Implications. *Clin Chim Acta* (1996):246:51–57.

Criqui, M.H., V. Vargas, J.O. Denenberg, et al. Ethnicity and Peripheral Arterial Disease: The San Diego Population Study. *Circulation* (2005):112:2703–2707.

Cushman, M., R.A. Cantrell, L.A. McClure, et al. Estimated 10-Year Stroke Risk by Region and Race in the United States: Geographic and Racial Differences in Stroke Risk. *Ann Neurol* (2008):64:507–513.

Dahlof, B., L.H. Lindholm, L. Hansson, B. Schersten, T. Ekbom, and P.O. Wester. Morbidity and Mortality in the Swedish Trial in Old Patients with Hypertension (STOP-Hypertension). *Lancet* (1991):338:1281–1285.

Danesh, J., and S. Lewington. Plasma Homocysteine and Coronary Heart Disease: Systematic Review of Published Epidemiological Studies. *J Cardiovasc Risk* (1998):5:229–232.

Danesh, J., P. Whincup, M. Walker, et al. Low Grade Inflammation and Coronary Heart Disease: Prospective Study and Updated Meta-Analyses. *BMJ* (2000):321:199–204.

Danesh, J., J.G. Wheeler, G.M. Hirschfield, et al. C-Reactive Protein and Other Circulating Markers of Inflammation in the Prediction of Coronary Heart Disease. *N Engl J Med* (2004):350:1387–1397.

de Andrade, M., I. Thandi, S. Brown, A. Gotto, Jr., W. Patsch, and E. Boerwinkle. Relationship of the Apolipoprotein E Polymorphism with Carotid Artery Atherosclerosis. *Am J Hum Genet* (1995):56(6):1379–1390.

DeFrances, C.J., C.A. Lucas, V.C. Buie, and A. Golosinskiy. 2006 National Hospital Discharge Survey. *Natl Health Stat Report* (2008):1–20.

Diez-Roux, A.V., F.J. Nieto, C. Muntaner, et al. Neighborhood Environments and Coronary Heart Disease: A Multilevel Analysis. *Am J Epidemiol* (1997):146:48–63.

Farquhar, J.W., S.P. Fortmann, J.A. Flora, et al. Effects of Communitywide Education on Cardiovascular Disease Risk Factors. The Stanford Five-City Project. *JAMA* (1990):264:359–365.

Farquhar, J.W., N. Maccoby, P.D. Wood, et al. Community Education for Cardiovascular Health. *Lancet* (1977):1:1192–1195.

Fibrinogen Studies Collaboration, J. Danesh, S. Lewington, et al. Plasma Fibrinogen Level and the Risk of Major Cardiovascular Diseases and Nonvascular Mortality: An Individual Participant Meta-Analysis. *JAMA* (2005):294:1799–1809.

Figueroa, M.S., and J.I. Peters. Congestive Heart Failure: Diagnosis, Pathophysiology, Therapy, and Implications for Respiratory Care. *Respir Care* (2006):51:403–412.

Flora, J.A., E.W. Maibach, and N. Maccoby. The Role of Media Across Four Levels of Health Promotion Intervention. *Annu Rev Public Health* (1989):10:181–201.

Folsom, A.R., K.K. Wu, E. Shahar, and C.E. Davis. Association of Hemostatic Variables with Prevalent Cardiovascular Disease and Asymptomatic Carotid Artery Atherosclerosis. The Atherosclerosis Risk in Communities (ARIC) Study Investigators. *Arterioscler Thromb* (1993):13:1829–1836.

Folsom, A.R., J.H. Eckfeldt, S. Weitzman, et al. Relation of Carotid Artery Wall Thickness to Diabetes Mellitus, Fasting glucose and insulin, body size, and physical activity. Atherosclerosis Risk in Communities (ARIC) Study Investigators. *Stroke* (1994):25:66–73.

Ford, E.S., U.A. Ajani, J.B. Croft, et al. Explaining the Decrease in U.S. Deaths from Coronary Disease, 1980–2000. *N Engl J Med* (2007):356:2388–2398.

Fortmann, S.P., J.A. Flora, M.A. Winkleby, C. Schooler, C. Barr Taylor, and J.W. Farquhar. Community Intervention Trials: Reflections on the Stanford Five-City Project Experience. *Am J Epidemiol* (1995):142:576–586.

Freedman, D.S., D.F. Williamson, J.B. Croft, C. Ballew, and T. Byers. Relation of Body Fat Distribution to Ischemic Heart Disease. The National Health and Nutrition Examination Survey I (NHANES I) Epidemiologic Follow-up Study. *Am J Epidemiol* (1995):142:53–63.

Garg, P.K., L. Tian, M.H. Criqui, et al. Physical Activity During Daily Life and Mortality in Patients with Peripheral Arterial Disease. *Circulation* (2006):114:242–248.

Gillum, R.F. Epidemiology of Heart Failure in the United States. *Am Heart J* (1993):126:1042–1047.

Glantz, S.A., and W.W. Parmley. Passive Smoking and Heart Disease. Epidemiology, Physiology, and Biochemistry. *Circulation* (1991):83:1–12.

Goldman, L., and E.F. Cook. Reasons for the Decline in Coronary Heart Disease Mortality: Medical Interventions Versus Life-Style Changes. In: Higgins M.W., and R.V. Luepker, editors, *Trends in Coronary Heart Disease Mortality: The Influence of Medical Care.* New York, NY: Oxford University Press (1988):67–75.

Goldstein, L.B., and G.P. Samsa. Reliability of the National Institutes of Health Stroke Scale. Extension to Non-Neurologists in the Context of a Clinical Trial. *Stroke* (1997):28:307–310.

Goldstein, L.B., R. Adams, M.J. Alberts, et al. Primary Prevention of Ischemic Stroke: A Guideline from the American Heart Association/American Stroke Association Stroke Council: Cosponsored by the Atherosclerotic Peripheral Vascular Disease Interdisciplinary Working Group; Cardiovascular Nursing Council; Clinical Cardiology Council; Nutrition, Physical Activity, and Metabolism Council; and the Quality of Care and Outcomes Research Interdisciplinary Working Group: The American Academy of Neurology Affirms the Value of this Guideline. *Stroke* (2006):37:1583–1633.

Gornik, H.L., and M.A. Creager. Contemporary Management of Peripheral Arterial Disease: I. Cardiovascular Risk-Factor Modification. *Cleve Clin J Med* (2006):73(4 Suppl):S30–S37.

Greenwood, D.C., K.R. Muir, C.J. Packham, and R.J. Madeley. Coronary Heart Disease: A Review of the Role of Psychosocial Stress and Social Support. *J Public Health Med* (1996):18:221–231.

Hackam, D.G., and S.S. Anand. Emerging Risk Factors for Atherosclerotic Vascular Disease: A Critical Review of the Evidence. *JAMA* (2003):290:932–940.

Haheim, L.L., I. Holme, I. Hjermann, and P. Leren. Smoking Habits and Risk of Fatal Stroke: 18 Years Follow Up of the Oslo Study. *J Epidemiol Community Health* (1996):50(6):621–624.

Hakim, A.A., H. Petrovitch, C.M. Burchfiel, et al. Effects of Walking on Mortality Among Nonsmoking Retired Men. *N Engl J Med* (1998):338:94–99.

Haldeman, G.A., J.B. Croft, W.H. Giles, and A. Rashidee. Hospitalization of Patients with Heart Failure: National Hospital Discharge Survey, 1985 to 1995. *Am Heart J* (1999):137(2):352–360.

Hankey, G.J. Review: Statins Prevent Stroke and Reduce Mortality. *Evid Based Med* (2008):13:113.

Hankey, G.J., P.E. Norman, and J.W. Eikelboom. Medical Treatment of Peripheral Arterial Disease. *JAMA* (2006):295:547–553.

Hanna, E.Z., S.P. Chou, and B.F. Grant. The Relationship Between Drinking and Heart Disease Morbidity in the United States: Results from the National Health Interview Survey. *Alcohol Clin Exp Res* (1997):21:111–118.

Haugen, S., I.P. Casserly, J.G. Regensteiner, and W.R. Hiatt. Risk Assessment in the Patient with Established Peripheral Arterial Disease. *Vasc Med* (2007):12:343–350.

He, Y., L. Tai Hing, L. Liang Shou, et al. The Number of Stenotic Coronary Arteries and Passive Smoking Exposure from Husband in Lifelong Non-Smoking Women in Xi'an, China. *Atherosclerosis* (1996):127:229–238.

Heald, C.L., F.G. Fowkes, G.D. Murray, and J.F. Price. Risk of Mortality and Cardiovascular Disease Associated with the Ankle-Brachial Index: Systematic Review. *Atherosclerosis* (2006):189:61–69.

Heinrich, J., L. Balleisen, H. Schulte, G. Assmann, and J. van de Loo. Fibrinogen and Factor VII in the Prediction of Coronary Risk. Results from the PROCAM Study in Healthy Men. *Arterioscler Thromb* (1994):14:54–59.

Hendrix, S.L., S. Wassertheil-Smoller, K.C. Johnson, et al. Effects of Conjugated Equine Estrogen on Stroke in the Women's Health Initiative. *Circulation* (2006):113:2425–2434.

Hennekens, C.H., S. Satterfield, and P.R. Herbert. Treatment of Elevated Blood Pressure to Prevent Coronary Heart Disease. In: Higgins, M.W., and R.V. Luepker, editors, *Trends in Coronary Heart Disease Mortality: The Influence of Medical Care.* New York, NY: Oxford University Press (1988):103–108.

Heron, M.P., D.L. Hoyer, S.L. Murphy, J. Xu, K.D. Kochanek, and B. Tejada-Vera. *Deaths: Final Data for 2006.* National Vital Statistics Reports. Hyattsville, Maryland. National Center for Health Statistics (2009).

Higgins, M.W., et al. Mortality from Coronary Heart Disease and Related Causes of Death in the United States, 1950–85. In: Higgins, M.W., and R.V. Luepker, editors, *Trends in Coronary Heart Disease Mortality: The Influence of Medical Care.* New York, NY: Oxford University Press (1988):279–297.

Hirsch, A.T., L. Hartman, R.J. Town, and B.A. Virnig. National Health Care Costs of Peripheral Arterial Disease in the Medicare Population. *Vasc Med* (2008):13:209–215.

Hjermann, I., B. Velve, I. Holme, and P. Leren. Effect of Diet and Smoking Intervention on the Incidence of Coronary Heart Disease. Report from the Oslo Study Group of a Randomised Trial in Healthy Men. *Lancet* (1981):2:1303–1310.

Hokanson, J.E., and M.A. Austin. Plasma Triglyceride Level is a Risk Factor for Cardiovascular Disease Independent of High-Density Lipoprotein Cholesterol Level: A Meta-Analysis of Population-Based Prospective Studies. *J Cardiovasc Risk* (1996):3:213–219.

Howard, G., R. Prineas, and C. Moy. Racial and Geographic Differences in Awareness, Treatment, and Control of Hypertension: The Reasons for Geographic and Racial Differences in Stroke Study. *Stroke* (2006):37:1171–1178.

Hu, F.B., M.J. Stampfer, G.A. Colditz, et al. Physical Activity and Risk of Stroke in Women. *JAMA* (2000):283:2961–2967.

Humphrey, L.L., R. Fu, K. Rogers, M. Freeman, and M. Helfand. Homocysteine Level and Coronary Heart Disease Incidence: A Systematic Review and Meta-Analysis. *Mayo Clin Proc* (2008):83:1203–1212.

Hunt, S.A., W.T. Abraham, M.H. Chin, et al. ACC/AHA 2005 Guideline Update for the Diagnosis and Management of Chronic Heart Failure in the Adult: A Report of the American College of Cardiology/American Heart Association Task Force on Practice Guidelines (Writing Committee to Update the 2001 Guidelines for the Evaluation and Management of Heart Failure): Developed in Collaboration with the American College of Chest Physicians and the International Society for Heart and Lung Transplantation: Endorsed by the Heart Rhythm Society. *Circulation* (2005):112:e154–e235.

Indian Health Service. *Inter-Tribal Heart Project (ITHP) Manual of Operations.* Bemidji, MN. Indian Health Service (1992).

Jackson, G., C.R. Gibbs, M.K. Davies, and G.Y. Lip. ABC of Heart Failure. Pathophysiology. *BMJ* (2000):320:167–170.

Jenkins, C.D. Epidemiology of Cardiovascular Diseases. *J Consult Clin Psychol* (1988):56:324–332.

Kannel, W.B. Incidence and Epidemiology of Heart Failure. *Heart Fail Rev* (2000):5:167–173.

Kawachi, I., D. Sparrow, A. Spiro, 3rd, P. Vokonas, and S.T. Weiss. A Prospective Study of Anger and Coronary Heart Disease. The Normative Aging Study. *Circulation* (1996):94:2090–2095.

Kawachi, I., G.A. Coditz, F.E. Speizer, et al. A Prospective Study of Passive Smoking and Coronary Heart Disease. *Circulation* (1997):95:2374–2379.

Keil, U., L.E. Chambless, A. Doring, B. Filipiak, and J. Stieber. The Relation of Alcohol Intake to Coronary Heart Disease and All-Cause Mortality in a Beer-Drinking Population. *Epidemiology* (1997):8:150–156.

Kim, H., Y. Friedlander, W.T. Longstreth, Jr., K.L. Edwards, S.M. Schwartz, and D.S. Siscovick. Family History as a Risk Factor for Stroke in Young Women. *Am J Prev Med* (2004):27:391–396.

King, A.C., R.W. Jeffery, F. Fridinger, et al. Environmental and Policy Approaches to Cardiovascular Disease Prevention Through Physical Activity: Issues and Opportunities. *Health Educ Q* (1995):22:499–511.

Kleindorfer, D., P. Panagos, A. Pancioli, et al. Incidence and Short-Term Prognosis of Transient Ischemic Attack in a Population-Based Study. *Stroke* (2005):36:720–723.

Knowles, J.W., T.L. Assimes, J. Li, T. Quertermous, and J.P. Cooke. Genetic Susceptibility to Peripheral Arterial Disease: A Dark Corner in Vascular Biology. *Arterioscler Thromb Vasc Biol* (2007):27:2068–2078.

Kostis, J.B., B.R. Davis, J. Cutler, et al. Prevention of Heart Failure by Antihypertensive Drug Treatment in Older Persons with Isolated Systolic Hypertension. SHEP Cooperative Research Group. *JAMA* (1997):278:212–216.

Kovar, M.G., M.I. Harris, and W.C. Hadden. The Scope of Diabetes in the United States Population. *Am J Public Health* (1987):77:1549–1550.

Krueter, M.W. PATCH: Its Origin Basic Concepts and Links to Contemporary Public Health Policy. *J Health Educ* (1992):23:135–139.

Kung, H.C., D.L. Hoyer, J. Xu, and S.L. Murphy. Deaths: Final Data for 2005. *Natl Vital Stat Rep* (2008):56:1–120.

Labarthe, D.R., M. Eissa, and C. Varas. Childhood Precursors of High Blood Pressure and Elevated Cholesterol. *Annu Rev Public Health* (1991):12:519–541.

Lam, T.H., L.J. Liu, E.D. Janus, C.P. Lau, and A.J. Hedley. Fibrinogen, Angina and Coronary Heart Disease in a Chinese Population. *Atherosclerosis* (2000):149:443–449.

Lasater, T., D. Abrams, L. Artz, et al. Lay Volunteer Delivery of a Community-Based Cardiovascular Risk Factor Change Program: The Pawtucket Experiment. In: Matarazzo, J.D., S.M. Weiss, J.A. Herd, N.E. Miller, S.M. Weiss, editors, *Behavioral Health: A Handbook of Health Enhancement and Disease Prevention*. New York, NY: John Wiley & Sons (1984):1166–1170.

Lee, I.M., C.H. Hennekens, K. Berger, J.E. Buring, and J.E. Manson. Exercise and Risk of Stroke in Male Physicians. *Stroke* (1999):30:1–6.

Leeder, S., S. Raymond, H. Greenberg, H. Liu, and K. Esson. *A Race Against Time: The Challenge of Cardiovascular Disease in Developing Economies*. New York, NY:Columbia University (2004).

Lefebvre, R.C., L. Linnan, S. Sundaram, and A. Ronan. Counseling Strategies for Blood Cholesterol Screening Programs: Recommendations for Practice. *Patient Educ Couns* (1990):16:97–108.

Levy, R.I. Primary Prevention of Coronary Heart Disease by Lowering Lipids: Results and Implications. *Am Heart J* (1985):110:1116–1122.

Lewington, S., R. Clarke, N. Qizilbash, R. Peto, R. Collins, and Prospective Studies Collaboration. Age-Specific Relevance of Usual Blood Pressure to Vascular Mortality: A Meta-Analysis of Individual Data for One Million Adults in 61 Prospective Studies. *Lancet* (2002):360:1903–1913.

Li, C., G. Engstrom, B. Hedblad, G. Berglund, and L. Janzon. Risk Factors for Stroke in Subjects with Normal Blood Pressure: A Prospective Cohort Study. *Stroke* (2005):36:234–238.

Libbey, J.E., T.L. Sweeten, W.M. McMahon, and R.S. Fujinami. Autistic Disorder and Viral Infections. *J Neurovirol* (2005):11:1–10.

Lin, H.J., P.A. Wolf, M. Kelly-Hayes, et al. Stroke Severity in Atrial Fibrillation. The Framingham Study. *Stroke* (1996):27:1760–1764.

Liu, L., J.A. Nettleton, A.G. Bertoni, D.A. Bluemke, J.A. Lima, and M. Szklo. Dietary Pattern, The Metabolic Syndrome, and Left Ventricular Mass and Systolic Function: The Multi-Ethnic Study of Atherosclerosis. *Am J Clin Nutr* (2009).

Lloyd-Jones, D., R. Adams, and M. Carnethon, et al. Heart Disease and Stroke Statistics—2009 Update: A Report from the American Heart Association Statistics Committee and Stroke Statistics Subcommittee. *Circulation* (2009):119:480–486.

Ma, J., A.R. Folsom, S.L. Melnick, et al. Associations of Serum and Dietary Magnesium with Cardiovascular Disease, Hypertension, Diabetes, Insulin, and Carotid Arterial Wall Thickness: The ARIC Study. Atherosclerosis Risk in Communities Study. *J Clin Epidemiol* (1995):48:927–940.

MacMahon, S. Blood Pressure and the Prevention of Stroke. *J Hypertens Suppl* (1996):14:S39–S46.

Mann, D.L. Mechanisms and Models in Heart Failure: A Combinatorial Approach. *Circulation* (1999):100:999–1008.

Mann, D.L., and M.R. Bristow. Mechanisms and Models in Heart Failure: The Biomechanical Model and Beyond. *Circulation* (2005):111:2837–2849.

Maresca, G., A. Di Blasio, R. Marchioli, and G. Di Minno. Measuring Plasma Fibrinogen to Predict Stroke and Myocardial Infarction: An Update. *Arterioscler Thromb Vasc Biol* (1999):19:1368–1377.

Mayo Foundation for Medical Education and Research. *Coronary Artery Disease Treatment.* Mayo Clinic: Arizona. Available at http://www.mayoclinic.org/coronary-artery-disease/treatment. html. Accessed June 30, 2009.

McDermott, M.M. The Magnitude of the Problem of Peripheral Arterial Disease: Epidemiology and Clinical Significance. *Cleve Clin J Med* (2006):73(4 Suppl):S2–S7.

McQueen, D.V., and J. Siegrist. Social Factors in the Etiology of Chronic Disease: An Overview. *Soc Sci Med* (1982):16:353–367.

Mittelmark, M.B., R.V. Luepker, D.R. Jacobs, et al. Community-Wide Prevention of Cardiovascular Disease: Education Strategies of the Minnesota Heart Health Program. *Prev Med* (1986):15:1–17.

Morgenstern, L.B., M.A. Smith, L.D. Lisabeth, et al. Excess Stroke in Mexican Americans Compared with Non-Hispanic Whites: The Brain Attack Surveillance in Corpus Christi Project. *Am J Epidemiol* (2004):160:376–383.

Myint, P.K., R.N. Luben, N.J. Wareham, et al. Combined Work and Leisure Physical Activity and Risk of Stroke in Men and Women in the European Prospective Investigation into Cancer-Norfolk Prospective Population Study. *Neuroepidemiology* (2006):27:122–129.

National Center for Health Statistics. Health, United States, 2008. Centers for Disease Control and Prevention, editor. Hyattsville, MD: U.S. Department of Health and Human Services (2009).

National Heart Lung and Blood Institute (NHLBI). *Incidence and Prevalence: 2006 Chart Book on Cardiovascular and Lung Diseases.* Bethesda, MD: National Institutes of Health (2006).

National Heart Lung and Blood Institute (NHLBI). *Third Report of the Expert Panel on Detection, Evaluation, and Treatment of High Blood Cholesterol in Adults (ATP III Final Report).* Rockville, MD: National Institutes of Health (2002).

National Research Council. *Diet and Health: Implications for Reducing Chronic Disease Risk.* Washington, DC: National Academy Press (1989).

New York State Healthy Heart Program. *Eight Approaches in Community Intervention: An Interim Report.* Albany, NY: New York State Department of Health (1992).

Newman, A.B., D.S. Siscovick, T.A. Manolio, et al. Ankle-Arm Index as a Marker of Atherosclerosis in the Cardiovascular Health Study. Cardiovascular Heart Study (CHS) Collaborative Research Group. *Circulation* (1993):88:837–845.

Nieto, F.J., E. Adam, P. Sorlie, et al. Cohort Study of Cytomegalovirus Infection as a Risk Factor for Carotid Intimal-Medial Thickening, a Measure of Subclinical Atherosclerosis. *Circulation* (1996):94:922–927.

Nygard, O., J.E. Nordehaug, H. Refsum, P.M. Ueland, M. Farstad, and S.E. Vollset. Plasma Homocysteine Levels and Mortality in Patients with Coronary Artery Disease. *N Engl J Med* (1997):337:230–236.

Nygard, O., S.E. Vollset, H. Refsum, et al. Total Plasma Homocysteine and Cardiovascular Risk Profile. The Hordaland Homocysteine Study. *JAMA* (1995):274:1526–1533.

Oldridge, N.B., G.H. Guyatt, M.E. Fischer, and A.A. Rimm. Cardiac Rehabilitation After Myocardial Infarction. Combined Experience of Randomized Clinical Trials. *JAMA* (1988):260:945–950.

Ostchega, Y., R. Paulose-Ram, C.F. Dillon, Q. Gu, and J.P. Hughes. Prevalence of Peripheral Arterial Disease and Risk Factors in Persons Aged 60 and Older: Data from the National Health and Nutrition Examination Survey 1999–2004. *J Am Geriatr Soc* (2007):55:583–589.

Papadakis, S., and I. Moroz. Population-Level Interventions for Coronary Heart Disease Prevention: What Have We Learned Since the North Karelia Project? *Curr Opin Cardiol* (2008):23:452–461.

Pearson, T.A., G.A. Mensah, and R.W. Alexander. Markers of Inflammation and Cardiovascular Disease: Application to Clinical and Public Health Practice. A Statement for Healthcare Professionals from the Centers for Disease Control and Prevention and the American Heart Association. *Circulation* (2003):107:499–511.

Petrea, R.E., A.S. Beiser, S. Seshadri, M. Kelly-Hayes, C.S. Kase, and P.A. Wolf. Gender Differences in Stroke Incidence and Poststroke Disability in the Framingham Heart Study. *Stroke* (2009):40:1032–1037.

Powell, K.E., and S.N. Blair. The Public Health Burdens of Sedentary Living Habits: Theoretical But Realistic Estimates. *Med Sci Sports Exerc* (1994):26:851–856.

Pradhan, A.D., S. Shrivastava, N.R. Cook, N. Rifai, M.A. Creager, and P.M. Ridker. Symptomatic Peripheral Arterial Disease in Women: Nontraditional Biomarkers of Elevated Risk. *Circulation* (2008):117:823–831.

Prineas, R.J., A.R. Folsom, and S.A. Kaye. Central Adiposity and Increased Risk of Coronary Artery Disease Mortality in Older Women. *Ann Epidemiol* (1993):3:35–41.

Puska, P., J. Tuomilehto, A. Nissinen, et al. The North Karelia Project: 15 Years of Community-Based Prevention of Coronary Heart Disease. *Ann Med* (1989):21:169–173.

Rafnsson, S.B., I.J. Deary, and F.G.R. Fowkes Peripheral Arterial Disease and Cognitive Function. *Vasc Med* (2009):14:51–61.

Rasmusson, K.D., J.A. Hall, and D.G. Renlund. The Intricacies of Heart Failure. *Nurs Manage* (2007):38:33–40; quiz 40–41.

Ridker, P.M., and N. Rifai, editors. *C-Reactive Protein and Cardiovascular Disease*. MediEdition: St. Laurent, Canada (2006).

Ridker, P.M., M.J. Stampfer, and N. Rifai. Novel Risk Factors for Systemic Atherosclerosis: A Comparison of C-Reactive Protein, Fibrinogen, Homocysteine, Lipoprotein(a), and Standard Cholesterol Screening as Predictors of Peripheral Arterial Disease. *JAMA* (2001):285:2481–2485.

Rifkind, B.M. High-Density Lipoprotein Cholesterol and Coronary Artery Disease: Survey of the Evidence. *Am J Cardiol* (1990):66:3A–6A.

Rosamond, W., K. Flegal, G. Friday, et al. Heart Disease and Stroke Statistics—2007 Update: A Report from the American Heart Association Statistics Committee and Stroke Statistics Subcommittee. *Circulation* (2007):115:e69–e171.

Rossouw, J.E., G.L. Anderson, R.L. Prentice, et al. Risks and Benefits of Estrogen Plus Progestin in Healthy Postmenopausal Women: Principal Results From the Women's Health Initiative Randomized Controlled Trial. *JAMA* (2002):288:321–333.

Sacco, R.L., R. Gan, B. Boden-Albala, et al. Leisure-Time Physical Activity and Ischemic Stroke Risk: The Northern Manhattan Stroke Study. *Stroke* (1998):29:380–387.

Sacco, R.L., R. Adams, G. Albers, et al. Guidelines for Prevention of Stroke in Patients with Ischemic Stroke or Transient Ischemic Attack: A Statement for Healthcare Professionals from the American Heart Association/American Stroke Association Council on Stroke: Co-Sponsored by the Council on Cardiovascular Radiology and Intervention: the American Academy of Neurology affirms the value of this guideline. *Stroke* (2006):37:577–617.

Safar, M.E., P. Priollet, F. Luizy, et al. Peripheral Arterial Disease and Isolated Systolic Hypertension: The ATTEST Study. *J Hum Hypertens* (2009):23:182–187.

Sallis, J.F., N. Owen, and E. Fisher. Ecological Models of Health Behavior. In: Glanz, K., B.K. Rimer, F.M. Lewis, editors, *Health Behavior and Health Education: Theory, Research, and Practice*. San Francisco, CA: Jossey-Bass Publishers (2002):462–484.

Schmid, T.L., M. Pratt, and E. Howze. Policy as Intervention: Environmental and Policy Approaches to the Prevention of Cardiovascular Disease. *Am J Public Health* (1995):85:1207–1211.

Schooler, C., J. Farquhar, S. Fortmann, et al. Synthesis of Findings and Issues from Community Prevention Trials. *Ann Epidemiol* (1997):7:S54–S68.

Selvin, E., and T.P. Erlinger. Prevalence of and Risk Factors for Peripheral Arterial Disease in the United States: Results from the National Health and Nutrition Examination Survey, 1999–2000. *Circulation* (2004):110:738–743.

Sempos, C., R. Fulwood, C. Haines, et al. The Prevalence of High Blood Cholesterol Levels Among Adults in the United States. *JAMA* (1989):262:45–52.

Sharrett, A.R., W. Patsch, P.D. Sorlie, G. Hess, M.G. Bond, and C.E. Davis. Associations of Lipoprotein Cholesterols, Apolipoproteins A-I and B, and Triglycerides with Carotid Atherosclerosis and Coronary Heart Disease. The Atherosclerosis Risk in Communities (ARIC) Study. *Arterioscler Thromb* (1994):14:1098–1104.

Simons-Morton, D.G., B.G. Simons-Morton, G.S. Parcel, and J.F. Bunker. Influencing Personal and Environmental Conditions for Community Health: A Multilevel Intervention Model. *Fam Community Health* (1988):11:25–35.

South Carolina Department of Health and Environmental Control. *Final Report: The South Carolina Cardiovascular Disease Prevention (CVD) Project*. Columbia, SC: Department of Health and Environmental Control (1991).

Stamler, J., D. Wentworth, and J.D. Neaton. Is Relationship Between Serum Cholesterol and Risk of Premature Death from Coronary Heart Disease Continuous and Graded? Findings in 356,222 Primary screenees of the Multiple Risk Factor Intervention Trial (MRFIT). *JAMA* (1986):256:2823–2828.

Stampfer, M.J., M.R. Malinow, W.C. Willett, et al. A Prospective Study of Plasma Homocyst(e)ine and Risk of Myocardial Infarction in US Physicians. *JAMA* (1992):268:877–881.

Steenland, K. Passive Smoking and the Risk of Heart Disease. *JAMA* (1992):267:94–99.

Steg, P.G., D.L. Bhatt, P.W. Wilson, et al. One-Year Cardiovascular Event Rates in Outpatients with Atherothrombosis. *JAMA* (2007):297:1197–1206.

Thom, T., N. Haase, W. Rosamond, et al. Heart Disease and Stroke Statistics—2006 Update: A Report from the American Heart Association Statistics Committee and Stroke Statistics Subcommittee. *Circulation* (2006):113:e85–e151.

U.S. Department of Health and Human Services (USDHHS). *Physical activity and Health: A Report of the Surgeon General*. Atlanta, GA: USDHHS Centers for Disease Control and Prevention, National Center for Chronic Disease Prevention and Health Promotion (1996).

U.S. Department of Health and Human Services (USDHHS). *Healthy People 2000: National Health Promotion and Disease Prevention Objectives*. Washington, D.C.: USDHHS (1991).

U.S. Department of Health and Human Services (USDHHS). *The Health Consequences of Smoking: Cardiovascular Disease. A report of the Surgeon General*. Rockville, MD: USDHHS Public Health Service, Office on Smoking and Health (1983).

U.S. Department of Health and Human Services (USDHHS). HHS Announces Initiative to Reduce the Incidence of Stroke in Stroke Belt States. Washington, D.C: USDHHS. Available at http://www.hhs.gov/news/press/2004pres/20040805.html. Accessed August 5, 2004.

U.S. Preventive Services Task Force (USPSTF). Guide to Clinical Preventive Services: An Assessment of the Effectiveness of 169 Interventions. *Report of the U.S. Preventive Services Task Force.* Baltimore, MD: Williams & Wilkins (1989).

Uemura, K., and Z. Pisa. Trends in Cardiovascular Disease Mortality in Industrialized Countries Since 1950. *World Health Stat Q* (1988):41:155–178.

UK Prospective Diabetes Study (UKPDS) Group. Intensive Blood-Glucose Control with Sulphonylureas or Insulin Compared with Conventional Treatment and Risk of Complications in Patients with Type 2 Diabetes (UKPDS 33). *Lancet* (1998):352:837–853.

Vidula, H., L. Tian, K. Liu, et al. Biomarkers of Inflammation and Thrombosis as Predictors of Near-Term Mortality in Patients with Peripheral Arterial Disease: A Cohort Study. *Ann Intern Med* (2008):148:85–93.

Viscoli, C.M., L.M. Brass, W.N. Kernan, P.M. Sarrel, S. Suissa, and R.I. Horwitz. A Clinical Trial of Estrogen-Replacement Therapy After Ischemic Stroke. *N Engl J Med* (2001):345:1243–1249.

Wannamethee, S.G., and A.G. Shaper. Lifelong Teetotallers, Ex-Drinkers and Drinkers: Mortality and the Incidence of Major Coronary Heart Disease Events in Middle-Aged British Men. *Int J Epidemiol* (1997):26:523–531.

Wassertheil-Smoller, S., S.L. Hendrix, M. Limacher, et al. Effect of Estrogen Plus Progestin on Stroke in Postmenopausal Women: The Women's Health Initiative: A Randomized Trial. *JAMA* (2003):289:2673–2684.

Wattanakit, K., A.R. Folsom, E. Selvin, J. Coresh, A.T. Hirsch, and B.D. Weatherley. Kidney Function and Risk of Peripheral Arterial Disease: Results from the Atherosclerosis Risk in Communities (ARIC) Study. *J Am Soc Nephrol* (2007):18:629–636.

Wattanakit, K., A.R. Folsom, E. Selvin, et al. Risk Factors for Peripheral Arterial Disease Incidence in Persons with Diabetes: The Atherosclerosis Risk in Communities (ARIC) Study. *Atherosclerosis* (2005):180:389–397.

Wendel-Vos, G.C., A.J. Schuit, E.J.M. Feskens, et al. Physical Activity and Stroke. A Meta-Analysis of Observational Data. *Int J Epidemiol* (2004):33:787–798.

Williams, R.B., Jr. Psychological Factors in Coronary Artery Disease: Epidemiologic Evidence. *Circulation* (1987):76:I117–I123.

Wilson, P.W., J.M. Hoeg, R.B. D'Agostino, et al. Cumulative Effects of High Cholesterol Levels, High Blood Pressure, and Cigarette Smoking on Carotid Stenosis. *N Engl J Med* (1997):337:516–522.

Wing, S., E. Barnett, M. Casper, and H.A. Tyroler. Geographic and Socioeconomic Variation in the Onset of Decline of Coronary Heart Disease Mortality in White Women. *Am J Public Health* (1992):82:204–209.

Wing, S., M. Casper, W. Riggan, C. Hayes, and H.A. Tyroler. Socioenvironmental Characteristics Associated with the Onset of Decline of Ischemic Heart Disease Mortality in the United States. *Am J Public Health* (1988):78:923–926.

Woo, D., J. Khoury, M.M. Haverbusch, et al. Smoking and Family History and Risk of Aneurysmal Subarachnoid Hemorrhage. *Neurology* (2009):72:69–72.

World Health Organization (WHO). *The Global Burden of Disease: 2004 Update.* Geneva, Switzerland: World Health Organization (2008).

Yancy, C.W. Heart Failure in Blacks: Etiologic and Epidemiologic Differences. *Curr Cardiol Rep* (2001):3:191–197.

Young, J.B. The Global Epidemiology of Heart Failure. *Med Clin North Am* (2004):88:1135–1143, ix.

CHAPTER 14

CANCER
(ICD-10 C00-C97)

Ross C. Brownson, Ph.D. and
Corinne Joshu, Ph.D, M.P.H.

Introduction

Cancer is now the leading cause of death among persons under the age of 85, and the second leading cause of death overall in the United States, accounting for an estimated 1.4 million new cases and 560,000 deaths in 2007 (Table 14.1) (American Cancer Society 2008a). Cancer has a complex set of "upstream" causes and "downstream" consequences (Figure 14.1), The lifetime probability of developing cancer is now estimated at one in two for men and one in three for women (American Cancer Society 2007a). Cancer death rates increased steadily since 1930, when nationwide mortality was first compiled. A sharp rise in lung cancer rates was the main reason for this increase (Figures 14.2a and 14.2b). Cancer death rates began declining in the early 1990s, and by 2002, rates were 14% lower in men and 7% lower in women compared to peak rates in 1990 and 1991, respectively. The most recent U.S. data show declines in overall incidence and mortality, yet with some large regional variations (Jemal et al. 2008). The declines are greater among young persons, thus forecasting a continued decline in cancer mortality in the coming decade.

Rates of cancer vary by age and sex. Although cancer occurs more frequently with advancing age, it is also the second leading cause of death due to disease among U.S. children aged 1 – 14 (American Cancer Society 2007a). Men have a 45% lifetime probability of developing cancer and women have a 38% lifetime probability (Jemal et al. 2007).

Racial and ethnic groups are not affected equally by cancer (Figures 14.3a and 14.3b). African American men have the highest incidence rate of cancer and non-Hispanic white men have the next highest rate (19% lower than that of African American men) (Surveillance, Epidemiology, and End Results Program 2007a). African Americans have poorer survival than whites for almost all types of cancer at all stages of diagnosis (Jemal et al. 2007). In addition, African Americans are less likely to be diagnosed at an early and more treatable stage of cancer than whites. Mortality rates are more than twice as high for African Americans as compared to whites for several cancers including prostate, stomach, myeloma, uterine cervix, and cancers of the head and neck (Albano et al. 2007; Ghafoor et al. 2002).

Inequality among factors such as income, education, and access to health care may account for a substantial proportion of the excess cancer burden among the African American population (Ghafoor et al. 2002). Among African Americans, those with 12 years of education or less are at an increased risk for developing cancer (Albano et al. 2007). Higher cancer incidence and mortality rates among the socioeconomically disadvantaged

Table 14.1. Public Health Impact of Major Cancers, United States

Cancer Type (ICD-10 Code)	Number of New Cases[a]	Number of Deaths[a]	Five-Year Survival[b]	Number of Hospital Days[c]
All Sites (C00-C97)	1,437,180	565,650	66	9,420
Lung (C34)	215,020	161,840	16	1,002
Colon and Rectum (C18-C20, C26)	148,810	49,960	65	1,351
Breast (C50)	184,450	40,930	89	225
Pancreas (C25)	37,680	34,290	5	228
Prostate (C61)	186,320	28,660	98.5	252
Leukemia (C91-C95)	44,270	21,710	49	508
Non-Hodgkin's lymphoma (C82-C85,C96)	66,120	19,160	63	335
Bladder (C67)	68,810	14,100	82	213
Stomach (C16)	21,500	10,880	24	248
Skin-Melanoma (C43)	62,480	8,420	92	–
Oral Cavity (C00-C14)	35,310	7,590	60	–
Uterine Corpus (C54)	40,100	7,470	84	164
Uterine Cervix (C53)	11,070	3,870	73	55
Hodgkin's Disease (C81)	8,220	1,350	86	65

[a]Estimated for 2008 (American Cancer Society 2008a).
[b]Five-year relative survival rate (%) for 1996–2002 (Jemal et al. 2007).
[c]Number of days of care for discharges, hospital days in thousands, based on the 2004 National Hospital Discharge Survey (Kozak, De Frances, and Hall 2006).

are the result of several factors. These include a higher prevalence of major cancer risk factors such as cigarette smoking, poor nutrition, and inadequate access to health care, which can delay cancer diagnosis and treatment. Many of these factors are consequences of living in poverty. African Americans account for 25% of those living in poverty and 15% of the uninsured, but only 13% of the total U.S. population (DeNavas-Walt, Proctor, and Lee 2006).

People of Hispanic origin have approximately 32% lower incidence of cancer than non-Hispanic whites (Surveillance, Epidemiology, and End Results Program 2007a).

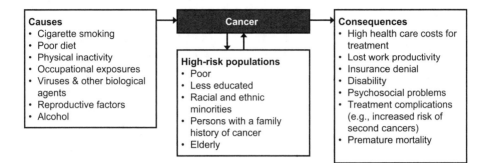

Causes
- Cigarette smoking
- Poor diet
- Physical inactivity
- Occupational exposures
- Viruses & other biological agents
- Reproductive factors
- Alcohol

Cancer

High-risk populations
- Poor
- Less educated
- Racial and ethnic minorities
- Persons with a family history of cancer
- Elderly

Consequences
- High health care costs for treatment
- Lost work productivity
- Insurance denial
- Disability
- Psychosocial problems
- Treatment complications (e.g., increased risk of second cancers)
- Premature mortality

Figure 14.1. Cancer: causes, consequences, and high–risk populations.

Those cancers that are higher among the Hispanic population tend to be associated with infectious etiologies, such as cancers of the cervix (e.g., human papilloma virus), stomach (e.g., *Helicobacter pylori*), and liver (e.g., Hepatitis B and C viruses), which may be the consequence of poor sanitary conditions and lack of preventive services (Howe et al. 2006). This Hispanic population makes up around 30% of the nation's uninsured and 25% of those living in poverty (DeNavas-Walt, Proctor, and Lee 2006). Like the African American population, they are also more likely to be diagnosed at later stages and less likely to be screened. Cancer risk among Latinos also varies by country origin (Howe et al. 2006). For example, Cubans are less likely to live below the poverty level and be

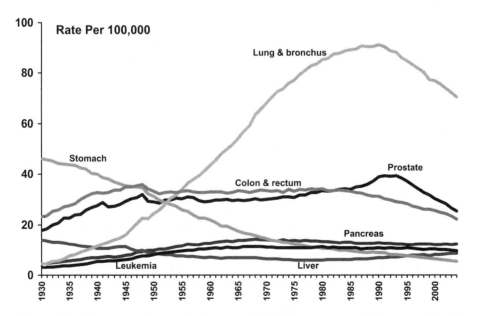

Figure 14.2a. Cancer mortality rates by site, men, United States, 1930–2004. Rates are adjusted to the age distribution of the 2000 U.S. standard population. *Sources*: U.S. Mortality Public Use Data Tapes 1960–2002, U.S. Mortality Volumes 1930–1959, National Center for Health Statistics, Centers for Disease Control and Prevention 2005, American Cancer Society 2008 (American Cancer Society 2008b).

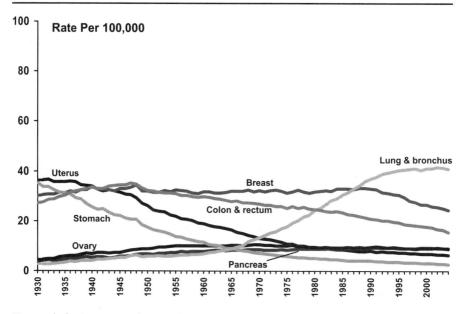

Figure 14.2b. Cancer mortality rates by site, women, United States, 1930–2004. Rates are adjusted to the age distribution of the 2000 U.S. standard population. *Sources*: U.S. Mortality Public Use Data Tapes 1960–2002, U.S. Mortality Volumes 1930–1959, National Center for Health Statistics, Centers for Disease Control and Prevention 2005, American Cancer Society 2008 (American Cancer Society 2008b).

obese than Puerto Ricans and Mexicans. Thus, future prevention efforts may need to target country of origin rather than generalizing to the entire Hispanic population.

The economic impact of cancer is enormous. The estimated direct medical costs of cancer in 2002 were $61 billion (Brown and Yabroff 2006). Indirect costs such as lost work productivity were estimated at $111 billion in 2002. Between 1995 and 2004, the overall costs of treating cancer increased by 75% (National Cancer Institute 2005). In contrast to the huge cost of cancer treatment, the total national resources dedicated to early detection activities, such as screening for breast, cervical, and colorectal cancer, are considerably smaller. The allocation of national resources to the primary prevention of cancer (e.g., tobacco control, dietary intervention) is even smaller.

Pathophysiology

Cancer occurs as a result of alterations in the mechanisms that control normal cell behavior. Cancer cells are different than normal cells as they (1) acquire inappropriate growth properties and (2) generally lose their ability to serve the functions they normally have in a given tissue.

Cancer is a diverse group of diseases characterized by uncontrolled growth and spread of these abnormal cells. Tumors, or abnormal enlargements of tissue, may be either benign or malignant. Benign tumors are generally innocuous and slow growing, whereas malignant tumors (commonly called cancers) contain abnormal genetic material and grow more rapidly. The principal danger of a cancer is its tendency to invade neighboring

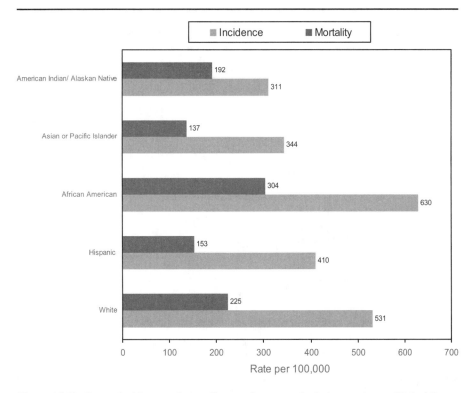

Figure 14.3a. Cancer incidence and mortality rates by race and ethnic group, men, United States, 2004. Rates are adjusted to the 2000 U.S. standard population. Hispanic and non-Hispanic are not mutually exclusive from white, African American, American Indian/Alaska Native, and Asian or Pacific Islander. *Source*: Surveillance, Epidemiology, and End Results (SEER) Program (Surveillance, Epidemiology, and End Results Program 2007a, 2007b).

tissues or organs, or to metastasize and to grow in other areas of the body. If this spread remains untreated, cancer cells invade vital organs or cause dysfunction by displacing normal tissue.

Different cancer types have widely varying induction periods—that is, the time between exposure to cancer-causing agents and cancer occurrence. For example, the induction period for some types of leukemia may be as short as a few years, compared with induction periods as long as four or five decades for some types of bladder cancer.

Cancers are classified according to their organ or tissue of origin (site code) and according to their histologic features (morphology code). The most widely used classification schemes are the *International Statistical Classification of Disease and Related Health Problems, Tenth Revision* (ICD-10) (WHO 2005) and the *International Classification of Diseases for Oncology* (ICD-O-3) (WHO 2000). The existence of hundreds of cancer varieties is readily apparent with 43 organs of origin and multiple histologic types for each organ (Giordano 2006).

In addition to being grouped by site and histologic features, cancers are classified according to their stage at diagnosis, or the extent to which the cancer has grown locally or invaded other tissues or organs. Cancer cells may remain at their original site (local stage),

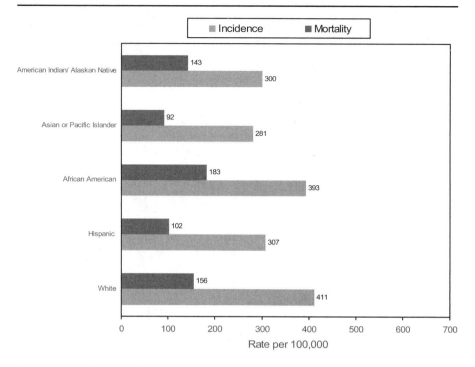

Figure 14.3b. Cancer incidence and mortality rates by race and ethnic group, women, United States, 2004. Rates are adjusted to the 2000 U.S. standard population. Hispanic and non-Hispanic are not mutually exclusive from white, African American, American Indian/Alaska Native, and Asian or Pacific Islander. *Source*: Surveillance, Epidemiology, and End Results (SEER) Program (Surveillance, Epidemiology, and End Results Program 2007a, 2007b).

spread to an adjacent area of the body (regional stage), or spread (metastasize) throughout the body (distant stage).

Cancer registries collect detailed information on cancer patients through hospitals and medical clinics (see also Chapter 3). Cancer registry data have many valuable uses, such as evaluation of cancer incidence patterns, cancer risk factors, effects of prevention and early detection efforts, survival patterns, and treatment effects. In the United States, the National Cancer Institute's Surveillance, Epidemiology, and End Results (SEER) Program has collected population-based data on newly diagnosed cancers since 1973 (Ries et al. 2007). The SEER Program is designed to accomplish four goals: (1) to assemble and report, on a periodic basis, estimates of cancer incidence, mortality, survival, and prevalence in the United States; (2) to monitor annual cancer incidence trends to identify unusual changes in specific forms of cancer occurring in population subgroups defined by geographic and demographic characteristics; (3) to provide continuing information on trends over time in the extent of disease at diagnosis, trends in therapy, and associated changes in patient survival; and (4) to promote studies designed to identify factors amenable to cancer control interventions.

The Centers for Disease Control and Prevention (CDC) has established the National Program of Cancer Registries (NPCR) (Public Law 102-515) and has funded 45 states, the District of Columbia, and three U.S. territories to develop registries or to enhance current registries. These state cancer registries are designed to (CDC 2007a):

- Monitor cancer trends over time
- Determine cancer patterns in various populations
- Guide planning and evaluation of cancer control programs (e.g., determine whether prevention, screening, and treatment efforts are making a difference)
- Help set priorities for allocating health resources
- Advance clinical, epidemiologic, and health services research
- Provide information for a national database of cancer incidence

The NPCR provides cancer incidence information on 96% of the U.S. population.

Causes

Several studies have been conducted to estimate the proportion of overall cancer deaths due to various modifiable causes (Doll and Peto 1981; Miller 1992; Harvard Report on Cancer Prevention 1996; Danaei et al. 2005). The Harvard Center for Cancer Prevention (Harvard Report on Cancer Prevention 1996) and Danaei et al. (2005) provide a useful benchmark on which to base preventive efforts (Table 14.2). These findings suggest the following priorities for cancer prevention and control: (1) eliminating use of tobacco; (2) consuming a prudent diet that includes an abundant distribution of fruits and vegetables and achieves a balance between energy intake and regular physical activity; (3) reducing exposures to occupational carcinogens; (4) controlling exposures to microbial agents that may be sexually transmitted or transmitted by sharing contaminated needles or personal articles, or prevented by immunization; (5) limiting consumption of alcohol; and (6) avoiding overexposure to sunlight (Greenwald and Sondik 1986; Colditz, Baer, and Tamimi 2002; American Cancer Society 2007b).

In 1985, the National Cancer Institute set a goal of reducing cancer mortality by 50% by the year 2000 through the systematic application of existing cancer control technologies (Greenwald and Sondik 1986). Although this 50% goal was overly ambitious and was not achieved, it was extremely beneficial in focusing cancer control efforts at all levels of public health practice. More recently, the National Cancer Institute has launched the initiative: NCI Challenge Goal 2015. Several prevention strategies within this national plan are highly relevant for public health practice. For example, a strategy for cancer prevention is to "Apply new knowledge and best practices to rapidly increase the adoption of evidence-based cancer prevention interventions in public health and clinical practice settings" (National Cancer Institute 2007).

In addition to these goals by the National Cancer Institute, the US Public Health Service has established a variety of objectives related to cancer prevention and control in *Healthy People 2010* (USDHHS 2000). It has been noted that without a stronger U.S. commitment to cancer prevention, public health goals for cancer prevention are unlikely to be achieved (Bailar and Gornik 1997; Byers et al. 1999).

Prevention and Control

As noted by Alciati and Marconi (Alciati et al. 1995), public health agencies at the federal, state, and local levels are vital entities in translating cancer control technologies into

Table 14.2. Estimates of the Proportion of Cancer Deaths Attributed to Various Factors

Factor	Harvard (Harvard Report on Cancer Prevention 1996) Estimate (%)	Comparative Risk Assessment (Danaei et al. 2005) Estimate[a] (%)
Tobacco	30	21[b]
Adult diet/obesity	30	7
Sedentary lifestyle	5	2
Occupational factors	5	–
Family history of cancer	5	–
Viruses/other biologic agents	5	–
Perinatal factors/growth[c]	5	–
Reproductive factors	3	–
Alcohol	3	5
Socioeconomic status	3	–
Unsafe sex	–	3
Environmental pollution	2	1
Ionizing/ultraviolet radiation	2	–
Prescription drugs/medicine procedures	1	2
Salt/other food additives/ contaminants	>1	–
Indoor smoke from household use of solid fuels	–	<0.5

[a]Estimates for all cancers worldwide.
[b]Smoking only.
[c]Excess energy intake early in life and/or larger birth weight.

practice. The federal support for cancer control activities in state health agencies only began in 1986 when the National Cancer Institute initiated its Technical Development in Health Agencies Program. More comprehensive listings of evidence-based cancer control programs are found in Cancer Control P.L.A.N.E.T. (Cancer Control PLANET 2005), which provides comprehensive cancer control resources to public health officials, and *The*

Guide to Community Preventive Services: What Works to Promote Health? (Zaza, Briss, and Harris 2005), which provides systematic reviews of selected population-based interventions. Meissner, Bergner, and Marconi (1992) summarized internal and external factors contributing to success in controlling cancer in public health settings. Internal factors include (1) commitment of the organization's leadership to cancer control, (2) existence of appropriate data to monitor and evaluate programs, (3) appropriately trained staff, and (4) the ability to obtain funds for future activities. External factors include (1) successful linkages and coalitions, (2) an established cancer control plan, (3) access to outside health experts, (4) an informed state legislature, and (5) diffusion of initially successful programs to other sites. The linkages between etiology of cancer and cancer prevention and control interventions are highlighted in Figure 14.4 (Hiatt and Rimer 2006). Public health agencies that take all of the issues into account in Figure 14.4 are more likely to be successful in controlling cancer through evidence-based interventions.

Describing each cancer site in detail in this chapter would be impractical. Therefore, we have limited this discussion to cancers that have one or more of the following characteristics: (1) they account for a major proportion of all cancer cases, (2) they can be reduced through scientifically proven prevention and control measures, or (3) they are frequently encountered in public health practice. Because of their importance, cancers of the lung, colon and rectum, breast, and cervix are discussed in detail. Shorter descriptions are provided for prostate cancer, lymphoma, leukemia, bladder cancer, cancer of the oral cavity, and skin melanoma.

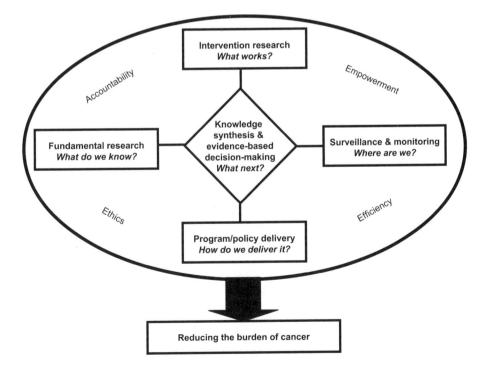

Figure 14.4. Framework for evidence-based cancer prevention and control. Cancer Epidemiology Prevention 3E by Schottenfeld (ed) Fig. 67-1 p. 1286 © 1996 by Oxford University Press, Inc. By permission of Oxford University Press, Inc.

LUNG CANCER
(ICD-10 C33-C34)

Significance

Lung cancer is the leading cause of cancer deaths in the United States, accounting for 29% of all cancer deaths in 2007, or a total of 160,390 deaths (Jemal et al. 2007). Lung cancer is also the most common cancer worldwide. This high mortality rate results from both a high incidence rate and a low survival rate: only 16% of U.S. lung cancer patients survive five years after diagnosis. There has been some improvement in lung cancer survival over the past half century as the survival rate for lung cancer was only 6% in the early 1950s (Spitz et al. 2006).

Pathophysiology

More than 90% of lung cancers are believed to originate in the basal cells of the lung epithelium, or the lining surfaces of the lung. A series of changes, over a period of years, occurs as lung cancer develops. These involve an increase in the number of cells, structural changes in certain epithelial cells that lead to abnormal function, appearance of patient signs and symptoms, and cancer spread. The major cell types of lung cancer are adenocarcinoma (approximately 38% of cases), squamous cell cancer (approximately 20% of cases), small cell cancer (approximately 13% of cases), and large cell cancer (approximately 5% of cases) (Ries et al. 2007). Lung cancer growth rates vary based on the cell type involved. Of the major cell types, small cell cancer appears to grow and spread the most rapidly.

Numerous genetic factors affect susceptibility to lung cancer. These are likely to involve a variety of cellular pathways including DNA repair, cell cycle, metabolism, and inflammation. Among the most studied genetic factors are the cytochrome P-450 enzymes (e.g., CYP1A1), which are known to metabolize many carcinogenic compounds (e.g., polycyclic aromatic hydrocarbons). The internal dose of tobacco smoke and other carcinogens to which the lung tissue is exposed is modulated by gene polymorphisms encoding for enzymes that affect activation and detoxification of cancer-causing chemicals (Spitz et al. 2006).

Descriptive Epidemiology

Because lung cancer is so strongly associated with cigarette smoking, its descriptive epidemiology is largely explained by smoking patterns and trends.

High-Risk Populations

Although lung cancer mortality rates remain 1.8 times higher among men than among women, lung cancer surpassed breast cancer as the leading cause of cancer deaths in women in 1987. Mortality rates are 1.1 times higher among African Americans than among whites. This racial difference is due to large differences in mortality between

African American and white men. Rates are nearly identical in African American and white women. Lung cancer mortality rates are approximately 60% lower among people of Hispanic origin than among non-Hispanics. Lung cancer rates increase with age, with 60 years being the average age of diagnosis. People of lower socioeconomic status are at higher risk for lung cancer.

Geographic Distribution

Lung cancer tends to cluster in areas with high smoking rates. In the United States, lung cancer rates are generally highest in the southern and lower Midwestern states. Kentucky has the highest lung cancer death rate followed by West Virginia and Arkansas. Utah has by far the lowest mortality rate, followed by Hawaii and New Mexico. Worldwide, lung cancer is most common in developed countries in North America and Europe (especially Eastern Europe) (Parkin et al. 2005).

Time Trends

The lung cancer mortality rate in the United States increased dramatically over the past 60 years, from 7 per 100,000 in 1940 to 53 per 100,000 in 2004 (Ries et al. 2007). The major increase in lung cancer mortality rates in men occurred from 1940 to 1979. In the 1980s, the rate of increase slowed, and from 1991 to 2003, male lung cancer mortality rate has declined 1.9% per year (American Cancer Society 2007b). In contrast, a sharp increase in lung cancer mortality rates was observed among women in the 1960s, although female lung cancer mortality rates are now approaching a plateau.

Causes

Modifiable Risk Factors

The strongest risk factor for lung cancer is cigarette smoking (Table 14.3). The association between smoking and lung cancer is one of the most widely studied and clearly defined relationships in chronic disease epidemiology. The relative risk of lung cancer due to current smoking is approximately 23 for men and 13 for women (Thun and Henely 2006), although this difference has been lessening over time as women have begun smoking more cigarettes per day and have started smoking at increasingly younger ages.

Exposure to lung carcinogens in the workplace increases lung cancer risk. Asbestos exposure among nonsmokers accounts for a relative risk of about five (Saracci 1987). When asbestos exposure is combined with cigarette smoking, the risk increases markedly to approximately 50-fold. Occupational exposure to radon accounts for a 20-fold increase in lung cancer risk (Lubin et al. 1994). Radon also interacts with smoking to greatly increase the risk. Increases in lung cancer risk have also been documented for exposure to inorganic arsenic, polycyclic hydrocarbons, chloromethyl ethers, chromium, and nickel (Spitz et al. 2006).

Exposure to radon gas in the home, especially in combination with cigarette smoking, may increase the risk of lung cancer. In addition, exposure to secondhand tobacco smoke (also called environmental tobacco smoke), elevates lung cancer risk slightly in

Table 14.3. Modifiable Risk Factors for Lung Cancer, United States

Magnitude	Risk Factor	Best Estimate (%) of Population-Attributable Risk (Range)
Strong (relative risk >4)	Cigarette smoking	82
	Occupation[a]	13 (10–20)
Moderate (relative risk 2–4)	None	–
Weak (relative risk <2)	Residential radon exposure	–
	Environmental tobacco smoke exposure	2 (–)
	5 or more servings of fruits and vegetables per day[b]	–
	Residence near large city for 10+ years	–

[a]Includes occupational exposures to asbestos, aluminum, beryllium, bis(chloromethyl) ether and chloromeythl ether, cadium, chromium, coke, mustard gas, radon, silica or sulfuric acid mist.
[b]Eating 5 or more servings of fruits and vegetables per day reduces risk.
Note: Data compiled from references (Miller 1992; U.S. Environmental Protection Agency 1992; Colditz, Baer, and Tamimi 2000; Rothenberg et al. 1987).

nonsmokers (i.e., a 20% excess risk associated with being married to a smoker) (Alberg and Samet 2003). Among dietary factors, the most consistent association is that between a low intake of fresh fruits and vegetables and higher risk of lung cancer (Spitz et al. 2006). Intake of high dose supplements of beta-carotene have been shown to increase lung cancer risk in smokers (World Cancer Research Fund/American Institute for Cancer Research 2007).

Population-Attributable Risk

An estimated 82% of lung cancer deaths are attributable to cigarette smoking (Table 14.3). The smoking-associated attributable risk is 88% among men and 72% among women (USDHHS 2004). Occupational exposures are estimated to contribute to an additional 13% of lung cancers. Extrapolations from risks among underground miners indicate that exposure to indoor radon may account for up to 10% of lung cancer deaths (Lubin and Boice 1989), although quantifying this risk factor accurately is extremely difficult. Exposure to environmental tobacco smoke accounts for approximately 2% of U.S. lung cancer cases (U.S.EPA 1992).

Prevention and Control

Prevention

Numerous interventions address primary prevention of lung cancer. Smoking cessation drastically reduces the risk of lung cancer, although a former smoker's risk does not drop back to that of a lifetime nonsmoker (USDHHS 2004). Smoking is usually adopted early in life; therefore, prevention of tobacco use among youth is critical to the overall goal of reducing smoking prevalence (see Chapter 5). Workers exposed to lung carcinogens (e.g., asbestos workers, uranium miners) should also be targeted for intervention, since many of their exposures interact with smoking to increase dramatically the risk of lung cancer. Dietary changes to increase consumption of fresh fruits and vegetables may decrease lung cancer risk. These changes are consistent with dietary guidelines discussed in other sections and chapters.

Evidence-based interventions can be found in numerous sources. Among these, *The Guide to Community Preventive Services: What Works to Promote Health* uses a systematic review process to highlight effective approaches (Zaza et al. 2005). Numerous effective interventions exist for tobacco control. These are also embodied in CDC's *Best Practices for Comprehensive Tobacco Control* (CDC 2007).

Screening

Several randomized trials have assessed the role of chest x-rays and examination of cells in the sputum (sputum cytology) in detecting lung cancer in the early stages. While these tests are able to detect early lesions, trials have not demonstrated a reduction in lung cancer mortality. Another test, low-dose spiral CT scanning, is undergoing testing in randomized trials to determine whether improved detection by CT will result in reduced lung cancer mortality (Manser 2004). Although this test can find lung cancer at an earlier stage, it has not yet been shown to reduce mortality in the long run.

Treatment

Lung cancer treatment is largely determined by the cell type and stage at diagnosis. Treatment options include surgery, radiation therapy, and chemotherapy. Lung cancer mortality could be reduced by an estimated 7% through early application of existing state-of-the-art treatments (Greenwald and Sondik 1986).

Examples of Evidence-Based Interventions

Public health interventions that are likely to affect lung cancer rates include the National Cancer Institute's *American Stop Smoking Intervention Study* (ASSIST) for Cancer Prevention (National Cancer Institute 2005a), the CDC's *National Tobacco Control Program* (CDC 2007c), and dedicated state tobacco taxes, such as those in California and Massachusetts (see Chapter 5) (Bal et al. 1990; Kohl 1996). A common element to all these programs involves a comprehensive approach, using price increases (e.g., through excise taxes), clean indoor air laws, mass media campaigns, restricting youth access, and providing low- or no-cost smoking cessation services.

Areas of Future Research

First, we must determine and apply effective smoking prevention and cessation techniques that target high-risk and/or difficult-to-reach populations such as youth, minorities, the economically disadvantaged and heavy smokers. Second, we need to further examine the roles of risk factors such as occupational exposures and residential radon exposure and their interactions with cigarette smoking. Third, we need to further evaluate the role of dietary factors in the prevention of lung cancer. Finally, we need to identify and refine efficacious methods for detecting lung cancer in its early stages.

COLORECTAL CANCER (ICD-10 C18-C21)

Significance

Cancer of the colon and rectum, also known as colorectal cancer, is the third leading cause of cancer death in men and women. It accounts for 10% of all cancer deaths in the United States. In 2007, approximately 79,130 new cases of colon and rectum cancer were diagnosed in men and 74,630 new cases in women. The overall five-year survival rate for colorectal cancer is 64%, with a rate of 90% for cancers identified in the local stage (Jemal et al. 2007).

Pathophysiology

Colon cancer develops from mucosal colonic polyps. The two most common histological types of polyps are adenomas and hyperplastic (Cappell 2005). The predominant cell type seen in colorectal cancer is adenocarcinoma. While only around 10% of adenomas progress into cancer, several factors increase the likelihood including larger size (greater than or equal to 1cm in surface diameter), multiplicity, degree of dysplasia, and villous histology (Giovannucci and Kana 2006).

A history of colorectal cancer in a first-degree relative elevates risk. A recent meta-analysis found the pooled relative risk for developing colon cancer was 4.25 (95% Confidence Interval: 3.01–6.08) times higher in those with more than one relative with colorectal cancer as compared to those without an affected relative (Johns and Houlston 2001). In addition to several low-penetrance genes, there are two main inherited, autosomal, dominant disorders known to predispose individuals to colorectal cancer: familial adenomatous polyposis (FAP) and hereditary nonpolyposis colorectal cancer (HNPCC) (Giovannucci and Kana 2006). FAP is very rare and characterized by multiple adenomas, usually 100 at the minimum, that turn cancerous if left untreated. HNPCC is also rare, accounting for 1%–5% of colon cancer, which occurs at an earlier age, approximately the mid-40s. In HNPCC, adenomas are uncommon, but more likely to have characteristics associated with progressing to cancer.

Descriptive Epidemiology

High-Risk Populations

Colorectal cancer mortality is 43% higher for men than for women and 41% higher for African Americans than for whites (National Cancer Institute 2007a). The incidence of colorectal cancer rises sharply after age 50, when 90% of colorectal cancers develop (Giovannucci and Kana 2006). The mean age at diagnosis is 73 years for colon cancer and 67 years for rectum cancer (National Cancer Institute 2007a). Medical conditions associated with colon cancer include inflammatory bowel disease (e.g., ulcerative colitis, Crohn's disease) (Giovannucci and Kana 2006; USDHHS 1996) and noninsulin dependent diabetes (Giovannucci and Kana 2006; Johns and Houlston 2001).

Geographic Distribution

In the United States, rates of colorectal cancer are highest in the Northeast, Midwest, and Western states (U.S. Cancer Statistics Working Group 2006). Worldwide, colorectal cancer rates are highest in developed countries in North America, Western Europe, Australia/New Zealand, and Japan (Parkin et al. 2005). Migration studies of populations that have moved from low-risk to high-risk areas have shown an increase in risk within the first generation. This suggests that environmental and lifestyle factors influence the development of colorectal cancer.

Time Trends

From 1995 to 2004, colorectal cancer mortality rates have been declining in the United States, though rates remain the lowest among whites (Surveillance, Epidemiology, and End Results Program 2007a). Colorectal incidence rates have also declined among all races except American Indian/Alaska Natives, which have experienced an annual percent increase of 6.4% per year from 2000 to 2004.

Causes

Modifiable Risk Factors

Few modifiable risk factors for colorectal cancer have been firmly characterized, despite many epidemiologic studies (Table 14.4). Physical activity has consistently been shown to have an inverse relationship with colorectal cancer risk. This may be due in part because it reduces body mass, a risk factor for colorectal cancer, but physical activity appears to confer at least some independent benefit. Recent studies have also shown an increase in colorectal cancer risk among tobacco users.

Considerable attention has focused on the relationship between diet and colorectal cancer. Although the precise dietary components and biologic mechanisms are not clearly understood, increased risk of colorectal cancer has been associated with a diet high in fat and carbohydrates. While red meat intake increases risk, protein from fish or poultry may decrease risk. Increased folate intake may also be protective against colorectal cancer,

Table 14.4. Modifiable Risk Factors for Colorectal Cancer, United States

Magnitude	Risk Factor	Best Estimate (%) of Population-Attributable Risk
Strong (relative risk >4)	None	–
Moderate (relative risk 2–4)	None	–
Weak (relative risk <2)	Physical inactivity[a]	26 (17–35)
	Age >50 not screened with appropriate method	17
	Obesity[b]	27 (0–43)
	No dietary milk or calcium supplement on most days	13
	3+ red meat servings per week	9
	Alcohol consumption[c]	<1
	Multivitamin use[d]	–
	Aspirin use[d]	–

[a]Includes occupational and recreational physical activities, population activity prevalence estimated for adults 45–64 years.
[b]BMI greater than 30.
[c]Two or more drinks per day.
[d]Use of multivitamin and/or aspirin may decrease risk (Giovannucci and Kana 2006).
Note: Data compiled from references (Ballard-Barbash et al. 2006, Lee and Oguma 2006).

especially among those with high alcohol intake. While a diet low in vegetables and fiber was previously thought to reduce risk, most recent work has shown a weak or nonexistent relationship to colorectal cancer. Studies of diet and colorectal cancer are confronted with many difficulties, including a high correlation between many dietary components and problems with subjects' ability to recall past dietary practices.

Population-Attributable Risk

Up to half of colorectal cancer cases may be related to obesity and physical inactivity (Table 14.4). Within this proportion, estimates suggest that 27% of colorectal cancer may be related to obesity and 26% to physical inactivity (Ballard-Barbash et al. 2006; Colditz, Baer, and Tamimi 2000; Lee and Oguma 2006). An estimated 17% of colorectal cancer cases may be related to a lack of routine screening (Colditz, Baer, and Tamimi 2000).

Prevention and Control

Prevention

Current evidence suggests that primary prevention strategies that improve diet and reduce sedentary behavior could reduce colorectal cancer incidence. Although the relationship of diet to colorectal cancer is not completely understood, some dietary recommendations can be made, such as limiting intake of high-fat foods, red meat, and alcohol. Further, increasing physical activity and maintenance of a healthy weight can also reduce risk (see Chapters 6 and 7).

Multiple complementary strategies are needed to achieve diet- and activity-related cancer prevention goals. These include routine provision of nutrition education and physical activity in schools as part of comprehensive health education, improved school lunch menus, and routine nutrition counseling by health professionals.

Screening

The principal screening tests for early detection of colorectal cancer are fecal occult blood testing, sigmoidoscopy, double contrast barium enema, and colonoscopy. Each of these screening tests has limitations. These limitations include the presence of false positive and false negative results in occult blood testing, the lower sensitivity of sigmoidoscopy and barium enema, and the higher risk, cost, and patient burden associated with colonoscopy.

The U.S. Preventive Services Task Force recommends one of the following testing schedules beginning at age 50: an annual fecal occult blood test, sigmoidoscopy or double contract barium every five years, or colonoscopy every 10 years (American Cancer Society 2007c; Agency for Healthcare Research and Quality 2006). All positive tests should be followed up with a colonoscopy. At a physician's recommendation, people at higher risk of colorectal cancer (e.g., a personal or strong family history of colorectal cancer or polyps, chronic inflammatory bowel disease, or a family history of FAP or HNPCC) may require more frequent screening, beginning at an earlier age. Some studies suggest colorectal incidence could be reduced by 60–70% and mortality by up to 80% with widespread screening. However, only approximately 50% of those aged 50 or older currently receive colorectal screening.

Treatment

Surgery is the most common method of treating colorectal cancer. After treatment, colorectal cancer patients need to be followed closely, because they are at a high risk of having recurrent or new cancers in the colon and rectum.

Examples of Evidence-Based Interventions

The CDC has a broad colorectal cancer initiative focused on screening (CDC 2007d). One program of the initiative is the "Screen for Life: National Colorectal Cancer Action Campaign," a multimedia effort to increase awareness of colorectal cancer and screening among those 50 years and older, offering materials in both English and Spanish. Recently, a three-year demonstration project began in five cities to screen low-income individuals with inadequate or no health insurance for colorectal cancer. In addition to these programs, the initiative monitors national screening rates and promotes health care provider awareness and research.

Areas of Future Research

Additional epidemiologic and clinical research is needed to better define the risk of colorectal cancer related to specific dietary factors. Long-term prospective studies currently under way should help clarify the relationship between diet and colorectal cancer risk. In addition to focusing on increasing screening behavior for secondary prevention, programs that encourage healthy changes in diet and reduction in sedentary behavior can serve as important tools for primary prevention of colorectal cancer.

BREAST CANCER
(ICD-10 C50)

Significance

Breast cancer is the most common cancer type among women in the United States and the second leading cause of cancer death (Jemal et al. 2007). It is estimated there were 178,480 new cases and 40,460 deaths in 2007. Worldwide, breast cancer is the second most common cancer and the fifth among cancer deaths (Colditz, Baer, and Tamimi 2006). Breast cancer rarely occurs in men, with 12,270 prevalent U.S. cases in 2004 (National Cancer Institute 2007a). Approximately one of every eight women will develop breast cancer at some time during her lifetime. The overall five-year survival rate for breast cancer is 88%, with a range of survival from 27% for distant-stage cancer to 98% for local-stage cancer.

Pathophysiology

Breast cancer develops as cells lose their normal regulatory control, and transition from carcinoma insitu, to noninvasive cancer, to invasive cancer, and finally metastatic disease. The predominant cell type of breast cancer is adenocarcinoma (approximately 95% of cases). Among invasive tumors, the number of lymph nodes involved is the best prognostic indicator of survival. Hormones, both endogenous and exogenous, play a role in breast cancer pathogenesis as they increase cell proliferation in the breast and the opportunity for random genetic errors during cell division deaths (Colditz, Baer, and Tamimi 2006). Proliferation is mediated by hormone receptors. Estrogen and progesterone receptors are often present in breast cancer tumors. When receptors are present above a certain threshold value, the tumor is considered receptor-positive. Receptor-positive women respond better to hormonal therapy and show increased survival rates.

Women with a first-degree relative with breast cancer have a 1.5 – 3 times increased risk of developing the disease. Mutations in BRCA1 (breast cancer 1) and/or BRCA2 (breast cancer 2) may correspond up to 80% lifetime risk of developing breast cancer (Easton et al. 1993). These germ line mutations likely account for 2% – 5% of all breast cancers. Additionally, women with a diagnosis of benign breast disease are also at an increased risk of breast cancer, though some types of benign breast lesions may be precursor lesions rather than a marker of risk (Colditz, Baer, and Tamimi 2006). Women with the greatest mammographic density, the overall percentage of dense tissue in the breast, have four to six times the risk of developing breast cancer as compared to women with little or no density.

Descriptive Epidemiology

High-Risk Populations

Although the incidence of breast cancer is higher in whites, mortality rates are 35% higher among African American women than among white women (Jemal et al. 2007). Women of higher socioeconomic status are at higher risk of developing breast cancer, which may explain some of the differences in incidence rates between white and African American women (Colditz, Baer, and Tamimi 2006). Differences in mortality may be due in part to the tendency for African American women to be diagnosed at later stages of the disease. Mortality also increases with age, with 58% of deaths from breast cancer occurring among women who are 65 years of age and older (National Cancer Institute 2007a).

Geographic Distribution

Breast cancer mortality rates in the United States are generally higher in Eastern states and lower in Western states. The District of Columbia has the highest, and Hawaii has the lowest breast cancer mortality rate (Surveillance, Epidemiology, and End Results Program 2007b). Breast cancer rates show wide international variations, with the highest rates being in North America and northern Europe and the lowest in Asia (Colditz, Baer, and Tamimi 2006). However, breast cancer incidence has been increasing in both high- and low-risk countries. Changes in lifestyle, as well as screening practices, may impact these rates.

Time Trends

Mortality due to breast cancer remained relatively stable in the first half of the 1900s. Between 1973 and 1990, breast cancer mortality rates increased 2% among U.S. women overall and 21% among African American women (USDHHS 1995). However, between 1990 and 2004, mortality rates decreased 38% overall, yet only 19% among African American women (Surveillance, Epidemiology, and End Results Program 2007b). Breast cancer incidence rates in the United States rose sharply throughout the 1980s, in part due to the increase in use of mammography screening. Recently, this trend has reversed as incidence rates have decreased from 132 per 100,000 in 1990 to 124 per 100,000 in 2004.

Causes

Modifiable Risk Factors

Through numerous epidemiologic studies, an array of modifiable breast cancer risk factors has been established (Table 14.5). Despite the large number of risk factors, few are strongly associated with the development of breast cancer, and no single factor or combination of factors can predict the occurrence of breast cancer in any one individual.

The risk associated with reproductive variables—never having children, being of a late age at first birth, having an early menarche, having a late menopause—is related to the hormonal environment to which the breast is exposed (e.g., during pregnancy or during a

Table 14.5. Modifiable Risk Factors for Breast Cancer, United States

Magnitude	Risk Factor	Best Estimate (%) of Population-Attributable Risk (Range)
Strong (relative risk >4)	None	
Moderate (relative risk 2–4)	Ionizing radiation	–
Weak (relative risk <2)	Never having children	5 (1–9)
	First full-term pregnancy after age 30	7 (1–13)
	Obesity after menopause	11 (4–37)
	Weight gain since age 18[a]	4
	Alcohol consumption	– (3–10)
	Physical inactivity	– (17–26)
	High caloric or high fat diet	–
	Lack of breast-feeding	18
	Postmenopausal hormone use	2 (1–6)
	Current use of oral contraception[b]	– (0–2)

[a] Among postmenopausal women.
[b] Prevalence estimate for women 40–44 years.
Note: Data compiled from references (Ballard-Barbash et al. 2006; Lee and Oguma 2006; Lacey, Colditz, and Schottenfeld 2006; Marshall and Freudenheim 2006).

long menstrual history) (USDHHS 1996; Colditz, Baer, and Tamimi 2006). Conversely, lactation is associated with a 4.3% decrease in risk for every 12 months of breast-feeding (Collaborative Group on Hormonal Factors in Breast Cancer 2002).

Energy intake and expenditure also impact breast cancer risk. In Western populations, body fat is associated with an increased risk among postmenopausal women and decreased risk among premenopausal women (Colditz, Baer, and Tamimi 2006). Physical activity has an inverse, dose–response affect on breast cancer risk.

Investigation of endogenous hormones have shown an increased risk of breast cancer among premenopausal women with high blood levels of insulin-like growth factor I (IGF-I) and among postmenopausal women with high blood estrogens. Exogenous hormones, such as oral contraceptive and postmenopausal hormones have generally shown little or no increased risk of breast cancer (Colditz, Baer, and Tamimi 2006). However, current and recent users of oral contraceptives may have a slight elevation in risk, though these women tend to be younger with a low absolute risk. Likewise, current users of postmenopausal hormones and those with the longest duration of use are also at an increased risk of breast cancer, though this risk is mitigated if hormone use has stopped for five or more years, regardless of previous duration.

Several dietary factors have also been examined in relation to breast cancer risk. Current evidence regarding fat and fruit and vegetable intake has been inconclusive or unsupportive of a relationship to breast cancer risk (Colditz, Baer, and Tamimi 2006). However, beta-carotene and folate intake do appear to be protective against breast cancer. Moderate-to-heavy alcohol consumption is associated with an increased risk of breast cancer (Longnecker 1994). High intake of folic acid may protect against the risk associated with alcohol intake (Zhang et al. 2003).

Population-Attributable Risk

Several established risk factors each account for relatively small proportions of overall breast cancer incidence (Table 14.5).

Prevention and Control

Prevention

Although challenging, there is sufficient evidence that the risk of breast cancer could be reduced by maintaining healthy weight (especially after menopause), being physically active, breast-feeding, and perhaps avoiding alcohol use. However, given the small attributable risk for these factors, and challenges in making changes, public health practitioners should also focus attention on secondary prevention—that is, early detection.

Screening

Several large studies have demonstrated that clinical breast examination by a physician or nurse and mammography screening (i.e., low-dose breast x-rays) are effective methods for the early detection of breast cancer in women over age 50 (Agency for Healthcare Research and Quality 2006; Colditz, Baer, and Tamimi 2006). Women in these studies had a 25–30% lower risk of dying from breast cancer when screened with mammography. While the evidence for women in their 40s is less clear, both the American Cancer Society and the U.S. Preventive Services Task Force recommend annual mammography and clinical breast examination beginning at age 40 (American Cancer Society 2007c; Agency for Healthcare Research and Quality 2006). Neither group recommends breast self-examination (BSE) due to insufficient evidence of its effectiveness and potential for false-positive results. In addition, the American Cancer Society recently expanded their screening recommendations to include breast magnetic resonance imaging (MRI) for women with a 20–25% or greater lifetime risk of developing breast cancer (Saslow et al. 2007).

Although there remains scientific controversy regarding the benefits versus the risk of screening women in their 40s, there is convincing evidence of the effectiveness of mammography for women age 50–69 years (Agency for Healthcare Research and Quality 2006). The decision to screen women under age 50 is commonly considered in relation to risk; for example, women with a family history of breast cancer may be screened more frequently. The prevalence of annual mammography screening among U.S. women age 40 and older more than doubled—from under 30% in 1987 to 70% in 2000 (American Cancer Society 2007c). While mammography rates have been lower among Hispanic women as compared to non-Hispanic whites and African Americans, they have increased slightly, from approximately 62% in 2000 to 65% in 2003 (Smith, Cokkinides, and Eyre 2007). However, the prevalence of mammography screening remains lower among women with no health insurance, with less education, or living below the poverty level (National Center for Health Statistics 2006; Swan et al. 2003).

Treatment

Depending on the stage of cancer and the patient's medical history, breast cancer treatment may require lumpectomy (local removal of the cancer), mastectomy (surgical removal of the breast), radiation therapy, chemotherapy, or hormone therapy. Two or more treatment methods are often used in combination. Cancer support groups such as the American Cancer Society's Reach to Recovery Program can provide valuable information and emotional support to breast cancer patients.

Examples of Evidence-Based Interventions

The Breast and Cervical Cancer Mortality Prevention Act of 1990 established the largest public health application of breast cancer control technology (Henson, Wyatt, and Lee 1996). This initiative guided the CDC in creating the National Breast and Cervical Cancer Early Detection Program (NBCCEDP), which provides breast and cervical cancer screening to low-income, uninsured, and underserved women in all 50 states, the District of Columbia, five U.S. territories, and 12 American Indian/Alaska Native tribes or tribal organizations (Division of Cancer Prevention and Control 2007). As of 1991, the NBCCEDP has served more than three million women and diagnosed over 30,000 breast cancers. Since 2000, women in the program have access to treatment through the state-based Medicaid insurance program. Program components include screening and diagnostic services, partnerships, professional development, mammography quality assurance, and evaluation.

Areas of Future Research

Several possible risk factors for breast cancer—diet, alcohol use, physical inactivity, and postmenopausal hormone use—would be amenable to primary prevention. Therefore, research should concentrate on improving diet and activity behavior at a population level. Other modifiable risk factors, like reproductive timing and breast-feeding duration, are influenced by social norms and may be affected by policy interventions such as support for childcare, breast-feeding in the workplace, and/or longer maternity leaves (Colditz, Baer, and Tamimi 2006).

Tamoxifen and other chemopreventive agents can be effective primary prevention strategies for high-risk women. However, additional research is needed to identify the criteria for determining which women will most benefit from these treatments (Colditz, Baer, and Tamimi 2006). Future research should also focus on determining the precise roles of endogenous hormones, as well as additional genetic, behavioral, and environmental risk factors in breast cancer. Additionally, the efficacy of new detection methods, such as the MRI and digital mammography, should be further explored.

CERVICAL CANCER (ICD-10 C53)

Significance

Invasive cancer of the uterine cervix, commonly known as cervical cancer, accounted for 11,150 new cases and 3,670 deaths among women in the United States in 2007 (Jemal et al. 2007). In situ cervical cancer—that is, detected in the earliest, premalignant stage—is much more common, accounting for about 55,000 U.S. cases per year. Cervical cancer is the 16th most common cancer in the United States; yet, it is the second most common cancer among women worldwide, with an estimated 493,000 incident cases in 2002 (Parkin et al. 2005). The overall five-year survival rate for cervical cancer is 73%; however, survival approaches 100% for cervical cancers detected in situ.

Pathophysiology

Due to advances in molecular biology, researchers now identify cervical cancer as a multi step process. As described later in this chapter, nearly all cases of cervical cancer are believed to result from persistent infection with one of about 15 genotypes of carcinogenic human papillomavirus (HPV) (Schiffman et al. 2007). There are four major steps in cervical cancer development: (1) infection of metaplastic epithelium at the cervical transformation zone, (2) viral persistence, (3) progression of persistently infected epithelium to cervical precancer, and (4) invasion through the basement membrane of the epithelium.

It is believed that early stages of cervical cancer are characterized by dysplasia, or the presence of cells that are altered in size, shape, and organization. Preclinical, preinvasive changes in the cervix are called cervical intraepithelial neoplasia (CIN). These early cervical cancer changes can easily be detected through the Pap test. The Pap test involves collecting and analyzing a small sample of cells from the cervix. Clinical manifestations of cervical cancer may involve bleeding or other vaginal discharges. The major cell types observed for invasive cervical cancer are squamous cell cancer (approximately 69% of cases) and adenocarcinoma (approximately 25% of cases) (Ries et al. 2007).

Descriptive Epidemiology

High-Risk Populations

Cervical cancer incidence increases sharply until age 45 and peaks around that age. The incidence of cervical cancer is 54% higher among African Americans as it is among whites, and mortality rates are approximately two times higher among African Americans (Ries et al. 2007). Elevated cervical cancer rates are also observed for Hispanics, American Indians, and Hawaiian natives. Women of lower socioeconomic status are at higher risk of cervical cancer. Several religious groups—Catholic nuns, Amish, Mormons, and Jews—have very low rates of cervical cancer, probably because of marital and sexual risk factors.

Geographic Distribution

Cervical cancer mortality rates in the United States are generally higher in southeastern states and lower in western (Rocky Mountain) and upper midwestern states. The District of Columbia has the highest rate, and Minnesota and Massachusetts have the lowest cervical cancer mortality rates (Ries et al. 2007). Internationally, cervical cancer incidence rates are highest in Africa and parts of Central and South America (Parkin et al. 2005).

Time Trends

Incidence and mortality rates of invasive cervical cancer have been decreasing steadily over the past 50 years. From 1950 to 2004, cervical cancer incidence and mortality in the United States have shown a larger annual percent decrease than have any other major cancer among women (Ries et al. 2007). However, this decline has been due to squamous cell carcinoma, and there is concern that cervical adenocarcinoma rates have risen in the past few decades in several countries, including the United States (Schiffman and Hildesheim 2006).

Causes

Modifiable Risk Factors

The primary risk factor for cervical cancer is infection with HPV—it is now accepted to be the central, necessary cause of virtually all cases of cervical cancer (Schiffman and Hildesheim 2006). There are likely over 100 types of HPV. About 30 of these are transmitted by sexual contact, and approximately 20 of these are causally related to cervical cancer. The relative risk estimate for HPV-DNA and cervical cancer was estimated at 158 (95% CI = 113 to 221) in the IARC multicenter study (Munoz et al. 2003), among the highest effect sizes observed for any human cancer (Bosch and de Sanjose 2003).

There are other established risk factors for cervical cancer including long-term use of hormonal contraceptives, cigarette smoking, five or more pregnancies, and several sexual risk factors: partners with greater than six other sexual partners and HPV infection in a male partner (Bosch and de Sanjose 2003).

Population-Attributable Risk

Estimates of attributable risk for HPV infection and cervical cancer range from 90% to 98%, suggesting that nearly all cases of cervical cancer are due to HPV infection.

Prevention and Control

Prevention

Several behavioral changes will reduce the risk of cervical cancer. These include limiting the number of sexual partners, delaying intercourse until a later age, avoiding sexually transmitted diseases, and eliminating cigarette smoking.

Recently, a vaccine has been approved by the U.S. Food and Drug Administration to prevent infection with the two types of HPV that cause approximately 70% of cervical cancers, and the two types of HPV that cause 90% of genital warts (National Cancer Institute 2007b). The approved vaccine provides protection against infection with these HPV types for at least five years. How long the protection lasts is under study, as are guidelines for its use among children.

Screening

The principal screening test for cervical cancer over the past five decades has been the Pap test—it is the oldest and most established early detection test (Hiatt et al. 2002). Decreases in cervical cancer incidence and mortality over the past 50 years are mainly the result of early detection due to widespread use of the Pap test (Agency for Healthcare Research and Quality 2006). Despite the availability and frequent use of the Pap test, subgroups of high-risk women—for example, those of lower education and income—either have never been screened or are screened infrequently. Pap testing is especially important in these high-risk groups and in women who no longer see a physician for obstetric needs.

There is debate about the optimal screening protocol for Pap testing. For example, the U.S. Preventive Services Task Force recommends that Pap tests should begin with the onset of sexual activity and should be repeated at least every three years (Agency for Healthcare Research and Quality 2006). An annual Pap test is recommended until three normal tests; then screening every two to three years is called for (American Cancer Society 2007c). The American Cancer Society recommends that Pap testing begin approximately three years after onset of sexual activity, but no later than 21 years of age.

The role of persistent HPV infection in cervical cancer etiology and advances in HPV typing are causing reexamination of screening practices (Holcomb and Runowicz 2005; Wright 2007). It has been suggested that over the next several years, screening for cervical cancer will switch from cytology-based detection (Pap testing) to testing for high-risk types of HPV (Wright 2007).

Treatment

Depending on the stage at diagnosis, cervical cancer is usually treated by surgery or radiation or both. In situ cancers can be treated by cryotherapy (cell destruction by extreme cold), electrocoagulation (cell destruction by intense heat), or local surgery.

Examples of Evidence-Based Interventions

The National Cancer Institute and the CDC began funding a series of cervical cancer research and application projects in 1985 (National Institutes of Health 1991). Most of these projects sought to increase the use of the Pap test in high-risk populations through "in-reach," or increasing use in women who attend clinics, and "outreach," or offering community-wide screening programs.

In addition, the CDC is sponsoring large-scale cervical cancer screening projects as part of the Breast and Cervical Cancer Mortality Prevention Act of 1990 (Henson, Wyatt, and Lee 1996). Early results from this program have shown higher rates of CIN among younger women and invasive cervical cancer in older women (Lawson et al. 1998).

Areas of Future Research

Further research into the causes of cervical cancer will lead to increased opportunities for primary prevention. A better understanding of the interaction between multiple risk factors is also needed. Given the high rates of cervical cancer mortality among minority and economically disadvantaged women, better targeting of proven cervical cancer control technologies is clearly needed.

PROSTATE CANCER (ICD-10 C61)

Significance

Cancer of the prostate is the most common cancer among men in the United States, accounting for 218,890 new cases in 2007 (Jemal et al. 2007). Prostate cancer is the second leading cause of cancer deaths in U.S. men, after lung cancer. Approximately one of every six men will develop prostate cancer over his lifetime (American Cancer Society 2007b). The incidence of prostate cancer is rising worldwide, but this is due at least partially to increased screening.

Descriptive Epidemiology

African-American men have the highest incidence of prostate cancer in the world, with an incidence that is 55% higher than that among white men in the United States (Ries et al. 2007). The incidence of prostate cancer in Asian countries is much lower, but Asian immigrants to the United States experience rates closer to those for U.S. men, suggesting that environmental factors, including nutrition, may play a role in etiology. The lifetime risk of prostate cancer among African-American men is now estimated at one in five. The median age of incidence is 68 years of age, and the five-year survival rate for prostate cancer is 98%. Latent (subclinical) prostate cancer affects an increasing proportion of men at each decade of life.

Causes

The causes of prostate cancer are largely unknown. Both environmental and familial factors may contribute to increased risk. The only conclusive risk factors are not modifiable, and include older age, being African American, and family history of prostate cancer (Platz and Giovannucci 2006). Hormonal factors are being extensively studied. Prostate cancer is hormonally dependent, and steroid hormones such as testosterone and dihydrotestosterone are suspected to play a role in pathogenesis.

Growing epidemiologic evidence suggests higher prostate cancer risk associated with a diet high in red and processed meat and dairy products. A family history of prostate cancer in a first-degree relative appears to double the risk, suggesting that interactions between genetic factors and environmental exposures may be important. In addition, suspected environmental factors include occupational exposure to cadmium and work in rubber manufacturing and farming.

Prevention and Control

Because its causes are not clearly understood, prostate cancer is not currently amenable to primary prevention. The U.S. Preventive Services Task Force concluded that the evidence is insufficient to recommend for or against routine screening using prostate-specific antigen (PSA) testing or digital rectal examination (Agency for Healthcare Research and Quality 2006). In contrast, the American Cancer Society recommends that men at average risk begin screening at age 50 by annual digital rectal examination and measurement of PSA in serum (American Cancer Society 2007c). PSA screening is now widely adopted with 75% of American men 50 and older reporting having had a PSA test (Sirovich, Schwartz, and Woloshin 2003). Research continues intensively on ways to improve the specificity of PSA and how to screen for other molecules that are markers of early prostate cancer.

LYMPHOMA
(ICD-10 C81-C85)

Significance

Lymphomas are cancers that affect lymphocytes, primarily in the lymph nodes, spleen, and thymus. Lymphomas are generally classified as either Hodgkin's lymphoma (HL) or non-Hodgkin's lymphoma (NHL). Hodgkin's disease and NHL are considered separately because they have distinct epidemiologic patterns, biological behavior, and histologic features.

Distribution

In 2007, an estimated 63,190 persons were diagnosed with NHL and 18,660 deaths (Jemal et al. 2007). NHL is the fifth most common cancer in the United States in terms of new cases (Jemal et al. 2007). The incidence of NHL is higher among men compared with women and is higher among whites compared with African Americans. Age-specific incidence and mortality rates increase with increasing age. The U.S. incidence rate for NHL has almost doubled since the 1970s (Hartge et al. 2006). While much of the increase in NHL rates is associated with HIV-related cancers, it is difficult to determine whether the AIDS epidemic explains all of this increase.

In contrast, the overall incidence of NHL has decreased since 1975 annual percent change (APC -0.2), particularly among the elderly (National Cancer Institute 2007a). However, there has been a slight increase among females since the mid-1990s. In 2007, it was estimated that there would be 8,190 new cases and 1,070 deaths from HL (Jemal et al. 2007). The incidence has been higher among whites than African Americans, and among males than females (Mueller and Grufferman 2006). The age distribution of HL is bimodal; one peak in early adulthood, and a second after age 60. The leading cause of death among long-term HL survivors is second malignancies.

In the United States, for each case of HL, there are almost eight cases of NHL. For each HL death, there are 14 NHL deaths. The five-year survival rates for NHL (63%) and HL (86%) are also markedly different.

Causes

The causes of the lymphomas are not well understood, in part because of the diversity of histologic forms of cancer in these diagnoses. People with immune system disorders, organ transplant patients, and persons undergoing treatment with immunosuppressive drugs are at increased risk of NHL (Hartge et al. 2006). NHL is extremely high in persons with HIV infection with relative risk estimates ranging from 50 to100. There is also some evidence that exposure to certain herbicides and pesticides elevates NHL risk, including phenoxy acid-based herbicides (such as 2,4-dichloro-phenoxyacetic acid) and chlorophenols.

An infectious origin has been suggested for Hodgkin's disease on the basis of its epidemiologic features, age at onset, and spatial clustering. Current evidence indicates the Epstein-Barr virus is a causal factor in a considerable proportion of HL cases (Mueller and Grufferman 2006).

Prevention and Control

Because the causes of NHL and Hodgkin's disease are not fully understood, clear prevention strategies are unavailable. Given the growing evidence of an association between pesticide use and NHL, however, prudent use of these chemicals is warranted. No screening tests are yet available for the early detection of NHL or HL. While the 5-year survival for HL is high, treatment for HL appears to result in the high rate of fatal secondary malignancies (Mueller and Grufferman 2006). The development of effective treatments that do not lead to secondary cancers is an important area for future research.

LEUKEMIA
(ICD-10 C91-C95)

Significance

Leukemia comprises a variety of cancers that arise in the bone marrow, lymph nodes, and/or other lymphoid tissue with immune function. Leukemia affects both children and adults and accounts for about 33% of cancers among children (2,400 new cases per year) and 2% of adult cancer cases (25,900 new cases per year). There are four main types of leukemia: acute myeloid (including acute monocytic) leukemia, acute lymphocytic leukemia, chronic lymphocytic leukemia, and chronic myeloid leukemia. In the United States, acute lymphocytic leukemia accounts for 73% of leukemia cases among children (American Cancer Society 2007b). The most common leukemia types among adults are acute myeloid leukemia and chronic lymphocytic leukemia.

From a public health standpoint, leukemia is important not only for its health impact on the population, but also because of the frequency of public inquiries regarding leukemia and the emotional nature of these inquiries and the media impact. State and local health departments respond to over 1,000 inquiries per year about suspected cancer clusters (Thun and Sinks 2004). These inquiries frequently concern apparent spatial clustering of childhood leukemia cases. Use of an established protocol aids in response to these concerns about cancer clusters (Kingsley, Schmeichel, and Rubin 2007).

Descriptive Epidemiology

Leukemia is 62% more common among men in the United States than among women and is slightly more common in whites than in African Americans (Ries et al. 2007). Among adults, leukemia mortality has declined slightly over the past 30 years. In contrast, survival among children due to acute lymphocytic leukemia has increased dramatically (58–87%) over the past few decades as the result of improvements in therapy.

Causes

The major causes of leukemia are unknown; however, several risk factors have been identified, including genetic abnormalities such as Down syndrome, exposure to ionizing radiation, and workplace exposure to benzene and other related solvents (USDHHS 1996; Linet, Devassa, and Morgan 2006). Adult T-cell leukemia is strongly associated with infection by human T-lymphotrophic virus, type I in endemic areas (Blattner 1993). Increasing evidence suggests that cigarette smoking is a causative risk factor for some forms of leukemia (Brownson, Novotny, and Perry 1993). Some studies have suggested that residential exposure to magnetic fields among children and occupational exposure among adults may increase risk, but more recent literature suggests that the evidence for magnetic fields as a risk factor is weak (Linet, Devesa, and Morgan 2006).

Prevention and Control

Because the causes of leukemia are largely undetermined, primary prevention is difficult. Reducing occupational and environmental exposures to radiation and leukemogenic chemicals and eliminating cigarette smoking may reduce leukemia incidence. Because symptoms often appear late, diagnosing leukemia early is difficult and no routine screening test exists.

BLADDER CANCER (ICD-10 C67)

Significance

Bladder cancer is the most common cancer of the urinary tract, accounting for 67,160 new cases and 7,550 deaths in the United States in 2007 (American Cancer Society 2007b).

Descriptive Epidemiology

Bladder cancer is more than four times more common among men than among women. Bladder cancer incidence is higher among whites than among African Americans, particularly for males where rates for white males are twice those for African American males (Ries et al. 2007). Incidence has been relatively stable over the past few decades.

Causes

Cigarette smoking is probably the best-established cause of bladder cancer. Bladder cancer risk for a smoker is approximately two to three times that of a nonsmoker, and smoking is estimated to account for 50–65% of cases in men and 20–30% of cases in women (Silverman et al. 2006). More than 40 occupational groups and exposures have been associated with bladder cancer, yet only a few of these are well established. Among these, increased risks are also associated with occupational exposures to aromatic amines and other chemicals in the textile, rubber, and leather industries. Several other occupations have been associated with an increased risk of bladder cancer, including truck drivers, leather workers, painters, printers, and aluminum workers. Occupational exposures are estimated to account for 5–25% of bladder cancer cases in men and 8–11% of cases in women. Studies are currently under way to better understand other risk factors, in particular the roles of genetic susceptibility in relation to bladder cancer risk.

Prevention and Control

Primary prevention of bladder cancer should focus on eliminating cigarette smoking and minimizing exposure to hazardous chemicals in the workplace. Currently, no routine screening test is available for early detection of bladder cancer.

ORAL AND PHARYNGEAL CANCER
(ICD-10 C00-C14)

Significance

Cancer of the oral cavity—that is, lip, salivary gland, mouth, and throat— accounted for an estimated 34,360 new cases and 7,550 U.S. deaths in 2007. In parts of Asia, oral cancer rates per 100,000 range from 4.6 in Thailand to 12.6 in India, due to behaviors such as smoking and the use of smokeless tobacco (e.g., betal nut or miang chew) (Petersen 2003).

Descriptive Epidemiology

Oral cancer mortality rates are 2.7 times higher among men in the United States than among women and 1.5 times higher among African Americans than among whites (National Cancer Institute 2007a). The overall five-year survival rate for oral cancer in the United States is 59%, although survival for cancer diagnosed in the local stage is 82%.

Causes

The use of tobacco in any form—cigarettes, cigars, and pipes, as well as the use of chewing tobacco and snuff—substantially elevates the risk of cancer of the tongue, mouth, and pharynx (Mayne, Morse, and Winn 2006). Cigarette smokers have a 3 – 12 times greater risk of oral cancer than do nonsmokers. Excessive alcohol consumption is also associated with cancer of the oral cavity. Smoking and drinking are independent risk factors for oral cancer and also interact synergistically to multiply risk. For example, among heavy smokers (i.e., more than 40 cigarettes per day) who consume at least 30 drinks per week, oral cancer is increased 38-fold (Blot et al. 1988). Fruit and vegetable intake, as well as certain nutrients like vitamin C and carotene/carotenoid have been shown to have an inverse relationship with oral cancer risk.

Prevention and Control

Oral and pharyngeal cancers are largely preventable. Oral cancer death rates could be reduced significantly through primary prevention and early detection. Eliminating smoking and smokeless tobacco use and reducing heavy alcohol consumption would substantially reduce oral cancer incidence. In addition, measures to reduce sun exposure (see section on Melanoma of the Skin) should be taken to reduce the risk of lip cancer. The U.S. Preventive Services Task Force concluded there is insufficient evidence to recommend oral cavity examination as there are little data regarding the sensitivity and specificity of this method (Agency for Healthcare Research and Quality 2006). The Task Force recommends clinicians remain alert to the increased potential for oral cancers among patients that use tobacco and alcohol and to counsel patients to cease smoking and limit alcohol intake. In contrast, the American Cancer Society recommends examination of the oral cavity for abnormal lesions as part of periodic health examinations (American Cancer Society 2007c).

MELANOMA OF THE SKIN
(ICD-10 C43)

Significance

Over 1,000,000 cases of skin cancer occurred in 2007; most were highly curable basal or squamous cell cancers (Jemal et al. 2007). A small fraction of the total cases, but the vast majority of deaths, were due to malignant melanoma of the skin. Melanoma accounted for an estimated 65,050 new cases and 10,850 deaths in the United States in 2007 (Jemal et al. 2007).

Descriptive Epidemiology

Melanoma mortality increases with age, and men have a higher risk than women. Melanoma incidence is almost 30 times more common among whites than among African Americans (Ries et al. 2007). From 1995 to 2004, melanoma among whites increased faster than nearly any other major cancer type (annual percent change = 1.8) (Ries et al. 2007). The five-year survival for melanoma is 91% (National Cancer Institute 2007a). Melanoma incidence rates increase with increasing ambient solar ultraviolet B radiation, although the pattern is not entirely consistent due in part to confounding of latitude with skin pigmentation (e.g., darker skin in the South than North) (Gruber and Armstrong 2006).

Causes

Sun exposure accounts for an estimated 90% of melanoma cases (Gruber and Armstrong 2006). Recreational sun exposure, especially intense, repeated, blistering overdoses during childhood, increase risk for melanoma. Risk is highest among fair-skinned people who sunburn easily. A family history of melanoma increases the risk by two to eight times. Both benign acquired nevi (e.g., moles) and atypical nevi (e.g., moles with irregular pigmentation and borders) are markers of increased melanoma risk and precursors of melanoma in some cases.

Prevention and Control

Prevention of melanoma should include avoiding all forms of ultraviolet radiation exposure, including the sun during peak exposure periods (10:00 a.m.-4:00 p.m.), wearing protective clothing, and wearing sunscreen (Agency for Healthcare Research and Quality 2006). However, wearing sunscreen alone could increase risk of melanoma if it also increases the amount of time spent in the sun. Recent research suggesting benefits from moderate sun exposure may lead to confusing messages for the public.

The U.S. Preventive Task Services Force concluded there is insufficient evidence to recommend routine screening; they suggest clinicians should be aware of suspicious skin lesions and evaluate them by following the "ABCD" criteria: Asymmetry, Border irregularity, Color variability, and Diameter greater than 6 mm (Agency for Healthcare Research and Quality 2006). Some organizations, such as the American Cancer Society, recommend that adults should perform monthly skin self-examinations, especially those people with heavy occupational or recreational sun exposure or with other significant risk factors (Gruber and Armstrong 2006).

Resources

American Cancer Society, Inc., 1599 Clifton Rd., NE, Atlanta, GA 30329-4251, 800-ACS-2345, http://www.cancer.org.

Division of Cancer Prevention and Control, Centers for Disease Control and Prevention, 4770 Buford Hwy, MS K-52, Atlanta, GA 30341-3724, 1-800-CDC-INFO, E-mail: cdcinfo@cdc. gov, http://www.cdc.gov/cancer.

Guide to Community Preventive Services, Community Guide Branch, National Center for Health Marketing (NCHM), Centers for Disease Control and Prevention, 1600 Clifton Road NE, Mailstop E-69, Atlanta, GA 30333, http://www.thecommunityguide.org/index.html.

National Cancer Institute, Cancer Information Service, 9000 Rockville Pike, Bldg. 31, Rm. 11A48, Bethesda, MD 20892-2590, 800-4-CANCER, E-mail: cancergovstaff@mail.nih.gov, http://www.cancer.gov.

World Health Organization: Cancer, Avenue Appia 20, 1211 Geneva 27, Switzerland, Telephone: + 41 22 791 21 11, http://www.who.int/cancer/en.

Suggested Reading

Colditz, G.A., M. Samplin-Salgado, C.T. Ryan, et al. Harvard Report on Cancer Prevention. Vol 5: Fulfilling the Potential for Cancer Prevention: Policy Approaches. *Cancer Causes Control* (2002):13(3):199–212.

Harvard Report on Cancer Prevention. Vol 1: Causes of Human Cancer. *Cancer Causes Control* (1996):7(Suppl)1:S3–59.

National Cancer Institute (NCI). *NCI Challenge Goal 2015. Eliminating the Suffering and Death Due to Cancer.* Available at: http://www.cancer.gov/aboutnci/archive/2015. Accessed November 11, 2007.

Schottenfeld, D., and J. F. Fraumeni, Jr., editors. *Cancer Epidemiology and Prevention* (3rd ed.). New York: Oxford University Press (2006).

Zaza, S., P.A. Briss, and K.W. Harris, editors. *The Guide to Community Preventive Services: What Works to Promote Health?* New York: Oxford University Press (2005).

References

Agency for Healthcare Research and Quality (AHRQ). *The Guide to Clinical Preventive Services* 2006: Recommendations of the U.S. Preventative Services Task Force. Rockville, MD; Agency for Healthcare Research and Quality (2006). AHRQ Publication 06-0588.

Albano, J.D., E. Ward, A. Jemal, et al. Cancer Mortality in the United States by Education Level and Race. *J Natl Cancer Inst* (2007):99(18):1384–1394.

Alberg, A.J., and J.M. Samet. Epidemiology of Lung Cancer. *Chest* (2003):123(1 Suppl):21S–49S.

Alciati, M., J. Marconi, P. Greenwalk, B. Kramer, and D. Weed. The Public Health Potential for Cancer Prevention and Control. In: Greenwald, P., B. Kramer, and D. Weed, editors, *Cancer Prevention and Control.* New York: Marcel Dekker (1995) pp. 435–449.

American Cancer Society. *American Cancer Society Guidelines for the Early Detection of Cancer* (2007). Atlanta, GA: (2007c).

American Cancer Society. *Cancer Facts & Figures 2006.* Atlanta, GA: American Cancer Society (2007a).

American Cancer Society. *Cancer Facts & Figures 2007.* Atlanta, GA: American Cancer Society (2007b).

American Cancer Society. Cancer *Facts & Figures 2008.* Atlanta, GA: American Cancer Society (2008a).

American Cancer Society. *Cancer Statistics 2008: A Presentation from the American Cancer Society* (2008b).

Bailar, J.C., 3rd, and H.L. Gornik. Cancer Undefeated. *N Engl J Med* (1997):336(22):1569–1574.

Bal, D.G., K.W. Kizer, P.G. Felten, H.N. Mozar, and D. Niemeyer. Reducing Tobacco Consumption in California. Development of a Statewide Anti-Tobacco Use Campaign. *JAMA* (1990):264(12):1570–1574.

Ballard-Barbash, R., C. Friedehreich, M. Slattery, and I. Thune. Obesity and Body Composition. In: Schottenfeld, M., and J.F. Fraumeni, Jr., editors, *Cancer Epidemiology and Prevention* (3rd ed.). New York: Oxford University Press (2006) pp. 422–448.

Blattner, W. T-Cell Lymphotrophic Viruses and Cancer Causation. In: deVita, V.T., S. Hellman, and S.A. Rosenberg, editors, *Cancer: Principles and Practice of Oncology.* Philadelphia, PA: Lippincott (1993).

Blot, W.J., J.K. McLaughlin, D.M. Winn, et al. Smoking and Drinking in Relation to Oral and Pharyngeal Cancer. *Cancer Res* (1988):48(11):3282–3287.

Bosch, F.X., and S. de Sanjose. Chap. 1: Human Papillomavirus and Cervical Cancer—Burden and Assessment of Causality. *J Natl Cancer Inst Monogr* (2003):(31):3–13.

Brown, M. L., and K. R. Yabroff. Economic Impact of Cancer in the United States. In: Schottenfeld, M., and J.F. Fraumeni, editors, *Cancer Epidemiology and Prevention* (3rd ed.). New York: Oxford University Press (2006) pp. 202–214.

Brownson, R.C., T.E. Novotny, and M.C. Perry. Cigarette Smoking and Adult Leukemia. A Meta-Analysis. *Arch Intern Med* (1993):153(4):469–475.

Byers, T., J. Mouchawar, J. Marks, et al. The American Cancer Society Challenge Goals. How Far Can Cancer Rates Decline in the U.S. by the Year 2015? *Cancer* (1999):86(4):715–727.

Cancer Control PLANET. Links resources to comprehensive cancer control. National Cancer Institute; Centers for Disease Control and Prevention; American Cancer Society; Substance Abuse and Mental Health Services; Agency for Healthcare Research and Quality. 2005. Available at http://cancercontrolplanet.cancer.gov/index.html. Accessed March 17, 2007.

Cappell, M.S. From Colonic Polyps to Colon Cancer: Pathophysiology, Clinical Presentation, and Diagnosis. *Clin Lab Med* (2005):25(1):135–177.

Centers for Disease Control and Prevention (CDC). *National Program of Cancer Registries.* 2007. Centers for Disease Control and Prevention, National Center for Chronic Disease Prevention and Health Promotion, Division of Cancer Prevention and Control. Available at http://www.cdc.gov/cancer/npcr/npcrpdfs/0607_npcr_fs.pdf. Accessed November 18, 2007a.

Centers for Disease Control and Prevention (CDC). *Best Practices for Comprehensive Tobacco Control Programs—2007.* Atlanta, GA: Centers for Disease Control and Prevention, National Center for Chronic Disease Prevention and Health Promotion, Office on Smoking and Health (2007b).

Centers for Disease Control and Prevention (CDC). *National Tobacco Control Program.* 2007. Centers for Disease Control and Prevention, National Center for Chronic Disease Prevention and Health Promotion, Office on Smoking and Health. Available at http://www.cdc.gov/tobacco/tobacco_control_programs/stateandcommunity/index.htm#about. Accessed November 24, 2007c.

Centers for Disease Control and Prevention (CDC). *Colorectal Cancer Initiatives.* Atlanta, GA: Centers for Disease Control and Prevention, National Center for Chronic Disease Prevention and Health Promotion, Division of Cancer Prevention and Control (2007d).

Colditz, G.A., K.A. Atwood, K. Emmons, et al. Harvard Report on Cancer Prevention. Vol. 4: Harvard Cancer Risk Index. Risk Index Working Group, Harvard Center for Cancer Prevention. *Cancer Causes Control* (2000):11(6):477–488.

Colditz, G.A., H.J. Baer, and R.M. Tamimi. Breast Cancer. In: Schottenfeld, D., and J. F. Fraumeni, Jr., editors, *Cancer Epidemiology and Prevention* (3rd ed.). New York: Oxford University Press (2006) pp. 995–1012.

Colditz, G.A., M. Samplin-Salgado, C.T. Ryan, et al. Harvard Report on Cancer Prevention. Vol. 5: Fulfilling the Potential for Cancer Prevention: Policy Approaches. *Cancer Causes Control* (2002):13(3):199–212.

Collaborative Group on Hormonal Factors in Breast Cancer. Breast Cancer and Breastfeeding: Collaborative Reanalysis of Individual Data from 47 Epidemiological Studies in 30 Countries, Including 50,302 Women with Breast Cancer and 96,973 Women without the Disease. *Lancet* (2002):360(9328):187–195.

Danaei, G., S. Vander Hoorn, A.D. Lopez, C.J. Murray, and M. Ezzati. Causes of Cancer in the World: Comparative Risk Assessment of Nine Behavioural and Environmental Risk Factors. *Lancet* (2005):366(9499):1784–1793.

DeNavas-Walt, C., B. Proctor, and C. Lee. *Income, Poverty, and Health Insurance Coverage in the United States: 2005.* Washington, D.C.: U.S. Census Bureau (2006).

Doll, R., and R. Peto. *The Causes of Cancer. Quantitative Estimates of Avoidable Risks of Cancer in the United States Today.* New York: Oxford University Press. (1981).

Easton, D.F., D.T. Bishop, D. Ford, and G.P. Crockford. Genetic Linkage Analysis in Familial Breast and Ovarian Cancer: Results from 214 Families. The Breast Cancer Linkage Consortium. *Am J Hum Genet* (1993):52(4):678–701.

Ghafoor, A., A. Jemal, V. Cokkinides, et al. Cancer Statistics for African Americans. *CA Cancer J Clin* (2002):52(6):326–341.

Giordano, T.J. Morphologic and Molecular Classification of Human Cancer. In: Schottenfeld, D., and J. F. Fraumeni, Jr., editors, *Cancer Epidemiology and Prevention* (3rd ed.). New York: Oxford University Press (2006) pp. 10–20.

Giovannucci, E., and W. Kana. Cancers of the Colon and Rectum. In: Schottenfeld, D., and J. F. Fraumeni, Jr., editors, *Cancer Epidemiology and Prevention* (3rd ed.). New York: Oxford University Press (2006) pp. 809–829.

Greenwald, P., and E. Sondik. *Cancer Control Objectives for the Nation: 1985–2000.* NIH, Bethesda, MD: U.S. Department of Health and Human Services, National Institutes of Health (1986) NIH Publication 86-2880.

Gruber, S.B., and B.K. Armstrong. Cutaneous Ocular Melanoma. In: Schottenfeld, D., and J. F. Fraumeni, Jr., editor, *Cancer Epidemiology and Prevention* (3rd ed.). New York: Oxford University Press (2006) pp. 1196–1229.

Hartge, P., P.M. Bracci, S.S. Wang, et al. Non-Hodgkin's Lymphoma. In: Schottenfeld, D., and J. F. Fraumeni, Jr., editors, *Cancer Epidemiology and Prevention* (3rd ed.). New York: Oxford University Press (2006):898–918.

Harvard Report on Cancer Prevention. Vol. 1: Causes of Human Cancer. *Cancer Causes Control* (1996):7(Suppl)1:S3–59.

Henson, R.M., S.W. Wyatt, and N.C. Lee. The National Breast and Cervical Cancer Early Detection Program: A Comprehensive Public Health Response to Two Major Health Issues for Women. *J Public Health Manage Pract* (1996):2(2):36–47.

Hiatt, R.A., C. Klabunde, N. Breen, J. Swan, and R. Ballard-Barbash. Cancer Screening Practices from National Health Interview Surveys: Past, Present, and Future. *J Natl Cancer Inst* (2002):94(24):1837–1846.

Hiatt, R., and B. Rimer. Principles and Applications of Cancer Prevention and Control Interventions. In: Schottenfeld, D., and J.F. Fraumeni, Jr., editors, *Cancer Epidemiology and Prevention* (3rd ed.). New York: Oxford University Press (2006) pp. 1283–1291.

Holcomb, K., and C.D. Runowicz. Cervical Cancer Screening. *Surg Oncol Clin N Am* (2005): 14(4):777–797.

Howe, H.L., X. Wu, L.A. Ries, et al. Annual Report to the Nation on the Status of Cancer, 1975–2003, Featuring Cancer among U.S. Hispanic/Latino Populations. *Cancer* (2006):107(8):1711–1742.

Jemal, A., R. Siegel, E. Ward, T. Murray, J. Xu, and M.J. Thun. Cancer Statistics, 2007. *CA Cancer J Clin* (2007):57(1):43–66.

Jemal, A., M.J. Thun, L.A. Ries, et al. Annual Report to the Nation on the Status of Cancer, 1975–2005, Featuring Trends in Lung Cancer, Tobacco Use, and Tobacco Control. *J Natl Cancer Inst* (2008):100(23):1672–1694. [Advance Access published online on November 25, 2008] (DOI:10.1093/jnci/djn389). Available at http://jnci.oxfordjournals.org/cgi/content/full/100/23/1672.

Johns, L.E., and R.S. Houlston. A Systematic Review and Meta-Analysis of Familial Colorectal Cancer Risk. *Am J Gastroenterol* (2001):96(10):2992–3003.

Kingsley, B.S., K.L. Schmeichel, and C.H. Rubin. An Update on Cancer Cluster Activities at the Centers for Disease Control and Prevention. *Environ Health Perspect* (2007):115(1):165–171.

Kohl, H.K. An Analysis of the Successful 1992 Massachusetts Tobacco Tax Initiative. *Tob Control* (1996):5(3):220–225.

Kozak, L.J., C.J. DeFrances, and M. Hall. National Hospital Discharge Survey: 2004 Annual Summary with Detailed Diagnosis and Procedure Data. *Vital and Health Stat* (2006):13(162): 1–209.

Lacey, J.V., G.A. Colditz, and D. Schottenfeld. Exogenous Hormones. In: Schottenfeld, D., and J. Fraumeni Jr., editors, *Cancer Epidemiology and Prevention* (3rd ed.). New York: Oxford University Press (2006) pp. 468–488.

Lawson, H.W., N.C. Lee, S.F. Thames, R. Henson, and D. Miller. Cervical Cancer Screening among Low-Income Women: Results of a National Screening Program, 1991–1995. *Obstet Gynecol* (1998):92(5):745–752.

Lee, I.M., and Y. Oguma. Physical Activity. In: Schottenfeld, D., and J.F. Fraumeni, Jr., editors, *Cancer Epidemiology and Prevention* (3rd ed.). New York: Oxford University Press (2006) pp. 449–467.

Linet, M.S., S.S. Devesa, and G.J. Morgan. The Leukemias. In: Schottenfeld, D., and J.F. Fraumeni, Jr., editors, *Cancer Epidemiology and Prevention* (3rd ed.). New York: Oxford University Press (2006) pp. 841–871.

Longnecker, M.P. Alcoholic Beverage Consumption in Relation to Risk of Breast Cancer: Meta-Analysis and Review. *Cancer Causes Control* (1994):5(1):73–82.

Lubin, J.H., and J.D. Boice, Jr. Estimating Rn-Induced Lung Cancer in the United States. *Health Phys* (1989):57(3):417–427.

Lubin, J.H., J.D. Boice, Jr., C. Edling, et al. Radon and Lung Cancer Risk: A Joint Analysis of 11 Underground Miners Studies. Bethesda, MD: U.S. Department of Health and Human Services, National Institutes of Health (1994). NIH Publication 94-3644.

Manser, R. Screening for Lung Cancer: A Review. *Curr Opin Pulm Med* (2004):10(4):266–271.

Marshall, J.R., and J. Freudenheim. Alcohol. In: Schottenfeld, D., and J.F. Fraumeni, Jr., editors, *Cancer Epidemiology and Prevention* (3rd ed.). New York: Oxford University Press (2006) pp. 243–258.

Mayne, S.T., D.E. Morse, and D.M. Winn. Cancers of the Oral Cavity and Pharynx. In: Schottenfeld, D., and J.F. Fraumeni, Jr., editors, *Cancer Epidemiology and Prevention* (3rd ed.). New York: Oxford University Press (2006) pp. 674–696.

Meissner, H.I., L. Bergner, and K.M. Marconi. Developing Cancer Control Capacity in State and Local Public Health Agencies. *Public Health Rep* (1992):107(1):15–23.

Miller, A. Planning Cancer Control Strategies. *Chronic Dis Can.* Vol 13. (1992):13(1);S1–S40.

Mueller, N.E., and S. Grufferman. Hodgkin's Lymphoma. In: Schottenfeld, D., and J.F. Fraumeni, Jr., editors, *Cancer Epidemiology and Prevention* (3rd ed.). New York: Oxford University Press (2006) pp. 872–897.

Munoz, N., F.X. Bosch, S. de Sanjose, et al. Epidemiologic Classification of Human Papillomavirus Types Associated with Cervical Cancer. *N Engl J Med* (2003):348(6):518–527.

National Cancer Institute (NCI). *ASSIST: Shaping the Future of Tobacco Prevention and Control*. Tobacco Control Monograph No. 16. Bethesda, MD: U.S. Department of Health and Human Services, National Institutes of Health, National Cancer Institute (2005a). NIH Publication 05-5645.

National Cancer Institute (NCI). *Cancer Trends Progress Report—2005 Update*. National Cancer Institute. (2005) Available at http://progressreport.cancer.gov/doc_detail.asp?pid=1&did=2005&chid=25&coid=226&mid=. Accessed November 23, 2007.

National Cancer Institute (NCI). *NCI Challenge Goal 2015. Eliminating the Suffering and Death Due to Cancer*. (2007) Available at http://www.cancer.gov/aboutnci/archive/2015. Accessed November 11, 2007.

National Cancer Institute (NCI). *SEER Cancer Statistics Review, 1975–2004*. Ries, L., D. Melbert, M. Krapcho, et al., editors. Bethesda, MD: National Cancer Institute (2007a).

National Cancer Institute (NCI). *Cervical Cancer Prevention (PDQ)*. National Cancer Institute. (2007b) Available at http://www.cancer.gov/cancertopics/pdq/prevention/cervical/Patient/page2#Section_14. Accessed November 25, 2007.

National Center for Health Statistics (NCHS). *Health, United States, 2006, with Chartbook on Trends in the Health of Americans*. Hyattsville, MD: Centers for Disease Control and Prevention, National Center for Health Statistics (2006).

National Institutes of Health (NIH). *Cervical Cancer Control: Status and Directions*. Bethesda, MD: National Institutes of Health (1991). NIH Publication 91-3223.

Parkin, D.M., F. Bray, J. Ferlay, and P. Pisani. Global Cancer Statistics, 2002. *CA Cancer J Clin* (2005):55(2):74–108.

Petersen, P. *The World Oral Health Report 2003: Continuous Improvement of Oral Health in the 21st Century—The Approach of the WHO Global Oral Health Programme*. Geneva: WHO (2003).

Platz, E.A., and E. Giovannucci. Prostate Cancer. In: Schottenfeld, D., and J.F. Fraumeni, Jr., editors, *Cancer Epidemiology and Prevention* (3rd ed.). New York: Oxford University Press (2006) pp. 1128–1150.

Ries, L., D. Melbert, M. Krapcho, et al., editors, *SEER Cancer Statistics Review, 1975–2004*. Bethesda, MD: National Cancer Institute (2007).

Rothenberg, R., P. Nasca, J. Mikl, et al. Cancer. In: Amler, R., and H. Dull, editors, *Closing the Gap: The Burden of Unnecessary Illness*. New York: Oxford University Press (1987) pp. 30–42.

Saracci, R. The Interactions of Tobacco Smoking and Other Agents in Cancer Etiology. *Epidemiol Rev* (1987):9:175–193.

Saslow, D., C. Boetes, W. Burke, A.C. Rodriguez, and S. Wacholder. American Cancer Society Guidelines for Breast Screening with MRI as an Adjunct to Mammography. *CA Cancer J Clin* (2007):57(2):75–89.

Schiffman, M., P.E. Castle, J. Jeronimo, A.C. Rodriguez, and S. Wacholder. Human Papillomavirus and Cervical Cancer. *Lancet* (2007):370(9590):890–907.

Schiffman, M., and A. Hildesheim. Cervical Cancer. In: Schottenfeld, D., and J.F. Fraumeni, Jr., editors, *Cancer Epidemiology and Prevention* (3rd ed.). New York: Oxford University Press (2006) pp. 1044–1067.

Silverman, D., S. Devesa, L. Moore, and N. Rothman. Bladder Cancer. In: Schottenfeld, D., and J.F. Fraumeni, Jr., editors, *Cancer Epidemiology and Prevention* (3rd ed.). New York: Oxford University Press (2006):1101–1127.

Sirovich, B.E., L.M. Schwartz, and S. Woloshin. Screening Men for Prostate and Colorectal Cancer in the United States: Does Practice Reflect the Evidence? *JAMA* (2003):289(11):1414–1420.

Smith, R.A., V. Cokkinides, and H.J. Eyre. Cancer Screening in the United States, 2007: A Review of Current Guidelines, Practices, and Prospects. *CA Cancer J Clin* (2007):57(2):90–104.

Spitz, M.R., X. Wu, A. Wilkinson, and Q. Wei. Cancer of the Lung. In: Schottenfeld, D., and J.F. Fraumeni, Jr., editors, *Cancer Epidemiology and Prevention* (3rd ed.). New York: Oxford University Press (2006) pp. 638–658.

Surveillance, Epidemiology, and End Results Program. SEER Stat Database: Incidence–SEER 13 Regs Limited-Use, Nov 2006 Sub, 1992–2004. 2007a. National Cancer Institute, Division of Cancer Control and Population Sciences, Surveillance Research Program, Cancer Statistics Branch. Released April 2007, based on the November 2006 submission.

Surveillance, Epidemiology, and End Results Program. SEER Stat Database: Mortality—All COD, Public-Use with State, Total U.S., 1969–2004. 2007b. National Cancer Institute, Division of Cancer Control and Population Sciences, Surveillance Research Program, Cancer Statistics Branch, underlying mortality data provided by the National Center for Health Statistics. Available at www.cdc.gov/nchs. Released April 2007.

Swan, J., N. Breen, R.J. Coates, et al. Progress in Cancer Screening Practices in the United States: Results from the 2000 National Health Interview Survey. *Cancer* (2003):97(6):1528–1540.

Thun, M.J., and S.J. Henley. Tobacco and Cancer. In: Schottenfeld, D., and J.F. Fraumeni, Jr., editors, *Cancer Epidemiology and Prevention* (3rd ed.). New York: Oxford University Press (2006) pp. 217–242.

Thun, M.J., and T. Sinks. Understanding Cancer Clusters. *CA Cancer J Clin* (2004):54(5):273–280.

U.S. Cancer Statistics Working Group. *United States Cancer Statistics: 2003 Incidence and Mortality.* Atlanta, GA: U.S. Department of Health and Human Services, Centers for Disease Control and Prevention and National Cancer Institute (2006).

U.S. Department of Health and Human Services (USDHHS). Cancer Statistics Review. In: U.S. Department of Health and Human Services: NIH Publication; 96-2789.

U.S. Department of Health and Human Services (USDHHS). *Cancer Rates and Risks.* (4th ed.). Washington, D.C.: U.S. Department of Health and Human Services (1996) Publication 96–691.

U.S. Department of Health and Human Services (USDHHS). Division of Cancer Prevention and Control, National Centers for Chronic Disease Prevention and Health Promotion. National Breast and Cervical Cancer Early Detection Program. Atlanta, GA: Centers for Disease Control and Prevention, 2007.

U.S. Department of Health and Human Services (USDHHS). *Healthy People 2010*, Vol. II. Conference edition. Washington, D.C.: U.S. Department of Health and Human Services (2000).

U.S. Department of Health and Human Services (USDHHS). *The Health Consequences of Smoking: A Report of the Surgeon General.* Washington, D.C.: U.S. Department of Health and Human Services, Centers for Disease Control and Prevention (2004).

U.S. Environmental Protection Agency (EPA). *Respiratory Health Effects of Passive Smoking: Lung Cancer and Other Disorders.* Washington D.C.: U.S. Environmental Protection Agency (1992).

World Cancer Research Fund/American Institute for Cancer Research. *Food, Nutrition, Physical Activity, and the Prevention of Cancer: A Global Perspective.* Washington, D.C.: AICR (2007).

World Health Organization (WHO). *International Classification of Diseases for Oncology* (3rd ed.) Geneva: World Health Organization (2000).

World Health Organization (WHO). WHO's International Statistical Classification of Diseases and Related Health Problems, 2nd ed., 10th rev. [ICD-10] Geneva: World Health Organization (2005).

Wright, T.C., Jr. Cervical Cancer Screening in the 21st Century: Is It Time to Retire the PAP Smear? *Clin Obstet Gynecol* (2007):50(2):313–323.

Zaza, S., P.A. Briss, and K.W. Harris, editors. *The Guide to Community Preventive Services: What Works to Promote Health?* New York: Oxford University Press (2005).

Zhang, S.M., W.C. Willett, J. Selhub, et al. Plasma Folate, Vitamin B6, Vitamin B12, Homocysteine, and Risk of Breast Cancer. *J Natl Cancer Inst* (2003):95(5):373–380.

CHAPTER 15

CHRONIC RESPIRATORY DISEASES (ICD-10 E84, G47.3, J40-J47)

Henry A. Anderson, M.D. and Mark Werner, Ph.D.

Introduction

Chronic respiratory diseases include a broad range of conditions marked by variability in the range of symptoms, causative and exacerbating factors, and diagnostic criteria. The "upstream" causes and "downstream" consequences of chronic respiratory diseases are complex, and related to the specific type of disease (Figure 15.1). According to the Centers for Disease Control and Prevention's (CDC) National Center for Health Statistics, chronic lower respiratory diseases were the fourth leading cause of death in the United States in 2004, responsible for 5.1% of U.S. deaths (Miniño et al. 2007). Hospitalization is a frequent adverse outcome of a chronic respiratory disease diagnosis, with the average duration of a hospitalization of 4.6 days for chronic obstructive respiratory disease and 2.9 days for asthma and/or bronchitis in 2005 (HCUP 2007). Population-based national health surveys have found rates of observed and reported obstructive lung disease in the range of 6–9% (Mannino et al. 2000).

Significance

The primary consequence of chronic respiratory diseases that contributes to morbidity is dyspnea, or pathologic breathlessness (Stulberg and Adams 2000). Depending on the severity, dyspnea may result in restrictions ranging from inability to climb stairs to constant breathlessness and difficulty in sleeping. Effects of dyspnea include impaired respiratory tract clearance mechanisms, excessive mucus production, and reduced lung capacity, which likely contribute to more frequent, severe, and prolonged acute viral and bacterial respiratory infections (Mahler and Meija 1999). Dyspnea is also a common clinical feature in chronic nonpulmonary conditions such as heart disease, obesity, and muscular diseases. Cough, chest pain, excessive phlegm or sputum production, wheezing, and coughing of blood (or hemoptysis) are other commonly observed symptoms of respiratory disease (Mason et al. 2000). As is the case for dyspnea, these symptoms can manifest variously in different respiratory and nonrespiratory disorders.

Among the challenges of describing symptoms commonly observed in respiratory disease is that terminology can differ greatly among clinicians describing similar patterns of respiratory impairment. The use of the term chronic obstructive pulmonary disease (COPD) can describe sets of symptoms that are alternately described as chronic bronchitis, emphysema, and/or asthma; as such, assigning a definition based on clinical, physiologic, or pathologic criteria may be problematic (Figure 15.2). Clinicians may also use the

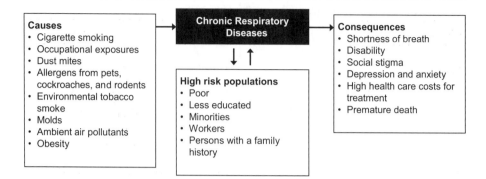

Figure 15.1. Chronic respiratory diseases: causes, consequences, and high-risk groups.

term COPD to describe nonspecific respiratory symptoms in cases where airflow impairment may be either absent or present. The ICD-9 and ICD-10 codes and the definitions used in this chapter are presented in Table 15.1.

Both cystic fibrosis (CF) and sleep apnea are chronic diseases affecting multiple systems with principal effects on the respiratory system. CF is an inherited disease characterized by excessive mucus production resulting in respiratory infections and pancreatic obstruction, and is a major source of severe chronic lung disease in children and an increasingly important cause of morbidity and mortality from chronic lung disease in young adults (Boucher, Knowles, and Yankaskas 2000). Obstructive sleep apnea (OSA) is characterized by sleep-disordered breathing associated with daytime symptoms such as excessive sleepiness and characterized by intermittent upper respiratory tract obstruction

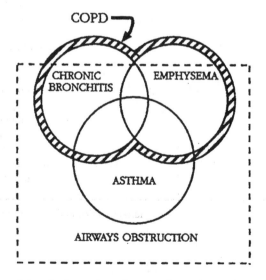

Figure 15.2. Schema of chronic obstructive pulmonary disease (COPD). COPD includes patients with chronic bronchitis and emphysema, and a subset of patients with asthma. Patients with COPD found outside the box for airways obstruction would have clinical or radiographic features of chronic bronchitis or emphysema.

Table 15.1. Definitions of Specific Chronic Respiratory Diseases

Disease	ICD-9	ICD-10	Definition
Asthma	493	J45–J46	Reversible airway obstruction with airway inflammation and increased airways responsiveness to a variety of stimuli
Bronchitis[a]	490–491	J40–J42	Excessive tracheobronchial mucus production associated with narrowing of the bronchial airways and cough
Emphysema[a]	492	J43	Alveolar destruction and associated airspace enlargement
Cystic fibrosis	277.00, 277.01	E84	Genetic disease with exocrine gland dysfunction resulting in pancreatic insufficiency, chronic progressive lung disease, and elevated sweat chloride production
Bronchiectasis	494	J47	Bronchial wall destruction
Pneumoconioses (and other externally induced alveolar diseases)	500–504; 506.4, 507.1, 507.8, 515, 516.3	J60–J67	Dust-, fume-, or mist-induced pneumoconiosis or lung injury (not immunologically mediated)
Sleep apnea	780.51, 780.53, 780.57	G47.3	Repetitive cessation of breathing during sleep

[a] Bronchitis and emphysema are the major conditions falling under the classification of chronic obstructive pulmonary disease.

(Caples, Gami, and Somers 2005). The condition has been estimated to be present in up to 5% of adults in Western countries (Young, Peppard, and Gottlieb 2002).

Pathophysiology

The diagnostic tests and associated criteria for definition differ among various chronic respiratory diseases. Chronic bronchitis is diagnosed by clinical signs and reported symptom history, whereas asthma and other forms of COPD are diagnosed by clinical evaluation and spirometric tests of lung function (GINA 2006; GOLD 2006). Emphysema is defined in histopathologic terms (i.e., study of lung tissue) and is diagnosed with certainty only with lung biopsy or autopsy, although computerized axial tomography (CT) scanning of the chest can be informative. A further complication is that the symptoms of gastroesophageal reflux, a digestive condition, can occasionally be similar to those of various airways diseases, and the two conditions are often confused (Guill 1995). One manifestation of the occupation-related pneumoconioses, or dust-induced lung conditions, is a fibrotic response to deposition of inorganic material. Diagnosis requires an exposure history and x-ray assessment (ILO 2002). In a heterogeneous group of lung disorders, interstitial lung diseases, the chest x-ray, and occasionally CT of the chest can assist in the evaluation and monitoring of disease status and are used in conjunction with other methods of assessing respiratory function, such as spirometry.

Spirometric testing is simple and inexpensive and is a sensitive and noninvasive method of assessing obstructive lung diseases as well as different fibrotic or restrictive lung diseases. Spirometry measures the expired volume as a function of time. Forced vital capacity (FVC) and forced expiratory volume in the first one sec (FEV1) are less variable than many other tests of lung function (Gold, W. 2000). Using the FVC or FEV1, or the ratio of FEV1 to FVC (FEV1/FVC), lung disorders can be categorized into those with airflow obstruction (FEV1/FVC less than 0.75) or restriction (FVC less than 80% of predicted) or into mixed disorders (decreases in both FEV1/FVC and FVC).

In addition to spirometry, other lung function tests can include measurement of total lung capacity, functional residual capacity, carbon monoxide diffusing capacity, and cardiopulmonary exercise testing. Assessment of lung function following bronchoprovocation with methacholine or histamine may indicate airway hyperreactivity and is sometimes performed if asthma is suspected but spirometry is inconclusive.

The chest radiograph is of most help in the clinical evaluation of chronic lung diseases. However, its role in the screening or epidemiologic study of lung diseases is limited by expense, feasibility, and technical considerations. A uniform method of chest radiograph interpretation has been developed by the International Labor Organization (ILO) for use in selected clinical settings (e.g., disability assessment for occupational lung disease) and for research purposes (ILO 2002). The system categorizes opacities and pleural changes on the chest radiograph by their shape, size, location, and density (ILO 2002). Physicians who obtain additional training in ILO interpretation of the chest x-ray and pass an examination are called B readers. Methods similar to the ILO scheme for the chest x-ray have not been developed for standardized interpretation of CT images of the chest.

This chapter not only discusses the two major chronic lung diseases, asthma and COPD, but also includes shorter descriptions of a variety of occupationally induced chronic lung diseases, including coal workers' pneumoconiosis (CWP), silicosis, asbestosis, byssinosis, and occupational asthma; lung diseases associated with exposure to organic dusts; and a diverse group of diseases resulting in fibrosis of the lung (i.e., interstitial lung disease), CF, and OSA.

ASTHMA (ICD-10 J45-J46)

According to results of the 2005 National Health Interview Survey (NHIS), approximately 7.6% of the general population currently has asthma (current prevalence), and 11.2% have received a diagnosis of asthma during their lifetime (lifetime prevalence) (CDC 2007). Although much effort has been made in recent years to develop standardized diagnostic criteria for asthma, estimates of asthma prevalence continue to vary with different data collection approaches, such as self-reported and physician-reported data. International asthma prevalence estimates vary widely, ranging from 2% in Albania to 15% in New Zealand (GINA 2006). In 2004, 3,816 people in the United States died from asthma (Miniño et al. 2007).

Significance

Asthma was responsible for an estimated 16.5 million ambulatory care visits in 2004 (Hing, Cherry, and Woodwell 2006). Appropriate medical management may limit the degree to which asthma affects productivity of children and adults; however, asthma remains a significant cause of missed days of work or school. In 2003, U.S. children missed an estimated 12.8 million days of school because of asthma (Akinbami 2006).

Pathophysiology

Historically, asthma has been classified into two categories: allergic or atopic (extrinsic) and nonallergic or nonatopic (intrinsic) asthma. Atopy is defined as the capacity to produce abnormal amounts of immunoglobulin E (IgE) in response to environmental allergen exposure. Between the two categories, asthma appears to be more commonly classified as allergic in children than in adults (Pearce, Pekkanen, and Beasley 1999). However, many individuals have asthmatic responses that are characteristic of both categories and the basis for this classification has been under question. The introduction of newer information about the role of genetics in asthma and observations of higher IgE levels in patients of all age groups has added weight to the proposal of a unifying hypothesis for both types of asthma (White and Kaliner 1991; Meyers, Larj, and Lange 2004).

Asthma primarily manifests itself in the airways, and patients with asthma show evidence of mucosal edema, epithelial disruption, infiltration with inflammatory cells, and excessive amounts of mucus in airways (Boushey et al. 2000). The development of the changes responsible for airway obstruction and hyperresponsiveness is primarily due to inflammatory responses in the airways of patients. In allergic asthma, IgE–antigen complexes bind to the membranes of various connective tissue cells, causing the release of signaling chemical agents responsible for an asthmatic response. Positive response to skin test batteries for common allergens is more prevalent among extrinsic asthmatics than among intrinsic asthmatics, and more common among asthmatics as a category than among people without asthma (Pearce, Pekkanen, and Beasley 1999).

Symptoms of asthma, such as intermittent wheezing or shortness of breath triggered by specific environmental exposures or exercise, frequently appear in children before the age of five years. About 50% of adults who were diagnosed with asthma as children no longer have the condition, with about half of these becoming totally symptom-free (Barbee and Murphy 1998). Conversely, about one-fourth of childhood asthma cases persist with a similar degree of severity into adulthood, and the remaining one-fourth may experience a temporary cessation in symptoms, with symptoms returning in adulthood (Sears 1991).

Descriptive Epidemiology

High-Risk Populations

Although there are a range of factors that are useful for describing the distribution of asthma and asthma-related adverse health outcomes among populations, the most important determinants of asthma and related morbidity and mortality are race/ethnicity, age, and sex. Racial disparities for asthma are found for a range of endpoints, most notably prevalence, mortality, and hospitalizations. Data from the 2005 NHIS (CDC 2007) found significantly higher values of current asthma prevalence for non-Hispanic African Americans than for non-Hispanic whites (9.9% versus 7.6%) (CDC 2007). When limited to children, the disparity was even more striking (13.0% versus 8.9%) (CDC 2007). Across all race groups, Hispanic ethnicity is not associated with higher asthma prevalence. As a subset of the Hispanic population, however, those of Puerto Rican descent have an asthma prevalence rate of 16.9% for all age groups and 19.9% among children of Puerto Rican descent. Asthma prevalence tends to be higher in children than adults. Data from the 2005 NHIS show higher prevalence among children versus adults for whites (8.9% versus 7.2%), African Americans (13.0 versus 8.4), and among Hispanics (8.6% versus 5.0%) (CDC 2007).

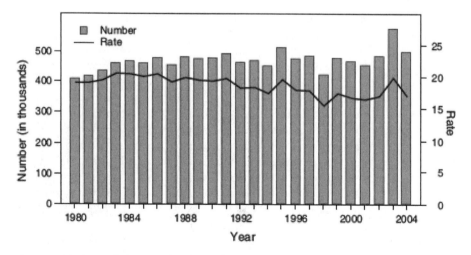

* - per 10,000 population. Age-adjusted to 2000 U.S. population
± - based on asthma as first-listed diagnosis

Figure 15.3. Number and rate* of asthma ± hospital discharges by year—United States, 1980–2004. Source: National Hospital Discharge Survey: National Center for Health Statistics.

For health care utilization, rates of inpatient hospitalization and emergency department use are significantly higher for African Americans than for whites. In 2004, the inpatient hospitalization rate for asthma among African Americans was 34 per 10,000 population compared to 10 per 10,000 for whites (Figure 15.3) (Akinbami 2007). The emergency department visit rate for asthma among African Americans and whites per 10,000 population was 201 and 44, respectively (Akinbami 2007). Differences in health care utilization for asthma by age, sex, and race are depicted in Figure 15.4. In 2003, the asthma mortality rate for non-Hispanic African Americans was three times higher compared to non-Hispanic whites (3.3 versus 1.1 per 1,000,000 population, respectively) (Akinbami 2007).

Among the striking features of the epidemiology of asthma is the observed trend by which prevalence shifts according to sex among age groups. By sex, asthma prevalence is higher in boys than in girls (Akinbami 2006). In 2005, asthma prevalence among boys and girls was 10.0% and 7.8%, respectively (CDC 2007). Among adults, however, this trend is reversed, with 2005 asthma prevalence rates for men and women of 5.1% and 9.2%, respectively (CDC 2007). This trend is borne out in health care utilization rates (inpatient admissions, emergency department visits, and ambulatory care visits) and for mortality rates. No clear explanation for this observation has emerged.

The degree to which the racial disparity in asthma prevalence and adverse health outcomes can be explained by socioeconomic differences is a subject of some controversy. Factors such as access to high-quality health care and housing conditions are likely to account for some of the racial disparities seen with asthma. Some ecologic studies of national databases indicate that controlling for family income can diminish or decrease the racial difference in asthma prevalence (Weitzman et al. 1992).

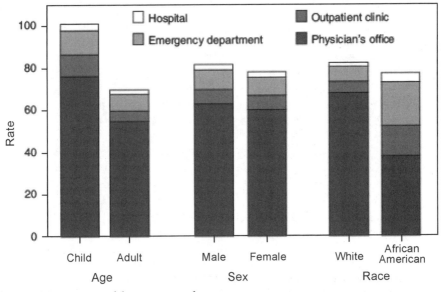

* per 100 persons with current asthma

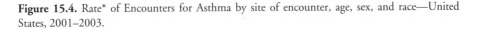

Figure 15.4. Rate* of Encounters for Asthma by site of encounter, age, sex, and race—United States, 2001–2003.

As described earlier, approximately 30% to 50% of the general population can be classified as atopic, and most asthmatics fall into this category (Pearce, Pekkanen, and Beasley 1999). Because of growing knowledge that atopy is strongly influenced by genetics, it follows that some aspects of asthma development may be under genetic control. Indeed, those with a family history of asthma have long been known to be at increased risk for developing the disease (Myers 1993).

Geographic Distribution

Data from the NHIS from 2001 to 2003 suggest that regional differences exist in the United States for asthma prevalence. Based on standard U.S. census regions, asthma prevalence is highest in the Northeast (8.1%), followed by the Midwest (7.5%), West (6.8%), and South (6.7%) (Moorman et al. 2007). Emergency department visit rate estimates from the National Hospital Ambulatory Medical Care Survey for the same period are highest in the Northeast (10.4 per 100 persons with current asthma), followed by the South (9.6), Midwest (8.7), and West (6.7) (Moorman et al. 2007).

Time Trends

Although the range of data sources available for asthma surveillance has changed over time, observed increases in patient encounter measures for asthma have been predicated by increased asthma prevalence in recent decades (Moorman et al. 2007). Based on survey responses regarding whether a family member had asthma in the past 12 months, asthma prevalence increased from 3.1% in 1980 to 5.6% in 1995. This increase occurred among all age, sex, and race subgroups. Although changes in survey questions make comparisons with newer national prevalence data problematic, prevalence rates from 1997 through 2003 appear to have stabilized. Data on asthma mortality suggest that death rates increased from 1980 through 1995 and have declined since 2000 (Moorman et al. 2007).

Seasonal trends have been consistently exhibited for both asthma morbidity and mortality. Asthma hospitalization rates reflect a seasonal variation whereby the highest rates occur in early spring and early fall, and are lowest in the summer (Weiss 1990). Studies on asthma mortality have suggested that asthma mortality in children and young adults may peak in summer, whereas mortality among older adults peaks in winter. Potential explanations for this observed seasonality include plant allergens, acute respiratory infections, cold weather, and air pollution. For school-age children, the onset of school in September has been found to contribute to increased emergency department visits for asthma (Silverman et al. 2005).

Causes

Modifiable Risk Factors

The bulk of the published literature on asthma epidemiology and risk factors has focused on the identification of asthma triggers—specific exposures that often precipitate symptoms in individuals with asthma. Common asthma triggers include dust mites, allergens from pets, cockroaches and rodents, environmental tobacco smoke, molds, ambient air pollutants, cold conditions, and exercise (GINA 2006). There are, by contrast, relatively few conclusive findings about what risk factors contribute to the development of the condition itself, and the factors that cause asthma remain largely unidentified (Taussig et al. 2003). As discussed in the previous section, atopic individuals are more likely to be diagnosed with asthma than others, and atopy is a significant risk factor for developing asthma. One study found that most people with asthma are atopic (Arbes et al. 2007). Children born to mothers with asthma have been found to be more likely to develop asthma than other children (GINA 2006). Although the relationship to atopy suggests that a strong genetic component among the factors related to the etiology of asthma, environmental factors appear to play a role as well. One longitudinal study in children found that although IgE levels in umbilical cord blood were not predictive of subsequent development of asthma, IgE blood levels in blood samples taken at age one year were predictive (Martinez et al. 1995). This finding suggests that exposures within the first year of life may be substantial contributors to the risk of developing asthma in childhood. Although exposures to dogs and cats in the home can be an asthma trigger for some people with asthma, results from studies on the effect of the presence of dogs and cats in the home environment on the development of asthma have been mixed. One longitudinal study found a decreased likelihood for developing wheezing among children without maternal asthma in homes with one or more indoor dogs, but no effect related to cats in the home (Remes et al. 2001). Another study found increased likelihood of cat sensitization and development of severe asthma among children reporting the presence of cats in the home before the age of two years (Melen et al. 2001). Although breast-feeding practices in childhood may also affect the risk of developing asthma in children, the results of studies on this question have also been mixed. In one longitudinal study, atopic children with asthmatic mothers were more likely to have asthma if they were exclusively breast-fed as infants (Wright et al. 2001). In the same study, however, exclusive breast-feeding was associated with reduced likelihood of recurrent wheeze in the first two years of life regardless of atopy status or whether the child's mother had asthma.

Environmental tobacco smoke has clearly been established as a risk factor for asthma exacerbations (Chilmonczyk et al. 1993; Witorsch and Witorsch 2000). There is also increasing evidence that exposure to environmental tobacco smoke may contribute to the development of asthma, both in adults and children (Gold, D. 2000; Jaakkola et al. 2003). For children, the risk associated with environmental tobacco smoke may be confounded by effects of maternal smoking that may have been incurred during pregnancy.

The relationship between asthma and obesity has received increased attention in recent years. Because obesity is associated with a generalized increase in inflammatory response, a causal role in asthma has been postulated (Beuther, Weiss, and Sutherland 2006). Increased incidence of asthma has been observed at higher rates among people with elevated body mass index (BMI) values (Ford et al. 2004). In children, the impact of obesity on incident asthma was shown to be more pronounced among girls than boys (Gold et al. 2003). Because of the possibility that reduced physical activity among people with asthma could contribute to the likelihood of obesity, the relationship between asthma and obesity is likely to be complex in nature.

Ambient air pollutants have been shown to be important asthma triggers (GINA 2006). Associations between asthma and exposure to ozone and particulate matter have been commonly observed, but other pollutants such as nitrogen dioxide and volatile organic compounds, and community traffic density and proximity to heavily traveled roads have also been found to be associated with adverse asthma-related health outcomes (Sarnat and Holguin 2007). The role of air pollution in the development of asthma is less certain. In a study of southern California schoolchildren, residence within 75 m of a major road was found to be associated with increased risk of lifetime asthma, with effects more pronounced in girls than in boys (McConnell et al. 2006). Among school-age children active in sports, incidence of asthma was found to be higher in children living in communities with high ozone concentrations than among other children (McConnell et al. 2002).

Population-Attributable Risk

The development of asthma clearly appears to be related to both genetic and environmental factors. As such, quantifying the relative contribution of genetics and environment is a difficult proposition. Specific genes related to atopy and asthma development have begun to be identified. Although it appears increasingly apparent that some specific environmental factors play a role in asthma development, there is a substantial amount of variability among individuals with asthma as to the triggers causing exacerbations. It is likely that the list of environmental and occupational exposures that may contribute to the development will be highly individual-specific as well.

Prevention and Control

Prevention

Because of the considerable uncertainty about how specific genetic and environmental factors contribute to the development of asthma at both the individual and population levels, there are few clear recommendations to offer by way of preventing the development of asthma. For potentially susceptible populations, such as siblings and children of people with asthma, there may be benefit in extending environmental control measures applied to the individual with asthma (such as limiting exposure to pets, pests, and mold) to other members of the household. For example, dust mites can be effectively controlled by encasing mattresses and pillows in airtight covers, washing bedding every week, and removing carpets. Given the increased evidence regarding environmental tobacco smoke and air pollutants as contributors to developing asthma, public policy efforts to ban smoking in public places and establish appropriate air pollutant restrictions for ozone and particulate matter may have benefit in reducing future asthma incidence and prevalence.

Rather than focus on poorly informed efforts on asthma prevention, public health activity on asthma has focused primarily on means by which individuals with asthma can reduce or eliminate exacerbations that may pose a threat to a patient's health or limit his or her quality of life. This has been effected by promoting regular interaction with appropriate health care providers, providing and disseminating guidance about appropriate use of control medications to patients and health care providers, and by educating patients about the nature of asthma as a chronic disease and how to identify and avoid asthma triggers that may cause exacerbations. Because environmental tobacco smoke is a known asthma trigger, efforts to discourage tobacco use in homes and other indoor environments or focusing smoking cessation efforts on people with asthma and their families may be worthwhile approaches to consider. Because influenza may have a considerable impact on asthma-related morbidity, it is recommended that people with asthma obtain a yearly flu shot. Whether people with asthma constitute a risk category on par with the elderly or other groups for targeting flu shots when resources are scarce remains an open question (Bueving, Thomas, and Wouden 2005). Exposure to ambient airborne particulates and irritants has been associated with asthma exacerbations and increased inpatient hospitalization and emergency department visit rates for asthma. In addition to efforts to decrease ambient concentrations of these pollutants, state and national public health alerts are issued when pollution concentrations exceed standards and could pose a threat to sensitive populations, including people with asthma.

Screening

Because effective management can minimize the frequency and severity of asthma exacerbations, applying a proper diagnosis to individuals who have asthma is an important step in controlling the disease and reducing asthma-related adverse health outcomes. However, mild to moderate cases of asthma may be difficult to diagnose, especially among young children. In such cases, symptoms can often be confused with recurrent respiratory infections or bronchitis, and, as such, may not be recognized as a chronic condition. Because of its impact on school attendance, as a major cause of hospitalization in children, and the preventable nature of asthma-related morbidity, the notion of population-based screening for asthma has received much attention as a potential intervention. Many organizations, including the American Thoracic Society, have refrained from endorsing such screening efforts because of the lack of evidence that such approaches result in measurable improvements in health outcomes (Gerald et al. 2007).

Population-based screening may be most effective in areas where there is likely to be a high prevalence of undiagnosed asthma and where access to high-quality care is likely to be available for newly diagnosed patients.

Treatment

The primary goal of asthma treatment is to control the condition and minimize exacerbations so as to avoid adverse asthma-related health outcomes. Most asthma medications can be described as controller medications or relief medications (GINA 2006). Controller medications are generally taken daily on a long-term basis to achieve control of inflammation. Common types of controller medications include inhaled corticosteroids such as fluticasone, leukotriene modifiers such as montelukast, and long-acting β2-agonists such as salmeterol. Reliever medications act quickly to address bronchoconstriction. These include rapid-acting β2-agonists and systemic glutocorticosteroids. Frequent use of reliever medications (e.g., on a daily basis) may signify that a patient's asthma is not being well controlled and his or her treatment plan should be reevaluated. Some medications in both classes are not recommended as stand-alone therapies, but are generally prescribed only when other controller medications are included in the patient's therapy plan.

Examples of Evidence-Based Interventions

Over the past decade, substantial effort has been made in designing, implementing, and evaluating public health interventions to address asthma. Common objectives for intervention efforts include educating patients about asthma, controlling exposure to triggers in the home and work environments, and enhancing communication across different parts of the health care system about patients with asthma. Sites where interventions have been implemented to address asthma include health care facilities (clinics, hospitals, emergency rooms), pharmacies, homes, schools, and workplaces. The focus of such interventions has ranged from patients and parents to teachers and health care providers, and effective programs have taken approaches such as modifying the home environment during pregnancy to reduce the likelihood of developing asthma in childhood (Custovic et al. 2001), assessing the quality of patients' interaction with pharmacists (Barbanel, Eldridge, and Griffiths 2003), and ensuring that health education messages are culturally appropriate for patients (Brotanek, Grimes, and Flores 2007). Coordinated efforts have been implemented to address asthma in tandem with related issues such as tobacco control and obesity. Guidelines have been established for asthma management and prevention at both the national and international levels, setting the stage for more uniform practices for the evaluation, dissemination, and adaptation of effective public health interventions for asthma (GINA 2006; NHLBI 2007).

Areas of Future Research

Risk factors for the development of childhood asthma have not been fully assessed, and further work to develop appropriate animal models for asthma research is needed (Coleman 1999). A broader description of the genetic determinants of asthma will help enable the identification of high-risk individuals for whom particular interventions to prevent asthma might be recommended. Although effective medications for asthma control exist, there remain concerns about long-term side effects such as growth restrictions in children for which more data are required. Although interventions to reduce exposure to asthma triggers in the home can be effective, the evidence to demonstrate their cost-effectiveness to the managed care community remains tenuous. Further data on the cost savings that may be associated with various approaches to home trigger reduction would be of great benefit.

CHRONIC OBSTRUCTIVE PULMONARY DISEASE (ICD-10 J40-J43)

COPD has been defined as a disease chiefly marked by airway obstruction that is not fully reversible (Rabe et al. 2007). The condition is usually progressive in nature and is associated with an abnormal inflammatory response of the lungs to noxious particles and gases (Shapiro et al. 2000). Conditions such as chronic bronchitis and emphysema that are obstructive in nature are frequently grouped together under the broader heading of COPD. Because there can be a significant overlap of symptoms and manifestations of different forms of COPD, distinctions among the various diagnoses within the broader COPD category can be difficult to make successfully.

Significance

In the 2000 NHIS, self-reported prevalence for chronic bronchitis (in the past 12 months) or emphysema (lifetime) was estimated at 6.0% (Mannino et al. 2002). By comparison, population projections based on spirometry data from physical examinations from the National Health and Nutrition Examination Survey (NHANES) from 1988 to 1994 place the prevalence of mild and moderate obstructive pulmonary disease at 6.9% and 6.6%, respectively (Mannino et al. 2000). This contrast (6.0% versus 13.5%) suggests that prevalence estimates based on self-reported data may constitute significant underestimates of actual COPD prevalence. There were an estimated 8 million physician office and hospital outpatient visits in the United States for COPD in 2000 (Mannino et al. 2002). In 2004, there were 773 deaths from chronic bronchitis and 13,639 deaths from emphysema in the United States (Miniño et al. 2007). For all health endpoints related to COPD, however, imprecise and variable definitions make the quantification of prevalence, morbidity, and mortality difficult.

A 1993 estimate of the economic costs of COPD in the United States was placed at $23.9 billion, including $14.7 billion for direct treatments and $9.2 billion for indirect morbidity and premature mortality and related lost future earnings (Sullivan et al. 2000). More than 70% of medical care costs were incurred by 10% of the affected population.

In addition to being a common primary diagnosis for hospitalization, COPD is the second most common comorbidity for inpatient hospitalizations. It was found to be present as a comorbid condition in 12% of hospital discharge records (Merrill and Elixhauser 2005).

Pathophysiology

Initial pathologic changes of COPD occur in the proximal and peripheral airways, lung parenchyma, and pulmonary vasculature (Hogg 2004). These pathologic changes consist of inflammatory responses and associated increases in goblet cell number and mucous gland size. This inflammation appears to be an amplification of normal inflammatory responses to toxic gases and particulates. This response is most commonly observed as ongoing exposure to tobacco smoke (Rabe et al. 2007).

Emphysema is best characterized by the destruction of the bronchioles, alveolar ducts, and alveoli that constitute gas exchange air spaces. The mechanism for this destruction is inflammatory in nature, most commonly resulting from ongoing exposure to tobacco smoke (Shapiro et al. 2000). The chief physiological result in emphysema is the obstruction of expiratory airflow and reduced gas transfer capacity. It is increasingly recognized that elastases play an important role in the pathophysiology of emphysema. Elastases are enzymes that digest and degrade elastin, an elastic substance that supports the structure of the lungs. It is theorized that exposure to toxic gases and particulates alters the balance between proteinase and antiproteinase activity in the lungs, resulting in the degradation of lung tissue that leads to the symptoms of emphysema (Shapiro et al. 2000).

In adults, the onset of COPD often begins with a moderate decline in lung function capacity before age 50 years. In many cases, COPD would be observable by spirometry, but medical attention may not be sought until symptoms such as dyspnea are observed. Among smokers, a characteristic cough may provide early evidence of the onset of COPD. In the typical case, the decline in lung function accelerates after the age of 50 years (Shapiro et al. 2000). As the disease progresses, the damage to the lung ultimately results in inadequate oxygen delivery. COPD is a common comorbid condition among patients presenting with cardiovascular disease and a range of other systemic conditions.

Descriptive Epidemiology

High-Risk Populations

Although describing the epidemiological burden of COPD is complicated by variable diagnostic criteria and differences between self-reported data and results from physical examinations, certain groups are at greater risk for COPD than others. Smokers and ex-smokers constitute the most distinct high-risk group for COPD, and the prevalence of tobacco smoking is the best predictor of COPD prevalence across the globe (GOLD 2006). The prevalence of COPD also increases with age, especially after the age of 40 years (Halbert et al. 2006). This increase in risk with age is due to both increased cumulative tobacco smoke exposure among smokers and a generally observed decline in lung function with age across populations. Although the U.S. death rate from COPD increased moderately among men from 1980 to 1998 (from 73 per 100,000 to 79 per 100,00), it increased markedly for women over the same period (from 20 per 100,000 to 50 per 100,000) (Mannino et al. 2002). This likely relates to observed increases in tobacco smoking among women in previous decades. Although observed COPD prevalence by sex closely follows expectations based on patterns of tobacco smoking, decline in lung function consistent with COPD appears to be more strongly affected by smoking in women than in men (Connett et al. 2003). Improvements in lung function upon tobacco cessation also appear to be greater among women than among men.

A small number of patients with COPD have a deficiency of the protein α_1-antitrypsin. The genetic variation leading to this deficiency is seen almost exclusively in Caucasians of northern European descent, and is estimated to be present in some degree in about 2–3% of the white population of the United States (Shapiro et al. 2000; Stoller and Aboussouan 2005). This protein acts to inhibit the destructive capabilities of the white blood cell elastase responsible for degradation of lung tissue, and deficiencies of α_1-antitrypsin have been associated with emphysema. Other high-risk groups may be defined based on low birthweight, respiratory infections in childhood, and occupational exposure to dusts (described later in this chapter).

Geographic Distribution

By state, COPD mortality rates have been shown to be higher in the western and Rocky Mountain states than elsewhere in the Unites States. Mortality data from 1997 showed the highest age-adjusted COPD mortality rates in Wyoming (32.2 per 100,000 population), Nevada (31.0), and Montana (29.2), whereas the lowest rates were found in Hawaii (10.9 per 100,000), Utah (15.6), and North Dakota (16.1) (Hoyert, Kochanek, and Murphy 1999). When compared with state-specific smoking-attributable mortality rates, the two sets of rankings were comparable except in western states such as Wyoming and Montana, where smoking-attributable mortality rates are low and overall COPD mortality rates are high (Weinhold 2000). Although theories regarding population migration, ambient air pollutants, and diagnostic differences have been postulated, this discrepancy has yet to be fully explained.

Time Trends

Although trends in overall COPD prevalence are difficult to detect, prevalence in men declined from 1980 to 1998 and increased among women over the same period (Mannino et al. 2002). Death rates increased from 1980 to 1998 across all race and sex groups. By 2000, the number of women dying from COPD in the United States exceeded the number of men dying from COPD—the first year such an observation was made (Mannino et al. 2002).

Causes

Modifiable Risk Factors

The most commonly encountered risk factor for the development of COPD is cigarette smoking. This risk is dose-related, and factors such as age of starting to smoke, total pack-years smoked, and current smoking status are all predictive of COPD mortality (GOLD 2006). As has been increasingly found for other smoking-related health outcomes, exposure to environmental tobacco smoke may also contribute to the risk of developing COPD (Eisner et al. 2005). Although expected declines in lung function with age may be more strongly affected by smoking in women than in men, the positive effect of smoking cessation on lung function is more pronounced in women (Connett et al. 2003).

Occupational exposure to organic and inorganic dusts and fumes may contribute to the development of COPD (Trupin et al. 2003). In an analysis of data from the NHANES, occupations found to be associated with an increased risk of developing COPD included records processing and construction trades workers (Hnizdo et al. 2002). There is growing literature that indoor pollution from the burning of biomass in poorly ventilated dwellings can contribute to the development of COPD, especially in developing countries (Ezzati 2005; Orozco-Levi et al. 2006). Although outdoor air pollution can contribute to COPD exacerbations, its role in the development of COPD remains unclear.

As evidenced by the role of α_1-antitrypsin deficiency in COPD susceptibility, genetics can be a significant risk factor for some portion of the population. In addition, there is some evidence that physician-diagnosed asthma increases one's risk of developing the irreversible airway obstruction seen in COPD (Silva et al. 2004).

Population-Attributable Risk

Cigarette smoking is by far the most commonly encountered risk factor for COPD, and estimates of the fraction of cases attributable to smoking range from 45% to 90% (Marsh et al. 2006). Environmental tobacco smoke in the home and work environments has been estimated to account for 9% and 7% of COPD cases, respectively (Eisner et al. 2005). A broader estimate for the fraction of COPD cases attributable to work based on NHANES data is 19% for cases arising in the general population and 31% for cases among non-smokers (Hnizdo et al. 2002).

Prevention and Control

Prevention

Because of the primacy of tobacco smoking as a risk factor for COPD, prevention of tobacco smoking is the single most important preventive activity to reduce the burden of COPD. Because the effect of tobacco smoking on COPD is dose-related, any reduction in smoking may bring about a reduction in related COPD morbidity. For ex-smokers, the rate of decline in FEV1 can approach the rate of lung function decline in nonsmokers; FEV1 does not appear to improve to the level of lung function seen in nonsmokers.

For individuals exposed to multiple risk factors, the effect of the collective set of risk factors appears to be additive. As such, identifying individuals with multiple risk factors, such as smoking and occupational exposures, may provide an important avenue for COPD prevention.

Screening

Because interventions aimed at reducing harmful exposures can be effective in slowing the progression of COPD, early detection of disease is beneficial for patients.

The primary mode of screening for COPD is to measure airflow obstruction with spirometry or peak airflow measurement. Because there is a large population that may be in the early stages of COPD without being aware of it, increasing awareness of the relationship between symptoms such as chronic cough and excessive sputum production and COPD may increase the fraction of patients who are appropriately diagnosed with COPD. Broad population-based screening should be limited to individuals at high risk for developing COPD, such as cigarette smokers. Screening for genetic markers for α_1-antitrypsin deficiency is available, but may best be limited to individuals for whom a genetic predisposition to the deficiency is suspected (de Serres and Blanco 2006).

Treatment

The most effective treatment for COPD is to avoid exposure to causative and exacerbatory agents, such as cigarette smoke, workplace dusts, and ambient air pollutants. Once COPD has been diagnosed, the objectives of disease management are to relieve symptoms, improve exercise tolerance and health status, and prevent and treat complications and exacerbations (GOLD 2006). A range of medications, such as inhaled bronchodilators and glucocorticosteroids, can help alleviate some of the symptoms of COPD. When the progression of disease results in decreased blood oxygen, supplemental oxygen therapy has been shown to increase survival (Shapiro et al. 2000). Pulmonary rehabilitation efforts such as exercise training and breathing retraining have been shown to decrease dyspnea, increase exercise tolerance, and improve patients' quality of life (Reis et al. 1995). Surgical approaches, such removal of emphysematous lung or lung transplantation, can be effective in increasing survival in selected circumstances. Vaccination for influenza viruses and other vaccine-preventable diseases is recommended for people diagnosed with COPD.

Examples of Evidence-Based Interventions

Effective tobacco control and prevention efforts (as discussed in a previous chapter) represent the most important avenue for interventions achieving a reduction in the burden of COPD. Policies prohibiting tobacco smoking in workplaces such as taverns and restaurants may decrease exposures that can precipitate COPD exacerbations. Governmental agencies such as the Occupational Safety and Health Administration (OSHA) and the Mine Safety and Health Administration (MSHA) have established enforceable occupational exposure limits to reduce harmful workplace exposures that may contribute to COPD development. The Environmental Protection Agency (EPA) and various state and local agencies have adopted emissions limits for ambient air pollutants. Public health and environmental agencies routinely issue alerts when air pollutant levels exceed guidelines to advise individuals with COPD and other high-risk groups to avoid activities that may increase the risk of an exacerbation.

Areas of Future Research

Although the primary risk factors for COPD are well established, differences in regional COPD mortality rates unexplained by tobacco smoking patterns may offer an opportunity to better understand the epidemiology of COPD. Additional studies of the cellular basis of COPD and identification of more sensitive and specific biochemical, genetic, and molecular markers of COPD may lead to better approaches for the diagnosis and control of COPD (Petty and Weinmann 1997). Additional epidemiologic studies assessing the interaction between cigarette smoking and exposures from environmental and occupational sources may aid in assessing the relative efficacy of various avenues for intervention. Longitudinal epidemiology studies may help identify and quantify risk factors that contribute to the development of COPD, either independently or in tandem with established COPD risk factors.

CYSTIC FIBROSIS (ICD-10 E84)

Significance

CF is an inherited disease characterized by excessive mucus production resulting in respiratory infections and pancreatic obstruction, and is a major source of severe chronic lung disease in children and an increasingly important cause of morbidity and mortality from chronic lung disease in young adults (Boucher, Knowles, and Yankaskas 2000). Although CF continues to result in premature death from lung, gastrointestinal, and endocrine diseases, major strides in screening and treatment in recent decades have improved patient outcomes and survival for patients with CF (Figure 15.5) (Strausbaugh and Davis 2007). There are an estimated 30,000 patients in the United States with CF, and current median survival for patients with CF is estimated at 36.5 years (CFF 2006).

Pathophysiology

The primary genetic defect associated with CF affects a transmembrane conductance regulator (CFTR) protein that acts as a chloride channel. This genetic defect has been localized to chromosome seven, and more than 1500 specific mutations have been identified and recorded. Levels of functional CFTR are substantially reduced in patients with CF, affecting ion transport in sweat ducts, airways, pancreatic ducts, and elsewhere. The severity and level of organ involvement in CF is directly related to tissue levels of CFTR. The primary manifestation of CF in the respiratory tract is abnormally thick and copious mucus in the airways that impairs microbial and mucociliary clearance. This often contributes to progressive cycles of respiratory infection and inflammation (Strausbaugh and Davis 2007). Impaired ion transport may result in depletion of periciliary liquid on airway surfaces, resulting in impaired clearance by both cough and ciliary mechanisms

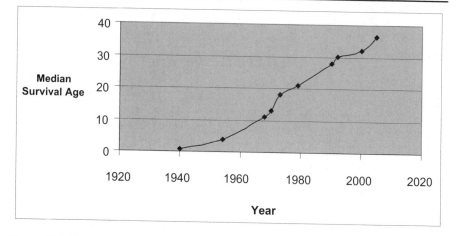

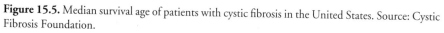

Figure 15.5. Median survival age of patients with cystic fibrosis in the United States. Source: Cystic Fibrosis Foundation.

(Boucher 2004). As more patients survive into adulthood, extrarespiratory effects such as CF-induced diabetes and fibrotic and cirrhotic liver disease are increasingly observed. Lung disease, however, remains the primary cause of morbidity and mortality from CF.

Descriptive Epidemiology

High-Risk Populations

CF is among the most common lethal genetic defects affecting Caucasians in the United States. Incidence varies greatly in the United States based on ethnicity, with incidence at 1:3,200 births for Caucasians, 1:15,000 births for African Americans, and 1:31,000 births for Asian Americans (Orenstein, Rosenstein, and Stern 2000). CF is inherited in an autosomal recessive fashion, and the estimates of the prevalence of the heterozygous form in individuals of Northern European descent ranges from 2% to 4% (Tsui and Buchwald 1991; Schulz et al. 2006). Individuals with the heterozygous form are not affected with CF.

A review of CF mortality records from ten countries found that the median age of death was consistently highest in the United States. Although increases in life span were observed in all ten countries over time, all ten showed a shorter life span for women with CF than for men with CF (Fogarty, Hubbard, and Britton 2000).

Causes

Risk for developing CF is based on genetics. However, there are several classes of specific mutations within the target gene that can lead to the condition, and there are observed differences in disease severity associated with the different classes (Strausbaugh and Davis 2007). Among patients with CF, observed FEV1 has been established as a marker for mortality risk (Kerem et al. 1992).

Prevention and Control

Prevention

Aside from genetic counseling and education for prospective parents, preventing CF is a difficult proposition. One promising avenue for research lies in the field of gene therapy. One approach in this regard would be to place a copy of the gene for normal CFTR in affected cells, resulting in production of normal CFTR. Although clinical trials have shown some early success, many hurdles remain to the use of gene therapy approaches in routine treatment of CF (Griesenbach, Geddes, and Alton 2006).

Screening

There is no family history of CF in more than 80% of individuals diagnosed with CF (Kerem et al. 1992). As such, newborn screening has been undertaken in many states to aid in early detection of CF. By 2003, newborn screening protocols for CF had been established in 13 states (Grosse et al. 2004). The most common method used for screening is measurement of immunoreactive trypsinogen on dried blood spots, with some states using a direct gene analysis approach for a second test in a two-tiered screening program. In 2004, CDC published findings from a workshop on newborn screening for CF, which included a recommendation that newborn screening for CF is justified as a population-based practice (Grosse et al. 2004). Among the reported benefits of early screening is the ability to begin nutritional interventions that may reduce the risk of growth failure and prolonged vitamin deficiency that can be associated with CF (Castellani 2003). Although no recommendation has been made to conduct carrier screening of the general population, screening and genetic counseling and education can be provided to family members or couples with a family history of CF and in women with CF and their spouses (Rosenfeld and Collins 1996).

SLEEP APNEA (ICD-10 G47.3)

Significance

Sleep apnea is defined as cessation of airflow at the nose or mouth during sleep (Bradley and Phillipson 2000). It is one of the leading causes of excessive daytime sleepiness in adults, and contributes to the development of several metabolic and cardiovascular conditions. OSA is most common form of the condition. In OSA, airflow is restricted because of occlusion at the oropharyngeal level, which leads to arousal and obstruction relief. The observed arousal does not always lead to complete awakening, but may interfere with sleep efficiency and contribute to daytime sleepiness.

Pathophysiology

Apnea is defined as a total cessation of airflow; hypopnea occurs when there is a decrease in airflow at the nose and mouth (Caples, Gami, and Somers 2005). A small number of apnea and hypopnea events occur in all people during sleep; the number of apneas and hypopneas considered abnormal depends on the population being tested and indications for testing. The frequency with which airflow reductions occur is termed the apnea–hypopnea index (AHI). The AHI is used as a quantitative characterization of the severity of OSA (Caples Gami, and Somers 2005). An AHI of five or more is indicative of mild OSA, whereas an AHI value of 15 or more indicates OSA of moderate severity.

Depending on the severity of the condition, sleepiness may be observed during passive activities (such as reading) or, in more severe cases, activities such as operating motor vehicles. In one study, individuals with OSA were found to be seven times more likely to have had an automobile accident than individuals without the syndrome (Young et al. 1997). Aside from daytime sleepiness, commonly observed symptoms of sleep apnea include snoring, poor memory, and impaired psychomotor function (Young, Peppard, and Gottlieb 2002).

Descriptive Epidemiology

High-Risk Populations

Estimates of the prevalence of OSA vary depending on the methodology used. Because obtaining an assessment of an individual's AHI requires an overnight visit to an appropriate sleep laboratory, data for measuring the prevalence of OSA can be scarce. Based on studies from three sleep cohorts involving in-laboratory polysomnography, prevalence estimates of 20% for mild OSA in adults and 7% for moderate OSA in adults were obtained (Young, Peppard, and Gottlieb 2002). These estimates were obtained from samples of predominately white men and women with a mean BMI of 25–28.

OSA has been implicated as a contributor to the development of a range of conditions, including hypertension, and cardiovascular and cerebrovascular diseases (Young, Peppard, and Gottlieb 2002). Specific outcomes such as acute myocardial infarction incidence and mortality (He et al. 1988; Hung et al. 1990) and stroke (Mooe et al. 2001) have been observed at increased levels among people with OSA. Injury-related outcomes observed with increased frequency in people with OSA include motor vehicle crashes and occupational injuries (Young, Peppard, and Gottlieb 2002).

Causes

Factors contributing to the development of OSA include excess body weight, smoking, nasal congestion, and habitual snoring (Wetter et al. 1994; Young, Peppard, and Gottlieb 2002). Other factors for which a causative role in the development of OSA is suspected include alcohol use and postmenopausal status.

Prevention and Control

Certain features of OSA, such as its high prevalence and its low recognition as a public health problem, have generated interest in using screening approaches to address the condition. Applying screening approaches to certain occupational populations such as long-distance truck drivers and hazardous duty personnel may be warranted (Baumel, Maislin, and Pack 1997). Concern about public safety led to the issuance of specific screening recommendations for OSA in commercial motor vehicles (Hartenbaum et al. 2006).

Application of continuous positive airway pressure (CPAP) via a nasal mask is the most effective means of therapy for OSA (Caples, Gami, and Somers 2005). In severe cases, surgery to remove soft palate tissue has been undertaken; however, the efficacy of surgical efforts to effectively address OSA remains controversial.

Examples of Evidence-Based Interventions

Addressing known risk factors such as body weight has been shown to reduce AHI in affected patients, and population-based weight reduction interventions may address diagnosed and undiagnosed cases of OSA. Increased awareness of OSA as a focus for attention in primary care settings and referral of individuals with suspected cases of OSA to sleep specialists may help reduce the burden of this condition.

INTERSTITIAL LUNG DISEASE (ICD-10 J80-J84)

Interstitial lung disease is associated with a variety of different agents and disorders (Table 15.2) (Crystal et al. 1981). Some are discussed in other sections of this chapter on occupational lung diseases and lung diseases associated with inhaling organic dust and fumes. Some cases of acute interstitial lung disease, such as those caused by medications, infections, or toxic gas inhalation, can evolve into a chronic form of interstitial lung disease. The lung interstitium that is affected by this disease includes the spaces between the pulmonary capillary cells and the pulmonary alveoli, the connective tissue surrounding blood vessels and bronchi, and the connective tissue of the pleura. Pulmonary fibrosis, alveolitis, and pneumonitis are other general terms sometimes used to describe this class of lung diseases.

During the initial assessment of individuals with interstitial lung disease, it is important to look for connective tissue disease or malignancy, and to consider medication use, symptom duration, and the history of exposure to different organic and inorganic dusts.

Table 15.2. Causes of Interstitial Lung Diseases[a]

Known Causes	Unknown Causes
Inorganic dusts	Idiopathic pulmonary fibrosis
Organic dusts	Collagen-vascular disease
Gases, fumes, vapors, aerosols	Sarcoidosis
Drugs	Histiocytosis X
Poisons	Goodpastures syndrome
Radiation	Wegener's granulomatosis
Infectious agents	Vasculitidies
Chronic pulmonary edema	Lymphocytic infiltrative disorders
Chronic uremia	

[a] Data from Crystal et al. (1981).

Progressive dyspnea is the most common presenting complaint. Pulmonary function testing, although it may show abnormalities with a restrictive defect with decreased functional vital capacity (FVC), is more helpful in following the course of the disease than in the initial diagnostic evaluation. The location and type of opacities on the chest radiograph can be helpful in diagnosing interstitial lung diseases (Coultas et al. 1994). A lung biopsy is sometimes required if the diagnosis remains in doubt or if the disease process is severe.

Descriptive Epidemiology

There are few studies on the epidemiology of interstitial lung diseases not related to specific agents or processes discussed in previous sections of this chapter. The ICD codes in this section are for causes unrelated to common occupational exposures. A major diagnostic challenge has been that individuals are characterized as having idiopathic interstitial fibrosis (essentially no identified cause) because a careful investigation of occult occupational exposures was not done. In a population-based registry in an urban county, the prevalence of interstitial lung disease in adults older than 18 years was 80.9 per 100,000 population in male, and 67.2 per 100,000 population in females (Mannino, Etzel, and Parrish 1996). Occupational and environmental causes were the most frequent in males (20.8 per 100,000) with idiopathic pulmonary fibrosis as the second most likely diagnosis (20.2 per 100,000). In women, pulmonary fibrosis was the most common diagnosis (14.3 per 100,000 individuals) with idiopathic pulmonary fibrosis second (13.2 per 100,000 individuals) (Mannino, Etzel, and Parrish 1996). In the same study, the incidence of pulmonary fibrosis in males was 31.5 per 100,000 per year and in females it was 26.1 per 100,000 per year. The most common incident diagnoses were pulmonary fibrosis and idiopathic pulmonary fibrosis, accounting for 46% of all diagnoses in men and 44% in women (Mannino, Etzel, and Parrish 1996). Sarcoidosis is a disease of unknown cause characterized by granulomas that most frequently affect the lung but can occur anywhere in the body. In the United States, the prevalence of sarcoidosis in whites is five per 100,000; in African Americans, it is approximately 40 per 100,000 (Thomas and Hunninghake 1987).

The age-adjusted mortality rates for idiopathic pulmonary fibrosis in 1991 were 51 per 1,000,000 in men and 27 per 1,000,000 for women (Iwai et al. 1994). Mortality rates were highest in the West and Southeast regions of the United States and lowest in the Midwest and Northeast.

Causes

Risk factors for developing most of the ICD-9 515–517 interstitial lung diseases are poorly understood. In an autopsy study on the risk factors for idiopathic pulmonary fibrosis, laundry workers, barbers, beauticians, painters, production metalworkers, and production woodworkers were at greater risk for developing the disease (Scott, Johnston, and Britton 1990). Other studies on environmental factors and idiopathic pulmonary fibrosis have found increased odds ratios for exposure to wood dust, textile dust, metal dust, and livestock (Hubbard et al. 1996; Mapel, Samet, and Coultas 1996; Baumgartner et al. 1997). Smoking has been found to be a risk factor for idiopathic pulmonary fibrosis in several studies (Scott, Johnston, and Britton 1990; Hubbard et al. 1996; Baumgartner et al. 1997). In a case-control study, a history of having ever smoked increased the risk for idiopathic pulmonary fibrosis by 60% (Hubbard et al. 1996). For the different inhaled agents that are known to cause interstitial lung disease (Table 15.2), it is not known why the disease will develop in some individuals but not in others with similar exposures.

Recently, occupational exposure to artificial food flavorings such as butter flavoring (diacetyl) applied to many different food products such as microwave popcorn has been associated with another rare lung condition (broncholitis obliterans) (Materna et al. 2007). Fortunately, such life-threatening illness is currently rare; however, the evolution of synthetic chemical use to include new settings requires vigilance, and the need to establish surveillance for illness associated with emerging industries and product use remains urgent.

Prevention and Control

For interstitial diseases that develop from inhaling organic or inorganic dusts or fumes, limiting or avoiding the exposure will minimize or prevent the disease. Many of the drug-induced and radiation-induced causes of interstitial disease are used in treating other, possibly life-threatening, diseases the patient may have and are, therefore, difficult to avoid. A trial of corticosteroids is often given in the initial management of the interstitial lung diseases of unknown etiology (Table 15.2), but the effectiveness of this treatment is not known (Mapel, Samet, and Coultas 1996). For many of the interstitial diseases, treatment is primarily supportive, treating the complications of respiratory and right heart failure. Preventive care should include flu and pneumococcal vaccines. Public health surveillance and clinician reporting of unusual diseases associated with occupational exposures is critical to early identification of emerging problems when intervention has the greatest potential for interrupting the emergence of disease.

OCCUPATIONAL LUNG DISEASES

This section covers coal workers' pneumoconiosis, silicosis, asbestosis, byssinosis, occupational asthma, and organic dust-related lung disease.

Significance

It is estimated that in 1999, 14 occupational illnesses generated $14.5 billion of health expenditures, including $2.2 billion attributed to COPD and $1.5 billion to asthma (Leigh, Yasmeen, and Miller 2003). One of the most common occupational lung diseases, occupational chronic bronchitis (see COPD above), along with the symptom of cough, is the least specific response to occupational exposures and is often the first indication of work-related pulmonary pathology. Given a sufficient dose and duration of exposure, nearly all respirable agents can contribute to the development or aggravation of chronic lung diseases. It is not uncommon to have multiple occupational lung diseases present in the same workforce or even the same person. This is especially true for occupational bronchitis and occupational asthma.

Many chronic occupational lung diseases are defined by the agent associated with the specific disease and often named after the agent (i.e., silica inhalation causes silicosis, asbestos fiber inhalation causes asbestosis). Several distinct pathological processes have been associated with exposure to specific respirable dusts present in the occupational environment. Only a few of these diseases result from acute exposures. Most, especially pneumoconiosis, result from multiple years of exposure and are associated with an important hallmark of the disease process known as the "disease latency period." This means disease does not appear immediately and typically at least 10 and commonly 20 or more years pass between first exposure and the recognition of clinical disease. Some of these diseases may first appear and even progress many years after exposure has ended.

Occupational dusts are classified as either inorganic (e.g., coal dust, silica, asbestos) or organic (e.g., cotton dust, grain dust, mold spores). The respiratory conditions associated with most inorganic dusts are called pneumoconioses and result from the direct effect of the dust on lung tissue. Chest x-ray is the primary diagnostic tool used to identify these diseases. Guidelines on how to classify chest radiographs for persons with pneumoconioses have been published by the World Health Organization International Labor Organization since 1950. These guidelines describe and codify the radiographic abnormalities of the pneumoconioses in a simple, reproducible manner using two sets of standard comparison films. The guidelines were issued in 1971 and 1980 and revised in 2000, and published in 2002 (ILO 2002). From 1968 to 1999, a total of 121,982 deaths from pneumoconiosis were recorded among U.S. residents (NIOSH 2004). The U.S. OSHA has established national permissible exposure limits for all inorganic dusts associated with disease.

Diseases resulting from exposure to most organic dusts are immunologically mediated. One exception to this latter classification is the condition related to cotton dust exposure; cotton dust is organic, but the condition is probably not immunologically mediated and is related to endotoxins present in the cotton dust.

Cigarette smoking increases the risk of lung disease in occupationally exposed workers. In most cases, the disease risks are additive—that is, the total disease risk is the sum of the risk from cigarette smoking and the risk from the occupational exposure. An exception to this is the multiplicative risk between asbestos exposure and cigarette smoking in the occurrence of lung cancer (discussed in Chapter 2).

The following sections briefly describe some important occupation-related chronic lung diseases.

COAL WORKERS' PNEUMOCONIOSIS (ICD-10 J60-J67)

CWP, first described in 1831 in a British coal miner, is known as black lung disease and is identified by a pattern of x-ray abnormalities and an exposure history. Through greater mechanization, coal production has increased while the workforce has declined. However, greater mechanization has led to dustier conditions. There are approximately 200,000 coal miners in the United States.

Between 1968 and 1999, 66,407 U.S. deaths occurred with CWP noted on the death certificates. Deaths have significantly declined from a high of 2,870 in 1972 to 1,003 in 1999. For the decade 1990–1999, more than three-fourths of all CWP decedents were residents of Pennsylvania, West Virginia, Virginia, and Kentucky. Pennsylvania alone accounted for about half of all CWP deaths in this period (NIOSH 2003). Mining machine operators had the highest proportionate mortality ratio (PMR) among occupations (NIOSH 2004). Although CWP has declined in the United States, the threat of CWP has significantly increased in developing countries seeking inexpensive sources of energy and where dust control measures are often rudimentary and regulatory frameworks ineffective. Since the enactment of the U.S. Black Lung compensation program in 1969, through 2004, approximately $41 billion has been paid for CWP benefits (GAO 2005).

Descriptive Epidemiology

The prevalence of CWP increases with increasing exposure to coal dust. In studies of CWP, years of mining are often used as a surrogate for dust exposure because information on dust exposure for individual miners is rarely complete.

CWP is classified as simple CWP if rounded opacities less than one cm are seen on the chest radiograph (ILO opacities "p," "q," or "r"; ILO 2002). It is typical for the opacities to first appear in the upper lung fields of the chest x-ray and then to progress to involve all lung fields. NIOSH maintains the National Study of Coal Workers' Pneumoconiosis (NSCWP). Data from that ongoing surveillance program shows that among U.S. underground coal miners with 25 or more years of mining surveyed between 1973 and 1978, 34% had simple CWP. The prevalence of simple CWP declined to 4% during survey years 1996–1999 (NIOSH 2004). It is uncommon in simple CWP for the radiographic abnormalities to progress after the individual has left the dusty environment. Complicated CWP often described as massive progressive fibrosis is often preceded by recurrent infection, especially tuberculosis. Radiographically, it is defined as small opacities and the presence of large opacities (greater than one cm) on the chest x-ray. Data from the national study suggest that the incidence of both simple and complicated CWP is declining, largely because dust standards in mines are being enforced (Figure 15.6) (Attfield and Castellan 1992; NIOSH 2003).

Chronic exposure to coal dust can lead to the development of chronic obstructive lung disease, even in the absence of radiographic changes (Oxman et al. 1993). Coal miners with chronic obstructive lung disease have increased rates of dyspnea, cough, and phlegm production. The magnitude of the deficit in lung function due to chronic coal dust exposure is between 150 and 450 mL over an average lifetime of work in a coal mine, with a smaller percentage of individuals having deficits of greater than one L (Lewis et al. 1996).

Causes

CWP is related to the total dust burden in the lungs. The type of coal (known as coal rank that is determined by the carbon content of the coal) is also important; the higher the rank, the greater the disease risk and dust biologic activity. Anthracite coal has the highest rank, followed by bituminous, subbituminous, and lignite. CWP is caused by respirable coal mine dust, (generally defined as dust particles less than five μm in aerodynamic diameter). Usually, 10 or more years of exposure to coal dust must have elapsed before CWP can be diagnosed by a chest x-ray. Coal dust also may contain other harmful mineral dusts, such as silica dust, which increase the risk of other chronic lung diseases such as silicosis. The radiographic appearance of silicosis can be indistinguishable from CWP. The risk of CWP diagnosed by x-ray increases with the higher rank of coal, in part

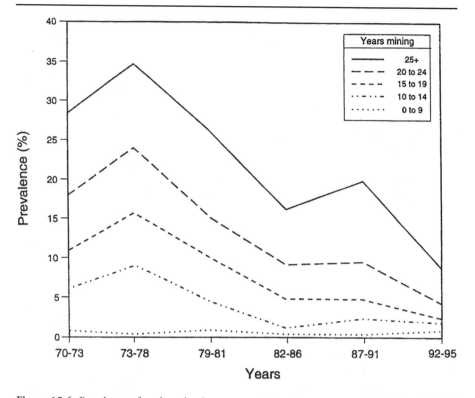

Figure 15.6. Prevalence of coal workers' pneumoconiosis, category one or higher, in the Coal Workers' X-ray Surveillance Program from 1970 to 1995, by tenure in coal mining.

explaining the higher occurrence in miners from the eastern coal-producing regions of the United States compared to western areas. Miners who work underground, where dust control is problematic, are at higher risk than aboveground/surface miners.

Risk factors for the development of chronic obstructive lung disease in coal miners are the duration and extent of dust exposure, prior dust exposure, and the presence of other risk factors for obstructive lung disease, especially cigarette smoking. The average lifetime coal dust exposure among coal miners with symptoms of chronic lung disease was found to result in a loss in lung function equivalent to that associated with smoking 20 cigarettes per day over a lifetime (Lewis et al. 1996). Coal miners working in jobs with higher silica exposure, such as surface coal mine drillers, are at higher risk for the development of chronic obstructive lung disease.

Prevention and Control

CWP can best be prevented by: reducing coal dust exposure in mines and the workplace; comprehensive industrial hygiene monitoring to measure dust suppression; educating workers about disease risk and safe work practices; and when excessive exposure circumstances are unavoidable, providing respiratory protection. Medical monitoring of coal miners is required, and periodic chest radiographs are intended to identify individuals who have CWP in its preliminary phases, thus enabling them to avoid further exposure and possibly preventing the disease's progression to more advanced stages. The use of the ILO pneumoconiosis grading system is critically important to allow quantification of changes over time and assessment of progression.

The Federal Coal Mine Health and Safety Act passed in 1969 and its amendments sets limits on the amount of respirable coal dust levels in the United States. For coal dust with less than 5% silica, the standard is two mg/m³. Although there is evidence that the current dust standards contributed to the decrease in the occurrence of CWP, the MSHA monitoring data from the 1980s through 1999 show little change in the level of coal dust exposure. More than 8% of the 794,000 samples exceeded the PEL and 26% exceed the National Institute for Occupational Safety and Health (NIOSH)–recommended respiratory dust standard of one mg/m³, which was recommend due to concerns that the current standard did not protect against other lung conditions (NIOSH 2003).

SILICOSIS (ICD-10 J62)

Silicons comprise almost 28% of the earth's crust. It is the crystalline forms that are most toxic. It exists as five polymorphs, the most common being quartz. Silica has many industrial applications. Occupational exposures occur worldwide and although the disease is decreasing in the developed countries it is increasing in developing countries. In the United States, excessive exposures continue and are most frequently found in small operations that are seldom visited by regulatory agencies. Chronic inhalation of respirable particles of crystalline silica is the cause of silicosis. Like CWP, silicosis is characterized by a predominance of small, rounded x-ray abnormalities in the upper lung fields indicative of fibrosis. The histopathologic hallmark is the formation of silicotic nodules containing birefringent particles. Also like CWP, silicosis can be divided into simple silicosis and complicated silicosis, or progressive massive fibrosis, based on the size of the opacities on the chest x-ray.

Unlike CWP, silicosis is also characterized as acute, accelerated, or chronic. Fortunately, acute silicosis is uncommon today and occurs after high levels of exposure as can occur in silica flour mills or in the now-outlawed use of silica for sandblasting. It is defined as silicosis that appears in less than five years from first exposure. The acute form is often life-threatening and characterized by pulmonary edema, accumulation of proteinaceous fluid within alveoli and interstitial inflammation. The most common form of the disease is chronic silicosis, which is defined as silicosis that appears 10 or more years after first exposure. In its initial phases, the disease is not associated with declines in lung function, although cough and phlegm production are common. Chronic exposure to silica dust can also result in chronic obstructive lung disease, even without the x-ray manifestations of silicosis (Cowie and Mabena 1991). The disease may slowly progress over 20 to 40 years to the point of respiratory failure. Individuals with silicosis are at increased risk of developing tuberculosis (Snider 1978). Based on analyses of nine studies showing increased rates of lung cancer, silica is now categorized as a probable human carcinogen by the International Agency for Cancer Research (Smith, Lopipero, and Barroga 1995; IARC 1997). Although deaths in the United States attributed to silicosis have decreased from more than 1,000 per year before 1971 to less than 200 in the late 1990s (NIOSH 2004), an estimated 2,000 cases of silicosis are diagnosed each year in the United States (Weeks, Levy, and Wagner 1991).

Descriptive Epidemiology

Hazardous exposure to respirable silica occurs in many different occupational settings including surface and underground mining of ores containing silica, surface drilling, ceramics manufacturing, stone cutting, construction, silica flour mills, foundries, cement production, abrasive manufacturing and use, and sandblasting. OSHA estimated that in 2003, two million workers were exposed to silica. As with CWP deaths, silicosis listed as a cause of death on a death certificate has declined from more than 1,000 annual deaths in the 1960s to less than 200 per year in the 1990s (NIOSH 2003). Pennsylvania alone accounted for nearly 18% of all reported silicosis deaths from 1990 to 1999. Construction and mining industries accounted for more than one-third of deaths with silicosis during that same period. Short-stay, nonfederal hospital-reported discharges listing silicosis decreased from approximately 6,000 per year in 1970 to 1,000 in 2000 (NIOSH 2003).

The prevalence of nonfatal silicosis in the United States is unknown. There are no national registries for the disease, and only a few states have surveillance requirements. By extrapolating from national mortality data, the Michigan state-based surveillance system and capture–recapture methodology estimated that from 1987 through 1996, 3,600–7,300 cases of silicosis occurred annually (Rosenman, Reilly, and Henneberger 2003). The U.S. Department of Labor estimated in 1980 that 59,000 of the workers who were then exposed to silica would eventually develop silicosis (Bates et al. 1992).

Silicosis is most prevalent among workers involved in the dry drilling or grinding of rock with high silica content and other activities that generate large quantities of respirable particles. Largely reflecting the exposed workforce, silicosis is nine times more common in men than in women and more common among African Americans than white males. The most common industrial environments where silicosis occurs among men are mines, foundries, quarries, and silica flour mills (NIOSH 2003). Among women, silicosis occurs most commonly in the ceramics industry.

Causes

Silicosis is caused by chronic inhalation of crystalline silica, which is present in quartz. A more toxic form of silica may be produced when quartz is heated or with freshly fractured quartz particles (Vallyathan et al. 1995). Foundry workers who are in occupations involving both heating and grinding quartz may be at greater risk of silicosis.

Prevention and Control

The most effective method for preventing silicosis is primary prevention—eliminating exposure to respirable silica—and, in settings where silica dust occurs, verifying exposure reduction and maintenance through an industrial hygiene monitoring program. A secondary line of defense is worker education and training, use of protective equipment and regulatory inspections and enforcement of existing work site standards. OSHA regulatory exposure limits for silica concentrations in the work environment were 0.1 mg/m³ from 1989 to 1993. In 1993, this limit was modified (and effectively raised) based on a formula with a default limit of five mg/m³ that is reduced as the silica content in a dust sample increases. NIOSH and ACGIH have recommended an exposure limit of 0.05 mg/m³. As with medical screening for conditions associated with other inorganic dusts, x-ray screening may identify individuals who have minimal disease, enabling these people to avoid additional exposure and possibly preventing progression to more advanced phases.

ASBESTOSIS (ICD-10 J61)

There are four main types of commercially used asbestos fiber, chrysotile (serpentine mineral), and the amphibole minerals amosite, crocidolite, and anthophyllite. Another fibrous amphibole, tremolite, is a frequent contaminant of chrysotile ores as well as ver- miculite. An estimated 27,500,000 workers were exposed to asbestos between 1940 and 1979 (American Thoracic Society 2004a). Asbestos was widely used in construction ma- terials, especially those used for insulation and acoustical products in many public, resi- dential, and commercial buildings. Most uses of asbestos have been eliminated and many countries, but not the United States, have banned all use of asbestos (Ramazzini position reference). Although its use in Europe, United States, and many other countries has sig- nificantly decreased, the production of asbestos has been growing. Raw fiber continues to be used in less-developed countries (LaDou 2004). Current concerns in the United States focus on the potential for exposure to widely distributed, in-place asbestos containing materials. The risk of adverse health effects from these sources of asbestos to workers or to building occupants depends on many factors, most specifically the status of the mate- rial—whether it is releasing asbestos fibers into the indoor environment, whether it is fre- quently disturbed, and how well contained fiber releases are from maintenance activities.

Adverse health effects from exposure to asbestos include pleural effusions, pleural thickening, and plaques with and without calcification, malignant mesothelioma, lung cancer, and asbestosis. Of these, asbestosis is the most prevalent chronic lung condition. Some researchers have suggested that asbestos exposure resulting in benign pleural disease can be associated with obstructive lung disease (Kilburn and Warshaw 1994), although these findings have been the subject of debate (Jones, Glindmeyer, and Weill 1995). Ap- proximately 10,000 asbestos-related deaths (from cancer or other diseases) occur in the United States each year (Bates et al. 1992).

In its early stages, asbestosis is often clinically characterized by dry rales, or whistling or crackling noises, at the end of each inspiration. Often, clinical signs and pulmonary function abnormalities appear before chest x-ray abnormalities become apparent. Eventually, diffuse fibrosis can result in decreased lung capacity, decreased gas exchange, and severe shortness of breath. The x-ray abnormalities evident in people with asbestosis are predominantly small, irregular opacities in the lower lung fields (ILO "s," "t," and "u"). In addition, pleural thickening or pleural plaques, often with calcification, can occur alone or in combination with asbestosis. Unlike CWP or silicosis, asbestosis deaths are continuing to increase, from less than 100 in 1968 to more than 1,250 annually in 1999 (NIOSH 2003).

Descriptive Epidemiology

In various surveys, between 6% and 40% of asbestos textile or insulation workers have detectable x-ray lung abnormalities. Results from the NHANES indicate that 2.3% of U.S. men and 0.2% of U.S. women have pleural thickening upon chest x-ray (Rogan et al. 1987). In a study of 17,800 insulation workers in the United States, asbestosis was identified as the cause of death in 7% of the workers who died (Selikoff, Hammond, and Seidman 1979). Asbestos had thousands of uses, each of which presented the possibility of exposure. Occupations and workers at risk span the life cycle of asbestos from removal from the ground to product manufacturing to installation of products to maintenance and removal, and finally disposal. Although most uses of asbestos in newly manufactured products in the United States have been eliminated, today's exposure threats come from the long life of asbestos-containing products still present in building materials, which may pose a risk to workers during maintenance, repair, renovation, and demolition. A long latency period usually exists between exposure and the development of asbestosis resulting in current cases seen today being a result of the legacy of exposures in the 1940s–1970s (Selikoff and Lee 1978).

Causes

Asbestosis is caused by exposure to airborne asbestos fibers. The magnitude of the risk of asbestosis depends on both the duration and the intensity of the exposure to asbestos dust. The more intense and prolonged the exposure, the greater the risk of developing the disease. Brief, but very heavy exposure can also cause the disease.

Asbestos is unique among the pneumoconiosis-causing agents. Nonoccupational exposure to family members of workers bringing dust home on their clothes and residence near mines and manufacturing facilities using asbestos have been associated with the occurrence of asbestos-associated disease (Anderson et al. 1976; NIOSH 1995).

Prevention and Control

Asbestosis can be prevented by eliminating exposure to asbestos. New asbestos-containing products have been largely eliminated from the work environment, but its release from existing materials must be controlled. Containment of asbestos in buildings may be initially less expensive than removal; however, containment is only a temporary solution, because product aging and deterioration will continue and ongoing maintenance and repair can result in a further release of asbestos and eventual enforced removal under U.S. EPA regulations. National legislation requires accreditation of contractors who work with asbestos and training for asbestos abatement workers to assure safety as well as prevent "bystander" exposure. Safe work practices include identifying materials that contain asbestos; implementing rigorous operating procedures, such as wetting asbestos-containing materials; and wearing a self-contained breathing apparatus.

X-ray and pulmonary function screening may also help in protecting workers. Results from these examinations can encourage the workers to avoid additional exposure, make them more aware of the need for strict work practices, and encourage them to participate in special health surveillance programs.

BYSSINOSIS (ICD-10 J66.0)

Byssinosis is both an acute and chronic airways disease caused by exposure to cotton dust. The acute phase of byssinosis is sometimes called "Monday morning syndrome," in which chest tightness and/or shortness of breath occurs when workers return to cotton dust exposure following a weekend or days off. Symptoms usually resolve the second day. Progression of the disease is characterized by chronic cough and a decline in lung function. After more than 10 years of exposure, overall pulmonary function is often seen to decline. Byssinosis is similar in pathology to chronic bronchitis. A grading system has been developed for byssinosis (Bouhuys et al. 1977). In the United States, approximately 500,000 workers are potentially at risk for byssinosis (Glindmeyer et al. 1991), although the disease is rarely fatal, claiming fewer than 10 lives in 1999 (NIOSH 2003).

Descriptive Epidemiology

The prevalence of byssinosis varies from a few percent to as high as 47% in some surveys (Zuskin et al. 1991). In 1970, it was estimated that approximately 35,000 workers in the cotton textile mills had byssinosis (Glindmeyer et al. 1991). Since regulation of cotton dust began in 1978, the degree of lung function impairment in cotton textile workers may have decreased (Glindmeyer et al. 1991). There is no evidence of sex or race differences in risk of developing byssinosis.

Causes

Byssinosis results from exposure to the dust of cotton, flax, or hemp. Much has been learned about the causal agent of byssinosis but the precise etiology is still being investigated. Evidence supports that it is not the cotton itself that is the causal agent but a bacterial endotoxin present in cotton dust (Rylander 2002). Among cotton workers, the risk is highest among workers involved in the initial stages of processing: opening, picking, carding, stripping, and grinding raw cotton.

Prevention and Control

The best way to prevent byssinosis is to avoid exposure to cotton dust. Cotton dust concentrations in the workplace must be kept below the U.S. OSHA's permissible exposure level. Another technique known as "cotton washing" is effective but may not be feasible on a large scale. Employers must treat the acute phase of byssinosis as a sentinel health event, using it as an opportunity to reduce exposure among other workers with early symptoms.

OCCUPATIONAL ASTHMA

Although the incidence of occupational respiratory diseases already discussed in this chapter is decreasing, occupational asthma is increasing and is rapidly becoming the most common occupational lung disorder in the developed countries (American Thoracic Society 2004b). Work-related asthma includes occupational asthma and asthma aggravated by work or the work environment, and is characterized by episodes of bronchoconstriction, airway inflammation, and airway hyperresponsiveness to agents or conditions present in the work environment. Primary occupational asthma is distinguished from exacerbations of existing asthma by the presence of a workplace sensitizing agent or acute exposure event and diagnosis by a specific case definition (Beach et al. 2007). The over-all prevalence of occupational asthma varies from region to region with estimates for the United States ranging between 10% and 23% of all adults with asthma (American Thoracic Society 2004b). In the United States, it was estimated that 15% of all asthma cases in the 1978 Social Security Disability Survey were occupationally related (Smith et al. 1989). Fifty percent to 90% of individuals with occupational asthma will continue to have symptoms even after being removed from the source of the exposure (Blanc 1987).

In diagnosing occupational asthma, it is important to establish the presence of airflow obstruction (Alberts and Brooks 1992). If the preliminary spirometry is normal, a repeat test, following inhalation challenge with methacholine or histamine, may be indicated. It may be difficult to establish that asthma is caused by an occupational exposure. The fact that initial symptoms may occur only at home or after work can be misleading (Blanc 1987). To document a change in airflow obstruction related to work, it may be helpful to measure the peak expiratory flow rate several times a day for two to three weeks. Skin testing with the suspected compound may also be of diagnostic value in selected cases. Specific inhalation challenge with the suspected compound is not routinely performed because it is expensive, time-consuming, not widely available, and carries the risk of a potentially serious reaction (Alberts and Brooks 1992; Chan-Yeung and Malo 1993).

Reactive airways dysfunction syndrome occurs hours after a single exposure to high levels of irritant gases and results in cough, wheezing, and shortness of breath (Alberts and Brooks 1992). Reactive airways dysfunction syndrome is not usually considered a form of occupational asthma because there is no latency period between the exposure and the de-velopment of symptoms. In occupational asthma, symptoms usually do not appear until a few weeks to as long as several years after the first exposure (Alberts and Brooks 1992). Byssinosis is another condition that may be confused with occupational asthma.

Descriptive Epidemiology

More than 250 causative agents have been associated with occupational asthma (American Thoracic Society 2004b), including a variety of materials of plant and animal origin, chem-icals, metals, biological enzymes, and drugs (Table 15.3). Several mechanisms have been identified that are associated with the development of work-related asthma; they include the following: sensitization; reactive airways dysfunction syndrome (associated with a single, high exposure to irritant agents with onset of symptoms within hours); nonimmunologic airway irritation of preexisting asthma; and poor indoor environments with biologic contaminants (American Thoracic Society 2004b). Agents are classified as high molecular weight com-pounds (less than 1,000 Da) or low molecular weight compounds (Chan-Yeung and Malo 1999). The high molecular weight compounds are proteins, polysaccharides, and peptides, which induce an allergic response by stimulating the production of specific IgE and some-times immunoglobulin G antibodies. Depending on the level of exposure, the prevalence of asthma from these compounds can be high. Asthma has been reported in 3% to 30% of animal handlers; 10% to 45% of workers exposed to biologic enzymes that are used, for ex-ample, in laundry detergents and other cleaning agents; 20% of bakers; and in 70% of flight crews dispersing sterile irradiated screwworm flies (Blanc 1987). Examples of the low molecu-lar weight compounds are isocyanates, wood dusts, metals, and drugs (Chan-Yeung 1990). An allergic response involving IgE occurs less frequently in the development of asthma from the low molecular weight compounds than from the high molecular weight compounds.

Table 15.3. Occupations at Risk for Occupational Asthma and the Probable Casual Agent[a]

Occupation	Causal Agent
Animal handlers, veterinarians, laboratory workers	Urine protein, dander
Bakers, millers	Wheat, rye, buckwheat, mites, hemicellulase, glucoamylase, papin, soybean
Chemical workers	Sulfonechloramides, azo dyes, ethylenediamine, anthraquinone
Coffee or tea workers	Green coffee, tea dust
Detergent workers	Proteases (*Bacillus subtilis*, esperases)
Electronics workers	Colophony, aminoethyl ethanolamine
Farmworkers	Animal antigens, vegetable dusts
Fishery and oyster workers	Crab, prawns, hoya, sea squirts
Grain handlers	Grain dust, insect debris dust
Insect handlers	Bee moth, cockroach, cricket, locust, river fly, screwworm fly, mealworm
Hairdresser	Sodium and potassium persulfate, henna
Leather workers	Formalin, chromium salts
Lumber and wood workers, carpentry, construction, sawmill, cabinetmaking	Wood dusts (western red cedar, redwood, iroko, oak, mahogany, Douglas fir, zebrawood)
Metalworkers	Platinum salts, nickel, chromium, cobalt, vanadium, tungsten carbide
Paper product workers	Natural glues
Pharmaceutical workers	Penicillins, cephalosporins, methyl dopa, spiramycin, tetracycline, pepcin, phenylglycine acid
Plastic workers, automobile repairmen, and painters	Diisocyanates (TDI, MDI), trimellitic anhydride, phthalic anhydride

[a]*Note:* Data from Chan-Yeung and Malo (1993).

Work-related asthma has been reported in 4% of workers exposed to the dust of western red cedar (Chan-Yeung, Lam, and Koener 1982), in 5% to 10% of workers exposed to toluene diisocyanate, in 29% to 40% of workers using epoxy resins, and in 70% of workers exposed to platinum salts in such processes as metallurgy and photography (Mapp et al. 2005).

Causes

Materials having known or suspected allergic properties account for the majority of cases of occupational asthma. Occupations with a high prevalence of these agents are listed in Table 15.3 (Chan-Yeung and Malo 1993). The risk of developing occupational asthma is usually related to the magnitude of exposure for many agents including western red cedar, toluene diisocyanate, baking products, and colophony fumes from soldering (Blanc 1987). Atopy, or allergy, is an important risk factor for developing asthma from the high molecular weight compounds but not for the low molecular weight compounds (Beach et al. 2007).

The risk for persistent symptoms in workers diagnosed with occupational asthma was examined in 125 western red cedar workers (Chan-Yeung, Lam, and Koener 1982). All workers who remained at work continued to have symptoms. Among workers who left the work, those who were older, had a longer duration of exposure, and had a longer duration of symptoms were at higher risk for having persistent symptoms. Workers who develop toluene diisocyanate–related asthma and continue to be exposed to the compound have been found to have continued deterioration in pulmonary function.

Prevention and Control

The only way to prevent occupational asthma is to avoid work and work sites where exposure to certain levels of agents occurs. Thus, it is important for facility managers to know what agents in their plant have been associated with asthma and to inform their workers and establish work practices that maintain exposures below known sensitization levels. Material safety data sheets need to include information on components that may cause or exacerbate asthma. Workers need to be educated and trained on proper handling of materials and avoiding spills. Improved ventilation and the use of respirators when exposures are likely can decrease the risk of disease. When sensitization occurs, often the only remedy for the affected worker is a transfer from the area of exposure. In cases where transfer is not possible, it is debatable whether the worker should be allowed to continue working with the suspected compound, even when protective measures are instituted (American Thoracic Society 2004b). Deaths have been recorded when sensitized individuals have been reexposed at the workplace. Desensitization before exposure has not been shown to be effective (Weeks, Levy, and Wagner 1991).

ORGANIC DUST-RELATED LUNG DISEASE (ICD-10 J66)

A variety of chronic lung conditions can develop following short-term or long-term exposure to organic dusts (hypersensitivity pneumonitis) or toxic gases such as nitrogen oxides produced from the storage or decay of organic material (silo fillers disease). Although agricultural workers are most frequently impacted (Bang et al. 2006), as with occupational asthma there are more than 200 agents known to cause hypersensitivity pneumonitis and among them industrial chemicals such as metal working fluids (Kreiss and Cox-Ganser 1997). In 2003, OSHA estimated that in 1996, 92,000 grain elevator and 68,000 grain mill employees working in approximately 5,200 grain elevator firms and 1,500 grain mill firms were impacted by the OSHA (2003) grain dust standard. Grain dust is a mixture of different grains, bacteria and fungus, mites, inorganic material, and herbicides and pesticides. Grain-handlers' disease, caused by inhaling grain dust, is characterized by a drop in lung function over a work shift and by changes that persist over a harvest season (James et al. 1986). Chronic grain dust exposure can result in chronic cough, phlegm, wheezing, and dyspnea, and a permanent decline in lung function. Pulmonary fibrosis may occur but is uncommon in workers with chronic grain dust exposure (James et al. 1986).

Farmer's lung is caused by inhaling spores from moldy hay and is characterized by repeated attacks of fever, chills, malaise, coughing, and breathlessness (do Pico 1992). The condition is a type of hypersensitivity pneumonitis or extrinsic allergic alveolitis that results from inhaling many different organic dusts. Most commonly, thermophilic actinomyces or other fungi are present. Testing patient serum for specific precipitating antibodies can help identify which organisms or agents may be contributing to the disease. In a well-controlled research setting, inhalation chamber challenges have been used to identify offending agents. Such testing is not a routine practice. The chronic form occurs in fewer than 5% of patients who develop the acute form of the disease (Speizer 1981). Lung function is abnormal in patients with the chronic form of the disease, with a decline in the FVC and a diffuse fibrosis on the chest x-ray.

Descriptive Epidemiology

Hypersensitivity pneumonitis is a rare disease with an increasing incidence and little is known about the distribution of the disease outside the agricultural sector (Bang et al. 2006). Some of the increase may be due to changes in agricultural practices and the movement to large-scale production of livestock in confined feeding operations (Van Essen and Auvermann 2005). Symptoms are often similar to asthma, COPD, and bronchitis, and initial acute attacks are often mistaken for pneumonia. No single clinical or laboratory test exists to establish the diagnosis. Chronic lung disease from inhaling of grain dust is probably more common, but relatively little is known about its epidemiologic patterns.

Causes

Those at risk for the disease from inhaling biologically active organic dusts include farmers, grain handlers, wood workers, bird breeders, mushroom workers, and animal handlers, including workers who clean pens and handle laboratory animals (Bang et al. 2006). Environments where water-based machining fluids are used have also been associated with hypersensitivity pneumonitis, probably due to aerosolization of bacteria or fungi growing in the fluids (Kreiss and Cox-Ganser 1997).

Prevention and Control

Agricultural dusts are regulated in the United States; the NIOSH has proposed a limit of four mg/m^3 for grain dust. The concern over dust levels in grain handling facilities has, in part, been due to the risk of explosions (2003). Improved design of grain elevators and livestock confinement spaces, proper ventilation, and education of farmworkers and rescue services can reduce the risk from dust and toxic gases (Speizer 1981). Self-contained breathing devices should be worn by workers entering closed or poorly ventilated spaces or tanks containing liquid manure. Diseases caused by molds can be minimized by proper grain storage techniques. A critical factor in control of disease is worker knowledge of the circumstances where exposures are likely to occur so that preventive precautions can be taken.

Resources

Centers for Disease Control and Prevention (CDC), http://www.cdc.gov

- National Asthma Control Program, http://www.cdc.gov/asthma
- National Institute for Occupational Safety and Health (NIOSH), http://www.cdc.gov/niosh
- Work-Related Lung Disease Surveillance System (WoRLD), http://www2.cdc.gov/drds/WorldReportData
- Agency for Toxic Substances and Disease Registries (ATSDR), http://www.atsdr.cdc.gov
- Toxicological Profiles, http://www.atsdr.cdc.gov/toxpro2.html
- Case Studies in Environmental Medicine, http://www.atsdr.cdc.gov/csem/csem.html

National Heart, Lung, and Blood Institute (NHLBI), http://www.nhlbi.nih.gov

- Lung Disease Information for Patients and the General Public, http://www.nhlbi.nih.gov/health/public/lung/index.htm
- Guidelines for the Diagnosis and Management of Asthma (EPR-3), http://www.nhlbi.nih.gov/guidelines/asthma

Global Initiative for Chronic Obstructive Lung Disease, http://www.goldcopd.com
Cystic Fibrosis Foundation, http://www.cff.org
American Lung Association, http://www.lungusa.org
National Sleep Foundation (Obstructive Sleep Apnea), http://www.sleepfoundation.org
Environmental Protection Agency (Asthma and Indoor Environments), http://www.epa.gov/asthma

Suggested Reading

Speizer, F.E., S. Horton, J. Batt, and A.S. Slutsky. Respiratory Diseases of Adults. In: Jamison, D.T., J.G. Breman, A.R. Measham, et al., editors, *Disease Control Priorities in Developing Countries*, 2nd ed. New York, NY: Oxford University Press (2006) pp. 681–694.
Chen, J.C., and D.M. Mannino. Obstructive, Occupational, and Environmental Diseases. Worldwide Epidemiology of Chronic Obstructive Pulmonary Disease. *Curr Opin Pulm Med* (1999)5(2): 93–99. Philadelphia, PA: Lippincott Williams and Wilkins.

Office of Disease Prevention and Health Promotion, Department of Health and Human Services. Healthy People 2010: Respiratory Diseases. Available at: http://www.healthypeople.gov/Document/HTML/Volume2/24Respiratory.htm. Accessed July 17, 2009.

Moorman, J., R. Rudd, C. Johnson, et al. National surveillance for asthma—United States, 1980–2004. *MMWR* (2007):56(SS08):1–14, 18–54.

Levy, B.S., G.R. Wagner, K.M. Rest, and J.L. Weeks, editors. *Preventing Occupational Disease and Injury (Second Edition)*. Washington, D.C.: American Public Health Association (2005).

Allies Against Asthma: A Program to Combine Clinical and Public Health Approaches to Chronic Illness (report on seven coalition-based efforts to improve pediatric asthma management). Available at http://www.rwjf.org/reports/npreports/zap.htm.

Morgan, M.T. *Environmental Health (3rd Edition)*. Florence, KY: Brooks Cole (2003). A comprehensive summary of the practices used in protecting the public from environmental health hazards.

References

Akinbami, L. State of Childhood Asthma, United States, 1980–2005. *Advanced Data from Vital Health Statistics* (2006):381:1–24.

Akinbami, L. *Asthma Prevalence, Health Care Use and Mortality: United States, 2003–2005, Health E-Stats*. National Center for Health Statistics (2007).

Alberts, W., and S. Brooks. Advances in Occupational Asthma. *Clin Chest Med* (1992):13:281–302.

American Thoracic Society. Diagnosis and Initial Management of Nonmalignant Disease Related to Asbestos. *Am J Respir Crit Care Med* (2004a):170:691–715.

American Thoracic Society. Guidelines for Assessing and Managing Asthma Risk at Work, School, and Recreation. *Am J Respir Crit Care Med* (2004b):169:873–881.

Anderson, H.A., S.M. Daum, R. Lilis, A.S. Fischbein, and I.J. Selikoff. Household-Contact Asbestos Neoplastic Risk. *Ann NY Acad Sci* (1976):271:311–323.

Arbes, S.J., P.J. Gergen, B. Vaughn, and D.C. Zeldin. Asthma Cases Attributable to Atopy: Results from the Third National Health and Nutrition Examination Survey. *J Allergy Clin Immunol* (2007):120:1139–1145.

Attfield, M., and R. Castellan. Epidemiological Data on US Coal Miners' Pneumoconiosis, 1960–1988. *Am J Public Health* (1992):82:964–970.

Bang, K., D. Weissman, G. Pinheiro, V. Antao, J. Wood, and G. Syamlal. Twenty-Three Years of Hypersensitivity Pneumonitis Mortality Surveillance in the United States. *Am J Ind Med* (2006):49:997–1004.

Barbanel, D., S. Eldridge, and C. Griffiths. Can a Self-Management Programme Delivered by a Community Pharmacist Improve Asthma Control? A Randomized Trial. *Thorax* (2003):58:851–854.

Barbee, R., and S. Murphy. Natural History of Asthma. *J Allergy Clin Immunol* (1998):102:S65–S72.

Bates, D., A. Gotsch, S. Brooks, P. Landrigan, J. Hankinson, and J. Merchant. Prevention of Occupational Lung Disease. *Chest* (1992):102:257S–276S.

Baumel, M., G. Maislin, and A. Pack. Population and Occupational Screening for Obstructive Sleep Apnea: Are We There Yet? *Am J Respir Crit Care Med* (1997):155:9–14.

Baumgartner, K., J. Samet, C. Stidley, T. Colby, and J. Waldron. Cigarette Smoking: A Risk Factor for Idiopathic Pulmonary Fibrosis. *Am J Respir Crit Care Med* (1997):155:242–248.

Beach, J., K. Russell, S. Blitz, et al. Systematic Review of the Diagnosis of Occupational Asthma. *Chest* (2007):131:569–578.

Beuther, D., S. Weiss, and E. Sutherland. Obesity and Asthma. *Am J Respir Crit Care Med* (2006):174:112–119.

Blanc, P. Occupational Asthma in a National Disability Survey. *Chest* (1987):92:613–617.

Boucher, R. New Concepts of the Pathogenesis of Cystic Fibrosis Lung Disease. *Eur Respir J* (2004):23:146–158.

Boucher, R., M. Knowles, and J. Yankaskas. Cystic Fibrosis. In: Mason, R., J. Murray, V. Broaddus, and J. Nadel, editors, *Murray and Nadel's Textbook of Respiratory Medicine*. Philadelphia, PA: WB Saunders Co. (2000).

Bouhuys, A., J. Schoenberg, G. Beck, and R. Schilling. Epidemiology of Chronic Lung Disease in a Cotton Mill Community. *Lung* (1977):154:167–186.

Boushey, H., D. Corry, J. Fahy, E. Burchard, and P. Woodruff. Asthma. In: Mason, R., J. Murray, V. Broaddus, and J. Nadel, editors, *Murray and Nadel's Textbook of Respiratory Medicine*. Philadelphia, PA: WB Saunders Co. (2000).

Bradley, T., and E. Phillipson. Sleep Disorders. In: Mason, R., J. Murray, V. Broaddus, and J. Nadel, editors, *Murray and Nadel's Textbook of Respiratory Disease*. Philadelphia, PA: WB Saunders Co. (2000).

Brotanek, J., K. Grimes, and G. Flores. Leave No Asthmatic Child Behind: The Cultural Competency of Asthma Education. *Ethn Dis* (2007):17:742–748.

Bueving, H., S. Thomas, and J. Wouden. Is Influenza Vaccination in Asthma Helpful? *Curr Opin Allergy Clin Immunol* (2005):5:65–70.

Caples, S., A. Gami, and V. Somers. Obstructive Sleep Apnea. *Ann Intern Med* (2005):142(3):187–197.

Castellani, C. Evidence for Newborn Screening for Cystic Fibrosis. *Paediatr Respir Rev* (2003):4:278–284.

Cystic Fibrosis Foundation (CFF). *CFF Patient Registry Annual Data Report to Center Directors, 2005*. Cystic Fibrosis Foundation (2006).

Chan-Yeung, M. Clinician's Approach to Determine the Diagnosis, Prognosis, and Therapy of Occupational Asthma. *Med Clin North Am* (1990):74:811–822.

Chan-Yeung, M., S. Lam, and S. Koener. Clinical Features and Natural History of Occupational Asthma Due to Western Red Cedar (*Thuja plicata*). *Am J Med* (1982):72:411–415.

Chan-Yeung, M., and J. Malo. Table of the Major Inducers of Occupational Asthma. In: Bernstein, I., M. Chan-Yeung, J. Malo, and D. Bernstein, editors, *Asthma in the Workplace*. New York, NY: Marcel Dekker (1993).

Chan-Yeung, M., and J. Malo. Natural History of Occupational Asthma. In: Bernstein, I., M. Chan-Yeung, J. Malo, and D. Bernstein, editors, *Asthma in the Workplace*, 2nd ed. New York, NY: Marcel Dekker (1999).

Chilmonczyk, B., L. Salmun, K. Megathlin, et al. Association between Exposure to Environmental Tobacco Smoke and Exacerbations of Asthma in Children. *N Engl J Med* (1993):328:1665–1669.

Coleman, R. Current Animal Models are not Predictive for Clinical Asthma. *Pulmon Pharmacol Therapeut* (1999):12:87–89.

Connett, J., R. Murray, S. Buist, et al. Changes in Smoking Status Affect Women More than Men: Results of the Lung Health Study. *Am J Epidemiol* (2003):157:973–979.

Coultas, D., R. Zumwalt, W. Black, and R. Sobonya. Epidemiology of Interstitial Lung Diseases. *Am J Respir Crit Care Med* (1994):150(4):967–972.

Cowie, R., and S. Mabena. Silicosis, Chronic Airflow Limitation, and Chronic Bronchitis in South African Coal Miners. *Am Rev Respir Dis* (1991):143:80–84.

Crystal, R., J. Gadek, V. Ferrans, J. Fulmer, B. Line, and G. Hunninghake. Interstitial Lung Disease: Current Concepts of Pathogenesis, Staging, and Therapy. *Am J Med* (1981):70:542–568.

Custovic, A., B. Simpson, A. Simpson, P. Kissen, and A. Woodcock. Effect of Environmental Manipulation in Pregnancy and Early Life on Respiratory Symptoms and Atopy During the First Year of Life: A Randomized Trial. *Lancet* (2001):358(9277):188–193.

Centers for Disease Control and Prevention (CDC). *National Health Interview Survey Data* (2007). Available at http://www.cdc.gov/asthma/nhis.

de Serres, F., and I. Blanco. Estimating the Risk for Alpha 1-Antitrypsin Deficiency among COPD Patients: Evidence Supporting Targeted Screening. *COPD* (2006):3:133–139.

do Pico, G. Hazardous Exposure and Lung Disease among Farm Workers. *Clin Chest Med* (1992):13:311–328.

Eisner, M., J. Balmes, P. Katz, L. Trupin, E. Yelin, and P. Blanc. Lifetime Environmental Tobacco Smoke Exposure and the Risk of Chronic Obstructive Pulmonary Disease. *Environ Health* (2005):4:7–11.

Ezzati, M. Indoor Air Pollution and Health in Developing Countries. *Lancet* (2005):366:104–106.

Fogarty, A., R. Hubbard, and J. Britton. International Comparison of Median Age at Death from Cystic Fibrosis. *Chest* (2000):117(6):1656–1660.

Ford, E., D. Mannino, S. Redd, A. Mokdad, and J. Mott. Body Mass Index and Asthma Incidence among USA Adults. *Eur Respir J* (2004):24:740–744.

Gerald, L., M. Sockrider, R. Grad, et al. An Official ATS Workshop Report: Issues in Screening for Asthma in Children. *Proc Am Thor Soc* (2007):4:133–141.

Glindmeyer, H., J. Lefante, R. Jones, R. Rando, H. Abdel Kader, and H. Weill. Exposure-Related Declines in the Lung Function of Cotton Textile Workers. *Am Rev Respir Dis* (1991):144:675–683.

Global Initiative for Asthma (GINA). *Global Strategy for Asthma Management and Prevention.* Global Initiative for Asthma (2006).

Global Initiative for Chronic Obstructive Respiratory Disease (GOLD). *Global Strategy for the Diagnosis, Management, and Prevention of Chronic Obstructive Pulmonary Disease.* Global Initiative for Chronic Obstructive Respiratory Disease (2006).

Gold, D. Environmental Tobacco Smoke, Indoor Allergens, and Childhood Asthma. *Environ Health Perspect* (2000):108(Suppl 4):643–651.

Gold, W. Pulmonary Function Testing. In: Mason, R., J. Murray, V. Broaddus, and J. Nadel, editors, *Murray and Nadel's Textbook of Respiratory Medicine.* Philadelphia, PA: WB Saunders Co. (2000).

Gold, D., A. Damokosh, D. Dockery, and C. Berkey. Body-Mass Index as a Predictor of Incident Asthma in a Prospective Cohort of Children. *Pediatr Pulmonol* (2003):36:514–521.

Griesenbach, U., D. Geddes, and E. Alton. Gene Therapy Progress and Prospects: Cystic Fibrosis. *Gene Ther* (2006):13(14):1061–1067.

Grosse, S., C. Boyle, J. Botkin, et al. Newborn Screening for Cystic Fibrosis: Evaluation of Benefits and Risks and Recommendations for State Newborn Screening Programs. *MMWR* (2004):53(RR13):1–36.

Guill, M. Respiratory Manifestations of Gastroesophageal Reflux in Children. *J Asthma* (1995):32:173–179.

Halbert, R., J. Natoli, A. Gano, E. Badamgarav, A. Buist, and D. Mannino. Global Burden of COPD: Systemic Review and Meta-Analysis. *Eur Respir J* (2006):28:523–532.

Hartenbaum, N., N. Collop, I. Rosen, et al. Sleep Apnea and Commercial Motor Vehicle Operators: Statement from the Joint Task Force of the American College of Chest Physicians, American College of Occupational and Environmental Medicine, and the National Sleep Foundation: Executive Summary. *J Occup Environ Med* (2006):48 Suppl:1–3.

Healthcare Cost and Utilization Project (HCUP). *HCUP Nationwide Inpatient Sample (NIS), 2005.* Healthcare Cost and Utilization Project Agency for Healthcare Research and Quality (2007).

He, J., M. Kryger, F. Zorick, W. Conway, and T. Roth. Mortality and Apnea Index in Obstructive Sleep Apnea: Experience in 385 Male Patients. *Chest* (1988):94:9–14.

Hing, E., D. Cherry, and D. Woodwell. National Ambulatory Medical Care Survey: 2004 Summary. *Advance Data from Vital and Health Statistics* (2006):374.

Hnizdo, E., P. Sullivan, K.M. Bang, and G. Wagner. Association between Chronic Obstructive Pulmonary Disease and Employment by Industry and Occupation in the US Population: A Study of Data from the Third National Health and Nutrition Examination Survey. *Am J Epidemiol* (2002):156(8):738–746.

Hogg, J. Pathophysiology of Airflow Limitation in Chronic Obstructive Respiratory Disease. *Lancet* (2004):364:709–721.

Hoyert, D., K. Kochanek, and S. Murphy. Deaths: Final Data for 1997. *National Vital Statistics Report* (1999):47(19):1–104.

Hubbard, R., S. Lewis, K. Richards, J. Britton, and I. Johnston. Occupational Exposure to Metal or Wood Dust and Aetiology of Cryptogenic Alveolitis. *Lancet* (1996):347(8997):284–289.

Hung, J., E. Whitford, R. Parsons, and D. Hillman. Association of Sleep Apnoea with Myocardial Infarction in Men. *Lancet* (1990):336(8710):261–264.

International Agency for Research on Cancer (IARC). *Monograph on the Evaluation of the Carcinogenic Risk of Chemicals to Humans: Silica, Some Silicates, Coal Dust, and Para-Aramid Fibres.* Lyon: International Agency for Research on Cancer (1997).

International Labour Office (ILO). Guidelines for the Use of ILO International Classification of Radiographs of Pneumoconioses. *Occupational Safety and Health Series* (No. 22). Geneva: International Labour Office (2002).

Iwai, K., T. Mori, N. Yamada, M. Yamaguchi, and Y. Hosoda. Idiopathic Pulmonary Fibrosis: Epidemiologic Approaches to Occupational Exposure. *Am J Respir Crit Care Med* (1994):150(3):670–675.

Jaakkola, M., R. Piipari, N. Jaakkola, and J. Jaakkola. Environmental Tobacco Smoke and Adult-Onset Asthma: A Population-Based Incident Case-Control Study. *Am J Public Health* (2003):93:2055–2060.

James, A., W. Cookson, G. Buters, S. Lewis, G. Ryan, R. Hockey, and A. Musk. Symptoms and Longitudinal Changes in Lung Function in Young Seasonal Grain Handlers. *Br J Ind Med* (1986):43:587–591.

Jones, R., H. Glindmeyer, and H. Weill. Review of the Kilburn and Warshaw Chest Article—Airways Obstruction from Asbestos Exposure. *Chest* (1995):107(6):1727–1729.

Kerem, E., J. Reisman, M. Corey, G. Canny, and H. Levison. Prediction of Mortality in Patients with Cystic Fibrosis. *N Engl J Med* (1992):326:1187–1191.

Kilburn, K., and R. Warshaw. Airways Obstruction from Asbestos Exposure: Effects of Asbestosis and Smoking. *Chest* (1994):106:1061–1070.

Kreiss, K., and J. Cox-Ganser. Metalworking Fluid-Associated Hypersensitivity Pneumonitis: A Workshop Summary. *Am J Ind Med* (1997):32:423–432.

LaDou, J. The Asbestos Cancer Epidemic. *Environ Health Perspect* (2004):112:285–290.

Leigh, J., S. Yasmeen, and T. Miller. Medical Costs of Fourteen Occupational Illnesses in the United States in 1999. *Scand J Work Environ Health* (2003):29:304–313.

Lewis, S., J. Bennett, K. Richards, and J. Britton. A Cross-Sectional Study of the Independent Effect of Occupation on Lung Function in British Coal Miners. *Occup Environ Med* (1996):53(2):125–128.

Mahler, D., and R. Meija. Dyspnea. In: Mason, R., J. Murray, V. Broaddus, and J. Nadel, editors, *Murray and Nadel's Textbook of Respiratory Medicine.* Philadelphia, PA: WB Saunders Co. (1999).

Mannino, D., R. Etzel, and R. Parrish. Pulmonary Fibrosis Deaths in the United States, 1979–1991. An Analysis of Multiple-Cause Mortality Data. *Am J Respir Crit Care Med* (1996):153(5):1548–1552.

Mannino, D., R. Gagnon, T. Petty, and E. Lydick. Obstructive Lung Disease and Low Lung Function in Adults in the United States: Data from the National Health and Nutrition Examination Survey, 1988–1994. *Arch Intern Med* (2000):160:1683–1689.

Mannino, D., D. Homa, L. Akinbami, E. Ford, and S. Redd. Chronic Obstructive Pulmonary Disease Surveillance—United States, 1971–2000. *MMWR* (2002):51(SS06):1–16.

Mapel, D., J. Samet, and D. Coultas. Corticosteroids and the Treatment of Idiopathic Pulmonary Fibrosis. *Chest* (1996):110(4):1058–1067.

Mapp, C., P. Boschetto, P. Maestrelli, and L. Fabbri. Occupational Asthma. *Am J Respir Crit Care Med* (2005):172:280–305.

Marsh, S., S. Aldington, P. Shirtcliffe, M. Weatherall, and R. Beasley. Smoking and COPD: What Really Are the Risks? *Eur Respir J* (2006):28:883–884.

Martinez, F., A. Wright, L. Taussig, C. Holberg, M. Halonen, and W. Morgan. Asthma and Wheezing in the First Six Years of Life. *N Engl J Med* (1995):332:133–138.

Mason, R., J. Murray, V. Broaddus, and J. Nadel, editors. *Murray and Nadel's Textbook of Respiratory Medicine*. Philadelphia, PA: WB Saunders Co. (2000).

Materna, B., J. Quint, J. Prudhomme, et al. Fixed Obstructive Lung Disease among Workers in the Flavor-Manufacturing Industry—California 2004–2007. *MMWR* (2007):56(16):389–393.

McConnell, R., K. Berhane, F. Gilliland, et al. Asthma in Exercising Children Exposed to Ozone: A Cohort Study. *Lancet* (2002):359:386–391.

McConnell, R., K. Berhane, L. Yao, et al. Traffic, Susceptibility and Childhood Asthma. *Environ Health Perspect* (2006):114(5):766–772.

Melen, E., M. Wickman, S. Nordvall, M. van Hage-Hamsten, and A. Lindfors. Influence of Early and Current Environmental Exposure Factors on Sensitization and Outcome of Asthma in Pre-School Children. *Allergy* (2001):56:646–652.

Merrill, C., and A. Elixhauser. *Hospitalization in the United States, 2002: HCUP Fact Book No. 6*. Rockville, MD: Agency for Healthcare Research and Quality (AHRQ) (2005).

Meyers, D., M. Larj, and L. Lange. Genetics of Asthma and COPD: Similar Results for Different Phenotypes. *Chest* (2004):126:105–110.

Miniño, A., M. Heron, S. Murphy, and K. Kochanek. Deaths: Final Data for 2004. *National Vital Statistics Report 55(19)*, National Center for Health Statistics (2007):55(19).

Mooe, T., K. Franklin, K. Holmström, T. Rabben, and U. Wiklund. Sleep-Disordered Breathing and Coronary Artery Disease: Long-Term Prognosis. *Am J Respir Crit Care Med* (2001):164(10):1910–1913.

Moorman, J., R. Rudd, C. Johnson, et al. National Surveillance for Asthma—United States, 1980–2004. *MMWR* (2007):56(SS08):1–14, 18–54.

Myers, D. Genetics of Atopic Allergy: Family Studies of Total Serum IgE Levels. In: Marsh, D., A. Lockhart, and S. Holgate, editors, *Genetics of Asthma*. Oxford: Blackwell Scientific (1993) 153–162.

National Heart, Lung, and Blood Institute (NHLBI). *Guidelines for the Diagnosis and Management of Asthma: National Asthma Education and Prevention Program Expert Panel Report 3*. National Heart, Lung, and Blood Institute, National Institutes of Health (2007).

National Institute for Occupational Safety and Health (NIOSH). *Report to Congress: Workers' Home Contamination Study Conducted Under the Workers' Family Protection Act*. Cincinnati, OH: National Institute for Occupational Safety and Health (1995).

National Institute for Occupational Safety and Health (NIOSH). *Work-Related Lung Disease Surveillance Report—2002*. Cincinnati, OH: National Institute for Occupational Safety and Health (2003).

National Institute for Occupational Safety and Health (NIOSH). *Worker Health Chartbook—2004*. Cincinnati, OH: National Institute for Occupational Safety and Health (2004).

Occupational Safety and Health Administration (OSHA) Grain Handling Facilities Standard. *Fed Regist* (2003):68:12,301–12,303.

Orenstein, D., B. Rosenstein, and R. Stern. Diagnosis of Cystic Fibrosis. In: Orenstein, D., B. Rosenstein, and R. Stern, editors, *Cystic Fibrosis Medical Care*. Philadelphia, PA: Lippincott, Williams and Wilkins (2000) pp. 21–54.

Orozco-Levi, M., J. Garcia-Aymerich, J. Villar, A. Ramirez-Sarmiento, J. Anto, and J. Gea. Wood Smoke Exposure and Risk of Chronic Obstructive Pulmonary Disease. *Eur Respir J* (2006):27:542–546.

Oxman, A., D. Muir, H. Shannon, S. Stock, E. Hnizdo, and H. Lange. Occupational Dust Exposure and Chronic Obstructive Pulmonary Disease. *Am Rev Respir Dis* (1993):148:38–48.

Pearce, N., J. Pekkanen, and R. Beasley. How Much Asthma is Really Attributable to Atopy? *Thorax* (1999):54:268–272.

Petty, T., and G. Weinmann. Building a National Strategy for the Prevention and Management of and Research in Chronic Obstructive Pulmonary Disease. *JAMA* (1997):277:246–253.

Rabe, K., S. Hurd, A. Anzueto, et al. Global Strategy for the Diagnosis, Management and Prevention of Chronic Obstructive Pulmonary Disease: GOLD Executive Summary. *Am J Respir Crit Care Med* (2007):176:532–555.

Reis, A., R. Kaplan, T. Limberg, and L. Prewitt. Effects of Pulmonary Rehabilitation on Physiologic and Psychosocial Outcomes in Patients with Chronic Obstructive Pulmonary Disease. *Ann Intern Med* (1995):122(11):823–832.

Remes, S., J. Castro-Rodriguez, C. Holberg, F. Martinez, and A. Wright. Dog Exposure in Infancy Decreases the Subsequent Risk of Frequent Wheeze but not of Atopy. *J Allergy Clin Immunol* (2001):108(4):509–515.

Rogan, W., B. Gladen, N. Ragan, and H. Anderson. U.S. Prevalence of Occupational Pleural Thickening: A Look at Chest X-rays from the First National Health and Nutrition Examination Survey. *Am J Epidemiol* (1987):126(5):893–900.

Rosenfeld, M., and F. Collins. Gene Therapy for Cystic Fibrosis. *Chest* (1996):109:241–252.

Rosenman, K., M. Reilly, and P. Henneberger. Estimating the Total Number of Newly-Recognized Silicosis Cases in the United States. *Am J Ind Med* (2003):44(2):141–147.

Rylander, R. Endotoxin in the Environment: Exposure and Effects. *J Endotoxin Res* (2002):8:241–252.

Sarnat, J., and F. Holguin. Asthma and Air Quality. *Curr Opin Pulm Med* (2007):13:63–66.

Schulz, S., S. Jakubiczka, S. Kropf, I. Nickel, P. Muschke, and J. Kleinstein. Increased Frequency of Cystic Fibrosis Transmembrane Conductane Regulator Gene Mutations in Infertile Males. *Fertil Steril* (2006):85:135–138.

Scott, J., I. Johnston, and J. Britton. What Causes Cryptogenic Fibrosin Alveolitis? A Case-Control Study of Environmental Exposure to Dust. *Br Med J* (1990):301(6759):1015–1017.

Sears, M. Epidemiological Trends in Bronchial Asthma. In: Kaliner, M., P. Barnes, and C. Persson, editors, *Asthma: Its Pathology and Treatment*. New York, NY: Marcel Dekker (1991) pp. 1–49.

Selikoff, I., E. Hammond, and H. Seidman. Mortality Experience of Insulation Workers in the United States and Canada, 1943–1976. *Ann NY Acad Sci* (1979):330:91–116.

Selikoff, I., and D. Lee, editors. *Asbestos and Disease*. New York, NY: Academic Press (1978).

Shapiro, S., G. Snider, et al. Chronic Bronchitis and Emphysema. In: Mason, R., J. Murray, V. Broaddus, and J. Nadel, editors, *Murray and Nadel's Textbook of Respiratory Medicine*. Philadelphia, PA: WB Saunders Co. (2000).

Silva, G., D. Sherrill, S. Guerra, and R. Barbee. Asthma as a Risk Factor for COPD in a Longitudinal Study. *Chest* (2004):126:59–65.

Silverman, R., K. Ito, L. Stevenson, and H. Hastings. Relationship of Fall School Opening and Emergency Department Asthma Visits in a Large Metropolitan Area. *Arch Pediatr Adolesc Med* (2005):159(9):818–823.

Smith, A., R. Castellan, D. Lewis, and T. Matte. Guidelines for the Epidemiologic Assessment of Occupational Asthma. *J Allergy Clin Immunol* (1989):84:794–805.

Smith, A., P. Lopipero, and V. Barroga. Meta-Analysis of Studies of Lung Cancer among Silicotics. *Epidemiology* (1995):6(6):17–24.

Snider, D. Relationship between Tuberculosis and Silicosis. *Am Rev Respir Dis* (1978):118:455–460.

Speizer, F. Epidemiology of Environmentally-Induced Chronic Respiratory Disease. *Chest* (1981):80:21S–23S.

Stoller, J., and L. Aboussouan. Alpha 1-Antitrypsin Deficiency. *Lancet* (2005):365:2225–2236.

Strausbaugh, S., and P. Davis. Cystic Fibrosis: A Review of Epidemiology and Pathobiology. *Clin Chest Med* (2007):28:279–288.

Stulberg, M., and L. Adams. Symptoms of Respiratory Disease and Their Management. In: Mason, R., J. Murray, V. Broaddus, and J. Nadel, editors, *Murray and Nadel's Textbook of Respiratory Medicine*. Philadelphia, PA: WB Saunders Co. (2000).

Sullivan, S., S. Ramsey, and T. Lee. Economic Burden of COPD. *Chest* (2000):117:5S–9S.

Taussig, L., A. Wright, C. Holberg, M. Halonen, W. Morgan, and F. Martinez. Tucson Children's Respiratory Study: 1980 to Present. *J Allergy Clin Immunol* (2003):111(4):661–675.

Thomas, P., and G. Hunninghake. Current Concepts of the Pathogenesis of Sarcoidosis. *Am Rev Respir Dis* (1987):135:747–760.

Trupin, L., G. Earnest, M. San Pedro, et al. Occupational Burden of Chronic Obstructive Respiratory Disease. *Eur Respir J* (2003):22:462–469.

Tsui, L.C., and M. Buchwald. Biochemical and Molecular Genetics of Cystic Fibrosis. *Adv Hum Genet* (1991):20:153–266, 311–312.

U.S. Government Accountability Office (U.S. GAO). *Federal Compensation Programs—Perspectives on Four Programs (Report to Congressional Questioners)*. Washington, D.C.: U.S. Government Accountability Office (2005).

Vallyathan, V., V. Castronova, D. Pack, et al. Freshly Fractured Quartz Inhalation Leads to Enhanced Lung Injury and Inflammation. *Am J Respir Crit Care Med* (1995):152:1003–1009.

Van Essen, S., and B. Auvermann. Health Effects from Breathing Air Near CAFOs for Feeder Cattle or Hogs. *J Agromed* (2005):10:55–64.

Weeks, J., B. Levy, and G. Wagner, editors. *Preventing Occupational Disease and Injury*. Washington, D.C.: American Public Health Association (1991).

Weinhold, B. Death Out West: The Link to COPD. *Environ Health Perspect* (2000):108:A350.

Weiss, K. Seasonal Trends in U.S. Asthma Hospitalizations and Mortality. *JAMA* (1990):263:2323–2328.

Weitzman, M., S. Gortmaker, A. Sobol, and J. Perrin. Recent Trends in the Prevalence and Severity of Childhood Asthma. *JAMA* (1992):268(19):2673–2677.

Wetter, D., T. Young, T. Bidwell, M. Safwan Badr, and M. Palta. Smoking as a Risk Factor for Sleep-Disordered Breathing. *Arch Intern Med* (1994):154(19):2219–2224.

White, M., and M. Kaliner. Mast Cells and Asthma. In: Kaliner, M., P. Barnes, and C. Persson, editors, *Asthma: Its Pathology and Treatment*. New York, NY, Marcel Dekker (1991) pp. 409–440.

Witorsch, R., and P. Witorsch. Review: Environmental Tobacco Smoke and Respiratory Health in Children: A Critical Review and Analysis of the Literature from 1969 to 1998. *Indoor Built Environ* (2000):9:246–264.

Wright, A., C. Holberg, L. Taussig, and F. Martinez. Factors Influencing the Relation of Infant Feeding to Asthma and Recurrent Wheeze in Childhood. *Thorax* (2001):56:192–197.

Young, T., J. Blustein, L. Finn, and M. Palta. Sleep-Disordered Breathing and Motor Vehicle Accidents in a Population-Based Sample of Employed Adults. *Sleep* (1997):20:608–613.

Young, T., P. Peppard, and D. Gottlieb. Epidemiology of Obstructive Sleep Apnea: A Population Health Perspective. *Am J Respir Crit Care Med* (2002):165:1217–1239.

Zuskin, E., D. Ivankovic, E. Schachter, and T. Witek Jr. Ten-Year Follow-Up Study of Cotton Textile Workers. *Am Rev Respir Dis* (1991):143(2):301–305.

CHAPTER 16

MENTAL DISORDERS (ICD-10 F00–F99)

Danny Wedding, Ph.D., M.P.H.

Introduction

Mental disorders are not as well understood as other leading causes of chronic disease morbidity and mortality, but they are clearly consequential and contribute significantly to the global burden of disease (Mathers and Loncar 2006). Heretofore, public health researchers have neglected these problems; however, the inclusion for the first time of a chapter in mental illness in the third edition of *Chronic Disease Epidemiology and Control* underscores growing awareness in public health about the importance of mental and emotional disorders.

Public Health Burden

Mental disorders are commonplace, and more than ten million adults in the United States have a serious mental disorder at any one time (Watanabe-Galloway and Zhang 2007). The most common disorders among people with serious mental illness are schizophrenia, bipolar disorder, and major depression.

Mental disorders are generally defined in the United States as those conditions classified as "Mental and Behavioural Disorders" (F00–F99) in the World Health Organization's *International Classification of Diseases* (ICD-10) or included in the *Diagnostic and Statistical Manual of the American Psychiatric Association* (DSM-IV). These disorders are listed in Table 16.1.

Alcohol use disorders are usually included as mental health condition; however, the magnitude of alcoholism as a public health problem is significant enough that this problem is discussed in Chapter 8 of this book and will not be included in this chapter. Likewise, although Alzheimer's disease and other dementias are included as mental disorders in the ICD-10, they are discussed in Chapter 17 (Neurological Disorders) of this text.

Mental disorders, including substance abuse, are leading causes of death, disability, and human suffering in the United States (Mokdad et al. 2004) and throughout the world (Ustun 1999). In a seminal study addressing the global burden of disease, Lopez and Murray (1998) noted that mental disorders fill five of the top ten causes of disability globally (see Table 16.2) and call for enhanced appreciation of the importance of mental disorders in all regions of the world. *Healthy People 2010* (USDHHS 2000) documents that in the United States, 22% of the population between 18 and 64 years met criteria for a diagnosis of a mental disorder or a co-occurring mental or addictive disorder in the past year; at least one in five children aged 9 to 17 years has a diagnosable mental disorder

Table 16.1. Comparison of ICD-10 and DSM-IV-TR Categories

ICD-10 Mental and Behavioral Disorders (F00–F99)

 F00–F09 Organic, including symptomatic, mental disorders

 F10–F19 Mental and behavioral disorders due to psychoactive substance use

 F20–F29 Schizophrenia, schizotypal, and delusional disorders

 F30–F39 Mood [affective] disorders

 F40–F49 Neurotic, stress-related, and somatoform disorders

 F50–F59 Behavioral syndromes associated with physiological disturbances and
   physical factors

 F60–F69 Disorders of adult personality and behaviour

 F70–F79 Mental retardation

 F80–F89 Disorders of psychological development

 F90–F98 Behavioral and emotional disorders with onset usually occurring in childhood
   and adolescence

 F99 Unspecified mental disorder

DSM-IV-TR categories

 1 Disorders usually first diagnosed in infancy, childhood, or adolescence

   1.1 Mental retardation

   1.2 Learning disorders

   1.3 Motor skills disorders

   1.4 Communication disorders

   1.5 Pervasive developmental disorders

   1.6 Attention-deficit and disruptive behavior disorders

   1.7 Feeding and eating disorders of infancy or early childhood

   1.8 Tic disorders

   1.9 Elimination disorders

   1.10 Other disorders of infancy, childhood, or adolescence

 2 Delirium, dementia, amnestic, and other cognitive disorders

   2.1 Delirium

   2.2 Dementia

   2.3 Amnestic disorders

   2.4 Other cognitive disorders

 3 Mental disorders due to a general medical condition not elsewhere classified

 4 Substance-related disorders

   4.1 Alcohol-related disorders

   4.2 Amphetamine (or amphetamine-like) related disorders

   4.3 Caffeine-related disorders

   4.4 Cannabis-related disorders

   4.5 Cocaine-related disorders

Table 16.1. (*continued*)

    4.6 Hallucinogen-related disorders

    4.7 Inhalant-related disorders

    4.8 Nicotine-related disorders

    4.9 Opioid-related disorders

    4.10 Phencyclidine (or phencyclidine-like)–related disorders

    4.11 Sedative-, hypnotic-, or anxiolytic-related disorders

    4.12 Other (or unknown) substance-related disorder

5 Schizophrenia and other psychotic disorders

6 Mood disorders

    6.1 Depressive disorders

    6.2 Bipolar disorders

7 Anxiety disorders

8 Somatoform disorders

9 Factitious disorders

10 Dissociative disorders

11 Sexual and gender identity disorder

    11.1 Sexual dysfunctions

    11.2 Paraphilias

    11.3 Gender identity disorders

12 Eating disorders

13 Sleep disorders

    13.1 Primary sleep disorders

    13.2 Parasomnias

    13.3 Other sleep disorders

14 Impulse-control disorders not elsewhere classified

15 Adjustment disorders

16 Personality disorders

at some time during the year, and 25% of elderly Americans experience mental disorders that are not specific to aging.

It is important to emphasize that comorbidity between mental and chronic disease is commonplace and may be normative for some conditions. For example, depression occurs in 40% to 60% of patients who have experienced a heart attack, and one in four people with cancer suffer from depression (APA 2003). Alcoholism or substance abuse may reflect an attempt to blunt the dysphoria and negative affect associated with depression. Medical and psychiatric comorbidity also has been well documented for adverse fetal experience (e.g., fetal exposure to alcohol) (Streissguth et al. 1996), cardiovascular disease, geriatric depression, and endocrine disorders (e.g., diabetes mellitus) (Eaton 2006). The significantly enhanced risk of diabetes and dyslipidemia found in people with

Table 16.2. The Leading Causes of Disability Worldwide

	Total YLDs[a] (million)	Percent of Total
All causes	472.7	
1. Unipolar major depression	50.8	10.7
2. Iron-deficiency anemia	22.0	4.7
3. Falls	22.0	4.6
4. Alcohol use	15.8	3.3
5. Chronic obstructive pulmonary disease	14.7	3.1
6. Bipolar disorder	14.1	3.0
7. Congenital anomalies	13.5	2.9
8. Osteoarthritis	13.3	2.8
9. Schizophrenia	12.1	2.6
10. Obsessive–compulsive disorders	10.2	2.2

[a]As measured by years of life lived with a disability.
Reprinted by permission from Macmillan Publishers Ltd: Lopez, A.D., and C.C.J.L. Murray. The Global Burden of Disease, 1990–2020. *Nat Med* (1998):4:1241–1243.

schizophrenia results from the weight gain that is so often associated with treatment with atypical antipsychotic medications such as clozapine and olanzapine (Newcomer and Haupt 2006).

Mental disorders also are intimately linked with social problems; two especially salient examples are war (Yehuda 2002) and poverty (Eisenberg 1997). Violence is also a particular problem for women throughout the world, and there is often a potentially lethal connection among anger, violence, and mental illness (Wyshak 2000).

Most people with mental disorders are not treated; Thornicoft (2007), in an article in *The Lancet*, compared mental illness with diabetes and noted that in Europe, mental illness affects 27% of the population each year, but 74% of these individuals receive no treatment; in contrast, only 8% of the population with diabetes mellitus went without care.

An emerging literature is linking mental illness with physical illness in both the United States and internationally. Sartorius (2007) has noted that people with schizophrenia are more likely to die from infectious diseases such as tuberculosis, and the prevalence of almost all other diseases is significantly greater in this population. Poor judgment is characteristic of diseases such as schizophrenia, and limitations in cognition and impaired decision-making abilities may result in risky behaviors such as unsafe sex practices and intravenous drug use, putting these patients at greater risk for communicable diseases such as human immunodeficiency virus (HIV). The only study to examine the prevalence of HIV in a general psychiatric population found an infection rate that was four times the occurrence of HIV infection in the general adult population in the United States; the groups at greatest risk were patients with substance abuse disorders, personality disorders, bipolar disorder, and posttraumatic stress disorder (Beyer et al. 2007). Likewise, Swartz et al. (2003) have estimated that 20% of persons with severe mental illness are infected with the hepatitis C virus. The false dichotomy between physical and mental illness (sometimes called the "Cartesian dichotomy" because of René Descartes' philosophy of mind/body dualism) continues to bedevil both medicine and public health, and it is clear that the burden of mental disorders will continue to be underestimated unless there is some appreciation for the contribution mental illness and addictions make to the burden of illness in the United States and in the world (Prince et al. 2007).

A major change that has occurred over the last decade is an enhanced appreciation for the fact that many people with mental illness *do* recover and go on to function effectively in society. Hopper et al. (2007) report on one of the few long-term prospective studies of schizophrenia conducted under the auspices of the World Health Organization. This project involved 69 investigators who studied more than a thousand individuals with schizophrenia sampled from 14 countries around the world. The study involved follow-up evaluations over periods as long as 26 years. The most important finding from this rigorous and well-designed investigation was that more than half of the subjects were rated as recovered at the end of the 12- to 26-year follow-up period.

Pathophysiology

There has been an explosion of information in the neurosciences that parallels the dramatic advances that have been made in genetics as a result of mapping the human genome. One consequence of this enhanced understanding of the brain is greater appreciation for the biological and genetic underpinnings for most mental disorders.

Biological explanations for mental illness have clearly become ascendant in twenty-first century psychiatry, and psychoactive medications are among the most widely prescribed medicines in the United States and other developed countries. Selective serotonin reuptake inhibitor and serotonin and norepinephrine reuptake inhibitor antidepressants are the third leading class of drugs sold in the United States (following statins and proton pump inhibitors), and 2004 sales approached $11 billion. Antipsychotic medications made up the fourth leading therapeutic class, with 2004 sales of over $9 billion. A single antidepressant medication, Zoloft, had sales in excess of $3 billion and showed an 8% increase in sales in 2004 (IMS Health 2005).

Many researchers (e.g., Valenstein 1998) have argued that the "chemical imbalance" hypotheses of mental illness are the result of a misguided attempt by psychiatry to emulate other branches of medicine in which the relationship among pathophysiology, etiology, and symptoms are more clearly established. Other investigators have pointed out that direct-to-consumer advertising campaigns have been largely responsible for widespread public acceptance of the belief that depression is caused by a lack of serotonin and the belief that this problem can be addressed by selective serotonin reuptake inhibitor antidepressants (Lacasse and Leo 2005). Currently, only the United States and New Zealand permit direct to consumer advertising for medication.

Like depression, the pathophysiology of schizophrenia is not well understood. The prevailing hypothesis—that schizophrenia results from an excess of dopamine—does a better job of explaining positive symptoms (e.g., hallucinations, delusions, disorganized thinking) than negative symptoms (e.g., passivity, lack of motivation and spontaneity, difficulty in making decisions). Although not as salient, negative symptoms may be more disabling than positive symptoms. While traditional antipsychotic medications such as haloperidol (Hadol) were effective in blocking the positive symptoms of the disease, they had little effect on negative symptoms. The development of clozapine (Clozaril), a new atypical antipsychotic, opened the door for more efficacious treatment and for a better, albeit not complete, understanding of the causes of schizophrenia.

More recent studies of the pathophysiology of schizophrenia have focused on the influence of the nicotinic receptor, glutamate, and glial cells. Anatomical studies have focused on the prefrontal cortex and limbic system, with particular focus on the hippocampus (Csernansky et al. 1997). High-definition neuroimaging technologies have dramatically enhanced our understanding of the neuroanatomical anomalies associated with schizophrenia.

Descriptive Epidemiology

Three major psychiatric epidemiological surveys have been conducted in the United States: the Epidemiologic Catchment Area (ECA) study (Robins 2001), the National Comorbidity Survey (NCS) (Kessler et al. 1994), and the National Comorbidity Survey Replication (NCS-R) (Kessler and Merikangas 2004). These surveys were generally consistent in finding that 12-month mental disorders were highly prevalent, with 26% to 30% of the population meeting criteria for at least one DSM-IV disorder. The three most prevalent disorders in the NCS-R were identical to the three most prevalent disorders identified in the NCS: specific phobia, social phobia, and major depressive disorder (Kessler et al. 2004).

High-Risk Populations

Genetic susceptibility has been well established for most mental disorders. One salient example is schizophrenia: having a first cousin with this disorder doubles one's risk; having a parent with the disorder increases risk 6-fold, while having a fraternal twin with diagnosis of schizophrenia increases risk for the disorder 17-fold. However, risk is not purely genetic. Although identical twins share 100% of their genes, someone with a twin with schizophrenia only has about a 50% chance of developing the disorder (Gottesman 1991). These data underscore the importance of understanding the complex interaction between genes and the environment.

The onset of schizophrenia typically occurs in the teen or early adult years, but onset before adolescence is rare. Men and women have approximately equal risk for schizophrenia, but women tend to have later onset, more prominent mood symptoms, and a better prognosis (APA 2000). Both anxiety disorders and mood disorders occur significantly more often in women than in men; in contrast, men are at higher risk for impulse-control disorders and substance use disorders. Lower levels of education are associated with higher risk for substance abuse (Kessler et al. 2004).

Depression is sometimes referred to as the "common cold of mental illness," a phrase that highlights the prevalence of this disorder. Depression is more common among these groups: women more than men (2.7:1 in the ECA study), adolescents more than adults and the elderly; less educated more than better educated; unemployed more than employed; and separated and/or divorced people more than single or married persons (e.g., people who were separated or divorced were shown in the ECA study to be almost three times more likely to be depressed) (Horwath, Cohen, and Weissman 2002).

The data linking mental disorders to ethnicity are complex and sometimes difficult to interpret. Riolo et al. (2005) conducted a large sample study of depression across ethnic groups and found that the prevalence of major depressive disorder was significantly higher in whites than in African Americans and Mexican Americans; in contrast, the opposite pattern existed for dysthymic disorder. Poverty was found to be a significant risk factor for major depressive disorder. Higher rates of depression have been documented in current and recent welfare recipients, and depression was shown to be associated with failure to move from welfare to work (Siefert et al. 2000).

Geographic Distribution

Considerable geographic variability exists in the degree of support people with mental illness receive across cities, states, regions, and countries. Psychiatric hospitalization in New York City, for example, has been shown to vary according to socioeconomic status and proximity to general hospitals with psychiatric beds; other predictors of psychiatric hospitalization included living in a poverty area, being African American, and living alone. This study found the highest hospital admission rates were concentrated in those areas of the city in which social and economic disadvantages were greatest (Almog et al. 2004).

Rates of HIV among people with severe mental illness vary dramatically across geographic regions in the United States, ranging from 4% to 23%. Rates of HIV were correlated with unsafe sexual practices, drug injection, and noninjected drug use, and women were as likely to be infected as men (Cournos and McKinnon 1997).

Most textbooks and the DSM-IV-TR estimate the lifetime prevalence of schizophrenia to be approximately 1% across countries; however, a meta-analysis of 1,712 estimates from 46 different countries yielded a median prevalence estimate of 4.0 per 1,000 for lifetime prevalence. This study did not identify sex differences or differences among urban, rural, and mixed sites; however, these investigators did find a higher incidence and prevalence for migrant workers, and prevalence estimates from less developed countries were significantly lower than the estimates found in both emerging and developed sites (Saha et al. 2005).

The prognosis for schizophrenia may be better in poorer countries. This belief is sometimes referred to as the "industrialization hypothesis." This theory maintains that "industrial economies and attendant life styles lead to poor support, intolerance, rejection, isolation, segregation and institutionalization of the severely mentally ill" (Jadhav et al. 2007).

Time Trends

The nineteenth century witnessed dramatic growth in asylums in both Europe and the United States, and many psychiatrists argued forcefully at the time that mental illness was increasing. However, the extant data are for prevalence rather than incidence, and the dramatic changes that occurred during the century can be attributed just as easily to the confluence of a number of social, political, and economic forces and events such as the suicide of Missouri Governor Thomas Reynolds in 1844. (Reynolds' unhappy death resulted in the establishment of Fulton State Hospital, the first psychiatric hospital built west of the Mississippi River.) Most authorities (Bresnahan et al. 2003; Warner 1995) believe the incidence of schizophrenia was either stable or slightly declining during the twentieth century.

Determinants

Modifiable Risk Factors

Many of the most salient risk factors for mental illness are genetic and therefore modifiable only through patient education, genetic counseling, and prudent decisions about childbearing (Figure 16.1). In children, twin and adoption studies have established clear evidence of the genetic risk associated with conduct disorder, attention-deficit/hyperactivity disorder, autism, and Tourette's disorder (Tsuang and Ming 2002). The genetic contribution to major psychiatric disorders such as schizophrenia and major depression is also unequivocal; for example, having a first-degree relative with major depression doubles or triples the risk that a child will be diagnosed with major depression. Having a parent (or parents) with mental illness clearly enhances risk for children due to the double burden of genetic susceptibility and the likelihood of atypical childhood experiences (e.g., parental neglect).

Lower socioeconomic status is a well-established risk factor, although at least part of the variance in SES studies results from "social drift" (i.e., people in upper SES groups are often unable to hold a job or manage money and therefore lose their privileged status). The quality of life in community neighborhoods is a substantial predictor of the mental health status of both children and families, and social inequality is clearly associated with community violence.

Nonadherence to medication is an especially important risk factor for people with schizophrenia. Although very few people with mental illness are dangerous, violence can and does occur, and, when it occurs, it is most often associated with a diagnosis of paranoid schizophrenia and a history of medication nonadherence (Swartz et al. 1998). The deteriorating mental state of a nonadherent patient is often exacerbated by alcohol or other drug abuse. These problems can be ameliorated somewhat by community interventions and the integration of treatment for mental illness and addictions.

Bipolar disorder is less common than major depression, although both are serious, commonplace, and devastating conditions. Bipolar disorder tends to occur in younger people, is more prevalent in urban populations, and—unlike major depression—occurs about equally in men and women. Social class and ethnicity are not significant predictors of bipolar disorder. Individuals who cohabit, divorce, or never marry are more likely to develop bipolar disorder than married individuals, and there is a dramatically higher prevalence rate for homeless people (Tohen and Angst 2002).

Additional risk factors for mental disorders include being male, divorced or separated, having a history of previous suicide attempts, a family history of suicide, a psychiatric dis-

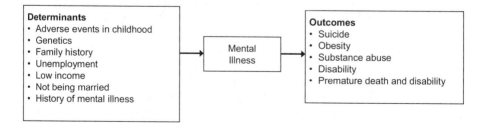

Figure 16.1. Determinants and health outcomes of mental illness.

order, a firearm in the home, or experiencing a recent stressful life event (Moscicki 1995). A team of Canadian researchers conducted a recent prospective cohort study to identify risk factors for depression in older men and identified the following seven risk factors: previous depressive episodes, birth outside Canada, low comorbidity, inadequate emotional support, few visits from children, depressed mood, and diurnal variation in mood. The risk of depression covaried with the number of risk factors present (Cole et al. 2008).

Major depressive disorder carries with it risk of chronicity, progressive disability, and premature death. Death is most likely to result from suicide, with the elderly being at greatest risk. The Sterling County Study examined the relationship between depression and smoking over a 40-year period and found that smoking increased the risk of depression threefold. In addition, those study participants who became depressed were more likely to start or continue smoking—and less likely to quit—than those who had never been depressed. As noted by Murphy et al. (2003), "when depression and smoking coexist, the quality and quantity of life are doubly assaulted" (p. 1668).

A previous history of a psychiatric disorder is a major risk factor for recurrence or the development of comorbid conditions. For example, a history of a previous diagnosis of dysthymic disorder is associated with a fivefold increase in risk, and a history of schizophrenia is associated with a threefold increase in risk for major depression (Horwath, Cohen, and Weissman 2002).

Population-Attributable Risk

Calculation or discussion of population-attributable risk (PAR) is relatively rare in mental health research, in part because of the multiple risk factors and poorly understood etiology involved in the development of diseases such as schizophrenia or poorly defined disorders such as attention-deficit/hyperactivity disorder. However, some researchers have attempted to parse out the PAR associated with some mental disorders, with the bulk of the research in this area focused on the relationship between suicide and depression.

Mortensen et al. (2000) attempted to delineate the risk factors for suicide in Denmark and the PAR associated with socioeconomic factors in an attempt to generate prevention strategies. They identified 811 cases of suicide and 79,871 controls and found that unemployment, low income, not being married, and a history of mental illness were all predictors of suicide. A history of mental illness was the strongest predictor, and the PAR associated with mental illness was 44.6%; the attributable risk associated with unemployment was 3.0%, while that associated with being single was 10.3%. The authors argue for better care for those patients admitted to the hospital and enhanced detection and treatment of mental disorders in the general population.

A more recent Danish study (Qin, Agerbo, and Mortensen 2003) replicated the findings by Mortensen showing that the highest attributable risk was the presence of a psychiatric disorder leading to hospitalization, followed by being single and being retired. A third study in Australia (Goldney et al. 2000) documented the relationship between clinical depression and suicidal ideation and estimated that the elimination of mood disorders would reduce suicidal ideation by approximately 47%.

Prenatal complications are a major risk factor for schizophrenia and account for as many as 22% of adult cases. Infants exposed to obstetrical complications at delivery are twice as likely to develop schizophrenia (Geddes and Lawrie 1995), and low birth weight has been unequivocally established as a risk factor for schizophrenia (Kunugi, Nanko, and Murray 2001).

Some researchers have attempted to examine the causal pathways between mental illness and violence, realizing that widespread public belief in this association plays a major role in maintaining the stigma associated with mental illness. One author (Monahan 1997) maintains "mental health status makes at best a trivial contribution to the overall level of violence in society." Another states "viewed in terms of attributable risk, the contribution made by those with schizophrenia to the level of recorded crime in the community is slender" (Wessely et al. 1994).

Evidence-Based Prevention and Control Measures

Primary Prevention

A number of common sense approaches to child development hold great promise for preventing or at least ameliorating a plethora of mental illnesses. These include enhancing social support, teaching parenting skills, improving early childhood education, and reducing if not eliminating school bullying. The absence of friends (loneliness), inept parenting, inadequate early education, and the failure to protect children from abuse all constitute risk factors for mental disorders. It is possible to enhance protective factors for children by promoting resilience, teaching social skills, and expanding a child's social network. The most successful primary prevention programs in mental health have a double focus—they work to reduce existing stressors and enhance the problem-solving competency of the children involved. As these children become more competent, they are better able to withstand and/or deal with those forces that would be likely to lead to deviancy, delinquency, or mental illness. The Institute of Medicine (1994) refers to primary prevention programs that target all children in a given classroom and/or community as universal interventions.

A meta-analysis of 177 primary prevention mental health programs for children and adolescents supported the general efficacy of these programs, demonstrating that they reduced problems, enhanced academic performance, increased general levels of competencies, and had a positive influence across multiple measures of functioning. Durlak and Wells (1997) note:

> Programs modifying the school environment, individually focused mental health promotion efforts, and attempts to help children negotiate stressful transitions yield significant mean effects ranging from 0.24 to 0.93. In practical terms, the average participant in a primary prevention program surpasses the performance of between 59% and 82% of those in a control group, and outcomes reflect an 8% to 46% difference in success rates favoring prevention groups. Most categories of programs had the dual benefit of significantly reducing problems and significantly increasing competencies (p. 115).

Screening and Early Detection

The Institute of Medicine refers to secondary prevention programs as indicated preventive interventions, and these often include screening and early detection. Durlak and Wells, cited above, extended their research using meta-analytical tools and examined indicated prevention programs targeting children and youth. This second study examined 130 evaluations of secondary prevention programs targeting youth who had been identified as at risk; most of these were school-based programs (Durlak and Wells 1998). This analysis also documented the efficacy of mental illness prevention programs, producing results that were both statistically and practically significant. "In practical terms, the average participant in a behavioral or cognitive-behavior intervention surpasses the performance of approximately 70% of those in the control group" (p. 790).

Teaching personal management and coping skills can significantly enhance the ability of individuals to cope with the stressors they experience in their lives. In turn, this new ability to cope with life's problems and demands can dramatically attenuate the likelihood of turning to substance abuse as a way to cope or developing a mental illness or disorder in response to stress.

The Center for Mental Health Services (CMHS) of the Substance Abuse and Mental Health Services (SAMHSA) has identified those programs in mental health and substance abuse prevention that hold the greatest promise in diminishing or preventing the development of a mental illness or a substance use disorder (Nitzkin and Smith 2004). The following programs are included:

- Universal screening of pregnant women for use of tobacco, alcohol, and illicit drugs
- Home visitation for selected pregnant women, and some children up to age 5
- Supplemental educational services for vulnerable infants from disadvantaged families
- Screening children and adolescents for behavioral disorders
- Screening adolescents for tobacco, alcohol, depression, and anxiety
- Screening adults for depression and anxiety, and use of tobacco and/or alcohol
- Psychoeducation to increase early ambulation of surgical patients and enhance adherence to prescribed regimens of care for patients with chronic diseases

The three practices with the most potential for reducing overall health care costs were (1) screening pregnant women for use of tobacco, alcohol, and illicit drugs, (2) screening for depression in persons with major chronic medical disease, and (3) psychoeducation for persons scheduled for major surgical procedures, persons with major chronic diseases, and selected other heavy users of health care services. The effect sizes for these preventive services in randomized controlled trials ranged from 5% to 30%; while modest, "the adverse consequences of the underlying disorders are such that the preventive services can be expected to pay for themselves in reduced health care costs and improved clinical and/or social outcomes."

Treatment, Rehabilitation, and Recovery

The *President's New Freedom Commission* (2001) has identified three obstacles that prevent Americans from getting good mental health care: stigma, unfair treatment limitations imposed by private health insurance companies, and a fragmented mental health service delivery system. In addition to calling for major reform of the U.S. health care system, this group underscored the importance of recovery and resilience, and the fact that recovery is possible.

Recovery refers to the process in which people are able to live, work, learn, and participate fully in their communities. For some individuals, recovery is the ability to live
a fulfilling and productive life despite a disability. For others, recovery implies the
reduction or complete remission of symptoms. Science has shown that having hope
plays an integral role in an individual's recovery.

Resilience means the personal and community qualities that enable us to rebound
from adversity, trauma, tragedy, threats, or other stresses—and to go on with life with
a sense of mastery, competence, and hope. We now understand from research that resilience is fostered by a positive childhood and includes positive individual traits, such
as optimism, good problem-solving skills, and treatments. Closely-knit communities
and neighborhoods are also resilient, providing supports for their members.

The treatments that have been shown in controlled studies to be effective for mental
illness and addictions vary across illness categories, and it is not possible to survey all treatments for all conditions within the confines of a chapter. However, the following general
principles apply (Lehman et al. 2004):

- Medications are effective for most [mental] illnesses . . . , and although they often
  have side effects, they are superior to psychosocial treatments alone in severe cases
  of many conditions.
- Combined treatments (medication plus psychosocial interventions) often produce
  the best results.
- Some psychotherapies are empirically supported, particularly cognitive–behavioral
  and interpersonal psychotherapies, and have equal efficacy vis-à-vis medication in
  mild-to-moderate cases of many conditions.
- Other psychosocial treatments (e.g., family education) and services (e.g., assertive
  community treatment (ACT) and supported employment for adults; multisys-
  temic treatment for children with conduct disorder) provide advantages for some
  conditions—particularly to promote rehabilitation and recovery in the most impaired individuals.

Examples of Public Health Interventions

There is growing interest in public health interventions in the disciplines of psychology,
psychiatry and social work, and an enhanced appreciation for the contributions public
health can make to the treatment of mental illness and addictions. Some of the most
promising interventions are listed below (Taylor et al. 2007):

- Screening and brief interventions delivered by primary care providers
- Employee assistance programs
- Workplace stress reduction programs
- Needle exchange
- Family education for the families of people with schizophrenia
- Respite care for family members providing demanding caregiving services
- Parent training

- Volunteering, especially in elderly volunteers
- Mass media campaigns that influence public attitudes about mental illness
- Participation in exercise to diminish the symptoms of depression
- Participation in groups such as Alcoholics Anonymous and Gamblers Anonymous

Assertive Community Treatment (ACT) is a stellar example of a cost effective treatment for persons with severe mental illness. ACT, developed as a way to respond to the needs of the large numbers of mentally ill people released from state psychiatric hospitals in the 1970s as a result of deinstitutionalization, is a team-based approach aimed at keeping clients connected with providers, reducing hospital admissions, and improving everyday functioning and quality of life. Assertive outreach, mobile treatment teams, and continuous treatment are essential components of ACT. Other important features include multidisciplinary staffing, integration of services, low client/staff ratios, home visits, a focus on ordinary problems in living, rapid access to services when required, and individualized treatment plans. This approach has been shown to be more effective than standard community care, hospital-based rehabilitation services, and typical case management. Multiple randomized clinical trials have documented that ACT, which targets the most expense high-end users of in-patient care, reduces the costs associated with hospital care at the same time it produces high levels of patient satisfaction (Marshall and Lockwood 1998).

It is clear that the needs of people with severe mental illness exceed the capacity of the mental health community to treat these needs. The Annapolis Coalition on the Behavioral Health Workforce has noted:

> Across the nation there is a high degree of concern about the state of the behavioral health workforce and pessimism about its future . . . . Most critically, there are significant concerns about the capability of the workforce to provide quality care. The majority of the workforce is uninformed about and unengaged in health promotion and prevention activities . . . . There is overwhelming evidence that the behavioral health workforce is not equipped in skills or in numbers to respond adequately to the changing needs of the American population (Annapolis Coalition 2007).

A public health approach to this workforce dilemma is having mental health services delivered by primary care providers, using the mental health workforce for consultation and support as is necessary. This collaborative care approach has been shown to be cost-effective in the treatment of depression, and it results in greater adherence to treatment goals and patient satisfaction (Hunkeler et al. 2000; Katon et al., 1995, 1996). This public health approach to chronic disease management that has been shown to be both efficient and effective (Wells et al. 2004). The integration of behavioral health services with primary care holds great promise as the most effective approach to addressing the mental health needs of the nation.

Areas of Future Research and Demonstration

Perhaps the most significant development in mental health in the past decade is the growing commitment to evidence-based practice. The fifth goal of the president's New Freedom Commission is that "excellent mental health care is delivered and research is accelerated," and it is difficult to receive NIH or SAMHSA funding without demonstrating a genuine commitment to evidence-based practice. Despite this commitment, it is increasing clear that much of what is taught in graduate programs in psychology, social work, and counseling programs is not relevant to the mental health needs of the communities in which many graduates will practice.

SAMHSA has promulgated five "tool kits" that support evidence-based practice: illness management and recovery, ACT, family psychoeducation, supported employment, and integrated dual diagnosis treatment for co-occurring disorders. More tool-kits are likely in the future. In addition, SAMHSA has developed a National Registry of Evidence-based Programs, and Practices (NREPP), a searchable database of interventions for the prevention and treatment of mental and substance use disorders designed to help consumers, agencies, organizations, and providers identify those practices for which a substantial evidentiary research base exists. Using the NREPP database, one can, for example, search for replicated programs offering mental health treatment for adolescents; such a search identifies six programs that have been rigorously evaluated and replicated at least once. NREPP classifies each program included in the database, in decreasing order of significance, as a model program, an effective program, or a promising program.

A parallel development has been the proliferation of practice guidelines for the treatment of mental and addictive disorders. For example, the Agency for Healthcare Research and Quality (AHRQ) homepage offers extensive information on evidence-based practice, outcomes and effectiveness, and clinical practice guidelines, including a link to the National Guidelines Clearinghouse (www.guidelines.gov), a remarkable repository of recommended guidelines for an enormous number of diseases and disorders, including mental illnesses and substance abuse. AHRQ also hosts an innovations exchange, a site where enthusiasts can share promising but still untested innovative practices. A similar resource is found in the Best Practices Registry for Suicide Prevention. It is likely that the coming years will see the continuing development and refinement of evidence-based practices, and the development of treatment methodologies that have grown out of rigorous randomized clinical trials.

Finally, it is likely that an ever-larger number of mental health professionals will seek out additional training in public health, and students will receive public health training to supplement their graduate education in one of the mental health professions. It is important to increase the number of individuals with both public health and mental health training in epidemiology, bioterrorism preparedness, and gerontology. Additional workforce training is especially important in gerontology if we are going to be able to adequately treat the mental health needs of the 71 million elderly adults projected to be living in the United States in 2030 (U.S. Census Bureau 2007).

Resources

Surgeon General's Report on Mental Health, http://www.surgeongeneral.gov/library/mentalhealth/home.html.
Mental Health: Culture, Race, Ethnicity, http://mentalhealth.samhsa.gov/cre/default.asp.
Presidents New Freedom Commission on Mental Health, http://www.mentalhealthcommission.gov.
The International Consortium in Psychiatric Epidemiology, http://www.hcp.med.harvard.edu/icpe.

National Institute of Mental Health: Psychiatric Epidemiology, http://www.mentalhealth.gov/ about/director/publications/psychiatric-epidemiology.shtml.

National Institute of Mental Health: Mental Health Topics, http://www.nimh.nih.gov/health/ topics/index.shtml.

National Alliance on Mental Illness, http://www.nami.org.

Mental Health America, http://www.nmha.org.

Suggested Reading

Kendler, K.S., and L.J. Eaves (Eds.). *Psychiatric Genetics.* Arlington, VA: American Psychiatric Publishing (2005).

New Freedom Commission on Mental Health. *Achieving the Promise: Transforming Mental Health Care in America: Final Report.* Rockville, MD: Department of Health and Human Services (2003). Publication SMA-03-3832.

Roberts, R.E., C.R. Roberts, and W. Chan. One year incidence of psychiatric disorders and associated risk factors among adolescents in the community. *J Child Psychol Psychiatry* 50 (2009):405–415.

Susser, E., S. Schwartz, A. Morabia, and E.J. Bromet. *Psychiatric Epidemiology: Searching for the Causes of Mental Disorders.* New York: Oxford University Press (2006).

Tsuang, M.T., and M. Tohen. *Textbook in Psychiatric Epidemiology.* New York: Wiley-Liss (2002).

Wang, P.S., O. Demler, and R. C. Kessler. The adequacy of treatment for serious mental illness in the United States. *Am J Public Health* (2002):92:92–98.

Wedding, D., P.H. DeLeon, and P. Olson. Mental Health Care in the United States. In: Olson, P. (Ed.) *Mental Health Systems Compared.* Illinois: Charles C. Thomas (2006).

References

Almog, M., S. Curtis, A. Copeland, and P. Congdon. Geographical Variation in Acute Psychiatric Admissions within New York City 1990–2000: Growing Inequalities in Service Use? *Social Science & Medicine* (2004):59:361–376.

American Psychiatric Association (APA). *Coexisting Severe Mental Disorders and Physical Illness.* Washington, D.C.: APA (2003). Available at http://www.psych.org/news_room/press_releases/ severementalillness0331.pdf.

American Psychiatric Association (APA). *Diagnostic and Statistical Manual of Mental Disorders, DSM-IV* (4th ed., 4th text rev.). Washington, D.C.: APA (2000).

Annapolis Coalition. *An Action Plan for Behavioral Health Workforce Development: A Framework for Discussion.* Rockville, MD: Department of Health and Human Services (2007). SAMHSA/ DHHS Publication 280-02-0302.

Ault, A. Generic Drugs: A Big Business Getting Bigger. *The Scientist* (2005):19:36.

Beyer, J.L, L. Taylor, K.R. Gersing, K. Ranga, and R. Krishnan. Prevalence of HIV Infection in a General Psychiatric Outpatient Population. *Psychosomatics* (2007):48:31–37.

Bresnahan, M., J. Boydell, R. Murray, and E. Susser. Temporal Variation in the Incidence, Course and Outcome of Schizophrenia. In: Murray, R.M., P.B. Jones, E. Susser, J. van Os, and M. Cannon, editors, *The Epidemiology of Schizophrenia.* Cambridge: Cambridge Univ. Press (2003).

Cournos, F., and K. McKinnon, HIV Seroprevalence among People with Severe Mental Illness in the United States: A Critical Review. *Clinical Psychology Review* (1997):17:259–269.

Csernansky, J.G., S. Joshi, L. Wang, et al. Hippocampal Morphometry in Schizophrenia by High Dimensional Brain Mapping. *Proc Natl Acad Sci USA* (1997):95(19):11406–11411.

Cole, M.G., J. McCusker, A. Ciampi, and E. Belzile. Risk Factors for Major Depression in Older Medical Inpatients: A Prospective Study. *Am J Geriatr Psychiatry* (2008):16:175–178.

Durlak, J.A., and A.M. Wells. Primary Prevention Mental Health Programs for Children and Adolescents: A Meta-Analytic Review. *Am Community Psychol* (1997):25:115–152.

Durlak, J., and A. Wells. Evaluation of Indicated Preventive Interventions (Secondary Prevention) Mental Health Programs for Children and Adolescents. *Am J Commun Psychology* (1998):26(5):775–802.

Eaton, W.W. *Medical and Psychiatric Comorbidity Over the Course of Life*. Washington, D.C.: American Psychiatric Publishing (2006).

Eisenberg, L. Psychiatry and Health in Low-Income Populations. *Compr Psychiatry* (1997):38(2):69–73.

Geddes, J.R., and S.M. Lawrie. Obstetric Complications and Schizophrenia: A Meta-Analysis. *Br J Psychiatry* (1995):67:786–793.

Goldney, R.D., D. Wilson, E. Dal Grande, L.J. Fisher, and A.C. McFarlane. Suicidal Ideation in a Random Community Sample: Attributable Risk Due to Depression and Psychosocial and Traumatic Events. *Aust N Z J Psychiatry* (2000):34:98–106.

Gottesman, I.I. *Schizophrenia Genesis: The Origins of Madness*. New York: W H Freeman (1991).

Hopper, K., G. Harrison, A. Janca, and N. Sartorius (Eds). *Recovery from Schizophrenia: An International Perspective: A Report from the WHO Collaborative Project, the International Study of Schizophrenia*. New York: Oxford Univ. Press (2007).

Horwath, E., R.S. Cohen, and M.M. Weissman. Epidemiology of Depressive and Anxiety Disorders. In: Tsuang, M.T. and M. Tohen, editors, *Textbook in Psychiatric Epidemiology* (2nd ed.). New York: Wiley-Liss (2002):389–426.

Hunkeler, E.M., J.F. Meresman, W.A. Hargreaves, et al. Efficacy of Nurse Telehealth Care and Peer Support in Augmenting Treatment of Depression in Primary Care. *Arch Fam Med* (2000):9:700–708.

Institute of Medicine. *Reducing Risks for Mental Disorders: Frontiers for Preventive Intervention Research*. Washington, D.C.: National Academy Press (1994).

Jadhav, S., R. Littlewood, A.G. Ryder, A. Chakraborty, S. Jain, and M. Barua. Stigmatization of Severe Mental Illness in India: Against the Simple Industrialization Hypothesis. *Indian J Psychiatry* (2007):49:189–194.

Katon, W., P. Robinson, M. Von Korff, et al. A Multifaceted Intervention to Improve Treatment of Depression in Primary Care. *Arch Gen Psychiatry* (1996):53:924–932.

Katon, W., M. Von Korff, E. Lin, et al. Collaborative Management to Achieve Treatment Guidelines: Impact on Depression in Primary Care. *JAMA* (1995):273:1026–1031.

Kessler, R.C., W.T. Chiu, L. Colpe, et al. The Prevalence and Correlates of Serious Mental Illness (SMI) in the National Comorbidity Survey Replication (NCS-R). In: Manderscheid, R.W. and J.T. Berry, editors, *Mental Health, United States, 2004*. Rockville, MD: Substance Abuse and Mental Health Services Administration (2004).

Kessler, R.C., K.A. McGonagle, S. Zhao, C.B. Nelson, M. Hughes, and S. Eshleman. Lifetime and 12-Month Prevalence of DSM-III-R Psychiatric Disorders in the United States. Results from the National Comorbidity Survey. *Arch Gen Psychiatry* (1994):51:8–19.

Kessler, R.C. and K.R. Merikangas. The National Comorbidity Survey Replication (NCS-R). *Int J Methods Psychiatr Res* (2004):13:60–68.

Kunugi, H., S. Nanko, and R.M. Murray. Obstetric Complications and Schizophrenia: Prenatal Underdevelopment and Subsequent Neurodevelopmental Impairment. *Br J Psychiatry* (2001):178(Suppl 40):s25–s29.

Lacasse, J.R., and J. Leo. Serotonin and Depression: A Disconnect between the Advertisements and the Scientific Literature. *PLoS Med* (2005):(12):e392.

Lehman, A.F., H.H. Goldman, L.B. Dixon, and R.C. Print. *Evidence-Based Mental Health Treatments and Services: Examples to Inform Public Policy*. Milbank Memorial Fund (2004).

Lopez, A.D., and C.C.J.L. Murray. The Global Burden of Disease, 1990–2020, *Nat Med* (1998):4:1241–1243.

Marshall, M., and A. Lockwood. Assertive Community Treatment for People with Severe Mental Disorders. *Cochrane Database of Systematic Reviews* (1998):(2):CD001089.

Mathers, C.D., and D. Loncar. Projections of Global Mortality and Burden of Disease from 2002 to 2030. *PLoS Med* (2006):3(11):e442.

Mental Health Commission. *President's New Freedom Commission on Mental Health* (2001). Available at http://mentalhealthcommission.gov/reports/FinalReport/FullReport.htm.

Mokdad, A.H., J.S. Marks, D.F. Stroup, and J.L. Gerberding. Actual Causes of Death in the United States, 2000. *JAMA* (2004):291:1238–1245.

Monahan, J. Clinical and Actuarial Predictions of Violence. In: Faigman, D., D. Kaye, M. Saks, and J. Sanders, editors, *Modern Scientific Evidence: The Law and Science of Expert Testimony* (1997):315.

Mortensen, P.B., E. Agerbo, T. Erikson, P. Qin, and N. Westergaard-Nielse. Psychiatric Illness and Risk Factors for Suicide in Denmark. *Lancet* (2000):355:9–12.

Moscicki, E.K. Epidemiology of Suicide. *Int Psychogeriatrics* (1995):7:137–148.

Murphy, J.M., N.J. Horton, R.R. Monson, N.M. Laird, A.M. Sobol, and A.H. Leighton. Cigarette Smoking in Relation to Depression: Historical Trends from the Stirling County Study. *Am J Psychiatry* (2003):160:1663–1669.

Newcomer, J.W., and D.W. Haupt. Schizophrenia, Metabolic Disturbance, and Cardiovascular Risk. *Medical and Psychiatric Comorbidity Over the Course of Life*. Arlington, VA: American Psychiatric Publishing (2006):331–349.

Nitzkin, J., and S.A. Smith. *Clinical Preventive Services in Substance Abuse and Mental Health Update: From Science to Services*. Rockville, MD: Center for Mental Health Services, Substance Abuse and Mental Health Services Administration (2004). DHHS Publication SMA 04-3906. Available at http://www.mentalhealthcommission.gov/reports/FinalReport/FullReport.htm.

Prince, M., V. Patel, S. Saxena, et al. No Health without Mental Health. *Lancet* (2007):370(9590): 859–877.

Qin, P., E. Agerbo, and P.B. Mortensen. Suicide Risk in Relation to Socioeconomic, Demographic, Psychiatric, and Familial Factors: A National Register–Based Study of All Suicides in Denmark, 1981–1997. *Am J Psychiatry* (2003):160:765–772.

Riolo, S.A., T.A. Nguyen, J.F. Greden, and C.A. King. Prevalence of Depression by Race/Ethnicity: Findings From the National Health and Nutrition Examination Survey III. *Am J Public Health* (2005):95:998–1000.

Robins, L.N., and D.A. Regier, editors, *Psychiatric Disorders in America: The Epidemiologic Catchment Area Study*, New York: Free Press (2001).

Saha, S., D. Chant, J. Welham, and J. McGrath. A Systematic Review of the Prevalence of Schizophrenia. *PLoS Med* (2005):2(5):e141.

Sartorius, N. Physical Illness in People with Mental Disorders. *World Psychiatry* (2007):6(1):3–4.

Siefert, K., P.J. Bowman, C.M. Heflin, S. Danziger, and D.R. Williams. Social and Environmental Predictors of Maternal Depression in Current and Recent Welfare Recipients. *Am J Orthopsychiatry* (2000):70:510–522.

Streissguth, A.P., H.M. Barr, J. Kogan, and F.L. Bookstein, *Understanding the Occurrence of Secondary Disabilities in Clients with Fetal Alcohol Syndrome (FAS) and Fetal Alcohol Effects (FAE), Final Report to the Centers for Disease Control and Prevention (CDC)*. Technical Report 96-06. Seattle: University of Washington, Fetal Alcohol and Drug Unit (1996).

Swartz, M.S., J.W. Swanson, V.A. Hiday, R. Borum, H.R. Wagner, and B.J. Burns. Violence and Severe Mental Illness: The Effects of Substance Abuse and Nonadherence to Medication. *Am J Psychiatry* (1998):155:226–223.

Swartz, M.S., J.W. Swanson, M.J. Hannon, et al. Five-Site Health and Risk Study Research Committee. Regular Sources of Medical Care among Persons with Severe Mental Illness at Risk of Hepatitis C Infection. *Psychiatr Serv* (2003):54(6):854–859.

Taylor, L., N. Taske, C. Swann, and S. Waller. *Public Health Interventions to Promote Positive Mental Health and Prevent Mental Health Disorders among Adults.* London: National Institute for Health and Clinical Excellence (2007).

Thornicroft, G. Most People with Mental Illness are Not Treated. *Lancet* (2007):307:807–808.

Tohen, M., and J. Angst. Epidemiology of Bipolar Disorder. In: Tsuang, M.T., et al., editors, *Textbook in Psychiatric Epidemiology* (2nd ed.). New York: John Wiley & Sons (2002).

Tsuang, M.T., and T.T. Ming. *Handbook in Psychiatric Epidemiology* (2nd ed.). New York: Wiley-Liss (2002).

U.S. Census Bureau. *International Database. Table 094. Midyear Population, by Age and Sex* (2007). Available at http://www.census.gov/population/www/projections/natdet-D1A.html.

U.S. Department of Health and Human Services (USDHHS). *Healthy People 2010* (2nd ed.). Washington, D.C.: U.S. Government Printing Office (2000).

Ustun, T.B. The Global Burden of Mental Disorders. *Am J Public Health* (1999):89:1315–1318.

Valenstein, E. *Blaming the Brain: The Truth about Drugs and Mental Health.* New York: Free Press (1998).

Warner, R. Time Trends in Schizophrenia: Changes in Obstetric Risk Factors with Industrialization. *Schizophr Bull* (1995):21(3):483–500.

Watanabe-Galloway, S., and W. Zhang. Analysis of U.S. Trends in Discharges from General Hospitals for Episodes of Serious Mental Illness, 1995–2002. *Psychiatric Services* (2007):58:496–502.

Wells, K., J. Miranda, M. L. Bruce, M. Alegria, and N. Wallerstein. Bridging Community Intervention and Mental Health Services Research. *Am J Psychiat* (2004):161(6):955–963.

Wessely, S., D. Castle, A.J. Douglas, and P.J. Taylor. The Criminal Career of Incident Cases of Schizophrenia. *Psychol Med* (1994):24:483–502.

Wyshak, G. Violence, Mental Health, Substance Abuse-Problems for Women Worldwide. *Health Care Women Int* (2000):21(7):631–639.

Yehuda, R. Post-Traumatic Stress Disorder. *N Engl J Med* (2002):346:108–114.

CHAPTER 17

NEUROLOGICAL DISORDERS (ICD-10 F00-F99, G00-G99, M00-M99, S00-T14)

Edwin Trevathan, M.D., M.P.H.

Introduction

Both developing countries and industrialized nations experience a major public health burden from chronic neurological conditions, which are a leading cause of lost productivity, disability, and premature death. Yet, until recently, the brain and central nervous system has been a "black box"—only visualized and studied extensively at autopsy in unusual and highly selected cases. With the routine use of brain imaging techniques (e.g., magnetic resonance imaging [MRI] scans) in industrialized nations, the "black box" has been opened by neuroscientists and by clinicians. Complex conditions are better understood, and classifications of neurological diseases are being changed—great news, but offering both opportunities and challenges for both epidemiologists and for public health professionals.

President George H. W. Bush declared the 1990s to be the "Decade of the Brain," (*Presidential Proclamation 6158* 1990) a gateway to the 21st century when views of neurological disease and brain function in our society would have both direct and indirect impact upon public health. Before the later half of the 20th century, most people viewed behavior, socialization, communication, and intelligence as matters of virtue (or lack thereof), personal style, individual choice, or even matters of religion or of the supernatural. Societies of developed countries in the 21st century generally understand the brain as the organ that determines the manifestations of communication, cognition, behavior, socialization, intelligence, and even personality. Therefore, disorders of the cerebral cortex are now more likely to be recognized as a disease; as a result public health officials have growing demands to address neurological disorders in the growing elderly population, and neurodevelopmental disorders among children. It is in this context of a growing societal interest in the brain and in its normal development, as well as its disease processes, that this chapter examines some of the more common neurological disorders from a public health perspective.

Chronic neurological disorders have neither received the attention of public health officials nor been the subject of intense epidemiological investigation and surveillance efforts, when compared with cancer and cardiovascular disease. Among the most common neurological disorders, such as Alzheimer's disease, Parkinson's disease, multiple sclerosis (MS), and the epilepsies, primary prevention efforts are either not possible or very limited because we have not identified sufficient modifiable risk factors.

Unintentional injuries resulting in traumatic brain injury and spinal cord injury offer significant opportunities for prevention. Likewise, the morbidity and loss of productivity caused by low back pain and carpal tunnel syndrome offer prevention opportunities yet to be fulfilled. The need for public health focused, epidemiological research to identify modifiable risk factors for Alzheimer's disease, Parkinson's disease, MS, and epilepsy should be emphasized, while opportunities for prevention of injuries and health promotion among people with disabilities should become a public health priority (see Table 17.1).

EPILEPSY (ICD-10 G40-G41)

Significance

The most common serious neurological disorder among children worldwide, (Editorial 1997; WHO 2003) epilepsy is the underlying condition that predisposes the individual to having repeated seizures. Operationally, epilepsy is defined as two or more seizures that are unprovoked. Excessive abnormal electrical discharges from cortical neurons and from specific structures adjacent to the cortex (e.g., the hippocampus) form the biological basis of seizures. Indeed, the manifestations of seizures are as varied as the functions of the cortex, defying simple rules for diagnosis, and often resulting in a delay in diagnosis of potentially serious epilepsy in some people, and the misdiagnosis of epilepsy among others (Duncan et al. 2006; Guerrini 2006).

Seizures that begin in a single region of the brain are classified as *partial seizures* and seizures that start all over both hemispheres at the beginning of the seizure are classified as *generalized seizures*. People with generalized seizures tend to have altered consciousness at the onset of their seizures, whereas people with partial seizures often do not have altered consciousness until the seizure has spread over a large enough portion of cortex to alter responsiveness (Duncan et al. 2006; Guerrini 2006).

Given the difficulties with accurate diagnosis of epilepsy noted among communities in both the United Kingdom (Chadwick and Smith 2002) and the United States, a few general observations regarding the diagnosis of epilepsy are important to note. First, the degree of alteration of conscious (or altered awareness) caused by a seizure is usually a function of the size of the cortical surface involved in the seizure; the larger the amount of cortex involved with the seizure, the greater the degree of altered awareness. If a large portion of the cortex is involved with the seizure, especially if both hemispheres are actively seizing, then consciousness is almost always impaired. Second, if the seizure starts in a single region of the brain, the manifestation of the seizure is a direct result of the disordered function of that brain region. For example, if the seizure starts in a region of the brain that normally moves the left thumb and fingers, then the seizure onset is manifested by twitching of the thumb and fingers on the left hand. Then, as the seizure spreads along the cortical surface, the seizure manifests those other cortical functions. For example, if the seizure starts in the area of brain that stores memories (e.g., the hippocampus within the temporal lobe), then the seizure onset is manifested by a sudden memory that emerges out of context—typically referred to as an *aura*. Seizures that begin in a specific region of the brain tend to be *stereotypic*, as that region of the brain when seizing has identical

Table 17.1. Neurological Diseases: Causes, Consequences, and High-Risk Groups

Disease	Causes	Consequences	High-Risk Groups
Epilepsy	Genetic factors Environmental exposures (often undefined) Cerebral malformations Trauma Encephalitis or meningitis Brain tumors or metastatic disease Hypoxic injury Strokes, vascular disease	Increased risk of premature death Increased risk of falls, burns, and/or drowning	Family history Central nervous system infections Cerebral malaria survivors Head injury Children with developmental delay Elderly with stroke
Parkinson's disease	Genetic factors Environmental triggers Viral infection Exposure to neurotoxins in the environment Occupational exposures to heavy metals	Motor impairment Cognitive decline Depression Increased long-term care needs Premature death	Family history Men Whites Certain occupations (e.g., teachers, health care workers, firefighters, farmers, welders)
Alzheimer's disease and other dementias	Genetic factors Long-term survival of chronic disease treatments Traumatic brain injury Multi-infarct strokes Diabetes, hypertension	Premature death Cognitive decline Increased long-term care needs Depression	Family history Elderly
Cerebral palsy	Prematurity Very low birthweight High birthweight Birth trauma (e.g., anoxia) Multiple births	Feeding difficulties Motor disability Social isolation	Premature births Twins and multiple births Family history Neonatal hyperbilirubinemia
Autism spectrum disorders	Genetic factors Potential environmental exposures	Social isolation Anxiety Impaired communication	Family history Males Premature births Advanced parental age

(continued on next page)

Table 17.1. (*continued*)

Disease	Causes	Consequences	High-Risk Groups
ALS	Genetic factors Exposures to lead, mercury, and other heavy metals	Progressive weakness Paralysis Respiratory impairment Premature death	Family history Men Older adults
MS	Genetic factors Viral or other infectious diseases	Intermittent motor, language, and/or cognitive impairment Long-term care needs Depression Premature death	Family history Females Young adults
Guillain-Barré syndrome	Genetic factors Autoimmune response triggered by a recent viral or bacterial infection	Temporary weakness and paralysis Respiratory failure Pneumonia Deep vein thrombosis	Family history Whites Living in northern latitudes
Tic disorders and Tourette syndrome	Genetic factors Potential environmental exposures	School failure—increased risk Social isolation Behavior problems	Family history Males
Traumatic brain injury and spinal cord injury	Falls Transportation-related injuries and automobile crashes Sports or recreation injuries Assaults Alcohol and drug use	Paralysis and death Cognitive deficits[a] Epilepsy[a] Dementia[a] Depression Complications of immobility Deep vein thrombosis	Alcohol and drug abusers Elderly Children and adolescents Men Lower social/economic persons Construction, farming, roofing, and logging occupations Motor cyclists Those who fail to wear seat belts

Table 17.1. (*continued*)

Disease	Causes	Consequences	High-Risk Groups
ADHD	Genetic factors Potential environmental exposures Some cases caused by brain injury (e.g., strokes, epilepsy, head injuries)	Poor self esteem Anxiety Conduct disorder Depression Sleep problems Substance abuse	Males
Carpal tunnel syndrome	Repetitive hand or wrist movements Wrist trauma Diabetes, hypothyroidism Pregnancy	Impaired hand use Lost income and job loss	Workers who engage in repetitive fine motor movements (e.g., typists). Food-processing workers, roofers, carpenters, and mill workers Pregnant women
Low back pain	Heavy lifting Abdominal obesity Cigarette smoking Premature menopause Genetic factors	Disability Lost income Time away from work	Occupations with heavy lifting (e.g., nursing, truck driving, warehouse, farm, lumber, construction workers, miners) Caregivers of disabled
Migraine and tension headaches	Genetic factors Depression Stress Environmental triggers (e.g., food)	School absence Lost income Time away from work Depression	Family history of headache Women Low social and economic class

[a] Complications of brain injury only.

characteristics at the beginning of each seizure, helping experienced clinicians make a diagnosis (Duncan et al. 2006; Guerrini 2006).

Clinicians often place excessive emphasis on the electroencephalogram (EEG) in the diagnosis of epilepsy. Unfortunately, the EEG is often normal between seizures—especially among people with partial seizures whose seizures start in areas of cortex folded far from the scalp. The history, taken by an experienced clinician who hypothesizes the location of the seizure onset from listening to the patient and the observers, can then, in combination with an EEG, make a diagnosis and minimize delays in proper treatment (Duncan et al. 2006; Guerrini 2006).

There are many types of epilepsy, each with different clinical manifestations and possible outcomes and comorbid conditions. For example, benign rolandic epilepsy tends to undergo spontaneous remission in almost all children who have this disorder but may also be associated with specific learning disorders (Panayiotopoulos et al. 2008). On the other end of the severity spectrum, Lennox-Gastaut syndrome is a profoundly severe epilepsy syndrome with children typically suffering multiple daily seizures that do not respond to treatment, and with almost universal intellectual disability and an increased risk of premature death (Shields 2004). The needs of people with severe epilepsy syndromes, who have high risk of severe disability, are great. Merging the populations of people with severe epilepsy syndromes and those with benign epilepsy to make general statements about epilepsy has oversimplified this heterogeneous class of disorders, impaired proper planning for services, and may delay public health needs for people with severe epilepsy.

Descriptive Epidemiology

The prevalence of epilepsy, using a variety of methods, has been estimated at about 6–9 per 1000 in developed countries of Europe, Asia, and in the United States. Using different methods, the prevalence of epilepsy in both Rochester, Minnesota, and in Atlanta, GA, has been estimated at approximately 7 per 1000; extrapolated to the total U.S. population, an estimated 2 million Americans have active epilepsy (Yeargin-Allsopp et al. 2008).

The highest incidence of new-onset epilepsy is among the very young and the elderly—important clues as to the two broad categories of etiologic factors. Between birth and age 65 years, the highest incidence occurs during the first year of life, with fairly high incidence during the first few years of life. Despite the fairly constant incidence of new-onset epilepsy between school-age and age 65 years, the prevalence remains fairly constant, as the new cases tend to equal those in the general population who experience spontaneous remission, as well as an increased mortality rate experienced by people with severe epilepsy. Beginning at age 65 years, the incidence of new-onset epilepsy rises sharply, as the aging population develops epilepsy as a secondary condition—associated largely from strokes and vascular disease, dementias, and cancer (Hauser, Annegers, and Rocca 1996).

That people with epilepsy have an increased risk of death, with elevated overall standardized mortality ratios (SMRs) on the order of 2.5, has been known for many decades. The SMRs are highest for childhood-onset symptomatic epilepsy syndromes such as Lennox-Gastaut syndrome and other severe epilepsy syndromes associated with other neurological conditions such as cerebral palsy and/or intellectual disability. The reasons for excessive mortality among people with epilepsy are only partially understood. Seizures causing falls, burns, and/or drowning are not rare, especially in developing countries where adequate seizure control is hampered by access to basic antiseizure drugs (Hughes 2009; Tomson, Nashef, and Ryvlin 2008).

"Sudden unexplained death in epilepsy" (SUDEP), which is most common among young adults with intractable epilepsy (seizures despite optimal antiseizure medication), has an incidence of about 2 to 10 per 1000 person-years—many times higher than the risk of sudden death among age-matched people in the general population without epilepsy. These deaths typically occur during sleep at night. SUDEP is not totally explained by coexisting pulmonary or cardiac disease but whether cardiac arrhythmias play a role is not clear. Available data strongly suggest that seizures themselves are directly linked to SUDEP, as there appears to be a dose–response relationship between the number of seizures per unit time and whether the patient has experienced previous status epilepticus. Regardless, experts agree that having no seizures on antiseizure medication significantly reduces the risk of SUDEP (Hughes 2009; Tomson, Nashef, and Ryvlin 2008).

Causes

Among infants and children who have onset of epilepsy, genetic risk factors are the most important class of risk factors. Some forms of epilepsy, such as childhood absence epilepsy, benign rolandic epilepsy, and juvenile myoclonic epilepsy are clearly genetic disorders, with probably a minimal role for environmental triggers (Lagae 2008). Still, other forms of epilepsy, such as partial epilepsy of mesial temporal lobe origin, are likely due to the combination of environmental triggers (mostly yet to be discovered) in a genetically predisposed individuals (Aronica and Gorter 2007). Much has been learned about susceptibility genes over the last few years, and gene–environmental interactions among genetically susceptible people will require much more study over the next several decades (Tan, Mulley, and Scheffer 2006).

In general, anything that damages, alters the structure, or inflames the cerebral cortex can cause epilepsy. Therefore, stroke, cerebral malformations, trauma, encephalitis, brain tumors or metastatic disease in the brain, and hypoxic injury to the cortex can all cause seizures and epilepsy. However, not all people who experience the same insult from a stroke or other injury to the cortex, or encephalitis, or tumor have seizures—raising the strong possibility that susceptibility genes play a role in these situations as well (Diaz-Arrastia et al. 2003).

Epilepsy associated with developmental regression during the first 18 months of life is a devastating feature of many different neurodevelopmental disorders (Blume 2004; Trevathan 2004). For those disorders that are well-known, a pattern of normal-appearing development preceding the regression typically occurs even when an obvious preexisting genetic, or even cortical structural abnormality occurs, as in the case of Rett syndrome. Over the last several years, vaccines occurring at or around the time of regression at 4–18 months have been blamed by some. However, the biologic plausibility of a vaccine-induced etiology is not very strong for almost all of these cases. For example, the myoclonic epilepsy and developmental regression (with encephalopathy) attributed by some in the 1980s to the pertussis vaccine is caused by the *SCN1A* gene mutation that causes severe myoclonic epilepsy of infancy (Dravet syndrome)—regardless of vaccine history (Berkovic et al. 2006).

Febrile seizures, especially febrile status epilepticus, are known to be associated with development of epilepsy—especially partial epilepsy of temporal lobe origin. However, most children with febrile seizures and febrile status epilepticus do not develop later epilepsy, and the relationship may be due to the underlying genes (or infections) causing the febrile seizures rather than the actual seizures themselves (Scheffer et al. 2007).

Prevention and Control

Several vaccines are likely effective in preventing epilepsy such as those that prevent *Hemophilus influenzae* meningitis, meningococcal meningitis, pertussis, and rubella, with their associated cortical inflammation and injury and/or cortical malformations (e.g., rubella) (Murthy and Prabhakar 2008). Folic acid fortification of the grain supply and preconception supplementation has significantly reduced the incidence of neural tube defects and associated hydrocephalus (from Chiari II malformations) (CDC 2008), but we do not know if other brain malformations that increase the risk of seizures have been reduced by folic acid fortification and supplementation. Prevention of congenital infections such as cytomegalovirus, herpes, and toxoplasmosis also prevents serious brain damage with associated intellectual disabilities and epilepsy. Prevention of head injuries likely could, and perhaps already does, have an impact upon the onset of epilepsy and associated neurological comorbidities—especially among adolescents. Among older adults opportunities for preventing cerebrovascular disease could have major impact on the prevention of associated epilepsy.

Perhaps the greatest untapped opportunity for prevention of the consequences of serious epilepsy is improved rapid diagnosis and appropriate early treatment for epilepsy—especially among children. Prevention of the excessive morbidity and mortality associated with status epilepticus by prompt treatment of prolonged seizures in emergency rooms and in communities should be a priority. Future epidemiological studies should emphasize the role of gene–environmental interactions and the identification of potentially modifiable risk factors for specific epilepsy syndromes.

PARKINSON'S DISEASE (ICD-10 G20)

Significance

Parkinson's disease is a common age-related neurodegenerative disorder that has growing worldwide impact as our population ages. The pathological marker for Parkinson's disease is a loss of pigmented neurons, especially with in the substantia nigra, with associated α-synuclean–positive inclusion bodies (Lewy bodies). Clinical manifestations of the neuronal loss within the substantia nigra and associated regions of the extrapyramidal system include a characteristic resting tremor, slowness in initiating movements, dystonia, and sometimes chorea, tics, and myoclonus. Most people with Parkinson's disease experience cognitive decline associated with dysfunction of prefrontal cortical regions. Depression commonly occurs among people with Parkinson's disease. People with Parkinson's disease also experience an increased risk of psychosis. Dementia occurs in up to 80% of people with advanced Parkinson's disease (Gelb, Oliver, and Gilman 1999).

Although we now know that the neuropathological basis of the classical features of Parkinson's disease is the unique neuronal loss within the substantia nigra and the targeted disruption of dopamine within the brain, Dr. James Parkinson's description from 1817 remains the foundation of Parkinson's disease diagnostic criteria. The presence of Parkinson's classic "pill-rolling" resting tremor, bradykinesia, rigidity, and postural instability usually make the diagnosis easy for most experienced clinicians. Standardized diagnostic criteria have been proposed (Gelb, Oliver, and Gilman 1999), and high-resolution MRI of the brain offers the potential to help distinguish Parkinson's disease from similar clinical conditions such as progressive supranuclear palsy, Alzheimer's disease, and basal ganglia vascular disease (Yekhlef et al. 2003).

Despite a well-understood pathophysiology, the discovery of susceptibility genes and hypothesized environmental triggers, the causes of Parkinson's disease are largely unknown (Yang, Wood, and Latchman 2009). With more effective treatment of symptoms, the degree of severity of disabling symptoms can be reduced in most people with Parkinson's disease (Lewitt 2008), but the needs of patients who are seeking greater participation and opportunities are growing. A comprehensive public health response requires better population-based data on Parkinson's disease outcomes, epidemiological research to identify potentially modifiable risk factors, and community-based programs that intersect our public health system with the medical needs of people with Parkinson's disease.

Descriptive Epidemiology

Within the United States alone, more than 1 million people currently have Parkinson's disease, and the prevalence is expected to triple over the next half-century as the population ages. The average age-adjusted incidence rate in the United States is approximately 20 per 100,000 per year. Among the 65- to 84-year-olds, the incidence is more than 500 per 100,000 per year and is very low before the age of 50 years. Rarely, Parkinson's disease occurs among people in their third decade. Several studies have reported that age-adjusted incidence and prevalence are higher among men than among women, and higher among whites than among African Americans. Studies from Rochester, MN, have not shown significant changes in the incidence over time (Tanner and Goldman 1996; Baldereschi et al. 2000).

Causes

A viral encephalitis epidemic in 1919, and a subsequent sequelae of parkinsonism provided the first demonstration that viral encephalitis can cause selective damage to the substantia nigra neurons. However, evidence that viral etiologies play a role in sporadic idiopathic Parkinson's disease has not been forthcoming (Tanner and Goldman 1996). In the early 1980s Parkinson's disease developed very rapidly among a few IV drug users who injected a synthetic compound, MPTP, with pharmacologic properties similar to heroin (Langston 1996). Pesticides have been of particular interest to investigators over the last few years, in part because of the similarities of some pesticides to MPTP. Farming or rural living has been identified as a possible risk factor for Parkinson's disease, adding potential support to the hypothesis that pesticide exposure may be causally linked to its development. Paraquat exposure in Taiwan and increased brain levels of dieldrin, as well as exposure to other herbicides, insecticides, alkylated phosphates, wood preservatives, and organochlorines, have all been reported to be associated with a higher risk of Parkinson's disease (Hatcher, Pennell, and Miller 2008).

Other than farming, some other occupations have been associated with a higher risk of Parkinson's disease. Teachers, health care workers, firefighters, and workers chronically exposed to heavy metals have had higher reported rates. However, these associations have not been consistently reported in all studies (Tanner and Goldman 1996). The prevalence among male welders has been reported significantly higher than among controls from the general population, and has been reproduced in several studies. The clinical features of Parkinson's disease among welders has been found to be indistinguishable from idiopathic Parkinson's disease, other than age of onset, suggesting that an exposure experienced by welders might be a risk factor for Parkinson's disease (Racette et al. 2005). The reason for higher risk among welders is unclear, but some authors have hypothesized that excessive exposure to solvents, pesticides, iron, copper, and/or manganese may play a role.

Genetic and hereditary susceptibility factors for Parkinson's disease have been important areas of research for several years. Twin studies have shown no difference in concordance between monozygotic and dizygotic twins. Some authors have suggested that the approximately 10% of people with Parkinson's disease who have one or more affected relatives may represent shared environmental influences rather than classic heritable disease. Genetic susceptibility to environmental neurotoxins could play an important etiologic role (Schapira 2006). Rare autosomal dominant forms have been found with linkage studies among large kindred's with Parkinson's disease, but it seems unlikely that these autosomal dominant or autosomal recessive genes contribute significantly to the burden of disease in the general population (Yang, Wood, and Latchman 2009; Schapira 2006).

Prevention and Control

There remains no primary treatment to reverse the degeneration of the substantia nigra neurons, although some experts have hypothesized that stem cell transplants may be effective. The functional status of people with Parkinson's disease can be improved with symptomatic therapy and with rehabilitation that takes the built environment into consideration. Replacing lost dopamine through administration of levodopa, and/or treatment of dopamine agonists (e.g., bromocriptine) can offer significant symptomatic relief. Unfortunately, over time, the dopamine agonists become less effective, and among some people with Parkinson's disease, long-term therapy with dopamine agonists can be associated with emergence of dyskinesias and/or psychiatric adverse effects (Lewitt 2008).

Genetic–environmental interactions, targeting environmental toxins requires additional study. Whether epigenetic mechanisms can play a role in Parkinson's disease is beginning to be discussed in the literature, and epidemiologists may soon need to consider epigenetic mechanisms in large-scale epidemiological studies.

ALZHEIMER'S DISEASE AND DEMENTING DISORDERS (ICD-10 G30-G32)

Significance

Dementia is a major public health problem, with growing dementia prevalence rates, that will demand a commiserate public health response. In concert with an aging population and improvements in the treatment of chronic diseases in industrialized nations, an increase in the prevalence of dementia is putting a burden upon not only those who have dementia, but also upon their caregivers within families and throughout communities. Previous generations typically regarded dementia in the elderly as an expected part of the aging process. But now that dementia is recognized by society as a brain disease, patients, families, and communities are demanding solutions to the problems associated with dementia. As treatments that can delay the onset of symptoms among those who are at high risk are developed and marketed, public health will need to play a role in ensuring that these technologies are utilized to benefit entire communities, while balancing health priorities and addressing major social determinants of disease, keeping in mind the growing impact of chronic dementia upon society.

Descriptive Epidemiology

The burden of dementing disorders upon society is enormous. Based upon 2000 census data, approximately 4.5 million people with Alzheimer's disease lived in the United States in 2000. The authors estimated that Alzheimer's disease occurs in about 5% of people between the ages of 65 and 74 years, about 17% of people between the ages of 75 and 84 years, and about 45% of people 85 years and older (Alzheimer's Association 2008). Assuming current trends, the prevalence will almost triple, with approximately 13.2 million having Alzheimer's disease in the United States by 2050, with estimates ranging from 11.3 million to 16 million (Ziegler-Graham et al. 2008). There is a slightly higher prevalence of Alzheimer's disease among women than among men (1.6:1) in several studies, and African Americans in the United States may have slightly higher prevalence rates of Alzheimer's disease than whites. The prevalence of Alzheimer's disease is high, but it reflects only about half of the overall burden of dementia from all causes upon society (Szekely et al. 2008).

About 20% of dementia is due to the effects of vascular disease—specifically small vessel cerebrovascular disease for which genetically mediated susceptibility combined with other factors such as diabetes mellitus, hypertension, and cigarette smoking seem to play a role. The incidence of vascular dementia is estimated to be about 4.2 per 1000 people older than 65 years each year (Knopman 2007).

Causes

Although the genetic risk factors for Alzheimer's disease have received considerable attention, probably less than 5% of Alzheimer's disease is associated with classic autosomal dominant inheritance, and there is considerable complexity in the genetic susceptibility for Alzheimer's disease. There is a strong association between the presence of the epsilon 4 (E4) allele of the apolipoprotein E (*APOE*) gene and late-onset Alzheimer's disease. The E4 allele has been associated with increased beta-amyloid deposition in susceptible brain regions associated with Alzheimer's disease (Bertram and Tanzi 2008).

Vascular disease appears to be a risk factor for Alzheimer's disease, but the relationship is complex as there is often coexistence of neuropathological findings of multi-infarct dementia and Alzheimer's disease in the same patients (Knopman 2007). Insulin resistance syndrome and associated conditions (e.g., hypertension, type 2 diabetes mellitus) are associated with age-related memory impairment and Alzheimer's disease. Raising plasma insulin to levels associated with insulin resistance causes increased levels of beta-amyloid and inflammatory agents—the very pathological findings known to impair memory associated with Alzheimer's disease. Therefore, the potential causal relationship between insulin resistance and AD seems biologically plausible (Craft 2006).

Low to moderate amounts of alcohol likely reduce the accumulation of cardiovascular pathology, as well as potentially exert a protective effect on cognitive function and reduce risk for dementia (Collins et al. 2009). Studies of cigarette smoking have not provided consistent results, with some studies showing no relationship, some studies showing a modest increase in risk, and still others suggesting a differential survival effect with smokers dying earlier and, therefore, having less time exposure to the risk of Alzheimer's disease with advanced age (Anstey et al. 2007). Although aluminum is a neurotoxin, and was previously hypothesized as being a risk factor for Alzheimer's disease, some experts have suggested that aluminum is not a likely causal risk factor for Alzheimer's disease (Doll 1993; Munoz 1998). The issue of whether aluminum might play a causal role in Alzheimer's disease is not yet settled, as some authors continue to argue that aluminum seems to play a role in amyloid aggregation and the potential pathogenic mechanisms of Alzheimer's disease (Drago, Bolognin, and Zatta 2008).

Prevention and Control

Considerable attention has been given to potential protective factors for Alzheimer's disease. Among those with the APOE E4 allele nonsteroidal anti-inflammatory drugs may be associated with reduced risk of Alzheimer's disease, but no protective effect has been consistently documented in the general population. The potential protective effect of nonsteroidal anti-inflammatory drugs in susceptible subpopulations may deserve additional study (Sano, Grossman, and Van Dyk 2008). Studies of hormone replacement therapy in women have not demonstrated a consistent impact on the risk of developing Alzheimer's disease (Sano et al. 2008).

Some people with Alzheimer's disease pathology do not have clinical diagnosis of dementia; the reasons why are not clear, but these protected individuals seem to have more cognitive reserve. Studies to determine whether individuals with relative protection from clinical dementia who have Alzheimer's disease pathology have common potentially protective characteristics may be helpful (Whitwell et al. 2007).

We will need to intervene in susceptible individuals before they have signs and symptoms of dementia if we are to significantly reduce the impact of Alzheimer's disease in the general population. Therefore, the use of genomics as a public health tool will be essential in identifying susceptible subpopulations. If we can delay the progression of Alzheimer's disease by five years or more, there would be a significant reduction in the prevalence of severe dementia—a major public health intervention. Future studies will need to consider the use of large-scale interventions in genetically susceptible individuals (Sloane et al. 2002).

CEREBRAL PALSY(ICD-10 G80-G83)

Significance

Cerebral palsy is an old term that is now used to describe a broad category of nonprogressive, but often changing with developmental stage, motor impairment syndromes due to abnormalities of brain structure and/or function with onset during early stages of brain development (Stanley, Blair, and Alberman 2000). The cerebral palsy syndromes each have different underlying neuropathology (Folkerth 2007). Most people with cerebral palsy have *spasticity*, or significant resistance to passive movement that becomes functionally worse as the velocity of movement increases. The spasticity alone can be limiting or disabling regardless of weakness, but typically the spasticity and weakness go hand in hand.

Between 18% and 45% of children with cerebral palsy have spastic diplegia, with *diplegia* referring to weakness of all four limbs, with the legs more severely affected than the arms. People with spastic diplegia typically have some trunk weakness and problems with balance. Infants with spastic diplegia often have normal or reduced muscle tone (resistance to passive movement) for the first few weeks or months of life and then develop obvious spasticity by the end of the first year (Stanley, Blair, and Alberman 2000). Spastic diplegia is a clinical diagnosis but often is associated with brain MRI abnormalities in the "watershed" region between the distribution of the anterior cerebral artery and the middle cerebral artery, and/or periventricular leukomalacia (Robinson et al. 2009).

Spastic hemiplegic cerebral palsy occurs in about a third of children with cerebral palsy and is characterized by hand and arm greater than leg weakness contralateral to the side of the brain lesion. Spastic hemiplegic cerebral palsy is often the result of an underlying intraventricular hemorrhage, or a (middle cerebral artery distribution) stroke that occurred during intrauterine life, or very early in the neonatal period.

Spastic quadriplegic cerebral palsy accounts for about 10%–30% of cases of cerebral palsy and is associated with severe impairment of both arms and legs—legs typically more severely affected. *Double hemiplegia* has been a term used to describe some people with quadriplegia whose arms bilaterally are more severely affected than their legs. Brain malformations are common causes of quadriplegia. Hypoxic–ischemic encephalopathy is a cause of a minority of cases of spastic quadriplegia cerebral palsy (Stanley, Blair, and Alberman 2000).

Cerebral palsy is often associated with intellectual disability. The frequency of associated intellectual disability and the severity of the intellectual disability is typically less with the types of cerebral palsy that involve smaller areas of cortical abnormality (e.g., spastic diplegia) and almost uniformly present and severe among those whose cerebral palsy is a reflection of widespread cortical dysfunction and/or damage (e.g., spastic quadriplegia). Coexisting morbidities including feeding problems, visual impairment, and epilepsy often exacerbate the level of disability and complicate the medical management and impair the community participation of people with cerebral palsy (Yeargin-Allsopp et al. 2008).

Descriptive Epidemiology

The prevalence of cerebral palsy among school-age children in recent reports has ranged from about 2–4 per 1000, with the majority of studies reporting a prevalence of about 2–3 per 1000. Boys are more likely to have cerebral palsy than are girls, with a sex ratio of 1.1:1 to 1.5:1. The relationship between race and the risk of cerebral palsy is complex. Studies in metropolitan Atlanta have demonstrated that African American children had lower prevalence rates of cerebral palsy than did white children if their birthweight was less than 2500 grams, but higher rates if their birthweight was 2500 grams or more. Cerebral palsy prevalence rates from three different states using a common methodology have recently been reported, with similar rates in Georgia, Wisconsin, and Alabama and an overall prevalence rate of 3.3 per 1000. The prevalence rate of cerebral palsy among 8-year-old children in 2002 in Georgia was 3.8 per 1000, higher than the rates reported from Georgia in the 1990s. Ongoing surveillance to determine if the increase is a trend is essential (Yeargin-Allsopp et al. 2008; Winter et al. 2002).

Causes

Prematurity is the most common risk factor for cerebral palsy. A bimodal distribution of birthweight among children with CP has been reported—one peak at about 1000 grams, and a second peak at about 3000 grams. About one-fourth of children with cerebral palsy were born weighing less than 1500 grams, compared with about 1% of the general population. About half of children with cerebral palsy were born weighing less than 2500 grams, compared with about 5% of the general population. Children from multiple births have a high risk of CP, primarily associated with their increased risk of prematurity. Death of a co-twin *in utero* is a significant risk factor for cerebral palsy. Children with cerebral palsy have higher rates of birth defects than do children in the general population (Yeargin-Allsopp et al. 2008; Allen 2008).

Prevention and Control

Cerebral palsy primary prevention largely depends upon efforts to prevent prematurity (Yeargin-Allsopp et al. 2008). Magnesium sulfate given to women at risk for preterm birth has been shown to offer neuroprotection to the fetus and has significant potential for reducing the rates of prematurity-associated cerebral palsy (Rouse et al. 2008). A recent Cochrane Collaboration analysis suggested that the number of at-risk women needed to treat to prevent one baby from having cerebral palsy is 63 (95% confidence interval 43–87) (Doyle et al. 2009).

Opportunities for secondary prevention abound. Children with cerebral palsy benefit from physical therapy and from improved nutrition that considers their higher caloric requirements. For some children, the treatment of epilepsy and/or the management of speech and language impairment can significantly improve quality of life and enhance community participation.

AUTISM SPECTRUM DISORDERS (ICD-10 F84)

Significance

Autism spectrum disorders, which include autistic disorder, Asperger's syndrome, and pervasive developmental disorder not otherwise specified are a heterogeneous group of developing brain disorders, or neurodevelopmental disorders. Each of these broad categories of autism spectrum disorders subsumes a large number of different disorders, that although quite different from one another, typically have three common characteristics: (1) abnormal language, (2) impaired reciprocal social interaction, and (3) abnormal behavior and restricted interests. People with autistic disorder have classic abnormalities of language, severe impairment of reciprocal social behavior, and severely restricted behaviors and interests. People with Asperger's syndrome have relative preservation of cognitive, language, and communication skills (Yeargin-Allsopp et al. 2008; Rapin and Tuchman 2006).

The known causes of autism spectrum disorders tend to share some common features—genetic predisposition to autism spectrum disorder even though the children may appear normal for the first few months of life and then experience autistic regression. The 4:1 male:female ratio has long informed experts of the underlying genetic influences. Twin studies have long demonstrated evidence of the strong genetic component for autism. Likewise, known genetic disorders such as fragile X syndrome, tuberous sclerosis, untreated phenylketonuria, Down's syndrome, and neurofibromatosis all have high rates of co-existing autism. Over the last two decades neuroscience research has clearly demonstrated that autism is not primarily caused by mechanisms that cause brain damage, but rather by intricate genetic influences that interact with environmental events, with resulting dysfunction of the widespread neural networks that interconnect language, social, emotional, and other regions of the cerebral cortex (Yeargin-Allsopp et al. 2008; Walsh, Morrow, and Rubenstein 2008; Rapin and Tuchman 2008).

Over the last few years, some parents who witness their normal-appearing children developmentally regress during the first two years of life, when vaccines are frequently administered, have blamed vaccines for their child's autism. Multiple studies have now been completed that have not demonstrated any causal relationship between autism and vaccines, and yet the concerns remain for some parents who find it difficult to believe that they witnessed a temporal relationship that was genetically driven and not caused by exposure to vaccines (Gerber and Offit 2009). Meanwhile, the number of studies documenting the genetic basis for autism has grown, so that now several new susceptibility genes have been determined over the last few years—susceptibility genes that will need to be studied further to investigate other possible gene–environmental interactions (Abrahams and Geschwind 2008).

Descriptive Epidemiology

The prevalence of autism spectrum disorders over the last few years, using *Diagnostic and Statistical Manual of Mental Disorders, Fourth Edition* diagnostic criteria have been reported at approximately 6 per 1000 school-aged children, or about 1 in 150 children (ADDMN 2007). All population-based studies have documented a significantly higher prevalence among boys than among girls. Debate exists regarding whether the prevalence of autism spectrum disorders now is higher than 20 years ago when the case definitions were different, and when societal beliefs regarding the origins of behavioral abnormalities were different, and when special education programs for children with autism spectrum disorders were more limited, or simply nonexistent (Yeargin-Allsopp et al. 2008; ADDMN 2007; Trevathan and Shinnar 2006). It will be very difficult, if not impossible, to determine whether the high prevalence rates of autism now are due only to increased recognition, although some of the increased prevalence seems to be clearly attributed to diagnostic substitution (Shattuck 2006). Regardless, it is now clear that autism spectrum disorders represent a common group of neurodevelopmental disorders that constitute a significant public health and educational concern in the United States and throughout the world.

Causes

Virtually all studies of autism spectrum disorders have demonstrated much higher rates among boys, typically with a male:female ratio of about 4:1 (Rapin and Tuchman 2008; Abrahams and Geschwind 2008; ADDMN 2007; Trevathan and Shinnar 2006).

Although most studies have not demonstrated a difference in autism prevalence between whites and African Americans, data from ongoing surveillance in metropolitan Atlanta has suggested that African-American children with autism spectrum disorders are more likely to have other comorbid developmental disabilities (Yeargin-Allsopp et al. 2003). An increase in autism prevalence rates among higher socioeconomic groups may have been confounded by enhanced diagnostic recognition among more affluent families, but some studies have continued to report higher rates among higher socioeconomic groups (Croen, Grether, and Selvin 2002).

Paternal age has recently received considerable attention as a risk factor for autism spectrum disorders (Croen, Grether, and Selvin 2002; Durkin et al. 2008). A variety of risk factors currently being investigated include various hormonal factors, immune mechanisms, and potential environmental toxins (Yeargin-Allsopp et al. 2008; Roberts et al. 2007). A flurry of discovery of new susceptibility genes has laid the groundwork for several years of future research in gene–environmental interactions (Abrahams and Geschwind 2008).

Prevention and Control

At present, there are no proven treatments for autism spectrum disorders. However, early identification of children with signs and symptoms of language delays/regression and so-cial impairment, and enrollment in early intervention programs before the age of three years seems to offer improved developmental outcomes in some children. Therefore, com-munity programs aimed at early diagnosis and intervention are currently a focus of public health, educational, and pediatric interventions.

Epidemiological research over the next few years will focus on gene–environmental interactions, while population-based surveillance must be sustained in order to monitor trends. As children with autism enter adulthood, addressing the transition needs and perhaps their unique health promotion needs will be important.

AMYOTROPHIC LATERAL SCLEROSIS AND MOTOR NEURON DISEASE (ICD-10 G12.2)

Significance

Amyotrophic lateral sclerosis (ALS) is the most common motor neuron disease worldwide. Also known as Lou Gehrig's disease, the pathological features of ALS are the slow, steadily progressive, and selective cell death of motor neurons in the spinal cord and the lower brain stem, whose axons innervate skeletal muscles of the body and the face and oral pharynx. In addition, ALS is also associated with some motor neuron loss in the primary motor area of the cerebral cortex —the precentral gyrus, whose neurons project to the spinal cord mo-tor neurons. The devastating clinical manifestations of the progressive cell death of spinal cord and precentral gyrus motor neurons are muscle wasting and weakness that typically starts in one location and then spreads throughout the affected limb, then typically crosses over to affect the contralateral limb, and them spreads throughout the body. Progressive weakness, paralysis, and death usually from respiratory failure typically occurs within about three years of the onset of symptoms (Rocha et al. 2005; Andrews 2009).

Descriptive Epidemiology

Several authors classify ALS into three separate forms—a variant of ALS primarily occurring in the western Pacific islands, a classic familial form of ALS, and a sporadic form of ALS. In the mid–twentieth-century epidemics of ALS were reported in Guam, New Guinea, and in the Kii Peninsula in the western Pacific. Further epidemics of ALS in the western Pacific have not been described. The western pacific variant of ALS has reported to have distinct pathological characteristics, and often co-occurs with a separate parkinsonism–dementia complex, suggesting that the Pacific variant of ALS may have separate etiologic risk factors. Some authors have suggested that a nut from a cycad tree in the western Pacific may serve as a toxin in susceptible individuals and be a risk factor for the western Pacific variant of ALS (Waring et al. 2004).

With the exception of the pockets of excessive rates of the western Pacific variant of ALS, the incidence rates of ALS have been fairly constant throughout the world. An incidence rate of about 2 per 100,000 per year has been reported in several different studies in the United States and elsewhere. The incidence of sporadic ALS in men is slightly higher than the incidence in women (about 1.2:1). The average age at diagnosis is 65 years of age. Population-based studies have demonstrated that the age-specific incidence rates increase with age (Waring et al. 2004; Turner et al. 2009). There are very few studies that have examined the racial and ethnic group-specific incidence rates

Over the last few years, slightly higher rates of ALS have been reported than several decades ago. Several factors may together account for these recent slightly higher rates in the United Kingdom—the aging population, the improved diagnosis and case ascertainment in more recent studies (as neurological diagnostic expertise has become more uniformly available), a possible loss of competing causes of death in susceptible cohorts, and possibly increased reporting of ALS on death certificates (Waring et al. 2004; Turner et al. 2009).

Other forms of motor neuron disease occur less frequently among infants as well as older children and adolescents. Spinal muscular atrophy is an autosomal recessive motor neuron disease, with a birth prevalence is approximately eight cases per 100,000 live births, and a high mortality during infancy and no known treatment. Death is caused by restrictive lung disease and respiratory failure (Lunn and Wang 2008).

Causes

Several genes have been identified for the familial forms of ALS, prompting many experts to hypothesize the presence of susceptibility genes for the sporadic forms of ALS. A gene for the familial form of ALS has been discovered on the X chromosome. Up to twenty percent of familial cases of ALS are due to mutations at the *SOD1* gene on chromosome 21 (Siddique and Siddique 2008; Rothstein 2009). Susceptibility genes for adult sporadic forms of ALS have been hypothesized as being those involved in the development of infantile spinal muscular atrophy, such as the *SMN* gene and the *neuronal apoptosis inhibitory protein (NAIP)* gene. Infantile spinal muscular atrophy is generally recognized as a genetic disorder caused by homozygous disruption of the survival motor neuron 1 (*SMN1*) gene (Lunn and Wang 2008; Siddique and Siddique 2008; Rothstein 2009; Sumner 2007).

Several studies have investigated the potential relationships between environmental exposures and development of sporadic ALS. An increased risk of ALS has been reported with high-level exposures to lead, mercury, and other heavy metals, with odds ratios in the range of 1.5 to 6.0. Occupations that are involved with heavy metal exposure, such as welding, have been reported to have an increased risk of ALS. In addition, the exposure to agricultural chemicals has also been reported to have an increased association with ALS. Some studies have investigated the relationship between electrical shock and exposures to electromagnetic fields. Many of these studies have some methodological limitations, including small sample size, selective reporting, recall bias, and inconsistent measurement of levels of exposures (Sumner 2007; Shaw and Höglinger 2008).

Low dietary intake of exogenous antioxidants has been hypothesized to increase the risk of ALS. A recently published report from Japan has suggested that a diet high in fruits and vegetables might offer some reduction in the risk of ALS (Okamoto et al. 2009).

Prevention and Control

Rehabilitation, good pulmonary care, and advances in mechanical ventilation have prolonged survival and improved the quality of life among people with motor neuron diseases, but unfortunately there is no effective treatment for the underlying disease process. Future epidemiological studies will need to examine the gene–environmental interactions among susceptible populations, and the role of diet in ALS deserves additional study.

MULTIPLE SCLEROSIS (ICD-10 G35)

Significance

MS is a demyelinating disease of the central nervous system characterized by abnormalities of the myelin sheath of axons, resulting in impaired transmission of electrical signals through axons; clinical symptoms are a reflection of the location of the damaged myelin within the brain and spinal cord. Typical symptoms at onset of the disease are highly variable but often include double-vision, tremor, weakness, sensory disturbances, bladder or bowel dysfunction, impaired balance and coordination, and problems with speech, language, and cognitive processing. MS typically has a stuttering course with overall reduced neurological functioning over time, but with short-term remissions and exacerbations (Noseworthy et al. 2000).

The pathological features of MS are white matter plaques that vary in age and in distribution in the brain and spinal cord. This scattering of MS lesions in time and place was noted by Charcot in the mid 1800s and led to the basic neurological principle that the clinical symptoms needed to involve different areas of the central nervous system and have onset in different time periods in order to make the clinical diagnosis. We now know that the demyelinating lesions in MS also involve the cortical regions (Stadelmann and

Bruck 2008; Kutzelnigg et al. 2005). More recently, standardized diagnostic criteria and the use of brain MRI imaging have greatly assisted diagnosis of MS (Fangerau et al. 2004; Polman et al. 2005).

Descriptive Epidemiology

MS, with onset typically in the early thirties, is the most common chronic progressive neurological disorder among adults between the ages of 20 and 50 years. Although the severity of the disease and the rate of progression vary considerably, the median survival following disease onset is approximately 30 years. Despite the prolong survival, compared with some other progressive neurological disorders, the contribution of MS to long-term disability and excessive morbidity is considerable. About half of people with MS will need assistance with walking within 15 years of diagnosis (Noseworthy et al. 2000; Debouverie et al. 2008). MS is significantly more common among women than men, and more common among whites than among African Americans within the United Kingdom. MS has been reported to be more common among those of upper socioeconomic groups, but whether reduced access to specialty care and early diagnosis of MS among lower socioeconomic groups underestimate the rates of MS is unknown (Noseworthy et al. 2000).

Little population-based surveillance data for MS exists in the United States outside of the Rochester, MN, medical record linkage system. The annual incidence of MS in Rochester has been estimated at about 6 per 100,000 (Wynn et al. 1990). The prevalence of MS in the United States and in other developed countries seems to be increasing, as-sociated with longer survival rates (Wynn et al. 1990: Gracia et al. 2009). There is some evidence that the incidence of MS is increasing as well in some studies—an increase that cannot be totally accounted for on the basis of improved diagnostic techniques, such as brain imaging with MRI (Alonso and Hernán 2008).

Causes

Classically, the MS prevalence and risk of death have increased with distance from the equator. The highest prevalence rates have been reported from the northern and north midwestern regions of the United States, northern Europe, Canada, as well as Australia and New Zealand. Whites also have higher rates of MS than Africans and African Americans and Asians. Incidence rates of MS have been reported lower in Africa and in Asia (Wynn et al. 1990; Kurtzke 1980). Migration studies have repeatedly shown that people migrating from a high-risk to a low-risk area before age 15 years seem to adopt the lower risk of their new regional home, while those people who migrate to lower risk areas as adults retain a higher risk of MS (Alter, Kahana, and Loewenson 1978). It seems unlikely that these results of migration studies are due totally to enhanced access to diagnostic services and technology in the more affluent and technologically advanced developed countries of the north compared with the developing countries near the equator.

Aggregation of MS cases within families and higher rates of MS among whites have long suggested a genetic susceptibility to MS. Population-based twin studies of MS have reported much higher concordance rates among monozygotic than among dizygotic twin pairs. The risk of non-twin siblings of MS cases has been found to be similar to the risk of MS among dizygotic twins (Ebers, Bulman, and Sadovnick 1986). Overall, the familial studies of MS have pointed to likely shared genes among affected family members rather than environmental factors, and that several genes likely contribute to MS susceptibility (Ramagopalan, Dyment, and Ebers 2008).

While the pace of discovery of susceptibility genes for many chronic diseases has been extremely rapid over the last decade, the identification of MS susceptibility genes has been relatively limited. Recent studies have suggested that epigenetic modifications of germline susceptibility might play an important role (Ramagopalan, Dyment, and Ebers 2008). Epigenetic interactions with major histocompatability complex may play important roles in MS (Chao et al. 2009). Whether genome-wide association studies will lead to other clues regarding the role of genetics in MS should be determined in the near future.

Because MS cases have tended to cluster in time and have varied with latitude, many investigators have focused on the roles of infectious diseases as risk factors for MS. Latent viral infections from childhood and early adolescence in genetically susceptible individuals that via unknown immunologic mechanisms initiate the disease process in early adulthood may be important in the pathogenesis of MS (Kurtzke 1980). For example, some authors have reported that rubella antibody titers are higher among patients with MS than among controls from the general population. The risk of MS seems to increase among people whose rubella infection occurred in later childhood or early adolescence. An oft-cited study is that of an epidemic of MS in the Faroe Islands a few years after World War II, following the arrival of British troops, consistent with the introduction of a new (but yet undetermined) infectious agent into the island population (Kurtzke 1980). Hypothesized, but not proven, associations between Epstein-Barr virus (EBV) (Jilek et al. 2008) and other viruses such as herpes simplex virus I and II (Alvarez-Lafuente et al. 2008), varicella zoster (Sotelo et al. 2008), mumps, and cytomegalovirus have been reported (Hernán et al. 2001). A possible association between chlamydia infection and the risk of MS has received some recent attention in the literature (Parratt et al. 2008). Many of these studies of associations with infectious diseases are complicated by both potential recall bias and by inconsistent laboratory procedures for measurement of the infectious exposures.

The well-established modulation of the immune system by sex hormones, along with the variation in MS incidence by sex, has prompted the investigation of sex hormones as potential modulating factors in MS. MS relapses have long been recognized as being rare during pregnancy. MS exacerbations are often seen among women with MS weeks after delivery (Lee and O'Brien 2008). No significant associations have been reported between oral contraceptives and MS.

Exacerbation of MS symptoms has been reported after cigarette smoking, and early cigarette smoking has been reported as a possible risk factor in case control studies from Canada and the United Kingdom. It is also appears that cigarette smoking worsens the long-term prognosis among people with MS (Sundström and Nyström 2008).

Prevention and Control

Despite focused clinical research and drug development strategies over several decades, a cure for MS does not exist. However, the clinical management of MS has improved considerably. Brain imaging techniques such as brain MRI have improved clinicians' ability to diagnosis and follow patients with MS. Treatments such as interferon beta have made long-term drug treatment of MS more tolerable with fewer adverse events than long-term or frequent treatment with steroids. Treatment of MS exacerbations with prednisone or adrenocorticotropic hormone remain common practice with short-term benefit but without impact on the long-term course of the disease. As the treatment regimens for MS have become more complex, treatment guidelines that can be uniformly and consistently followed by patients who maintain long-term compliance has become a challenge. Strategies for effective long-term treatment require coordination between the primary care medical home and neurologists, with effective utilization of nursing and health education (Noseworthy et al. 2000). The built environment and accessibility for people with motor disabilities is especially important for people who are disabled as a result of MS.

As with some other progressive neurological disorders, low concentrations of dietary antioxidants have been thought to be a potential risk factor by some authors. Although a protective role for vitamin D has been discussed in the literature (Brandes et al. 2009), the known variations in MS incidence by latitude could be an important confounding variable. Recent publications have highlighted the high rate of adverse health behaviors (e.g., smoking, lack of exercise) among people with MS, suggesting the need for targeted health promotion and chronic disease prevention activities (Khurana et al. 2009; Marrie et al. 2009).

Better population-based surveillance data and epidemiological research of potential risk factors, including gene–environmental interaction studies are needed to mount a public health response to MS in developing countries. The role of diet, hormonal factors, and latent viral infections with long-term immunologic responses will continue to be important areas of investigation.

GUILLAIN-BARRÉ SYNDROME (ICD-10 G61.0)

Significance

Guillain-Barré syndrome, long of interest to public health professionals, is an acute demyelinating disease of the peripheral nervous system affecting motor and sensory motor neurons throughout the body. The onset is characterized by progressive weakness over many hours to many days. Typically, the onset of weakness is accompanied by vague uncomfortable sensory complaints, with progression from the legs and arms to the trunk and chest muscles, then leading to requirements for mechanical ventilation. The rate of demyelination and associated clinical deterioration is often faster in children than among adults, with children recovering faster as well. Most people with Guillain-Barré syndrome have complete or near complete recovery of their weakness. However, short-term mortality and morbidity remains significant. Guillain-Barré syndrome is generally considered to result from an autoimmune response directed against the myelin sheath of peripheral nerves, typically triggered by a recent viral or bacterial infection, or less commonly a noninfectious agent (Asbury 2000; Burns 2008; Pritchard 2008). Standard case definitions for Guillain-Barré syndrome have improved both clinical research efforts and epidemic investigations.

Descriptive Epidemiology

The reported incidence of Guillain-Barré syndrome has varied considerably, with annual incidence rates ranging from less than 0.5 to more than 2 per 100,000. Some studies have reported higher incidence rates for men than for women and higher rates for whites than for African Americans (McGrogan et al. 2009).

Causes

Infections that trigger peripheral nerve myelin directed autoimmune responses have long been the focus of research and are thought to be the primary risk factors for Guillain-Barré syndrome. Gastrointestinal and upper respiratory infections a few weeks before onset of weakness are typical and are more common among Guillain-Barré syndrome cases than among controls. Campylobacter, Epstein-Barr virus, and cytomegalovirus have received the most attention from investigators. A few outbreaks of Guillain-Barré syndrome have been reported following epidemics of campylobacter gastroenteritis. Concern regarding the increased risk of Guillain-Barré syndrome following the swine flu vaccine in 1976 and 1977 received considerable attention. Of interest is that the studies of swine flu vaccine administered after 1977 and Guillain-Barré syndrome have not shown any association, suggesting that there was a unique immunologic reaction from the vaccine used in 1976 and 1977 that has not occurred since that time (McGrogan et al. 2009; Kuwabara 2004).

Prevention and Control

Prevention of infectious triggers of Guillain-Barré syndrome and control of epidemics of campylobacter are currently the best opportunities for primary prevention. Rapid diagnosis and supportive care, including respiratory care and mechanical ventilation if needed, remain the mainstay of treatment. If treated early in the course of the disease process, plasmapheresis or intravenous gamma globulin can shorten the course of the demyelinating disorder and may reduce the odds of requiring mechanical ventilation (Asbury 2000).

Vigilance on the part of public health officials and rapid response to potential epidemics of Guillain-Barré syndrome remains important.

TIC DISORDERS AND TOURETTE SYNDROME (ICD-10 F95)

Significance

Tics are stereotypic, purposeless, and sudden movements, that although may be transiently suppressed and resemble purposeful movement, are involuntary. Tics have been generally classified as simple and chronic. Simple tic disorders are those in which a single motor tic manifestation occurs in an individual such as an eyeblinks, jaw jutting movements, or throat clearing, without evolution of multiple different motor tic manifestations and without vocal tics. Chronic multifocal tic disorders manifest multiple different simple and complex motor tics, often accompanied by vocal tics that are most commonly noises such as snorts or consonant sounds, but may also be involuntary expletive speech (corprolalia). Simple tics often undergo spontaneous remission, especially among children, within a year of onset. Chronic multifocal tics, when in association with vocal tics, that last for greater than a year are typically lifelong in duration and are classified as Tourette syndrome. While most people with tics are not disabled, and often are not aware that their movements are abnormal, some people with Tourette syndrome are significantly impaired. Tourette syndrome is commonly associated with attention-deficit disorder and/or obsessive–compulsive disorder (Kuwabara 2004; Faridi and Suchowersky 2003; Kossoff and Singer 2001; Lombroso and Scahill 2008).

A major challenge for both clinical and epidemiological investigations is the lack of laboratory or radiographic diagnostic tests for tic disorders or Tourette syndrome. Furthermore, distinguishing Tourette syndrome from simple tic disorders using medical record review and self-reported data is difficult at best.

Descriptive Epidemiology

Tic disorders are very common among children, but the published estimates range considerably with the methods used. The prevalence of Tourette syndrome has been reported to be as low as 5 per 10,000, and as high as 3.8%. Overall, the best estimates for the prevalence of Tourette syndrome, including relatively mild cases are approximately 1% of the childhood population between the ages of 5 and 18 years old. Boys have a higher prevalence of Tourette syndrome than girls, with male:female ratios reported as high as 4.7:1. Tourette syndrome seems to occur worldwide (Robertson 2008).

Causes

Tourette syndrome has a strong familial predisposition, although parents are often diagnosed as a result of manifestations in their children, underscoring the likely underascertainment from medical record reviews (Faridi and Suchowersky 2003). The association of simple tics with Group A beta-hemolytic streptococci has been reported, but this association has been questioned as a causal factor for chronic tic disorders (Harris and Singer 2006).

Recently published evidence of linkage to the centromeric region of chromosome five in a single large family with Tourette syndrome has highlighted the potential for future genetic studies (Laurin et al. 2009).

Prevention and Control

There are no proven methods for preventing tic disorders or Tourette syndrome. Whether there is a causal relationship between streptococcal infections and tic disorders will require additional study, but current data suggest that streptococcal infections are highly unlikely to account for a significant percentage of Tourette syndrome cases (Harris and Singer 2006). Management of the behavioral and learning (attention-deficit) comorbid conditions is important, and public health professionals should be aware of the mental health needs of people with Tourette syndrome (Faridi and Suchowersky 2003; Kossoff and Singer 2001; Lombroso and Scahill 2008).

Future epidemiological studies of Tourette syndrome will need to address the potential factors (genetic and environmental) that might impact the severity of these tic disorders, with an emphasis on factors that may exacerbate tics in susceptible individuals.

TRAUMATIC BRAIN INJURY (ICD-10 S00-S09)

Significance

Traumatic brain injuries are common, associated with devastating long-term disability, and excessive mortality. About 1.4 million people experience traumatic brain injury each year in the United States, of which approximately 235,000 are hospitalized and 50,000 die. Up to 50% of all trauma deaths in the United States are associated with significant traumatic brain injury. Brain injury is the primary cause of death among one third to one half of all trauma-related deaths (Sosin, Sniezek, and Waxweiler 1995; Bruns and Hauser 2003; Thurman et al. 1999).

Descriptive Epidemiology

Differences in traumatic brain injury study methods make comparisons between studies difficult without careful consideration of inclusion and exclusion criteria for each study. The annual incidence of traumatic brain injury in the United States is approximately 180 to 250 per 100,000. Males and people living in lower socioeconomic regions tend to have higher rates. The very young, adolescents, young adults, and the elderly are also at higher risk for traumatic brain injury. The associated annual mortality rate in the United States decreased from 25 per 100,000 in 1979 to 19 per 100,000 in 1992 (Sosin, Sniezek, and Waxweiler 1995; Bruns and Hauser 2003; Thurman et al. 1999; Langlois et al. 2003).

Causes

The most common risk factors for traumatic brain injury are falls, transportation-related injuries and automobile crashes, sports or recreation injuries, and assaults. Alcohol and drug use are interactive risk factors for motor vehicle crashes leading to falls, transportation-related injuries and automobile crashes, sports or recreation injuries, and assaults. Workers in specific occupations such as construction, farming, roofing, and logging are at especially high risk of TBI (Bruns and Hauser 2003; Thurman et al. 1999; Langlois et al. 2003; Langlois, Rutland-Brown, and Wald 2006).

Prevention Control Measures

Primary prevention efforts for preventing traumatic brain injury include both modifications of the built environment and policy changes. Brain injury prevention through improved vehicle and road design, better separation between pedestrian walkways and major highways, prevention of falls (especially in the elderly), and prevention of work-related injuries are all important areas of intervention (Langlois, Rutland-Brown, and Wald 2006; Judge et al. 1993; Campbell et al. 1999; National Center for Injury Prevention and Control 2009).

Preventing falls and reducing brain injuries among the elderly begins with making living areas safer by (a) removing tripping hazards (e.g., throw rugs), (b) using non-slip mats in bathtubs and showers, (c) installing handrails on both sides of stairways, (d) installing grab bars next to toilets and in showers and tubs, (e) enhancing the lighting throughout homes, and (f) providing opportunities for regular physical activity. Preventing falls among children also requires making living areas safer by (a) installing window guards to keep young children from falling out of open windows, (b) using safety gates at the top and the bottom of stairs when young children are present, and (c) building surfaces on playgrounds made of shock-absorbing material such as hardwood mulch or sand (Mack, Sacks, and Thompson 2000). Building codes and policies that require and enforce these prevention measures offer opportunities for brain injury prevention (Thurman et al. 1999; National Center for Injury Prevention and Control 2009).

Policies that require and enforce the use of bicycle and motorcycle helmets, seatbelts, and speed limits have been proven to reduce serious head injuries. Children and parents should know that helmets should also be worn when playing contact sports (football, hockey, boxing, wrestling), using in-line skates or riding skateboards, batting or running bases in baseball or softball, riding a horse, or skiing and snowboarding (Thurman et al. 1999; National Center for Injury Prevention and Control 2009).

Especially important for prevention of brain injuries among young children are the consistent and proper use of booster seats when children outgrow their child safety seats (when they reach the weight of 40 pounds), the use of the booster seat until they reach a height of about four feet, nine inches when they can properly wear a lap/shoulder belt (National Center for Injury Prevention and Control 2009; CDC 1993).

Likewise public education efforts combined with policies that reduce alcohol- and drug-related crashes and injuries have been helpful, but can be improved.

SPINAL CORD INJURY (ICD-10 S10-S19)

Significance

According to the Spinal Cord Injury Information Network at the University of Alabama, Birmingham, about 12,000 Americans sustain a spinal cord injury each year. Estimates from several years ago suggested that in the United States about 200,000 people with some form of disability due to previous spinal cord injury. Recent estimates suggest that at least 400,000 Americans currently have a disabling condition due to a previous spinal cord injury (Spinal Cord Injury Facts and Figures 2009). The most common causes of spinal cord injury vary by age. Among people 65 years and older, most injury is caused by falls—many of which are preventable. Overall, the leading cause of spinal cord injury among people younger than 65 years is motor vehicle crashes. Sports and other recreational activities are responsible for about 20% of all spinal cord injury and are more common among adolescents and young adults (Spinal Cord Injury Facts 2009; SCI Facts 2009).

Secondary medical conditions and comorbidities are a major health issue for the developed world, where more people survive spinal cord injuries than in years past. Airway management problems, secondary pulmonary conditions and pneumonia, urinary tract infections, pressure sores, spasticity, deep vein thrombosis, osteoporosis, and scoliosis are all major secondary conditions that each has their own opportunities for secondary prevention efforts (Meyers et al. 2000). The annual cost to the United States for spinal cord injuries is estimated at $9.7 billion. The average lifetime cost for a typical 25-year-old person with spinal cord injuries varies by the severity (or spinal cord level) of the injury and has recently been estimated to be between $682,000 for an incomplete motor impairment and over $3 million for a complete high-cervical (C1–C4) injury (Spinal Cord Injury Facts 2009; Berkowitz et al. 1998).

Descriptive Epidemiology

The estimated incidence of spinal cord injuries in the United States every year is about 40 per million. The prevalence is estimated at 11–112 per 100,000, but recently emerging estimates suggest that these may be significant underestimates. Overall mortality from spinal cord injuries is very high but has declined considerably over the last several decades. The reduction in spinal cord injury–associated mortality rates, as well as the rising prevalence estimates of people living with disability is due in part to improvements in emergency medical services (especially emergency neurosurgical care), development of specialty centers for care, improved professional training, and reduction in the death rates from infections and other secondary conditions (Spinal Cord Injury Facts and Figures 2009; Spinal Cord Injury Facts 2009; DeVivo and Stover 1995).

Causes

SCI primarily occurs among adolescents and young adults. Over the last decade, approximately 75% of spinal cord injuries have occurred among males. Since 2005, about 42% have been the result of motor vehicle crashes, with falls (27.1%), violence (15.3%), and sports and recreational injuries (7.4%) also significantly contributing to the total burden. As for traumatic brain injury, alcohol and drug use significantly contribute to the risk of injury (Spinal Cord Injury Facts and Figures 2009; Spinal Cord Injury Facts 2009).

Prevention and Control

As noted in the prevention of traumatic brain injury, improving the built environment, promoting policies that improve safety, and prevention education for the community can all lead to improved primary prevention of SCI.

For those with spinal cord injuries, outcomes are better with skilled trauma care and with a well-coordinated emergency medical system—including emergency trauma center systems that cross state lines when saving time saves lives and improves outcomes. Emphasizing the coordination between public health surveillance, primary prevention programs, and emergency medical systems in any health care reform measures will enhance prevention efforts.

ATTENTION-DEFICIT HYPERACTIVITY DISORDER (ICD-10 F90)

Significance

Attention-deficit hyperactivity disorder (ADHD) is a heterogeneous group of common neurological conditions with onset during preschool years and characterized by problems with attention, impulsivity, and overactivity. Anxiety, conduct disorder, learning disorders, obsessive–compulsive disorder, epilepsy, tic disorders, depression, bipolar disorder, and sleep disorders all occur more commonly among children and adults with ADHD than in the general population. People with ADHD are more likely than their peers in the general population to have problems with substance abuse and to smoke cigarettes (Stein and Shin 2008; McClernon and Kollins 2008).

Neuroscience has clearly demonstrated that ADHD is a brain disorder and not simply a matter of poor behavior or a lack of discipline. Evidence from multiple studies has converged on the neural connections between the prefrontal cortex and the striatum of the brain (the caudate nuclei and the putamen) as areas of dysfunction among people with ADHD. Other studies have suggested that while the frontal and prefrontal areas of the brain are clearly implicated in the pathophysiology of ADHD that more posterior regions of the brain are involved as well. When performing cognitive tasks, people with ADHD tend to activate broader regions of the cortex than do people who have less difficulty focusing—probably explaining the tendency of people with ADHD to have problems with distraction (Brennan and Arnsten 2008; Durston 2003).

Descriptive Epidemiology

ADHD occurs in up to 2% to 7.5% of all school age children, and is estimated to impact about 2%–4% of adults in the United States. School-age boys are almost three times more likely to be diagnosed with ADHD as are girls. Trends in the true frequency of ADHD in the general population are difficult to determine, as the prevalence rates increase as community awareness is enhanced and as treatments for ADHD are made available and promoted. Regardless, it is clear that the prevalence rates of ADHD among school-aged children in the United States are much higher than 30 years ago. ADHD, once considered to be a disorder of childhood, is now known to occur commonly among adults—perhaps in as many as 4% of all adults (Stein and Shin 2008; Barbaresi et al. 2002).

Causes

The causal risk factors for ADHD in some children are obvious, especially when the prefrontal regions are rendered dysfunctional as a result of hypoxic–ischemic encephalopathy, strokes, intractable epilepsy, head injuries, encephalitis, or brain tumors. Yet, for the majority of people with ADHD, the cause is unknown, even though the brain mechanisms behind the disorder are fairly well understood (Stein and Shin 2008).

Susceptibility genes play some role in ADHD, at least for some subgroups of individuals affected. Fragile X syndrome, the most common genetic cause of intellectual disability, is also strongly associated with ADHD (Hagerman et al. 2009). Family, twin, adoption studies, and segregation analyses, as well as molecular genetic studies strongly suggest that both genetic and environmental factors contribute to the causes of ADHD. The relationship between genetically determined neurotransmitter dysregulation and abnormal attention and impulse control are only beginning to be discovered, and these areas of research may offer significant insights into the genetics and neurobiology of ADHD in the future (Todd and Neuman 2007; Kim et al. 2008; Faraone and Doyle 2001).

Prevention and Control

Primary prevention opportunities for ADHD are limited. However, given the high frequency of comorbid conditions among adolescents and adults who were diagnosed with ADHD as children, identification of children with ADHD identifies those who are at higher risk of cigarette smoking, substance abuse, depression, and other mental illnesses; therefore, opportunities for focused health promotion efforts should become an emphasis among public health professionals. The diagnosis and management of the child with ADHD has benefited in recent years by the development of consensus guidelines for diagnosis, evaluation, and treatment (Committee on Quality Improvement 2000; Committee on Quality Improvement 2001). Early diagnosis and treatment can prevent school failure, and improve long-term academic and social outcomes.

CARPAL TUNNEL SYNDROME (ICD-10 G56.0)

Significance

Carpal tunnel syndrome, caused by entrapment of the median nerve at the wrist as it passes under the transverse carpal ligament, is common and results in sensory changes (numb tingling, pain) and, eventually, weakness of the muscles of the hand. The most commonly diagnosed entrapment syndrome of peripheral nerves, carpal tunnel syndrome symptoms are exacerbated at night during sleep, and occur frequently among pregnant women and among workers who engage in repetitive fine motor movements of the fingers and wrists (e.g., typists). The diagnosis is made based upon typical history and exam findings consistent with an inflamed and dysfunctional median nerve distal to the wrist. The diagnosis is aided by abnormal median nerve conduction studies (Rempel et al. 1998).

Descriptive Epidemiology

There appears to be increased reporting and diagnosis of carpal tunnel syndrome over the last few decades, possibly with the introduction of improved diagnostic techniques. In Rochester, the adjusted annual increased rates increased from 258 per 100,000 in 1981–1985 to 424 in 2000–2005. One study from Sweden reported a prevalence of about 3.8% in the general population of adults (Atroshi et al. 1999; Gelfman et al. 2009).

Causes

Wrist trauma is strongly associated with development of carpal tunnel syndrome. However, other risk factors, such as diabetes, hypothyroidism, pregnancy, and repetitive hand or wrist movements, probably account for a higher proportion of cases. Food-processing workers, roofers, carpenters, and mill workers seem to have especially high rates of carpal tunnel syndrome. Office workers who spend long hours typing are likewise at high risk for carpal tunnel syndrome (Roquelaure et al. 2008). The increasing rates of obesity may contribute to the increasing rates of carpal tunnel syndrome (Farmer and Davis 2008).

Prevention and Control

Enhancing worker safety programs and training in ergonomics hazard prevention in the workplace can prevent carpal tunnel syndrome. Screening tools to identify workers at risk have been used by many industries, and enhance targeted ergonomic interventions that can prevent carpal tunnel syndrome. Prevention of obesity and early diagnosis and nonsurgical management of carpal tunnel syndrome can reduce morbidity and time lost from work.

LOW BACK PAIN (ICD-10 M54.5)

Significance

About two thirds of adults in the United States experience at some point in their lives low back pain. Low back pain is second only to upper respiratory track infections as a reason for adults visiting a physician in the United Kingdom (Deyo and Weinstein 2001).

Among people with acute low back pain, recovery usually occurs within a few weeks regardless of treatment. Low levels of pain and occasional disability persist from 3 to at least 12 months after onset of pain for some people with low back pain. Most people return to work one month after onset of low back pain, and about 90% of people return to work by three months after onset of low back pain. A majority of people with new-onset low back pain will have at least one recurrence within a year (Deyo and Weinstein 2001; Pengel et al. 2003). Because low back pain is so common, a small percentage of people who have longer-term pain and/or significant disability account for a significant burden of disability, morbidity, and lost productivity.

Descriptive Epidemiology

Approximately 2% of all workers in the United States report disabling back pain each year. Reported rates of low back pain are higher in lower socioeconomic classes (Karahan et al. 2009).

Causes

High-risk occupations include hospital nursing, prolonged truck driving, dock workers, warehouse workers, farm workers, lumber workers, miners, construction workers, and others who engage in frequent heavy lifting. Cigarette smoking, premature menopause, and abdominal obesity all increase the risk of low back pain (Deyo and Weinstein 2001; Pengel et al. 2003; Adera, Deyo, and Donatelle 1994; Shiri et al. 2008). Newer data suggest a genetic suscepti- bility to some low back pain associated with lumbar disc degeneration (Battié et al. 2007).

Prevention and Control

Concern has been raised by many investigators overtreatment of low back pain by physi- cians, with excessive numbers of MRI, and perhaps excessive numbers of low back surger- ies. A combination of exercises that strengthen the paraspinous and abdominal muscles, maintaining correct posture, and lifting objects properly can help prevent injuries (Deyo and Weinstein 2001; Pengel et al. 2003).

Improvements in the built environment can reduce the risk of low back pain among workers in high-risk populations. Improved ergonomic design in vehicles, high-risk work places, as well as education on lifting techniques and strength conditioning may further reduce risk of back injuries.

MIGRAINE AND TENSION-TYPE HEADACHE (ICD-10 G43-G44)

Significance

Almost everyone experiences headache at some time. Headaches are a very common rea- son for adolescents and adults to visit a physician. About one third of men and approxi- mately one half of women experience episodic tension-type headache. For most of these people, their headaches have minimal impact on their lives, but for the small percentage of people who have evolution of chronic daily headache, the degree of impairment and even disability can be significant. An estimated 20% of women and about 5%–10% of men experience migraine. Although most people with migraine do not experience disability, migraine attacks are more disabling and are more frequently associated with time from work. Children with migraine average twice as many days absent from school as children without migraine headaches (Schwartz et al. 1998; Mack 2009).

Descriptive Epidemiology

The International Headache Society diagnostic criteria for migraine has become the gold standard used by clinicians (IHS 2004). Yet the practical application of headache classifi- cation schemes in the general population is difficult, as the distinction between migraine and other types of headache is often blurred. Given these methodological issues, the aver- age annual incidence of severe headache has been estimated at 0.5%. Migraine typically presents in childhood or adolescence, with new onset of migraine after age 40 years being very rare. Migraine prevalence is two to four times higher among women than men and is twice as high among low-income populations. Exacerbation of migraine headaches during or after menopause is common among women (Mack 2009).

Causes

A positive family history, depression, epilepsy, female sex, and low socioeconomic status are all risk factors for migraine headaches (Haan et al. 2008; Martin and Lipton 2008; Bigal et al. 2007). Given the high frequency of maternal migraine history among people with migraine, a mitochondrial DNA pattern of inheritance has long been hypothesized. Recent reports have verified that two common mitochondrial DNA polymorphisms are highly associated with migraine headache, and likely account for a very high proportion of familial cases of migraine (Zaki et al. 2009). Depression and stress have long been known to be important risk factors for other types of headaches (Jensen and Stovner 2008).

Among people with headaches, especially migraine, specific triggers that precipitate headaches are well-defined and require that clinicians and patients become familiar with the triggers unique to each person affected. The most common triggers include onset of menses, dietary changes or specific foods (cheeses, chocolate, nuts), extreme fatigue, or variation in sleep patterns. Patient surveys have been developed to identify potential triggers in order to develop prevention strategies (Kelman 2007).

Prevention and Control

Among people with migraine headaches, a medical home, sustained care, and education that allows them to learn their own triggers with the help of their physician offer the best opportunity for improving quality of life and preventing headaches. Although chronic stress is a major contributor to episodic tension-type headache, prevention of chronic stress involves major upstream interventions to address the social determinants of health. Proper diet and regular adequate sleep are important for minimizing headaches among most people with migraine.

People with frequent migraine headaches often benefit from daily prophylactic treatment; medications such as propranolol, tricyclic drugs, cyproheptadine have all been helpful. Drugs that can abort migraine attacks if given early in the course of a headache, such as ergotamine tartrate and sumatriptan, can be helpful but require careful expert medical management in order to minimize adverse events (Gendolla 2008). Disabling episodic tension-type headache, especially among people with chronic daily headache, benefit from stress management and psychophysiological techniques such as biofeedback (Nestoriuc et al. 2008); treatment for coexisting depression is sometimes important for people with chronic daily headaches.

Resources

Alzheimer's Association, 17th Floor, 225 N Michigan Avenue, Chicago, IL 60601-7633, tel.: (866) 699-1246, (312) 355-8700, http://www.alz.org

Alzheimer's Foundation of America, 7th Floor, 322 8th Avenue, New York, NY 10001, http://www.alzfdn.org

Autism Society of America, Suite 300, 7910 Woodmont Avenue, Bethesda, MD 20814-3067, tel.: (301) 657-0881, http://www.autism-society.org

American Parkinson Disease Association, 135 Parkinson Avenue, Staten Island, NY 10305, tel.: (718) 981-8001, http://www.apdaparkinson.org

National Parkinson Foundation, Inc., 1501 NW 9th Avenue, Bob Hope Road, Miami, FL 33136-1494, tel.: (800) 327-4545, http://www.parkinson.org

Parkinson's Action Network, 1025 Vermont Ave, NW, Suite 1120, Washington, DC 20005, tel.: (800) 850-4726 or (202) 638-4101, http://www.parkinsonsaction.org

Parkinson's Disease Foundation (PDF), 1359 Broadway, Suite 1509, New York, NY 10018, tel.: (212) 923-4700, http://www.pdf.org

United Parkinson Foundation (UPF), 833 West Washington Boulevard, Chicago, IL 60607, tel.: (312) 733-1893

Muscular Dystrophy Association, 3300 East Sunrise Drive, Tucson, AZ 85718, tel.: (800) 572-1717, http://www.mda.org

National Multiple Sclerosis Society, 733 3rd Avenue, New York, NY 10017-3288, tel.: (212) 463-7787, http://www.nationalmssociety.org

Brain Injury Association, Inc., 1776 Massachusetts Avenue NW, Suite 100, Washington, DC 20036, tel.: (800) 444-6443, http://www.biausa.org

Paralyzed Veterans of America, Spinal Cord Research Foundation, 801 18th Street NW, Washington, DC 20006, tel.: (800) 555-9140, http://www.pva.org

Epilepsy Foundation of America, 8301 Professional Place, Landover, MD 20785-4951, tel.: (800) EFA-1000, (301) 459-3700, http://www.epilepsyfoundation.org

Citizens United for Research in Epilepsy (CURE), 730 N. Franklin Street, Suite 404, Chicago, IL 60654, info@cureepilepsy.org

Tourette Syndrome Foundation, 42-40 Bell Boulevard, Suite 205, Bayside, NY 11361-2820, tel.: (718) 224-2999, http://www.tsa-usa.org

National Headache Foundation, 2nd Floor, 428 W. Saint James Place, Chicago, IL 60614-2750, tel.: (800) 843-2256, (312) 388-6399, http://www.headaches.org

Suggested Reading

Banerjee, P.N., D. Filippi, and W.A. Hauser. The Descriptive Epidemiology of Epilepsy—A Review. *Epilepsy Res* (2009):85(1):31–45.

Brandt, T., L.R. Caplan, J. Dichgans, H. Diener, and C. Kennard, editors. *Neurological Disorders: Course and Treatment* (2nd ed.). Amsterdam/Boston: Academic Press (2003).

Bruns, J., and W.A. Hauser. The Epidemiology of Tramatic Brain Injury: A Review. *Epilepsia* (2003):44(Suppl 10):2–10.

Herbert, L.E., P.A. Scherr, J.L. Bienias, D.A. Bennett, and D.A. Evans. Alzheimer Disease in the U.S. Population: Prevalence Estimates using the 2000 Census. *Arch Neurol* (2003):60:1119–1122.

MacDonald, B.K., O.C. Cockerell, J.W.A.S. Sander, and S.D. Shorvon. The Incidence and Lifetime Prevalence of Neurological Disorders in a Prospective Community Based Study in the U.K. *Brain* (2000):123:665–676.

National Institute of Neurological Disorders and Stroke. Disorder Index (Descriptions of Over One Hundred Neurologic Disorders). Available from: http://www.ninds.nih.gov/disorders/disorder_index.htm. Accessed July 17, 2009.

Pengel, L.H.M., R.D. Herbert, C.G. Maher, and K.M. Refshauge. Acute Low Back Pain: Systematic Review of its Prognosis. *BMJ* (2003):327:323

Rowland, A.S., C.A. Lesesne, and A.J. Abramowitz. The Epidemiology of Attention-Deficit/Hyperactivity Disorder (ADHD): A Public Health View. *Mental Retardation and Developmental Disabilities Reviews* (2002):8:162–170.

Van den Eeden, S.K., C.M. Tanner, A.L. Bernstein, R.D. Fross, A. Leimpeter, D.A. Bloch, and L.M. Nelson. Incidence of Parkinson's Disease: Variation by Age, Gender, and Race/Ethnicity. *Am J Epidemiol* (2003):157(11):1015–1022.

World Health Organization (WHO). *Neurological Disorders: Public Health Challenges.* Geneva (2006).

References

Abrahams, B.S., and D.H. Geschwind. Advances in Autism Genetics: On the Threshold of a New Neurobiology. *Nature Reviews Genetics* (2008):9:341–355.

Adera, T., R.A. Deyo, and R.J. Donatelle. Premature Menopause and Low Back Pain. A Population-Based Study. *Ann Epidemiol* (1994):4(5):416–422.

Allen, M.C. Neurodevelopmental Outcomes of Preterm Infants. *Curr Opin Neurol* (2008):21(2): 123–128.

Alonso, A., and M.A. Hernán. Temporal Trends in the Incidence of Multiple Sclerosis: A Systematic Review. *Neurology* (2008):71(2):129–135.

Alter, M., E. Kahana, and R. Loewenson. Migration and Risk of Multiple Sclerosis. *Neurology* (1978):28:1089–1093.

Alvarez-Lafuente, R., M. García-Montojo, V. De Las Heras, et al. Herpesviruses and Human Endogenous Retroviral Sequences in the Cerebrospinal Fluid of Multiple Sclerosis Patients. *Mult Scler* (2008):14(5):595–601.

Alzheimer's Association. 2008 Alzheimer's Disease Facts and Figures. *Alzheimers Dement* (2008):4(2):110–133.

Andrews, J. Amyotrophic Lateral Sclerosis: Clinical Management and Research Update. *Curr Neurol Neurosci Rep* (2009):9(1):59–68.

Anstey, K.J., C. von Sanden, A. Salim, and R. O'Kearney. Smoking as a Risk Factor for Dementia and Cognitive Decline: A Meta-Analysis of Prospective Studies. *Am J Epidemiol* (2007):166(4):367–378.

Aronica, E., and J.A. Gorter. Gene Expression Profile in Temporal Lobe Epilepsy. *Neuroscientist* (2007):13(2):100–108.

Asbury, A.K. New Concepts of Guillain-Barré Syndrome. *J Child Neurol* (2000):15(3):183–191.

Atroshi, I., C. Gummesson, R. Johnsson, E. Ornstein, J. Ranstam, and I. Rosen. Prevalence of Carpal Tunnel Syndrome in the General Population. *JAMA* (1999):282:153–158.

Autism and Developmental Disabilities Monitoring Network Surveillance (ADDMN) Year 2002 Principal Investigators; Centers for Disease Control and Prevention. Prevalence of Autism Spectrum Disorders—Autism and Developmental Disabilities Monitoring Network, 14 Sites, United States, 2002. *MMWR Surveill Summ* (2007 Feb 9):56(1):12–28.

Baldereschi, M., A. Di Carlo, W.A. Rocca, et al. Parkinson's disease and parkinsonism in a longitudinal study: two-fold higher incidence in men. ILSA Working Group. Italian Longitudinal Study on Aging. *Neurology* (2000):55(9):1358–1363.

Barbaresi, W.J., S.K. Katusic, R.C. Colligan, et al. How Common is Attention-Deficit/Hyperactivity Disorder? Incidence in a Population Based Birth Cohort in Rochester, Minnesota. *Arch Pediatric and Adolescent Med* (2002):156:217–224.

Battié, M.C., T. Videman, E. Levalahti, K. Gill, and J. Kaprio. Heritability of Low Back Pain and the Role of Disc Degeneration. *Pain* (2007):131(3):272–280.

Berkovic, S.F., L. Harkin, J.M. McMahon, et al. De-novo Mutations of the Sodium Channel Gene SCN1A in Alleged Vaccine Encephalopathy: A Retrospective Study. *Lancet Neurol* (2006 Jun):5(6):488–492.

Berkowitz, M., P. O'Leary, D. Kruse, and C. Harvey. *Spinal Cord Injury: An Analysis of Medical and Social Costs.* New York: Demos Medical Publishing Inc. (1998).

Bertram, L., and R.E. Tanzi. Thirty Years of Alzheimer's Disease Genetics: The Implications of Systematic Meta-analyses. *Nat Rev Neurosci* (2008):9(10):768–778.

Bigal, M.E., R.B. Lipton, P. Winner, M.L. Reed, S. Diamond, and W.F. Stewart; AMPP Advisory Group. Migraine in Adolescents: Association with Socioeconomic Status and Family History. *Neurology* (2007):69(1):16–25.

Blume, W.T. Lennox-Gastaut Syndrome: Potential Mechanisms of Cognitive Regression. *Ment Retard Dev Disabil Res Rev* (2004):10(2):150–153.

Brandes, D.W., T. Callender, E. Lathi, and S. O'Leary. A Review of Disease-Modifying Therapies for MS: Maximizing Adherence and Minimizing Adverse Events. *Curr Med Res Opin* 2009):25(1):77–92.

Brennan, A.R., and A.F. Arnsten. Neuronal Mechanisms Underlying Attention Deficit Hyperactivity Disorder: The Influence of Arousal on Prefrontal Cortical Function. *Ann N Y Acad Sci.* (2008):1129:236–245.

Bruns, J., and W.A. Hauser. The Epidemiology of Traumatic Brain Injury: A Review. *Epilepsia* (2003):44(S10):2–10.

Burns, T.M. Guillain-Barré Syndrome. *Semin Neurol* (2008):28(2):152–167.

Campbell, A.J., M.C. Robertson, M.M. Gardner, R.N. Norton, and D.M. Buchner. Falls Prevention Over 2 Years: A Randomized Controlled Trial in Women 80 Years and Older. *Age and Aging* (1999):28:513–518.

Centers for Disease Control and Prevention (CDC). Use of Supplements Containing Folic Acid among Women of Childbearing Age—United States, 2007. *MMWR* (2008):11:57(1):5–8.

Centers for Disease Control and Prevention (CDC). Warning on Interaction between Air Bags and Rear-Facing Child Restraints. *MMWR* (1993):42(14):20–22.

Chadwick, D., and D. Smith. The Misdiagnosis of Epilepsy. *BMJ* (2002 Mar 2):324(7336):495–496.

Chao, M.J., S.V. Ramagopalan, B.M. Herrera, M.R. Lincoln, D.A. Dyment, A.D. Sadovnick, and G.C. Ebers. Epigenetics in Multiple Sclerosis Susceptibility: Difference in Transgenerational Risk Localizes to the Major Histocompatibility Complex. *Hum Mol Genet* (2009):18(2):261–266.

Collins, M.A., E.J. Neafsey, K.J. Mukamal, M.O. Gray, D.A. Parks, D.K. Das, and R.J. Korthuis. Alcohol in Moderation, Cardioprotection, and Neuroprotection: Epidemiological Considerations and Mechanistic Studies. *Alcohol Clin Exp Res* (2009):33(2):206–219.

Committee on Quality Improvement, Subcommittee on Attention-Deficit/Hyperactivity Disorder. Clinical Practice Guideline: Diagnosis and Evaluation of the Child with Attention-Deficit/Hyperactivity Disorder. *Pediatrics* (2000):105(5):1158–1170.

Committee on Quality Improvement, Subcommittee on Attention-Deficit/Hyperactivity Disorder. Clinical Practice Guideline: Treatment of the School-Aged Child with Attention-Deficit/Hyperactivity Disorder. *Pediatrics* (2001):108(4):1033–1044.

Craft, S. Insulin Resistance Syndrome and Alzheimer's Disease: Pathophysiologic Mechanisms and Therapeutic Implications. *Alzheimer Dis Assoc Disord* (2006):20(4):298–301.

Croen, L.A., J.K. Grether, and S. Selvin. Descriptive Epidemiology of Autism in a California Population: Who is at Risk? *J Autism Dev Disord* (2002):32:217–224.

Debouverie, M., S. Pittion-Vouyovitch, S. Louis, and F. Guillemin; LORSEP Group. Natural History of Multiple Sclerosis in a Population-Based Cohort. *Eur J Neurol* (2008):15(9):916–921.

DeVivo, M.J., and S.L. Stover. Long-Term Survival and Causes of Death. In: Stover, S.L., J.A. DeLisa, and G.G. Whiteneck, editors, *Spinal Cord Injury: Clinical Outcomes from the Model Systems.* Gaithersburg, MD: Aspen Publishers (1995):289–316.

Deyo, R.A., and J.N. Weinstein. Low Back Pain. *N Engl J Med* (2001):344:363–370.

Diaz-Arrastia, R., Y. Gong, S. Fair, et al. Increased Risk of Late Posttraumatic Seizures Associated with Inheritance of APOE epsilon4 Allele. *Arch Neurol* (2003):60(6):818–822.

Doll, R. Review: Alzheimer's Disease and Environmental Aluminum. *Age Ageing* (1993):22:138–153.

Doyle, L.W., C.A. Crowther, P. Middleton, S. Marret, and D. Rouse. Magnesium Sulfate for Women at Risk of Preterm Birth for Neuroprotection of the Fetus. *Cochrane Database Syst Rev* (2009 Jan 21):(1):CD004661.

Drago, D., S. Bolognin, and P. Zatta. Role of Metal Ions in the Abeta Oligomerization in Alzheimer's Disease and in Other Neurological Disorders. *Curr Alzheimer Res* (2008):5(6):500–507.

Duncan, J.S., J.W. Sander, S.M. Sisodiya, and M.C. Walker. Adult Epilepsy. *Lancet* (2006): 367(9516):1087–1100.

Durkin, M.S., M.J. Maenner, C.J. Newschaffer, et al. Advanced Parental Age and the Risk of Autism Spectrum Disorder. *Am J Epidemiol* (2008):168(11):1268–1276.

Durston, S. A Review of the Biological Basis of ADHD: What Have We Learned From Imaging Studies? Mental Retardation and Developmental Disabilities *Research Reviews* (2003):9(3): 184–195.

Ebers, G.C., D. Bulman, A.D. Sadovnick, et al. A Population-Based Study of Multiple Sclerosis in Twins. *N Engl J Med* (1986):64:808–817.

Editorial. Bringing Epilepsy Out of the Shadows. *BMJ* (1997):315:2–3.

Fangerau, T., S. Schimrigk, M. Haupts, et al. Multiple Sclerosis Study Group. Diagnosis of Multiple Sclerosis: Comparison of the Poser Criteria and the New McDonald Criteria. *Acta Neurol Scand* (2004):109(6):385–389.

Faraone, S.V., and A.E. Doyle. The Nature and Heritability of Attention-Deficit/Hyperactivity Disorder. *Child Adolesc Psychiatr Clin N Am* (2001):10(2):299–316.

Faridi, K., and O. Suchowersky. Gilles de la Tourette's Syndrome. *Can J Neurol Sci* (2003):30(Suppl 1):S64–S71.

Farmer, J.E., and T.R. Davis. Carpal Tunnel Syndrome: A Case-Control Study Evaluating its Relationship with Body Mass Index and Hand and Wrist Measurements. *J Hand Surg Eur Vol.* (2008):33(4):445–448.

Folkerth, R.D. The Neuropathology of Acquired Pre- and Perinatal Brain Injuries. *Semin Diagn Pathol* (2007):24(1):48–57.

Gelb, D.J., E. Oliver, and S. Gilman. Diagnostic Criteria for Parkinson's Disease. *Arch Neurol* (1999):56(1):33–39.

Gelfman, R., L.J. Melton, B.P. Yawn, P.C. Wollan, P.C. Amadio, and J.C. Stevens. Long-Term Trends in Carpal Tunnel Syndrome. *Neurology* (2009):72:33–41.

Gendolla, A. Early Treatment in Migraine: How Strong is the Current Evidence? *Cephalalgia* (2008):28(Suppl 2):28–35.

Gerber, J.S., and P.A. Offit. Vaccines and Autism: A Tale of Shifting Hypotheses. *Clin Infect Dis* (2009 Feb 15):48(4):456-461.

Gracia, F., L.C. Castillo, A. Benzadón, et al. Prevalence and Incidence of Multiple Sclerosis in Panama (2000-2005). *Neuroepidemiology* (2009):32(4):287–293.

Guerrini, R. Epilepsy in Children. *Lancet* (2006):367(9509):499–524.

Haan, J., A.M. van den Maagdenberg, O.F. Brouwer, and M.D. Ferrari. Migraine and Epilepsy: Genetically Linked? *Expert Rev Neurother* (2008):8(9):1307–1311.

Hagerman, R.J., E. Berry-Kravis, W.E. Kaufmann, et al. Advances in the Treatment of Fragile X Syndrome. *Pediatrics* (2009):123(1):378–390.

Harris, K., and H.S. Singer. Tic Disorders: Neural Circuits, Neurochemistry, and Neuroimmunology. *J Child Neurol* (2006):21(8):678–688.

Hatcher, J.M., K.D. Pennell, and G.W. Miller. Parkinson's Disease and Pesticides: A Toxicological Perspective. *Trends Pharmacol Sci* (2008):29(6):322–329.

Hauser, W.A., J.F. Annegers, and W.A. Rocca. Descriptive Epidemiology of Epilepsy: Contributions of Population-Based Studies from Rochester, Minnesota. *Mayo Clin Proc* (1996):71(6):576–586.

Headache Classification Subcommittee of the International Headache Society (IHS). The International Classification of Headache Disorders. *Cephalalgia* (2004): 24(Suppl 1):1–160.

Hernán, M.A., S.M. Zhang, L. Lipworth, M.J. Olek, and A. Ascherio. Multiple Sclerosis and Age at Infection with Common Viruses. *Epidemiology* (2001):12(3):301–306.

Hughes, J.R. A Review of Sudden Unexpected Death in Epilepsy: Prediction of Patients at Risk. *Epilepsy Behav* (2009):14(2):280–287.

Jensen, R., and L.J. Stovner. Epidemiology and Comorbidity of Headache. *Lancet Neurol* (2008):7(4):354–361.

Jilek, S., M. Schluep, P. Meylan, et al. Strong EBV-Specific CD8+ T-cell Response in Patients with Early Multiple Sclerosis. *Brain* (2008):131(Pt 7):1712–1721.

Judge, J.O., C. Lindsey, M. Underwood, and D. Winsemius. Balance Improvements in Older Women: Effects of Exercise Training. *Physical Therapy* (1993):73(4):254–265.

Karahan, A., S. Kav, A. Abbasoglu, and N. Dogan. Low Back Pain: Prevalence and Associated Risk Factors among Hospital Staff. *J Adv Nurs* (2009):65(3):516–524.

Kelman, L. The Triggers or Precipitants of the Acute Migraine Attack. *Cephalalgia* (2007):27(5):394–402.

Khurana, S.R., A.M. Bamer, A.P. Turner, R.V. Wadhwani, J.D. Bowen, S.L. Leipertz, and J.K. Haselkorn. The Prevalence of Overweight and Obesity in Veterans with Multiple Sclerosis. *Am J Phys Med Rehabil* (2009):88(2):83–91.

Kim, C.H., I.D. Waldman, R.D. Blakely, and K.S. Kim. Functional Gene Variation in the Human Norepinephrine Transporter: Association with Attention Deficit Hyperactivity Disorder. *Ann NY Acad Sci* (2008):1129:256–260.

Knopman, D.S. Cerebrovascular Disease and Dementia. *Br J Radiol* (2007):80(Spec No. 2):S121–S127.

Kossoff, E.H., and H.S. Singer. Tourette Syndrome: Clinical Characteristics and Current Management Strategies. *Paediatr Drugs* (2001):3(5):355–363.

Kurtzke, J.F. Epidemiologic Contributions to Multiple Sclerosis: An Overview. *Neurology* (1980):30:61–79.

Kutzelnigg, A., C.F. Lucchinetti, C. Stadelmann, et al. Cortical Demyelination and Diffuse White Matter Injury in Multiple Sclerosis. *Brain* (2005):128(Pt 11):2705–2712.

Kuwabara, S. Guillain-Barré Syndrome: Epidemiology, Pathophysiology, and Management. *Drugs* (2004):64(6):597–610.

Lagae, L. What's New in: "Genetics in Childhood Epilepsy". *Eur J Pediatr* (2008):167(7):715–722.

Langlois, J.A., S.R. Kegler, J.A. Butler, et al. Traumatic Brain Injury-Related Hospital Discharges: Results from a Fourteen State Surveillance System, 1997. *Morbidity and Mortality Weekly Reports* (2003):52(SS-04):1–18.

Langlois, J.A., W. Rutland-Brown, and M. Wald. The Epidemiology and Impact of Traumatic Brain Injury: A Brief Overview. *Journal of Head Trauma Rehabilitation* (2006):21(5):375–378.

Langston, J.W. The Etiology of Parkinson's Disease with Emphasis on the MPTP Story. *Neurology* (1996):47:S153–S160.

Laurin, N., K.G. Wigg, Y. Feng, P. Sandor, and C.L. Barr. Chromosome 5 and Gilles de la Tourette Syndrome: Linkage in a Large Pedigree and Association Study of Six Candidates in the Region. *Am J Med Genet B Neuropsychiatr Genet* (2009):150B(1):95–103.

Lee, M., and P. O'Brien. Pregnancy and Multiple Sclerosis. *J Neurol Neurosurg Psychiatry* (2008):79(12):1308–1311.

Lewitt, P.A. Levodopa for the Treatment of Parkinson's Disease. *N Engl J Med* (2008):359(23):2468–2476.

Lombroso, P.J., and L. Scahill. Tourette Syndrome and Obsessive-Compulsive Disorder. *Brain Dev* (2008 Apr):30(4):231–237.

Lunn, M.R., and C.H. Wang. Spinal Muscular Atrophy. *Lancet* (2008):371(9630):2120–2133.

Mack, K.J. New Daily Persistent Headache in Children and Adults. *Curr Pain Headache Rep* (2009):13(1):47–51.

Mack, M.G., J.J. Sacks, and D. Thompson. Testing the Impact Attenuation of Loose Fill Playground Surfaces. *Injury Prevention* (2000):6:141–144.

Marrie, R., R. Horwitz, G. Cutter, T. Tyry, D. Campagnolo, and T. Vollmer. High Frequency of Adverse Health Behaviors in Multiple Sclerosis. *Mult Scler* (2009):15(1):105–113.

Martin, V.T., and R.B. Lipton. Epidemiology and Biology of Menstrual Migraine. *Headache* (2008):48(Suppl 3):S124–S130.

McClernon, F.J., and S.H. Kollins. ADHD and Smoking: From Genes to Brain to Behavior. *Ann NY Acad Sci* (2008):1141:131–147.

McGrogan, A., G.C. Madle, H.E. Seaman, and C.S. de Vries. The Epidemiology of Guillain-Barré Syndrome Worldwide. A Systematic Literature Review. *Neuroepidemiology* (2009):32(2):150–163.

Meyers, A., M. Mitra, D. Walker, N. Wilber, and D. Allen. Predictors of Secondary Conditions in a Sample of Independently Living Adults with High-Level Spinal Cord Injury. *Topics in Spinal Cord Injury Rehabilitation* (2000):6(1):1–7.

Munoz, D.G. Is Exposure to Aluminum a Risk Factor for the Development of Alzheimer's Disease? *Arch Neurol* (1998):55:737–739.

Murthy, J.M., and S. Prabhakar. Bacterial Meningitis and Epilepsy. *Epilepsia* (2008):49(Suppl 6):8–12.

National Center for Injury Prevention and Control, Centers for Disease Control and Prevention (CDC). Traumatic Brain Injury Prevention. Available at http://www.cdc.gov/TraumaticInjury/prevention.html. Accessed February 26, 2009.

Nestoriuc, Y., A. Martin, W. Rief, and F. Andrasik. Biofeedback Treatment for Headache Disorders: A Comprehensive Efficacy Review. *Appl Psychophysiol Biofeedback* (2008):33(3):125–140.

Noseworthy, J.H., C. Lucchinetti, B.G. Moses, and B.G. Weinshenker. Multiple Sclerosis. *New Eng J Med* (2000):343(13):938–952.

Okamoto, K., T. Kihira, G. Kobashi, et al. Fruit and Vegetable Intake and Risk of Amyotrophic Lateral Sclerosis in Japan. *Neuroepidemiology* (2009):32(4):251–256.

Panayiotopoulos, C.P., M. Michael, S. Sanders, T. Valeta, and M. Koutroumanidis. Benign Childhood Focal Epilepsies: Assessment of Established and Newly Recognized Syndromes. *Brain* (2008):131(Pt 9):2264–2286.

Parratt, J., R. Tavendale, J. O'Riordan, D. Parratt, and R. Swingler. Chlamydia Pneumoniae-Specific Serum Immune Complexes in Patients with Multiple Sclerosis. *Mult Scler* (2008):14(3):292–299.

Pengel, L.H.M, R.D. Herbert, C.G. Maher, and K.M. Refshauge. Acute Low Back Pain: Systematic Review of its Prognosis. *BMJ* (2003):327:323–328.

Polman, C.H., S.C. Reingold, G. Edan, et al. Diagnostic Criteria for Multiple Sclerosis: 2005 Revisions to the "McDonald Criteria". *Ann Neurol* (2005):58(6):840–846.

Presidential Proclamation 6158. Decade of the Brain (July 17, 1990). Available at http://www.loc.gov/loc/brain/proclaim.html. Accessed February 28, 2009.

Pritchard, J. What's New in Guillain-Barré Syndrome? *Postgrad Med J* (2008):84(996):532–538.

Racette, B.A., S.D. Tabbal, D. Jennings, L. Good, J.S. Perlmutter, and B. Evanoff. Prevalence of Parkinsonism and Relationship to Exposure in a Large Sample of Alabama Welders. *Neurology* (2005):64(2):230–235.

Ramagopalan, S.V., D.A. Dyment, and G.C. Ebers. Genetic Epidemiology: The Use of Old and New Tools for Multiple Sclerosis. *Trends Neurosci* (2008):31(12):645–652.

Rapin, I., and R.F. Tuchman. Autism: Definition, Neurobiology, Screening, Diagnosis. *Pediatr Clin North Am* (2008):55(5):1129–1146.

Rapin, I., and R.F. Tuchman. Where We Are: Overview and Definitions. In: Tuchman, R., and I. Rapin, editors, *Autism: A Neurological Disorder of Early Brain Development. International Review of Child Neurology Series*. London: MacKeith Press (2006):1–18.

Rempel, D., B. Evanoff, P.C. Amadio, et al. Consensus Criteria for the Classification of Carpal Tunnel Syndrome in Epidemiologic Studies. *Am J Public Health* (1998):88(10):1447–1451.

Roberts, E.M., P.B. English, J.K. Grether, G.C. Windham, L. Somberg, and C. Wolff. Maternal Residence Near Agricultural Pesticide Applications and Autism Spectrum Disorders among Children in the California Central Valley. *Environ Health Perspect* (2007):115(10):1482–1489.

Robertson, M.M. The Prevalence and Epidemiology of Gilles de la Tourette Syndrome. Part 1: The Epidemiological and Prevalence Studies. *J Psychosom Res* (2008):65(5):461–472.

Robinson, M.N., L.J. Peake, M.R. Ditchfield, S.M. Reid, A. Lanigan, and D.S. Reddihough. Magnetic Resonance Imaging Findings in a Population-Based Cohort of Children with Cerebral Palsy. *Dev Med Child Neurol* (2009):51(1):39–45.

Rocha, J.A., C. Reis, F. Simões, J. Fonseca, and J. Mendes Ribeiro. Diagnostic Investigation and Multidisciplinary Management in Motor Neuron Disease. *J Neurol* (2005):252(12):1435–1447.

Roquelaure, Y., C. Ha, G. Nicolas, et al. Attributable Risk of Carpal Tunnel Syndrome According to Industry and Occupation in a General Population. *Arthritis Rheum* (2008 Sep 15):59(9):1341–1348.

Rothstein, J.D. Current Hypotheses for the Underlying Biology of Amyotrophic Lateral Sclerosis. *Ann Neurol* (2009):65(Suppl 1):S3–S9.

Rouse, D.J., D.G. Hirtz, E. Thom, et al. Eunice Kennedy Shriver NICHD Maternal–Fetal Medicine Units Network. A Randomized, Controlled Trial of Magnesium Sulfate for the Prevention of Cerebral Palsy. *N Engl J Med* (2008):359(9):895–905.

Sano, M., D. Jacobs, H. Andrews, et al. A Multi-Center, Randomized, Double Blind Placebo-Controlled Trial of Estrogens to Prevent Alzheimer's Disease and Loss of Memory in Women: Design and Baseline Characteristics. *Clin Trials* (2008):5(5):523–533.

Sano, M., H. Grossman, and K. Van Dyk. Preventing Alzheimer's Disease: Separating Fact from Fiction. *CNS Drugs* (2008):22(11):887–902.

Schapira, A.H. Etiology of Parkinson's Disease. *Neurology* (2006):66(10 Suppl 4):S10–S23.

Scheffer, I.E., L.A. Harkin, B.E. Grinton, et al. Temporal Lobe Epilepsy and GEFS+ Phenotypes Associated with SCN1B Mutations. *Brain* (2007):130(Pt 1):100–109.

Schwartz, B.S., W.F. Stewart, D. Simon, and R.B. Lipton. Epidemiology of Tension-Type Headache. *JAMA* (1998):279:381–383.

SCI Facts. Christopher and Dana Reeve Foundation, Available at http://www.christopherreeve.org/site/c.ddJFKRNoFiG/b.4425921/k.ECD3/SCI_Facts.htm. Accessed February 28, 2009.

Shattuck, P.T. The Contribution of Diagnostic Substitution to the Growing Administrative Prevalence of Autism in U.S. Special Education. *Pediatrics* (2006):117(4):1028–1037.

Shaw, C.A., and G.U. Höglinger. Neurodegenerative Diseases: Neurotoxins as Sufficient Etiologic Agents? *Neuromolecular Med* (2008):10(1):1–9.

Shields, W.D. Diagnosis of Infantile Spasms, Lennox-Gastaut Syndrome, and Progressive Myoclonic Epilepsy. *Epilepsia* (2004):45(Suppl 5):2–4.

Shiri, R., S. Solovieva, K. Husgafvel-Pursiainen, et al. The Association between Obesity and the Prevalence of Low Back Pain in Young Adults: The Cardiovascular Risk in Young Finns Study. *Am J Epidemiol* (2008):167(9):1110–1119.

Siddique, N., and T. Siddique. Genetics of Amyotrophic Lateral Sclerosis. *Phys Med Rehabil Clin N Am* (2008):19(3):429–439.

Sloane, P.D., S. Zimmerman, C. Suchindran, P. Reed, L. Wang, M. Boustani, and S. Sudha. The Public Health Impact of Alzheimer's Disease, 2000-2050: Potential Implications of Treatment Advances. *Annu Rev Pub; Health* (2002):23:213–231.

Sosin, D.M., J.E. Sniezek, and R.J. Waxweiler. Trends in Death Associated with Traumatic Brain Injury 1979 Through 1992: Success and Failure. *JAMA* (1995):273:1778–1780.

Sotelo, J., A. Martínez-Palomo, G. Ordoñez, and B. Pineda. Varicella-Zoster Virus in Cerebrospinal Fluid at Relapses of Multiple Sclerosis. *Ann Neurol* (2008):63(3):303–311.

Spinal Cord Injury Facts and Figures. Spinal Cord Injury Information Network. Birmingham: University of Alabama (2008). Available at http://www.spinalcord.uab.edu/show.asp?durki=1 16979&site=4716&return=19775. Accessed February 28, 2009.

Spinal Cord Injury Facts. National Center for Injury Control and Prevention, Centers for Disease Control and Prevention. Available at http://www.cdc.gov/ncipc/factsheets/scifacts.htm. Accessed February 28, 2009.

Stadelmann, C., and W. Bruck. Interplay between Mechanisms of Damage and Repair in Multiple Sclerosis. *J Neurol* (2008):255(Suppl 1):12–18.

Stanley, F., E. Blair, and E. Alberman. *Cerebral Palsies: Epidemiology and Causal Pathways.* London: MacKeith Press (2000).

Stein, M.A., and D. Shin. Disorders of Attention: Diagnosis. In: Accardo, P.J., editor, *Capute & Accardo's Neurodevelopmental Disabilities in Infancy and Childhood*, Volume II. Baltimore, MD: Paul H. Brookes Publishing Co. (2008):639.

Sumner, C.J. Molecular Mechanisms of Spinal Muscular Atrophy. *J Child Neurol* (2007):22(8):979–989.

Sundström, P., and L. Nyström. Smoking Worsens the Prognosis in Multiple Sclerosis. *Mult Scler* (2008):14(8):1031–1035.

Szekely, C.A., J.C. Breitner, A.L. Fitzpatrick, T.D. Rea, B.M. Psaty, L.H. Kuller, and P.P. Zandi. NSAID Use and Dementia Risk in the Cardiovascular Health Study: Role of APOE and NSAID Type. *Neurology* (2008):70(1):17–24.

Tan, N.C., J.C. Mulley, and I.E. Scheffer. Genetic Dissection of the Common Epilepsies. *Curr Opin Neurol* (2006):9(2):157–163.

Tanner, C.M., and S.M. Goldman. Epidemiology of Parkinson's Disease. *Neurol Clin* (1996):(2):317–335.

Thurman, D., C. Alverson, K. Dunn, J. Guerrero, and J. Sniezek. Traumatic Brain Injury in the United States: A Public Health Perspective. *Journal of Head Trauma Rehabilitation* (1999):14(6):602–615.

Todd, R.D., and R.J. Neuman. Gene-Environment Interactions in the Development of Combined Type ADHD: Evidence for a Synapse-Based Model. *Am J Med Genet B Neuropsychiatr Genet* (2007):144B(8):971–975.

Tomson, T., L. Nashef, and P. Ryvlin. Sudden Unexpected Death in Epilepsy: Current Knowledge and Future Directions. *Lancet Neurol.* (2008 Nov):7(11):1021–1031.

Trevathan, E., and S. Shinnar. Epidemiology of Autism Spectrum Disorders. In: Tuchman, R., and I. Rapin, editors, *Autism: A Neurological Disorder of Early Brain Development. International Review of Child Neurology Series.* London: MacKeith Press (2006):20–38.

Trevathan, E. Seizures and Epilepsy among Children with Language Regression and Autistic Spectrum Disorders. *J Child Neurol* (2004 Aug):19(Suppl 1):S49–S57.

Turner, M.R., M.C. Kiernan, P.N. Leigh, and K. Talbot. Biomarkers in Amyotrophic Lateral Sclerosis. *Lancet Neurol* (2009):8(1):94–109.

Walsh, C.A., E.M. Morrow, and J.L.R. Rubenstein. Autism and Brain Development. *Cell* (2008):135:396–400.

Waring, S.C., C. Esteban-Santillan, D.M. Reed, U.K. Craig, D.R. Labarthe, R.C. Petersen, and L.T. Kurland. Incidence of Amyotrophic Lateral Sclerosis and of the Parkinsonism-Dementia Complex of Guam, 1950-1989. *Neuroepidemiology* (2004):23(4):192–200.

Whitwell, J.L., C.R. Jack Jr., J.E. Parisi, et al. Rates of Cerebral Atrophy Differ in Different Degenerative Pathologies. *Brain* (2007):130:1148–1158.

Winter, S., A. Autry, C. Boyle, and M. Yeargin-Allsopp. Trends in the Prevalence of Congenital Cerebral Palsy in Atlanta, Georgia. *Pediatrics* (2002):10:1220–1225.

World Health Organization (WHO). *WHO Global Campaign Against Epilepsy.* Geneva: ILAE/IBE/WHO (2003).

Wynn, D.R., M. Rodriguez, W.M. O'Fallon, and L.T. Kurland. A Reappraisal of the Epidemiology of Multiple Sclerosis in Olmsted County, Minnesota. *Neurology* (1990):40:780–786.

Yang, Y.X., N.W. Wood, and D.S. Latchman. Molecular Basis of Parkinson's Disease. *Neuroreport* (2009):20(2):150–156.

Yeargin-Allsopp, M., C. Boyle, K. van Naarden Braun, and E. Trevathan. The Epidemiology of Developmental Disabilities. In: Accardo, P.J., editor, *Capute & Accardo's Neurodevelopmental Disabilities in Infancy and Childhood*. Baltimore, MD: Paul H. Brookes Publishing Co. (2008):61–104.

Yeargin-Allsopp, M., C. Rice, T. Karapurkar, N. Doerberg, C. Boyle, and C. Murphy. Prevalence of Autism in a U.S. Metropolitan Area. *JAMA* (2003):289:49–55.

Yekhlef, F., G. Ballan, F. Macia, O. Delmer, C. Sourgen, and F. Tison. Routine MRI for the Differential Diagnosis of Parkinson's Disease, MSA, PSP, and CBD. *J Neural Transm* (2003):110(2):151–169.

Zaki, E.A., T. Freilinger, T. Klopstock, et al. Two Common Mitochondrial DNA Polymorphisms are Highly Associated with Migraine Headache and Cyclic Vomiting Syndrome. *Cephalalgia* (2009):29(7):719–728.

Ziegler-Graham, K., R. Brookmeyer, E. Johnson, and H.M. Arrighi. Worldwide Variation in the Doubling Time of Alzheimer's Disease Incidence Rates. *Alzheimers Dement* (2008):4(5):316–323.

CHAPTER 18

ARTHRITIS AND OTHER MUSCULOSKELETAL DISEASES (ICD-10 M00-M99)

Rosemarie Hirsch, M.D., M.P.H. and Marc C. Hochberg, M.D., M.P.H.

Introduction

Arthritis and other musculoskeletal diseases are the most common causes of physical disability in the United States (Kelsey and Hochberg 1988). According to the 2003–2005 National Health Interview Survey (NHIS), 21.6% of the U.S. population reported having doctor-diagnosed arthritis. By applying this prevalence to 2000 U.S. population figures, an estimated 46.4 million individuals are afflicted with arthritis (Hootman and Helmick 2006). Women are affected more often than men, and prevalence increases with increasing age in both groups (Figure 18.1) (Hootman and Helmick 2006). According to 2003–2005 NHIS data on the epidemiology of arthritis, 50.0% of all interviewees aged 65 years and older reported having doctor-diagnosed arthritis (Hootman et al. 2006).

Arthritis-attributable activity limitation, defined as limitation in any way in any usual activity because of arthritis or joint symptoms, was present in 8.8% of U.S. adults (18.9 million) according to 2003–2005 NHIS data (Hootman et al. 2006). Among those with doctor-diagnosed arthritis, 40.9% reported arthritis-attributable activity limitation. Groups with higher rates of arthritis-attributable activity limitation included older people, non-Hispanic blacks and Hispanics (compared with non-Hispanic whites), people with less than a high school education, and those who were obese (Body Mass Index $\geq$ 30 kg/m^2) or physically inactive (Hootman et al. 2006).

Musculoskeletal diseases such as arthritis are a heavy economic burden in the United States. The 2005 National Hospital Ambulatory Medical Care Survey estimated that musculoskeletal and connective tissue related disorders resulted in 80.6 million physician visits, and the National Hospital Discharge Survey estimated 761,000 hospitalizations with osteoarthritis and allied disorders as the primary diagnosis (Cherry, Woodwell, and Rechtsteiner 2007; DeFrances, Cullen, and Kozak 2007). The total cost of arthritis to the U.S. economy (including in- and out-patient care, medications, and lost productivity) in 2003 has been estimated at $128 billion, based on the Medical Expenditure Panel Survey (Yelin et al. 2003). Since the 2003 Medical Expenditure Panel Survey did not have a nursing home component, costs among nursing home residents were not included in this estimate. Total direct costs (i.e., medical expenditures) were $80.8 billion, averaging $1,752 per person with arthritis or related conditions, and total indirect costs (i.e., lost earnings) were $47 billion.

571

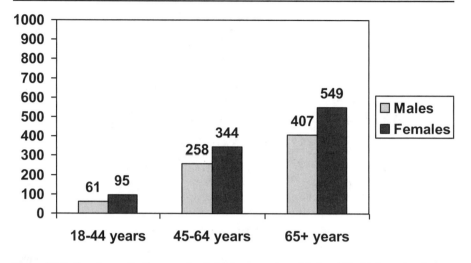

Figure 18.1. Prevalence of self-reported arthritis by age and sex, National Health Interview Survey, 2003. Data from Hootman and Helmick (2006).

More than 100 diseases make up the spectrum of arthritis and musculoskeletal disorders, with a variety of "upstream" causes and "downstream" consequences (Figure 18.2). Most of these diseases are uncommon, are of unknown cause, and allow little opportunity for primary or secondary prevention in the general population (Hochberg 1992). However, two disorders, osteoarthritis and osteoporosis, make up the vast majority of the disability and economic costs and are subject to primary and secondary prevention initiatives. The remainder of this chapter reviews the epidemiology of these conditions as well as the opportunities for their prevention and control. In addition, shorter descriptions are provided for two common types of inflammatory arthritis: rheumatoid arthritis and gout.

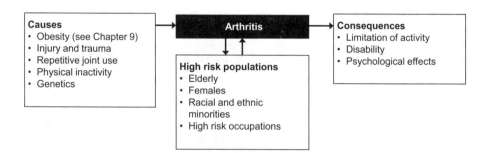

Figure 18.2. Arthritis: causes, consequences, and high-risk groups.

OSTEOARTHRITIS
(ICD-10 M15-M19)

Significance

The prevalence of osteoarthritis has been estimated in three national studies: the National Health Examination Survey (NHES), the First National Health and Nutrition Examination Survey (NHANES I, conducted from 1971 to 1975), and NHANES III (conducted from 1988 to 1994). The case definitions were based on x-ray changes in the hands and feet in NHES, on x-ray changes in knees and hips plus physician diagnosis in NHANES I, and on x-ray changes in the knees and physician examination plus symptoms in the hands in NHANES III. Overall, about one-third of adults aged 25 to 74 years had x-ray evidence of osteoarthritis involving at least one site. The prevalence of clinical osteoarthritis, based on both physician examination and symptoms, was 12.1% in adults aged 25 to 74 years in NHANES I (Lawrence et al. 1989). The prevalence of site-specific osteoarthritis follows: radiographic foot osteoarthritis in 22% of persons aged 25–74 years from NHES; radiographic hand osteoarthritis in 33% of persons aged 25–74 years from NHES; symptomatic hand osteoarthritis (based on modified American College of Rheumatology [ACR] classification criteria; physician examination plus symptoms) in 8% of those aged 60 years and older in NHANES III; and radiographic knee osteoarthritis in 37.4% and symptomatic knee osteoarthritis (x-ray changes plus symptoms) in 12.1% of those aged 60 years and older in NHANES III (Dillon et al. 2006, 2007; Lawrence et al. 1989).

Pathophysiology

Osteoarthritis is defined as a "heterogeneous group of conditions that lead to joint symptoms and signs that are associated with defective integrity of articular (joint) cartilage, in addition to related changes in the underlying bone and at joint margins" (Altman et al. 1986). The pathophysiological basis of osteoarthritis is a combination of biomechanical and biochemical alterations in the physical and chemical properties of articular cartilage that affects all the tissues of the joint, including the subchondral bone and synovium, and surrounding periarticular tissues. These biomechanically induced biochemical alterations lead to loss of cartilage in areas of increased load, thickening of underlying subchondral bone, formation of spurs or marginal osteophytes (evidence of repair), and a variable degree of inflammation. The clinical features of osteoarthritis, including pain, tenderness, bony and/or soft-tissue swelling, and decreased function, result from these biomechanical and morphologic alterations (Hochberg 1993).

Descriptive Epidemiology

High-risk groups

The incidence of osteoarthritis increases with advancing age (Hochberg 1991a, 1991b). Prevalence of osteoarthritis, as well as the proportion of cases with moderate or severe disease, also increases with age at least through ages 65 to 74 years (Hochberg 1991a). These findings are consistent with observations of excess mortality in older subjects with symptomatic osteoarthritis, possibly due to cardiovascular and gastrointestinal side effects from the use of nonsteroidal anti-inflammatory drugs (Hochberg 1989b).

Osteoarthritis is more common among men than among women younger than 45 years and more common among women than among men older than 54 years (Lawrence et al. 1989). Clinically, patterns of joint involvement also demonstrate sex differences, with women having on average more joints involved and more frequent complaints of morning stiffness and joint swelling; indeed, the syndrome of generalized osteoarthritis with Heberden's nodes (bony enlargements of the last joint of the fingers) is found most commonly in postmenopausal women. Among adults in the United States, knee osteoarthritis is more common among Blacks than among whites (Anderson and Felson 1988; Dillon et al. 2006). No racial differences have been noted for hip osteoarthritis in the United States; however, hip osteoarthritis is quite rare in Chinese and other Asian populations (Tepper and Hochberg 1993).

Other groups at higher risk of osteoarthritis include (1) people with a genetic predisposition, especially women with the syndrome of Heberden's and Bouchard's (bony enlargements of the middle joint of the fingers) nodes; (2) people with congenital or developmental disease of bones and joints, such as congenital hip subluxation (partial dislocation) with subsequent hip osteoarthritis; (3) people with previous inflammatory joint disease, such as gout or rheumatoid arthritis; and (4) people with metabolic diseases such as hyperparathyroidism (overactive parathyroid gland(s)), hypothyroidism (underactive thyroid gland), and articular chrondocalcinosis (calcium crystal deposition in cartilage).

Geographic distribution

Data from national surveys suggest that arthritis and associated disabilities are most prevalent in the south and least prevalent in the northeast (Hochberg, Ardey, and Diamond 1989a). Possible explanations for these patterns include a lower socioeconomic status and greater proportion of population employed in manual labor in the south. No specific studies have been conducted to determine reasons for these regional variations, however.

Time trends

No data are currently available on time trends in the prevalence of osteoarthritis in the United States.

Causes

Risk factors for the development of osteoarthritis have been the subject of many studies. They are generally considered in two broad categories; those that cause osteoarthritis through systemic mechanisms and those that cause osteoarthritis through local, predominantly biomechanical, mechanisms. Results will be summarized briefly here; readers are referred to the bibliography for more detailed reviews and citations to original studies.

Modifiable risk factors

The major modifiable risk factors for osteoarthritis are joint trauma, obesity, and repetitive joint usage (Table 18.1) (Hochberg 1991a, 1991b). A history of joint trauma is the

Table 18.1. Modifiable Risk Factors for Osteoarthritis,[a] United States

Magnitude	Risk Factor
Strong (relative risk >4)	Joint trauma
Moderate (relative risk 2–4)	Repetitive occupational usage
	Obesity
Weak (relative risk <2)	Muscle weakness
	Nutritional deficiencies

[a]Risk factors differ in their magnitude based on the site of osteoarthritis involved.

strongest risk factor for unilateral osteoarthritis at either the knee (Davis, Ettinger, and Neuhaus 1990) or the hip (Tepper and Hochberg 1993).

Obesity has been convincingly demonstrated to have a causal role in osteoarthritis of the knee. In cross-sectional studies, obesity as measured by body mass index is a strong risk factor for both unilateral and bilateral knee osteoarthritis in both sexes (Anderson and Felson 1988; Davis, Ettinger, and Neuhaus 1990). Furthermore, in longitudinal studies, obesity predicts the development of knee osteoarthritis in both sexes (Felson 1990). Weight loss decreases the risk of developing symptomatic knee osteoarthritis in women (Felson et al. 1992). Furthermore, weight loss reduces symptoms and functional impairment in patients with symptomatic knee osteoarthritis. Data regarding the association of obesity with both hand and hip osteoarthritis, however, are inconsistent (Gelber et al. 1999; Hochberg 1991a; Hochberg et al. 1991; Scott and Hochberg 1987; Tepper and Hochberg 1993).

Repetitive joint use, largely the result of occupational demands, is also associated with osteoarthritis. Numerous studies have demonstrated an excess of site-specific osteoarthritis in occupational groups with repetitive use of specific joints. Occupations requiring knee-bending have been associated with knee osteoarthritis in both retrospective and prospective studies (Anderson and Felson 1988; Felson 1990). Farming has been associated with hip osteoarthritis in several retrospective studies (Croft et al. 1992; Scott and Hochberg 1987). Avocational activities, including moderate running and many other sports activities, have not been associated with the development of osteoarthritis among people who have not had joint injuries. However, sports that include acute or repetitive joint impact or twisting (e.g., elbows and shoulders of baseball pitchers) have been associated with osteoarthritis (Felson et al. 2000; Panush 1990).

Other modifiable risk factors that may contribute to osteoarthritis include muscle weakness and nutritional deficiencies. Quadriceps muscle weakness has been associated with the development of radiographic and symptomatic knee osteoarthritis (Slemenda et al. 1997). Low intake of vitamin C has been shown to increase the risk of knee osteoarthritis progression and low intake of vitamin D has been associated with progression of knee and hip osteoarthritis (Felson et al. 2000). Studies addressing the association between estrogen replacement therapy and risk of osteoarthritis have produced conflicting findings (Felson et al. 2000).

In the studies of socioeconomic factors associated with osteoarthritis, having less than 12 years of formal education and having a low family income were each associated with a clinical diagnosis of osteoarthritis (Yelin and Felts 1990); however, neither factor was associated with the presence of knee or hip osteoarthritis diagnosed on the basis of x-ray criteria (Anderson and Felson 1988; Hannan et al. 1992; Tepper and Hochberg 1993).

Population-attributable risk

Although attributable risk estimates are not available for multiple sites of osteoarthritis, estimates for osteoarthritis of the knee are available (Felson 1990). These estimates indicate that repetitive occupational joint-bending and obesity account for large portions of knee osteoarthritis (32% and 24% respectively) in working men and women age 55-64 years old.

Prevention and Control

Prevention

Epidemiological considerations in the primary prevention of osteoarthritis have been reviewed elsewhere (Hochberg et al. 1991). On the basis of current knowledge of risk factors, avoiding joint trauma, preventing obesity, and modifying occupational-related joint stress through ergonomic approaches can all be recommended for the prevention of osteoarthritis. National recommendations include reducing obesity (Body Mass Index > 25.0 kg/m^2) to a prevalence of no more than 15% among adults, increasing the proportion of adults who perform physical activities that enhance and maintain muscular strength and endurance, and reducing the number of nonfatal unintentional injuries, especially those that are work related. Reduction of weight has been shown to reduce pain in symptomatic osteoarthritis of the knee (vide supra) (Felson et al. 1992).

Screening

Screening and early detection of osteoarthritis are not feasible at present.

Treatment

Multidisciplinary treatment of osteoarthritis is required (ACR 2000). This involves the use of nonpharmacological modalities such as physical therapy to maintain and improve joint range of motion and muscle strength, occupational therapy to maximize the patient's independent ability to perform activities of daily living including dressing, feeding, bathing, toileting, and grooming, patient education, weight loss, aerobic conditioning, and social support to increase self-efficacy. In patients whose symptoms are not adequately controlled by nonpharmacological modalities and over-the-counter analgesics, nonsteroidal anti-inflammatory drugs, including COX-2–selective inhibitors, and/or intra-articular corticosteroids or hyaluronans can be used to control symptoms of pain and stiffness. The potential role of nutritional supplements (e.g., glucosamine, chondroitin sulfate) or disease-modifying osteoarthritis drugs (e.g., doxycycline) have yet to be finalized (Brandt et al. 2005; Clegg et al. 2006). Surgery, especially total joint replacement, is indicated in patients with moderate-to-severe pain and/or limitation of physical activities that reduce their health-related quality of life despite medical therapy.

Increasing evidence indicates that people with arthritis are less physically active and less fit than their peers (CDC 1997). They can benefit significantly from conditioning exercise programs to improve both cardiovascular and musculoskeletal fitness without disease exacerbation or joint damage (Minor and Lane 1996), such as low-impact weight-bearing exercises (walking or resistance training for major muscle groups), water aerobics, or stationary bicycling, many of which are available in communities through the Arthritis Foundation Exercise Program and Aquatic Program.

RHEUMATOID ARTHRITIS (ICD-10 M05-06, M08)

Significance

Most studies in developed countries report a prevalence of 0.5%–1.0% in the adult population. The U.S. prevalence is 0.85% for whites age 35 years and older (Gabriel, Crowson, and Fallon 1999) and on the order of 2% for those age 60 years and older, based on data from NHANES III (Rasch et al. 2003). Studies in numerous populations have shown a progressive decline in rheumatoid arthritis incidence since the 1960s (Doran et al. 2002). This decline in incidence is also reflected as a decreasing prevalence in younger age groups in more recent decades (Helmick et al. 2008).

Pathophysiology

Rheumatoid arthritis is an autoimmune disease involving chronic inflammation. The inflammation begins in the synovial membranes of the joints and spreads to other joint tissues. The inflamed synovial tissue may invade and damage the cartilage in the joints and erode bone (pannus), leading to joint deformities. The usual clinical symptoms include stiffness, pain, and swelling of multiple joints, commonly the small joints of the hands and feet. The wrists, elbows, ankles, and knees are also typical sites of involvement. Although it primarily affects the joints, rheumatoid arthritis can also affect connective tissue throughout the body and can cause disease in a variety of organs, including the lungs, the heart, and the eyes.

Descriptive Epidemiology

In general, the prevalence of rheumatoid arthritis increases with age in both sexes. In addition, prevalence rates are two to three times greater among women than among men. No striking differences in morbidity rates have been noted between blacks and whites. Several Native American tribes, however, have a particularly high prevalence of rheumatoid arthritis, including the Yakima of central Washington State and the Mille-Lac Band of Chippewa in Minnesota. Asians, including Japanese and Chinese, appear to have lower prevalence rates than do whites (Alarcon 1995). The reasons for these differences are unknown, but they probably relate to both genetic and environmental factors.

Causes

Although the causes of rheumatoid arthritis are unknown, genetic factors play an important role in a person's predisposition to rheumatoid arthritis, and may contribute upwards of 60% to the risk of developing rheumatoid arthritis (MacGregor et al. 2000). The disease exhibits a higher concordance rate in monozygotic (identical) twins than in dizygotic (fraternal) twins (Silman 1994). In addition, the susceptibility to rheumatoid arthritis appears to be inherited as an autosomal-dominant trait in multicase families. Studies have demonstrated a strong association between rheumatoid arthritis and the "shared epitope," a sequence in the third hypervariable region of the HLA-DR β-chain (de Vries et al. 2002). This association crosses ethnic and racial boundaries, such as whites, the Yakima Indians of Washington State, and Israeli Jews and Koreans, but is not inclusive. The role of other major histocompatibility complex (MHC) genes and non-MHC genes in disease susceptibility has been suggested by several studies (Alarcon 1995; Begovich et al. 2004; Silman 1994).

Although there is a marked increase in the prevalence of rheumatoid arthritis in women, the underlying hormonal influences are not well understood. A protective effect of the use of oral contraceptives on the development of rheumatoid arthritis has been suggested by a number of studies (Silman 1994). However, a meta-analysis has failed to support this observation; the authors concluded that there may be some evidence of protection for severe forms of rheumatoid arthritis (Pladevall-Villa et al. 1996).

Environmental and infectious risk factors have been proposed but have yet to be substantiated. The only modifiable risk factor for rheumatoid arthritis is cigarette smoking, and smoking cessation may prevent disease onset (Criswell et al. 2006; Saag et al. 1997).

Rheumatoid arthritis is associated with excess mortality. Causes of death that are more frequent in rheumatoid arthritis patients include respiratory and infectious diseases and gastrointestinal disorders; the latter may be related to the use of nonsteroidal anti-inflammatory drugs. Although the proportionate mortality from cancer is reduced in rheumatoid arthritis, the actual incidence of and mortality from non-Hodgkin's lymphoma, Hodgkin's disease, and lung cancer is higher for these patients than for the general population (Mellemkjaer et al. 1996). Some of the excess mortality caused by gastrointestinal disorders may be related to the complications of therapy with nonsteroidal anti-inflammatory drugs for the arthritis. Low socioeconomic status, as measured by education level, is also associated with increased mortality and excess disability. Recent data suggest that patients treated with methotrexate and/or tumor necrosis factor blockers have reduced mortality compared with patients with similar disease severity not treated with these agents.

Prevention and Control

No screening or primary prevention measures are available at present, although avoidance of cigarette smoking or smoking cessation might be considered. Patients with rheumatoid arthritis have been treated with disease-modifying antirheumatic drugs such as hydroxychloroquine, leflunomide, methotrexate, sulfasalazine, azathioprine, and other immunosuppressive agents. Since 1999, new biologic disease-modifying medications have been introduced, such as tumor necrosis factor blockers (etanercept, infliximab, adalimumab), the interleukin 1 receptor antagonist anakinra, and other biologic response modifiers, such as abatacept and rituximab. The treatment approach has also moved toward early aggressive treatment, sometimes with multiple medications, followed by a step-down of medications once disease control is achieved, as opposed to the older paradigm of repeated use of monotherapy or step-up combination regimens (ACR 2002).

Because of the excess mortality from respiratory and infectious diseases among patients with rheumatoid arthritis, the single most important public health intervention available is immunization with pneumococcal vaccine, annual influenza vaccine, and tuberculosis screening before anticytokine or other biologic response modifier treatment (Winthrop et al. 2005). Growing evidence shows that participation in regular, moderate physical activity improves health status, emotional well-being, and physical fitness without aggravation of rheumatoid arthritis (Van Den et al. 2000).

GOUT (ICD-10 M10)

Significance

The most recent estimates of the prevalence of gout in the United States are based on 1996 NHIS participant responses to the question, "Have you had gout within the last year?" (Adams, Hendershot, and Marano 1999). The one-year period prevalence rates were 9.4 per 1000.

Based on comparable data from the 1969 NHIS, the prevalence rate of gout was 4.8/1000 and has increased in both sexes over a 27-year period (Wilder 1974). The increase in gout prevalence is the result of (1) a temporal increase in mean serum uric acid levels among men, (2) increased use of drugs known to produce secondary hyperuricemia, especially thiazide diuretics used by women; and (3) longer survival by people with gout. Also, part of the apparent increase may be artifactual and attributable to the incorrect diagnosis of individuals with joint pain and hyperuricemia who do not actually have gout. The most recent lifetime prevalence estimates of self-reported gout in adults from NHANES III were 38 per 1000 for men and 16 per 1000 for women (Kramer and Curhan 2002).

Pathophysiology

Gout is a metabolic disease characterized by recurrent attacks of acute arthritis, an increase in serum uric acid concentration (hyperuricemia), and deposition of sodium urate monohydrate crystals in and around joints. Because gout is relatively easy to diagnose, most reports of prevalence are based on self-reported physician diagnosis.

Descriptive Epidemiology

Prevalence rates for gout are nearly twice as high in men than in women. In addition, prevalence increases sharply with age for both sexes, and is greater among blacks than among whites over age 45 (Adams, Hendershot, and Marano 1999).

Table 18.2. Modifiable Risk Factors for Gout, United States

Magnitude	Risk Factor
Strong (relative risk >4)	None
Moderate (relative risk 2–4)	Hypertension
	Obesity
Weak (relative risk <2)	Alcohol
	Purine-rich foods

Causes

In addition to having hyperuricemia and being male, other risk factors for gout include high blood pressure, obesity, consumption of alcohol (especially beer), a high protein diet, renal disease, occupational and environmental lead exposure, and a family history of gout (see Table 18.2) (Choi et al. 2004a, 2004b; Hochberg et al. 1995; Roubenoff et al. 1991). Numerous family studies suggest a multifactorial inheritance and environmental factors probably contribute significantly to the familial aggregation.

Prevention and Control

The prevention of gout in people with asymptomatic hyperuricemia should include lifestyle modifications such as weight reduction, dietary changes, moderating or eliminating alcohol intake, and control of hypertension (without the use of thiazide diuretics) and hyperlipidemia. In addition, because of the known association of occupational lead exposure with gout, prevention efforts should also reduce such exposure in high-risk professions such as painting, plumbing, shipbuilding, and steel work.

Hyperuricemia is a known necessary risk factor for the development of gout and can be readily identified even in nonaffected people through automated multichannel analysis of serum specimens. The decision as to when to treat people with asymptomatic hyperuricemia is controversial. Several practical arguments against routine treatment include poor patient compliance, high costs, and adverse drug reactions. Furthermore, acute gout attacks are easily, inexpensively, and effectively treated with short courses of nonsteroidal anti-inflammatory drugs and/or glucocorticoids.

Medical treatment of gout is at the stage where recurrent attacks of arthritis may be prevented through long-term use of colchicine and through reversal of hyperuricemia with agents that either increase uric acid excretion or inhibit its production. The control strategies for gout should be employed in conjunction with treatment of associated conditions such as hypertension and hyperlipidemia.

OSTEOPOROSIS
(ICD-10 M80-M82)

Significance

Osteoporosis is a major public health problem in countries with aging populations. In 2004, the Surgeon General of the United States issued the first report on bone health and osteoporosis (DHHS 2004). This report contained six parts. Part 2 focused on the status of bone health in the United States while Parts 3 and 4 focused on strategies by individuals and health care professionals, respectively, to promote bone health.

For purposes of epidemiological studies, the World Health Organization (WHO) defined osteoporosis as a bone mineral density (BMD) value measured at the femoral neck or total hip of ≥2.5 standard deviations below the mean for normal young white women (WHO 1994). Based on data from the Third National Health and Nutrition Examination Survey (NHANES III), using this definition, there are an estimated 10 million women and 3 million men 50 year and older with osteoporosis in the United States (DHHS 2004; Looker et al. 1997). Approximately 1.5 million individuals experience fracture each year, with hip fractures accounting for about 300,000 of these (DHHS 2004). The annual direct costs for osteoporotic fractures ranged from $12.2 to $17.9 billion per year in 2002 for acute and chronic care (DHHS 2004).

Pathophysiology

Several definitions have been proposed for osteoporosis. The classic definition is "a systemic skeletal disorder characterized by low bone mass and microarchitectural deterioration of bone tissue, with a consequent increase in bone fragility and susceptibility to fracture (Consensus Development Conference 1991)." At a Consensus Conference sponsored by the National Institutes of Health in 2000, osteoporosis was defined as "a skeletal disorder characterized by compromised bone strength predisposing to an increased risk of fracture. Bone strength reflects the integration of two main features: bone density and bone quality. Bone density is expressed as grams of mineral per area or volume. . . . Bone quality refers to architecture, turnover, damage accumulation (e.g., microfractures) and mineralization" (NIH Consensus Statement 2000).

Concepts in the pathogenesis of osteoporosis have been reviewed recently with an emphasis on the complex interplay among genetics, hormones, nutrition, lifestyle, and environmental factors (Raisz 2005; Russell 2006). BMD in adulthood is determined in part by the amount of bone that is accrued by early to middle adult life and the rate of decline in bone mass during middle to late adult life. The clinical manifestations may include fractures of the spine, hip, wrist, or other areas of the skeleton (Cummings and Melton 2002). Indeed, fractures at almost all skeletal sites, except for the fingers, toes, face, and skull, are related to low BMD (Stone et al. 2003). Traditionally, fractures of the hip, spine, and wrist among older adults, especially when they occur in association with minimal or moderate trauma, have been considered as osteoporotic fractures. Many epidemiological studies have used fracture as a measure of osteoporosis because of the availability of data resources and the lack of access to technology to measure BMD. More recently, however, the availability of dual x-ray absorptiometry (DXA) for measurement of BMD has allowed the study of factors related to low BMD. Therefore, the epidemiology of osteoporosis is a combination of both the epidemiology of low BMD and the epidemiology of fracture.

Descriptive Epidemiology

High-Risk Groups

Osteoporosis is usually considered a disease of postmenopausal white women. Peak bone mass, usually achieved in the third decade, is lower in women than in men. On average, decline in bone mass occurs beginning in the fourth decade at a rate of 0.5% to 1.0% per year, with an accelerated rate of loss in the years immediately following menopause in women. Hence, the decline in bone mass in women proceeds from a lower baseline. In NHANES III, where BMD of the hip was measured as part of the examination, men had higher average BMD than women in every racial group reported; consequently, the prevalence of osteoporosis and osteopenia were lower in men than in women (Figure 18.3) (DHHS 2004). Not surprisingly, age-specific incidence rates for hip fracture are higher among women than among men through the ninth decade (Jacobsen et al. 1990a).

In western populations, whites have lower BMD, a higher prevalence of osteoporosis, (Figure 18.3), a greater rate of decline in BMD and a higher rate of nonspine and hip fractures than blacks (Cauley et al. 2005a, 2005b; DHHS 2004; George et al. 2003; Jacobsen et al. 1990b; Tracy et al. 2005). Age-specific incidence rates of hip fracture are about twice as high among white women as they are among black women, and most studies indicate a higher risk for hip fractures among white men than among black men. Mexican-American populations have lower hip fracture rates than whites but slightly higher rates than blacks (Bauer 1988). BMD is lower in Asians than in whites, but Asians may experience a lower incidence of hip fracture; this may be related to differences in geometry of the femoral neck between Asians and whites (Yano et al. 1985).

Twin and family studies suggest that genetic factors may explain as much as 85% of the variation in age-specific BMD in the population (Williams and Spector 2006). Genetics play the largest role in attainment of peak bone mass and probably also have a role in the rate of bone loss with aging or after menopause. The search for single-gene effects on BMD remains an active area of investigation. Allelic variations of the vitamin D receptor, type I collagen, estrogen receptor, and some cytokine genes, for example, are associated with BMD in some, but not all populations studied. Other candidate genes may also play important roles in the regulation of BMD, either alone or through an interaction with lifestyle factors.

Other factors associated with a high risk for osteoporosis and osteoporotic fractures are older age, low body weight, weight loss, physical inactivity, a history of a previous fracture after age 50 years, current smoking, excessive alcohol consumption, and recent use of oral glucocorticoids (Espallargues et al. 2001). Indeed, the WHO recently released the FRAX WHO Risk Assessment Tool that calculates an individual's 10-year cumulative risk of fracture based on knowledge of the person's age, sex, weight, height, history fracture, parental history of hip fracture, current smoking, current use of glucocorticoids, current use of alcohol, presence of rheumatoid arthritis or other causes of secondary osteoporosis, and BMD (www.shef.ac.uk/FRAX/).

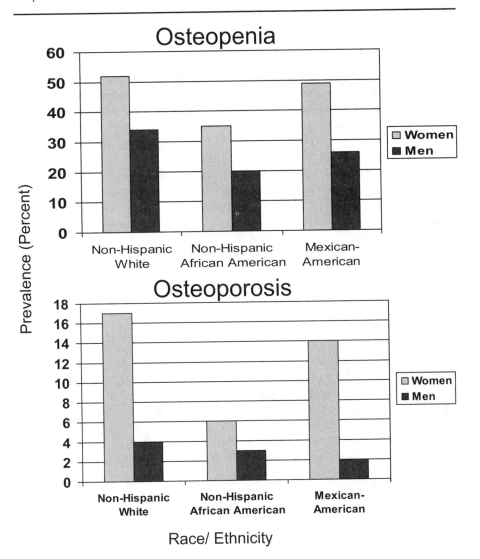

Figure 18.3. Age-adjusted prevalence of low bone density at the femoral neck by sex and race/ethnicity, ages 50 years and older, United States, 1988–1994 (NHANES III). Data from Looker et al. (1997).

Geographic Distribution

Internationally, the geographic distribution of osteoporosis has been studied principally based on rates of hip fractures. The highest age-adjusted rates of hip fracture are found in the Scandinavian countries, followed by the United States and western Europe; lower rates were reported in Latin America and Asia (Harvey et al. 2006). The highest age-adjusted rates of spine fractures also occurred in Scandinavia with lower rates in western European countries.

Jacobsen et al. (1990b) studied regional variations in hip fracture incidence among white women in the United States. By calculating age-specific rates of hip fracture at the county level, they identified a north–south gradient of increasing hip fracture occurrence, with a cluster of high incidence in the southeast. An analysis of data based on hospital discharge rates for hip fracture among Medicare recipients in 2001 confirmed that the highest rates occurred in the southeast and south central regions (Zingmond, Melton, and Silverman 2004).

Time Trends

As with geographic distribution, time trends in osteoporosis have been studied based on fracture rates. Hospital discharge rates for hip fractures among Medicare recipients increased during the last decade of the twentieth century but have largely stabilized since (Zingmond, Melton, and Silverman 2004). Data from a study in California suggest that hip fracture rates have increased in Hispanic women and men while they have declined in non-Hispanic white women from 1983 to 2000 (Zingmond, Melton, and Silverman 2004).

Causes

Modifiable Risk Factors

A number of lifestyle factors, medical conditions, and medications are associated with osteoporosis and osteoporotic fractures (Table 18.3) (DHHS 2004; Espallargues et al. 2001). While most of these are associated with osteoporosis as defined by low BMD, some are associated only with osteoporotic fractures because of their relationship with falls (e.g., reduced visual acuity, Parkinson's disease, excessive alcohol consumption). The

Table 18.3. Modifiable Risk Factors for Osteoporosis and Osteoporotic Fractures

Magnitude	Risk Factor
Strong (relative risk >4)	Immobility
	Low body weight and weight loss
	Current or recent use of glucocorticoids
Moderate (relative risk 2–4)	Current smoking
	Excessive alcohol intake
	Low calcium intake and/or low sunlight exposure
Weak (relative risk <2)	Current use of antidepressants
	Current use of proton pump inhibitors

risk factors for osteoporosis may act by either (1) interfering with the ability to produce a skeleton of optimal mass and strength during the period of growth and development or (2) increasing the rate of bone resorption and/or decreasing the rate of bone formation leading to a decline in BMD and deterioration of bone microarchitecture during adulthood. Recent studies have identified the molecular mechanisms involved in regulation of osteoclast and osteoblast development and function; these are the cells that are responsible for bone resorption and formation, respectively (Boyce and Xing 2007; Krishnan, Bryant, and MacDougald 2006; Raisz 2005).

Recently, a committee of the WHO has identified a set of risk factors that, in combination with BMD, can be used to predict a person's 10-year absolute risk for osteoporotic fracture (De Laet et al. 2005; Kanis et al. 2005). These risk factors were derived from a series of meta-analyses of data from population-based longitudinal cohort studies with fracture outcomes. The risk factors include age, sex, history of clinical fracture after age 50 years, parental history of hip fracture, current smoking, use of systemic glucocorticoids within the past year, excessive alcohol intake, and presence of rheumatoid arthritis as a prototype chronic systemic inflammatory disease. When results of BMD testing are not available, then body mass index can be used as a surrogate, as they are highly correlated. The WHO recently released FRAX: The Fracture Assessment Tool; it is anticipated that this will be approved by the Food and Drug Administration for incorporation into computer software so that an individual's 10-year risk can be calculated at the time of BMD testing. Until then, the practitioner will need to enter the femoral neck BMD results, as well as the answers to the risk factor questions, into the computer program to generate the 10-year cumulative probability of fracture.

Population-Attributable Risk

Elimination of risk factors, especially those that are more prevalent, has the potential to reduce the occurrence of low bone density and hip fracture. Table 18.4 presents calcula-

Table 18.4. Proportion of Hip Fractures Attributed to Various Modifiable Risk Factors, United States

Factor	Best Estimate (%)	Range (%)
Nonuse of hormone replacement	19	6–31
Thin body build	18	10.5–26
Cigarette smoking	10	4–16

Used with permission of the American College of Physicians, from Paganini-Hill, A., R.K. Ross, V.R. Gerkins, B.E. Henderson, M. Arthur, and T.M. Mack. Menopausal Estrogen Therapy and Hip Fractures. *Ann Intern Med* (1981):95:28–31; permission conveyed through Copyright Clearance Center, Inc. Paganini-Hill, A., A. Chao, R.K. Ross, and B.E. Henderson. Exercise and Other Factors in the Prevention of Hip Fracture: The Leisure World Study. *Epidemiology* (1991):2:16–25. Used with permission.

tions of population-attributable risk for hip fractures. Because of the lack of definitive studies, attributable risk estimates for osteoporosis are not available.

Prevention and Control

Prevention

The prevention of osteoporosis must focus on optimizing the attainment of peak bone mass during growth and development, and slowing the rate of bone loss with aging. Measures aimed at affecting peak bone mass must begin in childhood and adolescence. These include maintaining a nutritious diet with an adequate intake of calcium and vitamin D and an active lifestyle, with an emphasis on weight-bearing physical activities. Young women, in particular, should be discouraged from smoking cigarettes or participating in overly strenuous athletics that result in the development of amenorrhea (the "female athlete triad" of amenorrhea, low body weight, and low BMD; Beals and Meyer 2007). The ideal of extreme thinness, as typified by teenage actresses and models, also should be discouraged, and anorexia should be aggressively treated.

To slow bone loss, clinicians should discuss the use of hormone therapy beginning at or shortly after menopause. Again, weight-bearing exercise and adequate calcium and vitamin D intake should be encouraged, and smoking and heavy alcohol consumption should be discouraged.

Clinicians also should consider ways of addressing the risk factors for falling, particularly in older adults with low BMD. An environmental assessment to help older men and women "fall-proof" their living areas is helpful. This may include ensuring optimal lighting, installing appropriate and graspable hand rails on stairs and in the bathroom, checking throw rugs and extension cords, and placing "soft" corners on cabinets and furniture to minimize injuries if falls occur. In addition, attention to appropriate footwear to prevent tripping is important.

Screening

Evidence has emerged since the publication of the last edition of this volume indicating that BMD testing of all women aged 60 years and older is associated with significantly lower rates of osteoporotic fractures, including hip fractures (Kern et al. 2005; LaCroix et al. 2005). Measurement of BMD is now recommended in all postmenopausal women aged 65 years and older and in those aged 60 to 64 years with risk factors for fracture by the USPSTF (2002). The International Society of Clinical Densitometry (ISCD) recommends measurement of BMD in all postmenopausal women aged 65 years and older as well as men 70 years and older (www.iscd.org). The ISCD also recommends BMD testing in younger postmenopausal women and in adult men who have diseases or conditions and/or are taking medications that are associated with low BMD or increased rates of decline in BMD.

A number of algorithms and indices have been published that also can be used to identify women and men who should undergo measurement of BMD (Hochberg 2006). These should complement the clinical guidelines for measurement noted above rather than substitute for them. A review of recommendations for BMD testing was recently published (Hochberg 2006).

Treatment

Secondary prevention involves the prevention of fractures and treatment of persons with osteoporosis, defined based on low BMD. There are several medications that are approved by the Food and Drug Administration for the prevention and/or treatment of osteoporosis; these drugs work either by decreasing the rate of bone turnover (anticatabolic or antiresorptive agents) or increasing the rate of bone formation (anabolic agents). All of these drugs have been shown to reduce the risk of spine fractures in randomized placebo-controlled clinical trials; only some have been shown to reduce the risk of nonspine fractures, including hip fractures in these trials. A detailed discussion of these individual treatments is beyond the scope of this chapter; the reader is referred to a series of meta-analyses of osteoporosis therapies published in 2002 (Cranney et al. 2002) as well as more recent reviews included in the selected readings.

Prompt treatment of fractures and aggressive rehabilitation afterward, even among older patients, could greatly decrease long-term morbidity. Public health nursing services, physical therapy services, and support services in the home often enable recovering fracture patients to stay in their own homes.

Examples of Evidence-Based Interventions

A major arthritis public health initiative, The National Arthritis Action Plan: A Public Health Strategy, was developed in 1999 by the Centers for Disease Control and Prevention (CDC), the Arthritis Foundation, the Association of State and Territorial Health Officials, and 90 other organizations, and it outlines a national plan to reduce pain and disability and improve quality of life for people with arthritis. In 2007, CDC, the Arthritis Foundation, and other partners supported arthritis initiatives in 36 states, including arthritis public awareness efforts and evidence-based community self-management programs such as "People with Arthritis Can Exercise," the "Arthritis Self-Help Course,"' and "Arthritis Foundation Aquatics Program," and a health communications campaign "Physical Activity—The Arthritis Pain Reliever."

The Surgeon General's report identified a number of population-based public health interventions for improving bone health in the United States (DHHS 2004). These include programs to increase physical activity and reduce tobacco use, among others. One such program that was specifically highlighted was The National Bone Health Campaign, a multiyear national program created in 1998 by congressional mandate and conducted under the auspices of the CDC. The overall goal of the campaign is to encourage young girls to build and maintain strong bones by establishing lifelong healthy habits focused on calcium intake, physical activity, and avoidance of tobacco.

Areas of Future Research

The Surgeon General's report identified a number of key action steps as part of a National Action Plan for Bone Health. These include:

- Increasing awareness of the impact of osteoporosis and how it can be prevented and treated throughout the life span
- Changing the paradigm of preventing and treating fractures

- Continuing to build the science base on the prevention and treatment of osteoporosis
- Integrating health messages and programs on nutrition and physical activity relating to other chronic diseases.

Numerous areas for future research were described in the Surgeon General's report related to the epidemiology and impact of osteoporosis and fractures as well as the prevention and treatment of osteoporosis and related bone disease. The reader is referred to the report's sections for the individual recommendations (DHHS 2004).

Resources

National Arthritis Foundation: P.O. Box 19000, Atlanta, GA 30326, tel.: (800) 283-7800

National Arthritis, Musculoskeletal, and Skin Disease Information Clearinghouse: 9000 Rockville Pike, Box AMS, Bethesda, MD 20892, tel.: (301) 495-4484

National Osteoporosis Foundation: 2100 M Street, NW, Suite 602, Washington, DC 20037, tel.: (202) 223-2226

National Institute on Aging, Public Information Office, Office of Planning, Analysis, and Communication, Federal Building, Room 6C12, Bethesda, MD 20892, tel.: (301) 496-1752

Suggested Reading

Cummings S.R., F. Cosman, and S.A. Jamal. *Osteoporosis: An Evidence-Based Guide to Prevention and Management.* Philadelphia: American College of Physicians–American Society of Internal Medicine (2002).

Felson, D.T., R.C. Lawrence, P.A. Dieppe, et al. Osteoarthritis—New Insights, Part 1: The Disease and Its Risk Factors. *Ann Int Med* (2000):133:635–646.

Lane, N.E., and P.N. Sambrook, editors. *Osteoporosis and the Osteoporosis of Rheumatic Diseases.* Philadelphia: Mosby Elsevier (2006).

Sambrook, P.N., editor. Osteoporosis. *Rheum Dis Clin North Am.* (2006):32(4):617–780.

Silman, A.J., and M.C. Hochberg. *Epidemiology of Rheumatic Diseases* (2nd ed.). New York: Oxford University Press (2001).

References

Adams, P.F., G.E. Hendershot, and M.A. Marano. Current Estimates from the National Health Interview Survey, 1996. *Vital Health Stat* (1999):10(200). Available at: http://www.cdc.gov/nchs/data/series/sr_10/sr10_200.pdf.

Alarcon, G.S. Epidemiology of Rheumatoid Arthritis. *Rheum Dis Clin North Am* (1995):21:589–604.

Altman, R.D., E. Asch, D. Bloch, et al. Development of Criteria for the Classification and Reporting of Osteoarthritis: Classification of Osteoarthritis of the Knee. *Arthritis Rheum* (1986):29:1039–1049.

American College of Rheumatology Subcommittee on Osteoarthritis Guidelines. Recommendations for the Medical Management of Osteoarthritis of the Hip and Knee: 2000 Update. *Arthritis Rheum* (2000):43:1905–1915.

American College of Rheumatology Subcommittee on Rheumatoid Arthritis Guidelines. Guidelines for the Management of Rheumatoid Arthritis. *Arthritis Rheum* (2002):46:328–346.

Anderson, J.J., and D.T. Felson. Factors Associated with Osteoarthritis of the Knee in the First National Health and Nutrition Examination Survey (NHANES I): Evidence for an Association with Overweight, Race, and Physical Demands of Work. *Am J Epidemiol* (1988):128:179–189.

Bauer, R.L. Ethnic Differences in Hip Fracture: A Reduced Incidence in Mexican Americans. *Am J Epidemiol* (1988):127:145–149.

Beals, K.A., and N.L. Meyer. Female Athlete Triad Update. *Clin Sports Med* (2007):26:69–89.

Begovich, A.B., V.E. Carlton, L.A. Honigberg, et al. A Missense Single-Nucleotide Polymorphism in a Gene Encoding a Protein Tyrosine Phosphatase (PTPN22) is Associated with Rheumatoid Arthritis. *Am J Hum Genet* (2004):75:330.

Boyce, B.F., and L. Xing. Biology of RANK, RANKL, and Osteoprotegerin. *Arthritis Res Ther* (2007):9(Suppl 1):S1.

Brandt, K.D., S.A. Mazzuca, B.P. Katz, et al. Effects of Doxycycline on Progression of Osteoarthritis: Results of a Randomized, Placebo-Controlled, Double-Blind Trial. *Arthritis Rheum* (2005):52(7):2015–2025.

Cauley, J.A., L.Y. Lui, K.L. Stone, et al. Longitudinal Study of Changes in Hip Bone Mineral Density in Caucasian and African-American Women. *J Am Geriatr Soc* (2005a):53:183–189.

Cauley, J.A., L.Y. Lui, K.E. Ensrud, et al. Bone Mineral Density and the Risk of Incident Nonspinal Fractures in Black and White Women. *JAMA* (2005b):293:2102–2108.

Centers for Disease Control and Prevention (CDC). Prevalence of Leisure-Time Physical Activity Among Persons with Arthritis and Other Rheumatic Conditions—United States, 1990–1991. *MMWR* (1997):46:389–393.

Cherry, D.K., D.A. Woodwell, and E.A. Rechtsteiner. National Ambulatory Medical Care Survey: 2005 Summary. *Adv Data Vital Health Stat* (2007):(387). Available at: http://www.cdc.gov/nchs/data/ad/ad387.pdf.

Choi, H.K., K. Atkinson, E.W. Karlson, W. Willett, and G. Curhan. Alcohol Intake and Risk of Incident Gout in Men: A Prospective Study. *Lancet* (2004a):363:1277–1281.

Choi, H.K., K. Atkinson, E.W. Karlson, W. Willett, and G. Curhan. Purine-Rich Foods, Dairy and Protein Intake, and the Risk of Gout in Men. *N Engl J Med* (2004b):350(11):1093–1103.

Clegg, D.O., D.J. Reda, C.L. Harris, et al. Glucosamine, Chondroitin Sulfate, and the Two in Combination for Painful Knee Osteoarthritis. *N Engl J Med* (2006):354(8):795–808.

Consensus Development Conference. Prophylaxis and Treatment of Osteoporosis. *Osteoporos Int* (1991):1:114–117.

Cranney, A., G. Guyatt, L. Griffith, et al. IX: Summary of Meta-Analyses of Therapies for Postmenopausal Osteoporosis. *Endocrine Rev* (2002):23:570–578.

Criswell, L.A., K.G. Saag, T.R. Mikuls, et al. Smoking Interacts with Genetic Risk Factors in the Development of Rheumatoid Arthritis Among Older Caucasian Women. *Ann Rheum Dis* (2006):65:1163.

Croft, P., D. Coggon, M. Cruddas, and C. Cooper. Osteoarthritis of the Hip: An Occupational Disease in Farmers. *Br Med J* (1992):304:1269–1272.

Cummings, S.R., and L.J. Melton. Epidemiology and Outcomes of Osteoporotic Fractures. *Lancet* (2002):359:1761–1767.

Davis, M.A., W.H. Ettinger, and J.M. Neuhaus. Obesity and Osteoarthritis of the Knee: Evidence from the National Health and Nutrition Examination Survey (NHANES I). *Semin Arthritis Rheum* (1990):20:34–41.

DeFrances, C.J., K.A. Cullen, and L.J. Kojak. National Hospital Discharge Survey: 2005 Annual Summary with Detailed Diagnosis and Procedure Data. *Vital Health Stat* (2007):13(165). Available at: http://www.cdc.gov/nchs/data/series/sr_13/sr13_165.pdf.

De Laet, C., A. Oden, H. Johansson, O. Johnell, B. Jonsson, and J.A. Kanis. The Impact of the Use of Multiple Risk Indicators for Fracture on Case-Finding Strategies: A Mathematical Approach. *Osteoporos Int* (2005):16:313–318.

De Vries, N., H. Tijssen, P.L. van Riel, and L.B. van de Putte. Reshaping the Shared Epitope Hypothesis: HLA-Associated Risk for Rheumatoid Arthritis is Encoded by Amino Acid Substitutions at Positions 67–74 of the HLA-DRB1 Molecule. *Arthritis Rheum* (2002):46:921.

Dillon, C.F., E.K. Rasch, Q. Gu, and R. Hirsch. Prevalence of Knee Osteoarthritis in the United States: Arthritis Data from the Third National Health and Nutrition Examination Survey 1991–94. *J Rheumatol* (2006):33(11):2271–2279.

Dillon, C.F., R. Hirsch , E.K. Rasch, and Q. Gu. Symptomatic Hand Osteoarthritis in the United States: Prevalence and Functional Impairment Estimates from the Third U.S. National Health and Nutrition Examination Survey (1991–1994). *Am J Phy Med Rehabil* (2007):86:12–21.

Doran, M.F., G.R. Pond, C.S. Crowson, W.M. O'Fallon, and S.E. Gabriel. Trends in Incidence and Mortality in Rheumatoid Arthritis in Rochester, Minnesota over a Forty-Year Period. *Arthritis Rheum* (2002):46:625.

Espallargues, M., L. Sampietro-Colom, M.D. Estrada, et al. Identifying Bone-Mass Related Risk Factors for Fracture to Guide Bone Densitometry Measurements: A Systematic Review of the Literature. *Osteoporos Int* (2001):12:811–822.

Felson, D.T. The Epidemiology of Knee Osteoarthritis: Results from the Framingham Osteoarthritis Study. *Semin Arthritis Rheum* (1990):20(Suppl 1):42–50.

Felson, D.T., Y. Zhang, J.M. Anthony, et al. Weight Loss Reduces the Risk of Symptomatic Knee Osteoarthritis in Women: The Framingham Study. *Ann Intern Med* (1992):116:535–539.

Felson, D.T., R.C. Lawrence, P.A. Dieppe, et al. Osteoarthritis—New Insights, Part 1: The Disease and Its Risk Factors. *Ann Intern Med* (2000):133:635–646.

Gabriel, S.E., C.S. Crowson, and W.M. O'Fallon. The Epidemiology of Rheumatoid Arthritis in Rochester, Minnesota 1955–1985. *Arthritis Rheum* (1999):42:415–420.

Gelber, A.C., M.C. Hochberg, L.A. Mead, N.Y. Wang, F.M. Wigley, and M.J. Klag. Body Mass Index in Young Men and the Risk of Subsequent Knee and Hip Osteoarthritis. *Am J Med* (1999):107(6):542–548.

George, A., J.K. Tracy, W.A. Meyer, R.H. Flores, P.D. Wilson, and M.C. Hochberg. Racial Differences in Bone Mineral Density in Older Men. *J Bone Miner Res* (2003):18:2238–2244.

Hannan, M.T., J.J. Anderson, T. Pincus, and D.T. Felson. Educational Attainment and Osteoarthritis: Differential Associations with Radiographic Changes and Symptom Reporting. *J Clin Epidemiol* (1992):45:139–147.

Harvey, N., et al. The Epidemiology of Osteoporotic Fractures. In: Lane, N.E. and P.N. Sambrook, editors, *Osteoporosis and the Osteoporosis of Rheumatic Diseases: A Companion to Rheumatology* (1st ed.). Philadelphia: Mosby Elsevier (2006):1–13.

Helmick, C.G., D.T. Felson, R.C. Lawrence, et al. Estimates of the Prevalence of Arthritis and Other Rheumatic Conditions in the United States. *Arthritis Rheum* (2008):58:15–25.

Hochberg, M.C. Epidemiology of Osteoarthritis: Current Concepts and New Insights. *J Rheumatol* (1991a):18(Suppl 27):4–6.

Hochberg, M.C. Epidemiologic Considerations in the Primary Prevention of Osteoarthritis. *J Rheumatol* (1991b):18:1438–1440.

Hochberg, M.C. Arthritis and Connective Tissue Diseases. In: Thoene, J., editor, *Physician's Guide to Rare Diseases*. Montvale, NJ: Dowden Publishing Co (1992):907–959.

Hochberg, M.C. Osteoarthritis. In: Stobo, J.D., et al., editors, *Principles and Practice of Medicine* (23rd ed.). Norwalk, Conn: Appleton & Lange (1993).

Hochberg, M.C. Recommendations for Measurement of Bone Mineral Density and Identifying Persons to be Treated for Osteoporosis. *Rheum Dis Clin North Am* (2006):32:681–689.

Hochberg, M.C., S.L. Ardey, and E.L. Diamond. The Association of Self-Reported Arthritis with Disability: Data from the 1984 National Health Interview Survey Supplement on Aging (SOA). *Arthritis Rheum* (1989a):32(Suppl 4):S101.

Hochberg, M.C., R.C. Lawrence, D.F. Everett, and J. Cornoni-Huntley. Epidemiologic Associations of Pain in Osteoarthritis of the Knee. *Semin Arthritis Rheum* (1989b):18:4–9.

Hochberg, M.C., M. Lethbridge-Cejku, C.C. Plato, F.M. Wigley, and J.D. Tobin. Factors Associated with Osteoarthritis of the Hand in Males: Data from the Baltimore Longitudinal Study of Aging. *Am J Epidemiol* (1991):134:1121–1127.

Hochberg, M.C., J. Thomas, D.J. Thomas, L. Mead, D.M. Levine, and M.J. Klag. Racial Differences in the Incidence of Gout. *Arthritis Rheum* (1995):38:628–632.

Hootman, J.M., and C.G. Helmick. Projections of US Prevalence of Arthritis and Associated Activity Limitations. *Arthritis Rheum* (2006):54:226–229.

Hootman J., J. Bolen, C. Helmick, et al. Prevalence of Doctor-Diagnosed Arthritis and Arthritis-Attributable Activity Limitation—United States, 2003–2005. *MMWR* (2006):55:1089–1092 and Errata (2006):56:55.

Jacobsen, S.J., J. Goldberg, T.P. Miles, J.A. Brody, W. Stiers, and A.A. Rimm, et al. Hip Fracture Among the Old and Very Old: A Population-Based Study of 745,435 Cases. *Am J Public Health* (1990a):80:871–873.

Jacobsen, S.J., J. Goldberg, T.P. Miles, J.A. Brody, W. Stiers, and A.A. Rimm, et al. Regional Variation in the Incidence of Hip Fracture. *JAMA* (1990b):264:500–502.

Kanis, J.A., F. Borgstrom, C. de Laet, et al. Assessment of Fracture Risk. *Osteoporosis Int* (2005):16:581–589.

Kelsey, J.L., and M.C. Hochberg. Epidemiology of Chronic Musculoskeletal Disorders. *Ann Rev Public Health* (1988):9:379–401.

Kern, L.M., N.R. Powe, M.A. Levine, et al. Association between Screening for Osteoporosis and the Incidence of Hip Fracture. *Ann Intern Med* (2005):142:173–181.

Kramer, H.M., and G. Curhan. The Association between Gout and Nephrolithiasis: The National Health and Nutrition Examination Survey III, 1988–1994. *Am J Kidney Dis* (2002):40:37–42.

Krishnan, V., H.U. Bryant, and O.A. MacDougald. Regulation of Bone Mass by Wnt Signaling. *J Clin Invest* (2006):116:1202–1209.

LaCroix, A.Z., D.S. Buist, S.K. Brenneman, and T.A. Abbott, 3rd. Evaluation of Three Population-Based Strategies for Fracture Prevention: Results of the Osteoporosis Population-Based Risk Assessment (OPRA) Trial. *Med Care* (2005):43:293–302.

Lawrence, R.C., M.C. Hochberg, J.L. Kelsey, et al. Estimates of the Prevalence of Selected Arthritic and Musculoskeletal Diseases in the United States. *J Rheumatol* (1989):16:427–441.

Looker, A.C., E.S. Orwoll, C.C. Johnston, Jr., et al. Prevalence of Low Femoral Bone Density in Older US Adults from NHANES III. *J Bone Miner Res* (1997):12:1761–1768.

MacGregor, A.J., H. Snieder, A.S. Rigby, et al. Characterizing the Quantitative Genetic Contribution to Rheumatoid Arthritis Using Data from Twins. *Arthritis Rheum* (2000):43(1):30–37.

Mellemkjaer, L., M.S. Linet, G. Gridley, M. Frisch, H. Moller, and J.H. Olsen. Rheumatoid Arthritis and Cancer Risk. *Eur J Cancer* (1996):32A:1753.

Minor, M.A., and N.E. Lane. Recreational Exercise in Arthritis. *Rheum Dis Clin North Am* (1996):22:563–577.

Osteoporosis Prevention, Diagnosis, and Therapy. NIH Consensus Statement (2000):17(1):1–45.

Paganini-Hill, A., R.K. Ross, V.R. Gerkins, B.E. Henderson, M. Arthur, and T.M. Mack Menopausal Estrogen Therapy and Hip Fractures. *Ann Intern Med* (1981):95:28–31.

Paganini-Hill, A., A. Chao, R.K. Ross, and B.E. Henderson. Exercise and Other Factors in the Prevention of Hip Fracture: The Leisure World Study. *Epidemiology* (1991):2:16–25.

Panush, R.S. Does Exercise Cause Arthritis? Long-Term Consequences of Exercise on the Musculoskeletal System. *Rheum Dis Clin North Am* (1990):16(4):827–836.

Pladevall-Villa, M., G.L. Delclos, C. Varas, H. Guyer, J. Brugues-Tarradellas, and A. Anglada-Arisa. Controversy of Oral Contraceptives and Risk of Rheumatoid Arthritis: Meta-Analysis of Conflicting Studies and Review of Conflicting Meta-Analyses with Special Emphasis on Analysis of Heterogeneity. *Am J Epidemiol* (1996):144:1–14.

Raisz, J.G. Pathogenesis of Osteoporosis: Concepts, Conflicts, and Prospects. *J Clin Invest* (2005):115:3318–3325.

Rasch, E., R. Hirsch, R. Paulose-Ram, and M. Hochberg. Prevalence of Rheumatoid Arthritis in Persons 60 years of Age and Older in the U.S.: Effect of Different Methods of Case Classification. *Arthritis Rheum* (2003):48:917–926.

Roubenoff, R. Gout and Hyperuricemia. *Rheum Dis Clin North Am* (1990):16:539–550.

Roubenoff, R., M.J. Klag, L.A. Mead, K.-Y. Liang, A.J. Seidler, and M. C. Hochberg. Incidence and Risk Factors for Gout in White Men. *JAMA* (1991):266:3004–3007.

Russell, G. Pathogenesis of Osteoporosis. In: Lane, N.E. and P.N. Sambrook, editors, *Osteoporosis and the Osteoporosis of Rheumatic Diseases: A Companion to Rheumatology* (1st ed.). Philadelphia: Mosby Elsevier (2006):33–40.

Saag, K.G., J.R. Cerhan, S. Kolluri, K. Ohashi, G.W. Hunninghake, and D.A. Schwartz. Cigarette Smoking and Rheumatoid Arthritis Severity. *Ann Rheum Dis* (1997):56:463.

Scott, J.C., and M.C. Hochberg. Epidemiologic Insights into the Pathogenesis of Hip Osteoarthritis. In: Hadler, N.M., editor, *Clinical Concepts in Regional Musculoskeletal Illness*. Orlando, Fla: Grune & Stratton (1987):89–107.

Silman, A.J. Epidemiology of Rheumatoid Arthritis. *APMIS* (1994):102:721–728.

Slemenda, C., K.D. Brandt, D.K. Heilman, et al. Quadriceps Weakness and Osteoarthritis of the Knee. *Ann Intern Med* (1997):127(2):97–104.

Stone, K.L., D.G. Seeley, L.Y. Liu, et al. BMD at Multiple Sites and Risk of Fracture of Multiple Types: Long-Term Results from the Study of Osteoporotic Fractures. *J Bone Miner Res* (2003):18:1947–1954.

Tepper, S., and M.C. Hochberg. Factors Associated with Hip Osteoarthritis: Data from the National Health and Nutrition Examination Survey (NHANES I). *Am J Epidemiol* (1993):137:1081–1088.

Tracy, J.K., W.A. Meyer, R.H. Flores, P.D. Wilson, and M.C. Hochberg. Racial Differences in Rate of Decline in Bone Mass in Older Men: The Baltimore Men's Osteoporosis Study. *J Bone Miner Res* (2005):20:1228–1234.

U.S. Department of Health and Human Services. *Bone Health and Osteoporosis: A Report of the Surgeon General*. Rockville, MD: U.S. Department of Health and Human Services, Office of the Surgeon General (2004).

U.S. Preventive Services Task Force (USPSTF). Screening for Osteoporosis in Postmenopausal Women: Recommendations and Rationale. *Ann Intern Med* (2002):137:526–528.

Van Den Ende, C.H., T.P. Vliet Vlieland, M. Munneke, and J.M. Hazes. Dynamic Exercise Therapy for Rheumatoid Arthritis. *Cochrane Database Syst Rev* (2000):CD000322.

Wilder, M. Prevalence of Chronic Skin and Musculoskeletal Conditions, United States, 1969. *Vital Health Stat* (1974):10(92). Available at: http://www.cdc.gov/nchs/data/series/sr_10/sr10_092acc.pdf.

Williams, F.M.K., and T.D. Spector. The Genetics of Osteoporosis. In: Lane, N.E. and P.N. Sambrook, editors, *Osteoporosis and the Osteoporosis of Rheumatic Diseases: A Companion to Rheumatology* (1st ed.). Philadelphia: Mosby Elsevier (2006):14–21.

Winthrop, K.L., J.N. Siegel, J. Jereb, Z. Taylor, and M.F. Iademarco. Tuberculosis Associated with Therapy Against Tumor Necrosis Factor Alpha. *Arthritis Rheum* (2005):52:2968.

World Health Organization (WHO). Assessment of Fracture Risk and Its Application to Screening for Postmenopausal Osteoprosis. Geneva: WHO Technical Report Series (1994).

Yano, K., L.K. Heilbrun, R.D. Wasnich, J.H. Hankion, and J.M. Vogel. The Relationship between Diet and Bone Mineral Content of Multiple Skeletal Sites in Elderly Japanese-American Men and Women Living in Hawaii. *Am J Clin Nutr* (1985):42:877–888.

Yelin, E., M. Cisternas, A. Foreman, D. Pasta, L. Murphy, and C. Helmick. National and State Medical Expenditures and Lost Earnings Attributable to Arthritis and Other Rheumatic Conditions—United States 2003. *MMWR* (2007):56:4–7.

Yelin, E.H., and W.R. Felts. A Summary of the Impact of Musculoskeletal Conditions in the United States. *Arthritis Rheum* (1990):33:750–755.

Zingmond, D.S., L.J. Melton III, and S.L. Silverman. Increasing Hip Fracture Incidence in California Hispanics, 1983 to 2000. *Osteoporos Int* (2004):15:603–610.

CHAPTER 19

CHRONIC LIVER DISEASE (ICD-10 K70-77, E83, E83.1, E88, B15-19, C22-C22.9)

Adnan Said, M.D., M.S. and Jennifer Wells, M.D.

Introduction

"Liver disease" is a term that encompasses a broad range of clinical abnormalities, ranging from mild liver test abnormalities in asymptomatic individuals at one end of the spectrum to end-stage liver disease at the other. Liver conditions can present as acute and fulminant disease with rapid liver failure or as chronic liver disease that slowly progresses over decades. Commonly used liver tests include measurement of serum liver enzymes that signify inflammation of the liver (i.e., hepatitis) and bilirubin levels that are an indicator of liver function and the severity of liver disease (Schiff et al. 1999). Complications of advanced liver disease such as cirrhosis can present with complications such as gastrointestinal bleeding, accumulation of fluid in the abdominal cavity (ascites), and decreased cognitive and neuromuscular function (encephalopathy) (D'Amico et al. 1986).

The major causes of liver disease include excessive alcohol use, hepatitis infection, and less common metabolic abnormalities such as hemochromatosis and metabolic syndrome. Those persons at high risk for liver disease are those at high risk for alcohol abuse and hepatitis, including those with alcoholism, the poor and less educated, minorities, immigrants, and injection drug users. The epidemiology of liver disease—including the causes, consequences, and populations at high risk—is summarized in Figure 19.1 and described in detail below. Strategies for prevention and control are described in separate sections at the end of this chapter.

Significance

Chronic liver disease is an important drain on national health care resources with approximately 5.5 million people affected (Miller et al. 2006) in the United States and millions globally (Shepard et al. 2005). Over the past two decades, drastic changes in liver disease management have occurred, with development of antiviral therapies for chronic viral hepatitis and liver transplantation becoming a widely accepted procedure for patient with end-stage liver disease. Prevention of liver disease is integral to minimize the burden of advanced liver disease. Development of the hepatitis B vaccine is one of the most important medical advances in this field. However, stigmatization of patients with alcoholism and viral hepatitis is an impediment to this goal. Patients

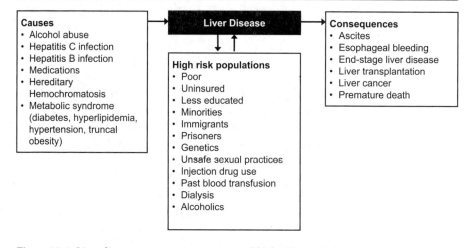

Figure 19.1. Liver disease: causes, consequences, and high-risk populations.

with liver disease often are socially disadvantaged and have poor access to health care. Improvement of services to prevent and treat alcoholism and reduce the transmission of viral hepatitis has improved over the past two decades but needs further support and dissemination.

Social and economic policies in the United States during the past century played a significant role on the incidence of chronic liver disease. Liver-related mortality was high before the 1920s, plummeting during the Prohibition, rising again during the Depression, with persistent increases through the time of World War II, peaking in the early 1970s (Terris 1967; Debakey et al. 1995).

In 2004, chronic liver disease and cirrhosis, based on the International Classification of Diseases, Tenth Revision (ICD-10), was reported to be the 12th leading cause of liver disease in the United States accounting for over 27,000 deaths (Heron 2007). This represented 1.1% of the total national mortality with an age-adjusted rate of death from chronic liver disease of 9.5/100,000 population, the lowest rate in U.S. history. This would indicate a decrease in liver disease death rates. When adding the impact of deaths from viral hepatitis as well as that from hepatocellular carcinoma to the above reported data, the numbers rise dramatically. In this context, liver disease accounts for approximately 46,000 deaths yearly (1.9%), thereby rising to the ninth cause of overall death (Kim et al. 2002). Trends for chronic liver disease mortality including viral hepatitis, liver cancer, and other causes from 1979 to 2005 are detailed in Figure 19.2.

The morbidity of liver disease is just as important given the effects on quality of life as well as the economic consequences. Direct medical cost related to chronic liver disease and cirrhosis, excluding patients with hepatitis C virus, is estimated in excess of $1.4 billion (Sandler et al. 2002). The health care costs for patients with hepatitis C virus (including liver transplantation) are in excess of $514 million annually (Kim et al. 2001), and when all aspects of liver disease are considered, the cost exceeds $3.4 billion/year (Sandler et al. 2002). Of those hospitalized, the mean length of stay is 5.9 days, with an average cost of $28,703 (Kim 2002). Trends in liver disease dis-

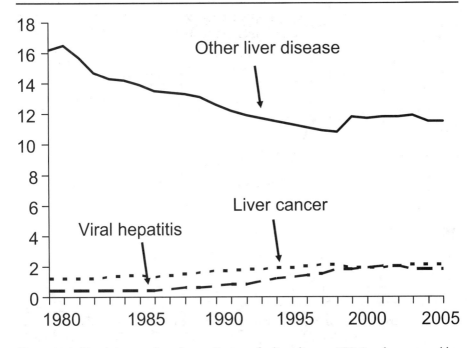

Figure 19.2. Trends in age-adjusted mortality rates for liver diseases. ICD-9 codes were used between 1979 and 1998 and ICD-10 codes from 1999 to 2005 (from CDC WONDER).

charges in community hospitals in the United States from 1979 to 2005 are shown in Figure 19.3.

Causes

Liver disease can be attributed to a multitude of causes (Schiff et al. 1999). Chronic liver disease is defined arbitrarily as liver disease that persists beyond 6 months from onset, and studies have demonstrated that up to 56% of persons with chronic liver disease may be completely asymptomatic (Zaman et al. 1990). This is an important factor to consider when studying the occurrence of new cases as well as the overall prevalence.

The most prevalent causes in the population include alcoholic liver disease, viral hepatitis, nonalcoholic fatty liver disease, hepatocellular carcinoma, and medication-related liver disease and occasionally less common genetic conditions such as hereditary hemochromatosis that leads to liver damage from iron overload. To investigate the epidemiology of liver disease, the Centers for Disease Control and Prevention (CDC), in collaboration with the National Institute of Diabetes and Digestive and Kidney Diseases, developed a surveillance program in which to record new instances of liver diagnoses made in the office of a gastroenterologist (Bell et al. 2001). Three U.S. counties, New Haven (Connecticut), Alameda (Oakland, California), and Multnomah (Portland, Oregon), were chosen. Preliminary analysis of the 725 patients enrolled indicated that the etiology of these patients' chronic liver disease included: hepatitis C virus, 42%; alcohol-related liver disease, 8%; hepatitis C virus and alcohol combined, 22%; nonalcoholic fatty liver disease, 10%; hepatitis B virus, 4%; other miscellaneous liver conditions (including autoimmune hepatitis,

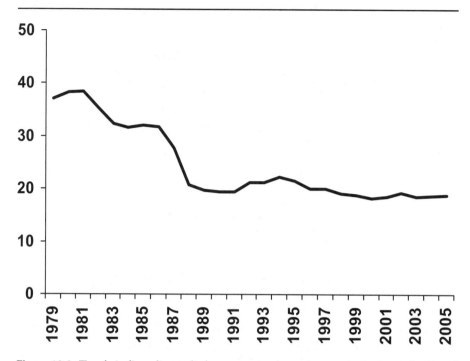

Figure 19.3. Trends in liver disease discharges among short-stay community hospitals: United States 1979–2005 (from Chiung and Chen 2007).

drug-induced liver disease, hemochromatosis, primary biliary cirrhosis, sclerosing cholangitis, hepatocellular carcinoma, and granulomatous liver disease), 8%; unknown etiologies, 6%. Based upon these results, it is estimated that the incidence of newly diagnosed chronic liver disease in referral practices is 67 per 100,000 in the population and that 150,000 new cases of chronic liver disease are diagnosed in gastroenterologists' offices yearly in the United States. This does not account for those patients who are solely managed by primary-care physicians (Kim 2002) and the majority that have not sought medical care yet. Etiology of chronic liver disease in nonreferral practices and the general population can varry considerably with higher attribution from alcohol and the combination of alcohol and hepatitis C compared to referral practices. The attributable risk for the leading risk factors for chronic liver disease in the U.S. population is presented in Table 19.1, using estimates of the prevalence of exposure and relative risk.

ALCOHOLIC LIVER DISEASE (ICD-10 K70–K70.9)

Significance

Chronic heavy alcohol use can lead to liver disease that manifests as fatty liver disease, alcohol-induced hepatitis, or cirrhosis, conditions that can overlap (Schiff et al. 1999)

Table 19.1. Risk Factors for Chronic Liver Disease: Estimates of Prevalence of Exposure, Relative Risk, and Population Attributable Risk[a]

Factor	Population Exposed	Prevalence (p) (%)	Relative risk (RR) (range)	Population attributable risk (range)* (%)
Chronic heavy alcohol use	15 million	5	10 (4–20)	31 (13–50)
Hepatitis C	4.1 million	1.4	12 (8–20)	13 (8–20)
Hepatitis B	1.25 million	0.4	10 (2.5–20)	4 (1–7)
Metabolic syndrome	6 million	2	4 (2–6)	6 (2–10)

[a]Population attributable risk = $p(RR - 1)/(1 + p(RR - 1))$.

(see Chapter 8: Alcohol Use). Alcohol-induced fatty liver can be seen in up to 90% of persons with alcoholism. It develops rapidly, in some studies after a weekend of binging. With alcohol cessation, it resolves quickly as well, within 2 weeks in some studies (Thaler 1977). Alcohol-induced fatty liver can progress to cirrhosis in 10%–15% of patients over long-term follow-up of 10 years or more (Sorensen et al. 1984). The risk increases with the amount of alcohol consumed over this duration.

With alcohol-induced hepatitis, the clinical spectrum ranges from a self-limited disorder to a severe life threatening illness with liver failure. With longitudinal follow-up, the risk of developing cirrhosis can be as high as 70% in patients with alcohol-induced hepatitis (Alexander et al. 1971; Diehl 1997). With cessation of alcohol intake, the changes of alcohol-induced hepatitis can be reversible except in the most severe cases.

Descriptive Epidemiology

Alcoholic liver disease is closely linked to per capita consumption of alcohol in populations. In an examination of trends in chronic liver disease mortality and socioeconomic determinants in the United States from 1935 to 1996, alcohol use, unemployment, and minority concentration were closely linked to liver disease mortality. A 10% decrease in per capita alcohol consumption has been associated with a 2.5% reduction in cirrhosis mortality with a lag time as short as one year (Singh and Hoyert 2000). In a European study a 1-liter increase in alcohol consumption per capita was associated with a 14% increase in cirrhosis mortality for men and 8% for women (Ramstedt 2001).

Along with alcohol consumption rates, death rates from alcohol-induced cirrhosis increased after the Prohibition in the United States from the 1930s to 1973, a peak of 14.9 deaths per 100,000 population (Terris 1967). Alcohol-related deaths have declined from the 1970s in the United States. From 1973 to 1997, age-adjusted death rates from cirrhosis and chronic liver disease decreased at an average annual rate of 3.0% for the entire population, by 2.6% for white men, 3.0% for white women, 4.1% for African-American men, and 4.8% for African-American women (Saadatmand et al. 2000).

Hospital discharges in the United States measured in short-stay community hospitals showed an upward trend in alcohol-induced liver disease and cirrhosis-related discharges between 1988 and 2005 (Chiung and Chen 2007). In the United States, this decreased mortality from alcoholic liver disease since the 1970s occurred despite increasing alcohol consumption rates until the 1980s. This paradox has been attributed to multiple causes including better health care, better nutrition, and increasing treatment of alcohol addiction (Mann et al. 1991; Holder and Parker 1992; Smart and Mann 1993; Kerr et al. 2000; Ramstedt 2001). Despite stable consumption rates, alcohol liver disease–induced mortality has increased in the United Kingdom and other parts of northern Europe. In England, the rate of alcohol cirrhosis–induced death rates increased from 2.8/100,000 in 1993 to 8.0/100,000 in 2000. These increases were seen in all ethnic groups, but the mortality rate in Asian men was 3.8 times that of white men (Fisher et al. 2002). In parts of Asia, including Japan, Korea, and China, the consumption of alcohol has increased steadily from the 1960s, and the proportion of liver disease attributed to alcohol has increased commensurately (Park et al. 1998). In Japan, the proportion of all liver diseases from alcohol increased from 5.1% in 1968 to 14.1% by 1986 (Hasumura and Takeuchi 1991).

Causes

The risk of alcohol-induced cirrhosis rises with the amount of alcohol consumed. The risk is increased with sustained intake of greater than 60 g/day in men and greater than 20 g/day in women, but the risk varies considerably (a single drink is 8–12 g in the United States). Only 6%–40% of people drinking to this level will eventually develop cirrhosis (Lelbach 1975; Bellentani et al. 1997; Corrao et al. 1997). The risk also increases with lifetime alcohol use (>100 kg in the Dionysos Italian population study) (Bellentani et al. 1997). The risk of death after alcohol-induced cirrhosis is diagnosed is much higher with continued drinking but improves significantly with abstinence. With continued drinking, the 5-year survival in patients with alcohol-induced cirrhosis is less than 30% but over 60% with abstinence and over 90% if they have compensated cirrhosis (Mandayam et al. 2004).

The wide variability in the risk of cirrhosis with alcohol intake is dependent upon poorly understood genetic factors, including polymorphisms in genes that influence alcohol metabolism and absorption, coexistence of other liver injurious agents (hepatitis C), iron overload (as seen in genetic hemochromatosis), and sex differences. Although alcohol abuse and cirrhosis-related deaths predominate in men worldwide including the United States, there is a growing proportion of women among heavy drinkers (Blume 1986). Women have a higher susceptibility to alcohol compared with men. The risk of cirrhosis develops with lower rates of drinking in women (20–60 g/day) compared with men (40–80 g/day), and cirrhosis develops with shorter duration of alcohol abuse in women. Multiple mechanisms are thought to underlie this susceptibility, including variations in alcohol distribution and levels in blood, gastric enzyme activity, first-pass metabolism, and sex hormone differences in endotoxin after exposure to alcohol (Frezza et al. 1990; Ikejima et al. 1998; Parlesak et al. 2000; Sato et al. 2001). Ethnic differences in alcohol use and alcohol-induced liver disease exist, with highest rates of alcoholic liver disease in Hispanic men, followed by black men and white men (Stinson et al. 2001). Part of this may be explained by continued high rates of heavy drinking in Hispanic populations compared with other ethnic groups (Caetano and Kaskutas 1995; Stinson et al.

2001). Differences in genetic predisposition, socioeconomic status, nutrition, and access to health care may all play a role but this has not been clarified.

Alcohol use is common in patients with hepatitis C virus infection, with some studies suggesting that as many as 60%–70% of hepatitis C virus–infected individuals consume as much as 40 g of alcohol per day (Loguercio et al. 2000). The association of alcohol abuse and viral hepatitis C infection is associated with higher rates of progression to cirrhosis, liver cancer, and cirrhosis-related death. Some studies suggest the association may be synergistic (Corrao and Arico 1998). Alcoholics with hepatitis C infection are at a higher risk of cirrhosis than non–hepatitis C–infected alcoholics (Ostapowicz et al. 1998; Degos 1999). Conversely, of patients infected with hepatitis C, those who consume alcohol heavily (>50 g/day) (Corrao and Arico 1998) have a higher risk of progression to cirrhosis than nondrinkers. The role of liver disease progression in hepatitis C–infected patients who consume alcohol occasionally and in lower to moderate amounts needs further study.

In addition, the contributing role of diabetes and obesity, which themselves are risk factors for liver disease, needs further clarification in alcohol-induced liver disease. Some studies have shown these to be independent risk factors (Naveau et al. 1997; Day 2000) while others have not (Bellentani et al. 1997). Obesity-related fatty liver disease may proceed along the same pathophysiological pathways of liver injury, as alcohol and the combination may have synergistic effects on liver damage. The association of diet, particularly of pork products, with beer drinking has been associated with liver disease in drinkers (Nanji and French 1985; Bode et al. 1998). Other studies have found protective effects of coffee drinking (Ruhl and Everhart 2005).

Prevention and Control

Viral Liver Disease

Chronic viral hepatitis is most often caused by hepatitis C and B. Hepatitis A and E cause acute self-resolving hepatitis. Hepatitis D only coinfects or superinfects persons infected with hepatitis B.

HEPATITIS A
(ICD-10 B15)

The hepatitis A virus is an RNA virus that spreads by feco-oral contact from contaminated food and water as well by person–person contact. It occurs in both sporadic cases and in epidemic outbreaks (60% of U.S. cases). It has been recently spread by contaminated green onions (Dentinger et al. 2001; Wheeler et al. 2005) imported from Mexico and strawberries from Guatemala. Contaminated food, particularly shellfish, is a usual source of contamination. Susceptible individuals are at risk for epidemic outbreaks, such as what occurred in Shanghai, which involved 290,000 people and was due to contaminated clams (Tang et al. 1991).

Significance

Hepatitis A causes an acute illness. The likelihood of developing symptomatic disease is age-dependent, with more than 70% of children being asymptomatic and the majority of adults and adolescents (>70%) developing symptomatic disease (Tong et al. 1995). The symptoms are nonspecific, including aches, fever, abdominal pain, and jaundice. The incubation period can last from 15 to 49 days; jaundice usually lasts 1–3 months.

Hepatitis A does not lead to chronic hepatitis except for very rare cases of relapsing forms, which ultimately resolve as well. Development of severe acute liver failure is also rare (<1%) but is more likely to occur in adults than in children and in those adults with underlying chronic liver disease such as from hepatitis C (Vento et al. 1998). Diagnosis is made by detection of serum hepatitis A antibody (HAV IgM subtype), which is positive by the onset of symptoms and detectable up to 6 months after onset of illness. After recovery, the individual usually develops lifelong hepatitis A antibody IgG subtype, rendering immunity from further attacks (Koff 1992; Schiff et al. 1999).

Descriptive Epidemiology

The incidence of hepatitis A is much higher in developing countries and occurs earlier in childhood (>95% are immune by adulthood), whereas in Europe and the United States, infection rates in children are lower, and adult symptomatic infection although not uncommon is decreasing. It is estimated that 33% of the U.S. population has been infected with the hepatitis A virus (Fiore et al. 2006; Brundage and Fitzpatrick 2006). Since there is no chronic infection, these individuals are now immune to the hepatitis A virus.

The incidence of hepatitis A in the United States has steadily decreased from the 1970s to 2006. The incidence of hepatitis A was 28/100,000 in 1970 in the United States, decreased to 13/100,000 by 1980, and remained steady until 1990 (Jajosky et al. 2006). This decrease was likely secondary to improved food handling and processing as well as epidemic management and vaccination. By 2006, only 32,000 estimated new infections occurred in the United States (Wasley et al. 2007). The decline in incidence between 1995 and 2005 is 88% (see Figure 19.4).

Causes

Risk factors associated with higher rates of hepatitis A virus infection included household crowding and poverty. International travel is a risk factor as well, particularly to countries where hepatitis A is endemic such as Mexico and Central/South America. Other risk factors include sexual and household contact with another person with hepatitis A, transmission in men who have sex with men, and illicit drug use (Jacobsen and Koopman 2004).

Prevention and Control

The disease can be prevented by improved sanitary conditions including treatment of water, avoidance of contaminated shellfish and food, and hand washing (Mbithi et al. 1992).

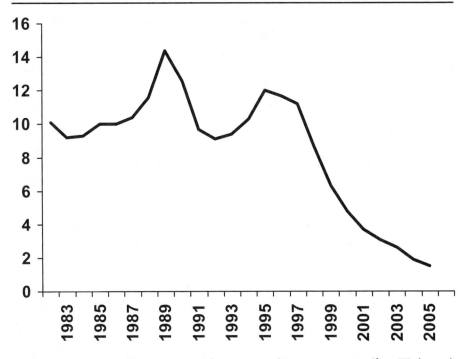

Figure 19.4. Incidence of acute hepatitis A by year: United States, 1982–2005 (from Wasley et al. 2007).

In epidemics, case and source finding and vaccination of exposed susceptible individuals are key to controlling epidemics.

Eventually, vaccination of children should decrease incidence further. Immunization for hepatitis A is now recommended universally for all children 12–23 months (since 2004) (Fiore et al. 2006) and those at higher risk of transmission (travelers to endemic areas, men who have sex with men, intravenous and non–intravenous drug users) (since 1996). A highly effective vaccine has been available since 1996 (Wasley et al. 2006).

HEPATITIS B
(ICD-10 B16, B18.0, B18.1)

Hepatitis B is a DNA virus belonging to the hepadnaviradiae family and is extremely prevalent globally (Schiff et al. 1999). The virus is spread by parenteral exposure to blood and body fluids. Due to a large prevalence in developing countries such as China (10%–20%), it is efficiently spread to neonates by vertical transmission and is the main modality of transmission in the developing world (Maynard 1990; Alter et al. 1990; Beasley et al. 1982). In the United States, which has a lower prevalence (estimated 1.25 million cases or 0.2%) and better access to perinatal care and childhood immunization, vertical transmission is less common than adult-to-adult transmission through sexual contact or illicit drug use.

Significance

In children and neonates, the acute infection is clinically silent in the majority. In adults, acute infection is symptomatic in 30%–50%. Hepatitis B acute infection has an incubation period of 1–4 months. Symptoms during the prodromal phase may be vague, including fatigue, aches, malaise, and abdominal pain. Jaundice can occur and can last from 4 to 12 weeks (Liaw et al. 1998).

With chronic infection, risk of developing cirrhosis and hepatocellular carcinoma increases with longer duration of infection. In endemic countries, the risk is highest in men older than 40 years (Fattovich et al. 1991; Liaw et al. 1998). Increased risk of progressive liver disease also depends upon the interaction between the host immune system and the virus. The risk is higher in those individuals with high levels of chronic viral replication with high levels of the virus in blood (Yang et al. 2002; Chen et al. 2006). The risk is reduced considerably in those individuals where the immune system successfully suppresses viral replication (Stevens et al. 1975; Tassopoulos et al. 1987).

Increased risk of progressive liver disease leading to cirrhosis and hepatocellular carcinoma also occurs with concurrent tobacco and alcohol use (Donato et al. 1997). The lifetime risk of cirrhosis and hepatocellular carcinoma is higher in individuals from endemic areas likely due to longer durations of infection (Beasley et al. 1982; Chen et al. 2006).

Descriptive Epidemiology

High rates of vertical transmission in developing countries result in high prevalence due to the high chances of developing chronic infection after exposure at this stage of life. In the United States, where most of the transmission is in adults, the lower rate of chronicity results in lower prevalence rates. The prevalence of chronic hepatitis B infection is estimated to be 1.25 million individuals in the United States, accounting for 5,000 estimated deaths yearly (Alter and Mast 1994). Globally, hepatitis B is a huge issue, with more than 350 million carriers and more than 1 million deaths from associated liver disease (Maynard 1990). The prevalence rates vary from 0.2% in the United States to 10%–20% in Southeast Asia and China.

The incidence of hepatitis B in the United States has decreased after peaking in the 1980s (Figure 19.5). The incidence of hepatitis B was 4.08/100,000 in the United States in 1970, peaked in 1980 to 8.39/100,000, and remained at 8.48/100,000 by 1990. Between 1995 and 2005, the incidence of acute hepatitis B declined by 79% to 1.8/100,000, the lowest ever reported. In the United States, 78,000 estimated new infections occurred in 2001, and this had dropped to 46,000 by 2006 (Wasley et al. 2007).

Declines were reported in all age groups but were most steep in children younger than 15 years (0.03/100,000) (Wasley et al. 2007). Universal hepatitis B vaccination has resulted in these reduced rates in children. High rates for hepatitis B continue among

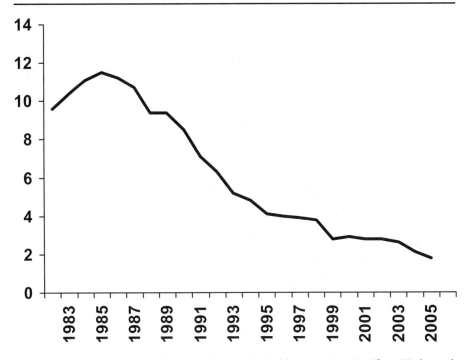

Figure 19.5. Incidence of acute hepatitis B by year: United States, 1982–2005 (from Wasley et al. 2007).

adults, particularly men aged 25–44 years, emphasizing the need to identify and vaccinate high-risk adults. The highest rate of hepatitis B was in the age group of 25–44 years (3.6/100,000), although between 1990 and 2005, this rate declined by 74% as well.

The rates for hepatitis B infection in men still predominated compared with women (2.3 vs. 1.4/100,000 in 2005). Rates were highest for blacks in 2005 (2.9/100,000) and similar in whites (1.1), Hispanics (1.1), and Asians (1.2).

Reductions in incidence have occurred due to a combination of universal vaccination of neonates and adolescents (younger than 18 years) and recommendation of vaccination of high-risk adults. Safer needle use practices in intravenous drug users as well as continued screening of blood products have also contributed to the reduction in adult to adult transmission (Jajosky et al. 2006).

Despite the decrease in incidence and prevalence of hepatitis B, the burden of disease has not decreased. The number of hospitalizations for hepatitis B–related liver disease has increased twofold over the last decade (Kim et al. 2004). This increased morbidity may due to increased access or increased numbers of patients with hepatitis B developing cirrhosis from chronic infection as well as increased influx of migrants with hepatitis B infection. It is estimated that 40,000 migrants with hepatitis B infection are admitted annually to the United States (Mast et al. 2006).

Causes

Reported risk factors in the United States include sexual behavior (32% multiple sex partners, 10% sexual contact with a person known to have hepatitis, 13% men who have sex with men), and injection drug use (15%). Hemodialysis was a risk factor in 0.3%, blood transfusion in 0.2%, and occupational exposure in 0.8% (Wasley et al. 2007) (see Figure 19.6).

The risk of developing chronic infection is dependent upon the age at which exposure occurs. Neonatal transmission results in chronic infection in 90% of nonvaccinated children (Stevens et al. 1975). In adults, however, acute infection results in chronic infection in only 5% (Beasley et al. 1982; Tassopoulos et al. 1987; Mast et al. 2006).

Prevention and Control

Hepatitis B is a vaccine-preventable disease. The vaccine has been available since the early 1980s, and the recent vaccine is more than 95% effective (Lai et al. 1993). The World Health Organization has recommended universal childhood vaccination worldwide. So far, 158 countries have incorporated hepatitis B vaccination in routine immunization, but coverage is far from universal, with 60% coverage (World Health Organization 2006). A comprehensive strategy to eliminate hepatitis B transmission has been introduced in the United States since 1991 and updated in 2006. Since 1991, vaccination has been recommended universally for all infants born in the United States as well for children younger than 18 years as a catch-up program. The catch-up program in the United States has reached 60% of children between 13 and 15 years old (Mast et al. 2005). In addition, all women seeking prenatal care are screened for hepatitis B infection, and for women

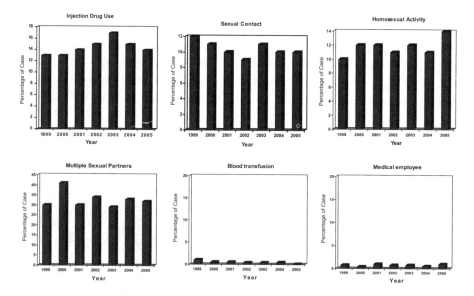

Figure 19.6. Trends in selected epidemiological characteristics among patients with acute hepatitis B by year: United States, 1999–2005 (from Wasley et al. 2007).

with hepatitis B, their infants are vaccinated and given prophylaxis with hepatitis B immunoglobulin at birth. Efficacy of this regimen is more than 95%. For adults at high risk, screening and vaccination are recommended. These include users of illicit drugs, those with multiple sexual partners, sex partners of persons with hepatitis B infection, solid organ recipients, dialysis patients, and health care workers among others.

In the United States, 56% of individuals attending dialysis were vaccinated against hepatitis B in 2002 (47% in 1997) as well as 90% of dialysis staff (CDC 1991). Hepatitis B incidence in 2002 was 0.12% in dialysis center patients (prevalence was 1%), a significant decline from 1982 when hepatitis B vaccination was first recommended for dialysis patients.

The efficacy of childhood vaccination is already seen in countries with a high rate of vertical and early childhood transmission. In Taiwan, where universal neonatal vaccination was introduced in 1986, the prevalence of hepatitis B in children younger than 15 years was 9.8% before this implementation and 1.2% in 2004 (Ni et al. 2007). The rate of hepatocellular carcinoma in children in Taiwan has also decreased by a third over this time period. In the United States, where hepatitis B transmission occurs mostly in adults, the results of universal childhood vaccination will have a considerably longer lag time before the benefits of vaccination are seen.

HEPATITIS C
(ICD-10 B17.1, B18.2)

Hepatitis C is an RNA virus belonging to the flavaviridae family that infects the liver (hepatotrophism) (Schiff et al. 1999). The virus is spread parenterally by breach of mucosal membranes and is efficiently spread by illicit drug use including intravenous drugs and intranasal cocaine and somewhat less efficiently by sexual transmission (Murphy et al. 2000). The surge in incidence of hepatitis C occurred in the 1970s and 1980s due to the transmission of the virus by these routes as well as by blood transfusion (Alter et al. 1989). Before the discovery of the hepatitis C viral genome for hepatitis C in 1989 (Choo et al. 1989), the safety of the blood supply was based on testing for elevated liver enzymes, and since chronic hepatitis C (called non-A non-B hepatitis before 1989) is often associated with normal liver enzymes, transfusion-associated transmission was not uncommon. With the discovery of the hepatitis C virus genome in 1989 and the development of an accurate antibody test thereafter (Kuo et al. 1989), the blood supply has become very safe, with the risk of transfusion-related hepatitis C estimated to be about 1/100,000 to 1/1,000,000 units transfused (Schreiber et al. 1996; Pomper et al. 2003).

Significance

After exposure to hepatitis C virus, chronic infection occurs in 70%–85%, with a minority clearing the virus within 6 months of exposure. Overall progression to cirrhosis is estimated to occur in 10%–20% of hepatitis C virus–infected patients over their lifetime (Freeman et al. 2001). Higher rates are seen with steady alcohol intake, in men, and with longer duration of infection as well as in individuals infected at older age (>40 years)

(Poynard et al. 1997). On average, it takes 20 years from initial hepatitis C virus infection to develop cirrhosis in these patients. Hepatocellular carcinoma develops at the rate of 1% per year in those with cirrhosis.

It is projected that a decline in the prevalence of infection from a peak of 2.7% in the 1990s to 1% by 2030 may occur (Armstrong et al. 2000). Despite the reduced incidence, the burden of disease due to hepatitis C is still rising due to its chronicity and the lag time from acquisition of infection to development of clinically significant liver disease. The death rate from hepatitis C virus has increased from 0.4 deaths/100,000 from hepatitis C virus (non-A non-B hepatitis) in 1982 to 1.8/100,000 in 2004 (CDC WONDER).

Morbidity and health care costs for hepatitis C virus are also increasing. Between 1991 and 2000, hepatitis C virus increased from 343 transplants in 1991 (12% of all transplants in the United States) to 1679 transplants by 2000 (37% of all liver transplants) (UNOS data). Data from the HealthCare Utilization project, which sampled hospitalizations at all nonfederal hospitals, showed that hepatitis C virus as the reason for hospitalization increased from under 10,000 admissions in 1991 to approximately 140,000 by 1998 (Kim 2002). The total charges linked with these hospitalizations also increased from US$39 million in 1991 to over a billion dollars by 1998. Hepatitis C virus also has a profound effect on quality of life in patients referred to health centers (Rodger et al. 1999; Hussain et al. 2001), some aspects of which are related to concurrent comorbid illnesses such as depression. In 1998, it was estimated that there were 317,000 outpatient visits for hepatitis C virus in the United States, resulting in costs of more than 24 million, with greater than 500 million spent on antiviral treatment (Sandler et al. 2002).

It is estimated that a twofold to fourfold increase in numbers of persons with hepatitis C virus infection for more than 20 years will occur between 1990 to 2015 (Armstrong et al. 2000; Davis et al. 2003). The increase in incidence of hepatocellular carcinoma in recent years (El-Serag and Mason 1999) is in a large part attributable to the hepatitis C virus epidemic. Consequently, it is projected that complications of cirrhosis will also increase, such as hepatocellular carcinoma (increase of 81%), hepatic decompensation (increase of 106%), and liver-related death (increase of 180%) (Davis et al. 2003). Even if every single hepatitis C patient is identified and treated, the number of cases with decompensated cirrhosis will decrease by only half after 20 years. Currently, most patients estimated to have hepatitis C virus infection do not know that they have the disease or do not have access to health care. As the proportion of those with cirrhosis increases and become clinically apparent, the burden on the health care system is expected to increase.

Descriptive Epidemiology

Hepatitis C is a reportable disease, but there is significant underreporting despite active surveillance programs (such as the National Notifiable Disease Surveillance System) (Wasley et al. 2007). The reasons for this are varied, but a large part of the problem is that acute hepatitis C is overwhelmingly asymptomatic and unnoticed. Furthermore, populations at risk for hepatitis C virus are socially and economically disadvantaged and often do not have seek nor have access to health care. Furthermore, national surveys such as National Health and Nutrition Examination Survey (NHANES) exclude populations with high prevalence of the disease such as incarcerated individuals and the homeless. Health care provider underreporting of diagnosed cases also occurs.

Hepatitis C leads to chronic disease, with spontaneous clearance occurring in only 15%–30% of cases after exposure. Consequently, the prevalence of the virus is high, with an estimated 4.1 million cases in the United States (NHANES 1999–2002) (Armstrong et al. 2006). The highest prevalence of infection was seen in the age group from 40 to 49 years, with men having a higher rate of infection than women (20% more likely) (Kim 2002). Blacks have a higher prevalence of infection (3.2%) than whites (1.5%), with Mexican Americans having intermediate rates (NHANES III) (Alter et al. 1999). Hepatitis C virus prevalence is higher in certain groups, including veterans (where the prevalence of hepatitis C virus antibody varies from 5% to 18%) (Briggs et al. 2001), the homeless (prevalence 40%) (Cheung et al. 2002), and incarcerated individuals (15%) (Weinbaum et al. 2003) and as high as 39% of men and 54% of women (Ruiz et al. 1999).

At the peak of the hepatitis C epidemic, 180,000 to 230,000 new cases were occurring yearly in the United States (Alter 1997; Williams 1999) in the mid-1980s. Since then, the incidence has declined to an estimated 20,000 new infections in 2005 in the United States (Wasley et al. 2007) (see Figure 19.7). The decrease in hepatitis C virus incidence is multifactorial (see Figure 19.8). Decline in transfusion-related hepatitis C virus started occurring after the introduction of the 1985 guidelines for selecting safer blood donors and sharply with the introduction of hepatitis C virus antibody testing of donated blood products starting in 1989. Safer needle practices and tattoo needle practices introduced to reduce HIV have also contributed to the reduced incidence. Declines have occurred in all groups. Persons ages 25–39 years have the highest incidence but have also had the greatest declines (Wasley et al. 2007), with a 92% decline in incidence of

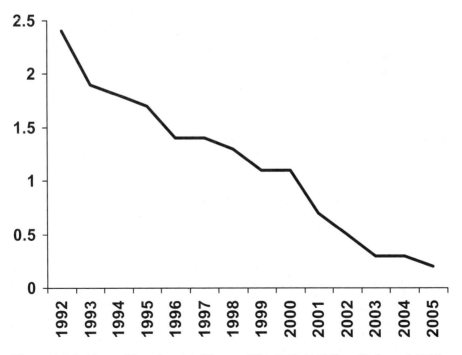

Figure 19.7. Incidence of Acute hepatitis C by year, USA, 1982–2005 (from Wasley et al. 2007).

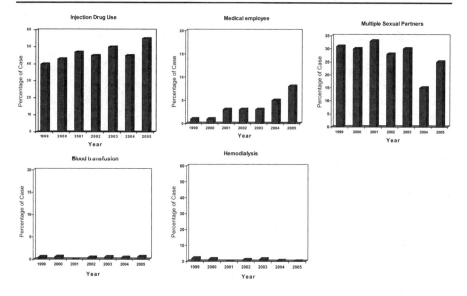

Figure 19.8. Trends in selected epidemiological characteristics among patients with acute hepatitis C by year: United States, 1999–2005 (from Wasley et al. 2007).

hepatitis C infection since 1992. The incidence is higher for men (0.26/100,000) than women (0.21/100,000), although this gap is narrowing. Declines in racial populations have occurred across the board. In 2005, rates were 0.36/100,000 in American Indians and Alaska natives and lowest in Asians (0.02). Rates of hepatitis C virus infection were similar in Hispanic and non-Hispanics.

Causes

Several large population studies have identified risk factors for hepatitis C virus infection. The largest of these, the NHANES III study, assessed prevalence in a random sample of 21,241 U.S. participants and had a hepatitis C virus prevalence of 1.8% (Alter et al. 1999). Risk factors included illicit drug use, number of sexual partners as well as weaker associations with socioeconomic markers such as poverty index, educational level, and marital status (Alter et al. 1999). Other population-based studies have found similar risk factors, with intravenous drug use being the strongest risk factor (Garfein et al. 1996). Other risk factors include blood transfusion or organ transplant before 1992, hemodialysis, and high-risk sexual behavior (Alter et al. 1989; Pereira et al. 1991; Geerlings et al. 1994).

Dialysis remains a risk factor despite universal infection control practices. In the national surveillance of dialysis-associated diseases in the United States in 2002, hepatitis C virus antibody was found in 7.8% of dialysis recipients, with an incidence rate of 0.34%. This is a decline of 25% since 1995. Hepatitis C virus testing was done in 2002 in 64% of centers. Hepatitis C virus routine testing with anti–hepatitis C virus antibody was recommended routinely every 6 months and at entry. Using disposable equipment in the dialysis machines has been associated with lower incidence of hepatitis C virus as well as by having a dedicated medication rooms (Finelli et al. 2005).

The incarcerated population has a high incidence and prevalence of hepatitis C virus infection. Risk factors in prison for viral hepatitis include illicit drug use in more than 50% preincarceration, but in as many as 3%–28% during incarceration as well (Weinbaum et al. 2003). Sexual activity in jail occurs in as many as 30% of inmates and is associated with high-risk sexual practices. Hepatitis C virus incidence is also higher in certain populations such as the veterans of foreign wars (5% prevalence).

Increase in progression toward severe liver disease has been shown with chronic alcohol intake, particularly moderate to severe alcohol intake (>50 g/day) (Poynard et al. 1997; Zarski et al. 2003). Older age at infection has also been associated with increased risk of progressive liver disease. Given the propensity of obesity and the metabolic syndrome to independently cause liver disease, the coexistence of obesity and the metabolic syndrome with hepatitis C virus has been investigated in preliminary studies. There is some evidence that with increased Body Mass Index (BMI) and features of the metabolic syndrome (diabetes, hypertension, hyperlipidemia, and truncal obesity), there is more rapid progression of liver disease in patients with hepatitis C virus (Zarski et al. 2003; Hourigan et al. 1999). In a large meta-analysis, steatosis (or fat in the liver) was independently associated with increased fibrosis and liver damage in hepatitis C (Leandro et al. 2006). In some analyses, male sex has been associated with increased fibrosis as well (Poynard et al. 1997; Leandro et al. 2006).

Prevention and Control

There is no vaccine available for hepatitis C virus. National recommendations issued in 1998 for prevention and control of hepatitis C virus infection include screening and testing blood donors, viral inactivation of plasma products, risk reduction counseling to reduce transmission in intravenous drug users, those at high risk of sexual transmission (multiple sex partners), and health care settings (infection control practices, dialysis).

Treatment is with interferon and ribavirin, antiviral agents that are associated with an average viral clearance rate of 50% and have to be taken for 24–48 weeks (Manns et al. 2001; Fried et al. 2002). The treatment can be difficult to tolerate (Younossi et al. 2007), and treatment candidates are patients who have risk of progressing to cirrhosis such as patients with elevated liver tests or presence of fibrosis on liver biopsy. Treatment has not been tested in a screening population. Treatment trials generally come from randomized controlled trials from teaching institutions and referral centers.

NONALCOHOLIC FATTY LIVER DISEASE (ICD-10 K76.0)

Recent attention has focused on a newly recognized epidemic called nonalcoholic fatty liver disease. It is believed that this condition may be the most common form of liver disease in the United States (Neuschwander-Tetri and Caldwell 2003). Nonalcoholic fatty liver disease is an umbrella term for hepatic steatosis (fat) of varying degree.

Significance

Although many patients have a benign course of bland fat deposition in the liver (fatty liver disease), there is a subset of patients who will develop inflammation and fibrosis and are called nonalcoholic steatohepatitis. These patients are at risk of progression to cirrhosis, liver failure, and hepatocellular carcinoma (Adams et al. 2005).

Nonalcoholic fatty liver disease is closely associated with the metabolic syndrome (truncal obesity, diabetes or insulin resistance, hyperlipidemia, hypertension) (Marchesini et al. 2003). The natural history of the condition remains poorly understood. Adams et al. (2005) published accounts of 420 patients diagnosed in Olmsted County, Minnesota, between 1980 and 2000 that were followed up for a mean of 7.6 years, culminating in 3,192 person-years of follow-up. Five percent of these patients developed cirrhosis over this relatively short follow-up; 3.1% developed liver-related complications. The mortality was 13% during the follow-up, significantly higher than the general population (relative risk 1.3). A longitudinal study describing 129 patients with biopsy-proven nonalcoholic fatty liver disease were compared with a matched reference population over 13.7 years. Those patients with more advanced nonalcoholic fatty liver disease (nonalcoholic steatohepatitis and fibrosis) were found to have end-stage liver disease in 5.4% as well as an increased mortality related to cardiovascular and liver-related causes. During the follow-up period, 69 of 88 patients (78%) developed diabetes or impaired glucose tolerance and 41% had progression of liver fibrosis. Those who had progressive liver damage were more likely to have had a significant amount of weight gain and were more insulin-resistant.

Descriptive Epidemiology

One of the few reported studies regarding incidence is a prospective, observational study from Japan (Hamaguchi et al. 2005). Using liver enzyme levels (alanine aminotransferase) and ultrasonography of the liver in patients without significant alcohol use, they found that at baseline, 812 of 4401 (18%) participants had nonalcoholic fatty liver disease. During the mean follow-up period of 414 ± 128 days, the authors observed 308 new cases (10%) of nonalcoholic fatty liver disease among 3147 participants who were disease-free at baseline.

The determination of prevalence, while still laden with challenges, has proven more feasible. Studies have been difficult, however, due to the need for an invasive liver biopsy for definitive diagnosis. As a result, most studies have elected to use either serum liver chemistries or radiological imaging as the surrogate diagnostic tool. Published reports have stated nonalcoholic fatty liver disease to be present in 3% to 23% (Clark et al. 2002) of the U.S. population. A recent study in which data collected as part of the NHANES from 1999 to 2002 (Ioannou et al. 2006) were compared with data collected by the same group from 1988 to 1994 (Clark et al. 2003). They reported a significant increase in the prevalence of nonalcoholic fatty liver disease. In the earlier study, the prevalence (and standard error) of nonalcoholic fatty liver disease based on elevated alanine aminotransferase, aspartate aminotransferase, or both was 3.4% (0.5), 2.7% (0.2), and 4.3% (0.3), respectively. The study from 1999 to 2002 reported levels nearly double at 7.3% (0.4), 3.6% (0.3), 8.1% (0.4) but is still felt to underrepresent the prevalence of nonalcoholic fatty liver disease in the United States due to the fact that many patients with hepatic steatosis have normal liver enzymes and may be overlooked. This was demonstrated by Browning et al. (2004) in a study of 2,287 participants of the Dallas Heart Study who were evaluated for liver steatosis (fat) by proton nuclear magnetic resonance spectroscopy and found 31% who met their criteria for diagnosis of nonalcoholic fatty liver disease. Of these patients, 79% were found to have a normal liver enzyme (alanine aminotransferase) level.

Increasingly, the pediatric population is being identified as part of this epidemic. There have been two population-based studies in the United States addressing this issue. Schwimmer et al. (2006) looked at 2450 obese adolescents between the ages of 12 and 18 years and found 3% to have abnormal alanine aminotransferase levels thought to be related to nonalcoholic fatty liver disease. More recently, a report was published by Schwimmer et al. in which autopsied specimens were reviewed in 742 pediatric victims of accidental death between the age of 2 and 19 years. They found an astounding 9.6% rate of fatty liver in these patients, with a pronounced age-related distribution of hepatic steatosis ranging from 0.7% for ages 2 to 4 years up to 17.3% for ages 15 to 19 years. The highest rate of fatty liver was seen in obese children (38%).

Nonalcoholic fatty liver disease affects persons of all ages and both sexes and has a worldwide distribution. Among both children and adults, nonalcoholic fatty liver disease increases with age, with highest occurrences in the fifth and sixth decade (Ruhl and Everhart 2004). Data from NHANES III showed nonalcoholic fatty liver disease based on elevated alanine aminotransferase levels peaked in the fifth decade among men and in the sixth decade among women (Ruhl and Everhart 2003). The comparison study of the same database by Ioannou had similar findings but with an unexplained striking reduction in the alanine aminotransferase levels of persons with further increasing age (Ioannou et al. 2006). Early descriptions of persons with nonalcoholic fatty liver disease showed a female preponderance to the condition; however, more recent studies in Japanese, Italian, and U.S. populations have consistently found men to be at increased risk (Bellentani et al. 1994; Ruhl and Everhart 2003; Shen et al. 2003).

Ethnic variation has been demonstrated repeatedly, with the Hispanic population being at the highest risk of fatty liver disease and blacks being at the lowest risk when compared with non-Hispanic whites. Asians also appear to be at decreased risk. A cross-sectional study of newly diagnosed cases of nonalcoholic fatty liver disease in the Chronic Liver Disease Surveillance Study was performed. Of the 742 persons evaluated, 159 (21.4%) had definite or probable nonalcoholic fatty liver disease: whites, 45%; Hispanics, 28%; Asians, 18%; African Americans, 3%; other races, 6%. Clinical correlates of nonalcoholic fatty liver disease (obesity, hyperlipidemia, diabetes) were similar among racial and ethnic groups, except that BMI was lower in Asians compared with other groups ($P<0.001$). Compared with the base population, Hispanics with nonalcoholic fatty liver disease were overrepresented (28% vs. 10%) and whites were underrepresented (45% vs. 59%) (Weston et al. 2005).

These racial and ethnic differences may be due to true genetic differences in risk of nonalcoholic fatty liver disease or due to cultural susceptibility in diet and lifestyle patterns. However, referral patterns and health care availability may influence results. The NHANES III avoids many biases that studies in certain populations may encounter. They too found Hispanics to have a higher prevalence of nonalcoholic fatty liver disease independent of BMI and demographic and metabolic factors, compared with non-Hispanic whites, while blacks continued to demonstrate lower prevalence of nonalcoholic fatty liver disease when adjusted for these factors (Ruhl and Everhart 2003, 2004).

Causes

Nonalcoholic fatty liver disease is associated with the metabolic syndrome, with diabetes, insulin resistance, and truncal obesity being the most closely linked correlates (Hamaguchi et al. 2005; Duvnjak et al. 2007). Secondary causes of nonalcoholic fatty liver disease include medications (such as steroids and tamoxifen), viruses, surgical procedures, rapid and excessive weight loss, and total parenteral nutrition. Gholam et al. (2007) published an article that identified nonalcoholic fatty liver disease in 89% of severely obese patients. The presence of non-alcoholic steatohepatitis and fibrosis (signifying more advanced liver damage from nonalcoholic fatty liver disease) was significantly less at 36% and 25%, respectively. In further subgroup analysis, hyperlipidemia, particularly low high-density lipoprotein, hyperglycemia, and insulin resistance were strongly associated with nonalcoholic fatty liver disease (Gholam et al. 2007).

Diabetes is known to be commonly linked with central obesity. Several studies have found the risk of diabetes in causing nonalcoholic fatty liver disease to be independent of the degree of obesity (Ruhl and Everhart 2003; Ogden et al. 2007). Insulin resistance itself is believed to be centrally related to the pathogenesis of nonalcoholic fatty liver disease (Neuschwander-Tetri and Caldwell 2003).

Prevention and Control

As described above, the potential for advanced liver disease in the form of cirrhosis and hepatocellular carcinoma is present in those patients with nonalcoholic fatty liver disease. Determining those at increased risk for progressive damage in nonalcoholic fatty liver disease as opposed to those with merely benign fatty liver disease is the principle target for much of today's research. Noninvasive markers in the determination of these two groups are also of utmost importance, given the magnitude of this condition in the otherwise healthy population. As society continues the trend toward obesity, so too will the trend of nonalcoholic fatty liver disease continue to rise, including the diagnosis of cirrhosis and associated hepatocellular carcinoma. Thus, many relatively new and evolving issues regarding nonalcoholic fatty liver disease will continue to be of interest for the coming years.

HEPATOCELLULAR CARCINOMA (ICD-10 C22.0)

Hepatocellular carcinoma is the fifth most common cancer worldwide, with an estimated 500 to 1 million deaths reported yearly (Parkin et al. 2005). According to the World Health Organization and other population-based cancer registries, it accounts for 5.6% of all cancers (7.5% in men and 3.5% in women) (World Health Organization Statistical Information System).

Significance

Hepatocellular carcinoma is rapidly fatal in the majority of patients; consequently, the prevalence, incidence, and mortality rates are very similar.

Descriptive Epidemiology

Hepatocellular carcinoma is more common in men than women worldwide. The sex disparity is noted to be more pronounced in endemic areas (2.1–5.7:1 male/female ratio), whereas intermediate- and low-incidence areas have progressively lower ratios (Bosch et al. 1999, 2005). Although not fully understood, these differences are theorized to be related to variations in viral hepatitis, alcohol abuse, toxins, and the trophic effect of androgens.

The hepatocellular carcinoma incidence in the United States is low compared with other countries in the developing world. However, there has been an increase in the incidence over the past few decades, from 1.4 per 100,000 in 1976–1980 to 2.4 per 100,000 in 1991–1995. Among black men, the incidence increased from 4 to 6.1, and in white men, from 1.7 to 2.8 per 100,000 in this study period. The steady rise was noted in nearly all age groups although younger men aged 40–60 years showed the steepest gains (El-Serag and Mason 1999). Parallel to these increases in incidence, there has been a 43% increase in mortality from primary liver cancers (El-Serag and Mason 1999).

Geographic distributions are associated with significant variety among the incidence rates of this cancer, even showing variation between ethnicities and regions within the same country. The age-adjusted incidence rates for hepatocellular carcinoma in developed versus developing countries is 8.7 for men and 2.9 for women per 100,000 compared with 17.4 for men and 6.8 for women per 100,000, respectively (World Health Organization Statistical Information System; Bosch et al. 2005). Some Asian and African regions have extraordinarily high rates, such as Mongolia (99 per 100,000) and the Gambia (39.6 per 100,000). In Austria, Europe, and the Americas, the rates are far less than 10 per 100,000 and with much less regional variability (Bosch et al. 2005).

Causes

Most hepatocellular carcinoma occurs in the setting of chronic liver disease and cirrhosis. Overall, 75%–80% of hepatocellular carcinoma can be related to persistent viral infections with either hepatitis B virus (50%–55%) or hepatitis C virus (25%–30%), which is further supported by the strong geographical correlation between the incidence of hepatocellular carcinoma and known prevalence of viral infections (Parkin et al. 2005). The risk associated with hepatitis B virus appears more profound in endemic regions where transmission often occurs vertically (at childbirth), and consequently, longer duration of infection is seen. In areas such as the United States, where most hepatitis B virus transmission occurs later in life by sexual transmission, the risk of hepatocellular carcinoma is much less (Sandler et al. 1983).

The risk of hepatitis C virus–related liver disease leading to hepatocellular carcinoma high in the United States due to the maturing of the hepatitis C epidemic of the 1970s and 1980s, leading to increased rates of hepatitis C–related cirrhosis at the current time. Any condition that can lead to cirrhosis is considered a risk for hepatocellular carcinoma. Alcohol, either alone or in combination with viral hepatitis, leads to a high risk for cirrhosis, although it is unclear whether alcohol is itself carcinogenic in addition to the risk of cirrhosis. Iron overload, autoimmune diseases, and nonalcoholic steatohepatitis are known to lead to hepatocellular carcinoma in individuals at the stage of cirrhosis. Rarer and debated causes would include aflatoxin exposure in parts of Africa, a mycotoxin that can may contaminate the diet, betel nut chewing, which is widespread in Asia, and tobacco use, which has be demonstrated in some studies as a risk factor (Kuper et al. 2000).

Prevention and Control

Protective measures include the prevention and treatment of diseases that cause cirrhosis, with the goal to delay or avoid the development of cirrhosis. Recent observational studies have also suggested that coffee may be protective, and a meta-analysis performed by Larsson et al. showed a 43% reduction of liver cancers occurred possibly due to antioxidant properties (Larsson and Wolk 2007). A remarkable decrease in hepatitis B virus infections has occurred with the introduction of the universal childhood hepatitis B vaccine in 1984 and the expectation is that there will be a long-term effect on the hepatocellular carcinoma rates (Chang et al. 1997).

Recent advances in treatment options have brought a new perspective to this condition traditionally considered a terminal illness with very poor outcomes, few treatment options, and a life expectancy of 6 months or shorter. Such advances include surgical resection, local ablation with alcohol, radiofrequency, chemoembolization, and liver transplantation (Bruix et al. 2001). Recent studies have shown hepatocellular carcinoma to be the leading cause in mortality from cirrhosis, as opposed to liver failure or nonmalignant liver-related conditions (Benvegnu et al. 2004). In response, health care providers have developed surveillance and treatment protocols that have dramatically improved survival in those patients diagnosed in the early stages of hepatocellular carcinoma (Sangiovanni et al. 2004; Bruix and Sherman 2005). Prevention of chronic liver disease such as with hepatitis B vaccination and reducing alcoholism and transmission of hepatitis C is still the most cost-effective way to deal with hepatocellular carcinoma.

HEMOCHROMATOSIS (ICD-10 E83.1)

Other causes of chronic liver disease include genetic conditions including metabolic liver disease (increased iron deposition in the liver and organs known as hemochromatosis, copper accumulation in the liver in Wilson's disease), cholestatic disorders (primary biliary cirrhosis, primary sclerosing cholangitis), autoimmune disorders, and drug-related liver disease (Schiff et al. 1999). Of these conditions, hereditary hemochromatosis is an autosomal recessive disorder with a prevalence of 1/200 to 1/250 in Caucasian populations in the United States and Europe. The most common genetic mutation is the *C282Y* mutation that results in excessive absorption of iron from the gut (Steinberg et al. 2001).

Significance

Organ overload, in time, can lead to cirrhosis, heart failure, diabetes, and hypogonadism. Organ damage is delayed in women compared with men due to menstrual iron loss (Adams 2006).

Descriptive Epidemiology

Despite the presence of the mutation for hemochromatosis, the penetrance is variable. In a large study in California using the Kaiser Permanente health clinic data of 41,038 individuals, 152 were homozygous for the *C282Y* mutation. Of these 152, only one had clinically evident disease (Beutler et al. 2002).

The yield of severe liver disease was similarly low in the Hemochromatosis and Iron Overload Screening Study, which screened 101,168 primary-care participants for iron overload (Adams et al. 2005). Three hundred thirty-three *C282Y* homozygotes were detected, and 75 had been previously diagnosed. Of the 302 *C282Y* homozygotes that underwent additional testing, 16% and 12% had increased levels of alanine aminotransferase and aspartate aminotransferase, respectively, compared with 11% and 8%, respectively, in controls. Of the 11 centrally reviewed liver biopsies, all showed increased liver iron concentrations, but only two had stage 3 or 4 fibrosis.

Prevention and Control

Based on these large population studies, U.S. Preventive Services Task Force recommended against the use of routine genetic screening for hereditary hemochromatosis in the asymptomatic general population (Whitlock et al. 2006). Family screening is effective due to higher pretest probability. It should be preformed with genetic testing if the proband is available for genetic testing.

References

Adams, L., J. Lymp, J. St. Sauver, et al. The Natural History of Nonalcoholic Fatty Liver Disease: A Population-Based Cohort Study. *Gastroenterology* (2005):129(1):113–121.

Adams, P.C. Review Article: The Modern Diagnosis and Management of Haemochromatosis. *Aliment Pharmacol Ther* (2006):23(12):1681–1691.

Adams, P.C., D.M. Reboussin, J.C. Barton, et al. Hemochromatosis and Iron-Overload Screening in a Racially Diverse Population. *N Engl J Med* (2005):352(17):1769–1778.

Alexander, J.F., M.W. Lischner, and J.T. Galambos. Natural History of Alcoholic Hepatitis. II. The Long-Term Prognosis. *Am J Gastroenterol* (1971):56(6):515–525.

Alter, H.J., R.H. Purcell, J.W. Shih, et al. Detection of Antibody to Hepatitis C Virus in Prospectively Followed Transfusion Recipients with Acute and Chronic Non-A, Non-B Hepatitis. *N Engl J Med* (1989):321(22):1494–1500.

Alter, M.J. Epidemiology of Hepatitis C. *Hepatology* (1997):26(3 Suppl 1):62S–65S.

Alter, M.J., and E.E. Mast. The Epidemiology of Viral Hepatitis in the United States. *Gastroenterol Clin North Am* (1994):23(3):437–455.

Alter, M.J., D. Kruszon-Moran, O.V. Nainan, et al. The Prevalence of Hepatitis C Virus Infection in the United States, 1988 Through 1994. *N Engl J Med* (1999):341(8):556–562.

Alter, M.J., S.C. Hadler, H.S. Margolis, et al. The Changing Epidemiology of Hepatitis B in the United States. Need for Alternative Vaccination Strategies. *JAMA* (1990):263(9):1218–1222.

Armstrong, G.L., M.J. Alter, G.M. McQuillan, and H.S. Margolis. The Past Incidence of Hepatitis C Virus Infection: Implications for the Future Burden of Chronic Liver Disease in the United States. *Hepatology* (2000):31(3):777–782.

Armstrong, G.L., A. Wasley, E.P. Simard, G.M. McQuillan, W.L. Kuhnert, and M.J. Alter. The Prevalence of Hepatitis C Virus Infection in the United States, 1999 Through 2002. *Ann Intern Med* (2006):144(10):705–714.

Beasley, R.P., L.Y. Hwang, C.C. Lin, et al. Incidence of Hepatitis B Virus Infections in Preschool Children in Taiwan. *J Infect Dis* (1982):146(2):198–204.

Bell, B.P., V.J. Navarro, M.M. Manos, et al. The Epidemiology of Newly-Diagnosed Chronic Liver Disease in the United States: Findings of Population-Based Sentinel Surveillance. *Hepatology* (2001):34(Part 2):468A.

Bellentani, S., G. Saccoccio, G. Costa, et al. Drinking Habits as Cofactors of Risk for Alcohol Induced Liver Damage. The Dionysos Study Group. *Gut* (1997):41(6):845–850.

Bellentani, S., C. Tiribelli, G. Saccoccio, et al. Prevalence of Chronic Liver Disease in the General Population of Northern Italy: The Dionysos Study. *Hepatology* (1994):20(6):1442–1449.

Benvegnu, L., M. Gios, S. Boccato, and A. Alberti. Natural History of Compensated Viral Cirrhosis: A Prospective Study on the Incidence and Hierarchy of Major Complications. *Gut* (2004):53(5):744–749.

Beutler, E., V.J. Felitti, J.A. Koziol, N.J. Ho, and T. Gelbart. Penetrance of 845G→A (*C282Y*) HFE Hereditary Haemochromatosis Mutation in the USA. *Lancet* (2002):359(9302):211–218.

Blume, S.B. Women and Alcohol. A Review. *JAMA* (1986):256(11):1467–1470.

Bode, C., J.C. Bode, J.G. Erhardt, B.A. French, and S.W. French. Effect of the Type of Beverage and Meat Consumed by Alcoholics with Alcoholic Liver Disease. *Alcohol Clin Exp Res* (1998):22(8):1803–1805.

Bosch, F.X. Global Epidemiology of Hepatocellular Carcinoma. In: K. Okuda, and E. Tabor, editors, *Liver Cancer*. New York: Churchill Livingston (1997):13–28.

Bosch, F.X., J. Ribes, J. Borràs, et al. Epidemiology of Primary Liver Cancer. *Semin Liver Dis* (1999):19(3):271–285.

Bosch, F.X., J. Ribes, R. Cleries, et al. Epidemiology of Hepatocellular Carcinoma. *Clin Liver Dis* (2005):9(2):191–211, v.

Briggs, M.E., C. Baker, R. Hall, et al. Prevalence and Risk Factors for Hepatitis C Virus Infection at an Urban Veterans Administration Medical Center. *Hepatology* (2001):34(6):1200–1205.

Browning, J.D., L.S. Szczepaniak, R. Dobbins, et al. Prevalence of Hepatic Steatosis in an Urban Population in the United States: Impact of Ethnicity. *Hepatology* (2004):40(6):1387–1395.

Bruix, J., and M. Sherman. Management of Hepatocellular Carcinoma. *Hepatology* (2005):42(5):1208–1236.

Bruix, J., M. Sherman, J.M. Llovet, et al. Clinical Management of Hepatocellular Carcinoma. Conclusions of the Barcelona-2000 EASL Conference. European Association for the Study of the Liver. *J Hepatol* (2001):35(3):421–430.

Brundage, S.C., and A.N. Fitzpatrick. Hepatitis A. *Am Fam Physician* (2006):73(12):2162–2168.

Caetano, R., and L.A. Kaskutas. Changes in Drinking Patterns among Whites, Blacks and Hispanics, 1984–1992. *J Stud Alcohol* (1995):56(5):558–565.

CDC. Hepatitis B Virus: A Comprehensive Strategy for Eliminating Transmission in the United States Through Universal Childhood Vaccination. Recommendations of the Immunization Practices Advisory Committee (ACIP). *MMWR Recomm Rep* (1991):40(RR-13):1–25.

CDC. CDC Wonder Web site. Available at http://wonder.cdc.gov.

Chang, M.H., C.J. Chen, M.S. Lai, et al. Universal Hepatitis B Vaccination in Taiwan and the Incidence of Hepatocellular Carcinoma in Children. Taiwan Childhood Hepatoma Study Group. *N Engl J Med* (1997):336(26):1855–1859.

Chen, C.J., H.I. Yang, J. Su, et al. Risk of Hepatocellular Carcinoma Across a Biological Gradient of Serum Hepatitis B Virus DNA Level. *JAMA* (2006):295(1):65–73.

Cheung, R.C., A.K. Hanson, K. Maganti, E.B. Keeffe, and S.M. Matsui. Viral Hepatitis and Other Infectious Diseases in a Homeless Population. *J Clin Gastroenterol* (2002):34(4): 476–480.

Chiung, M., and H-Y.Y. Chen. *Trends in Alcohol Related Morbidity among Short-Stay Community Hospital Discharges, United States, 1979–2005.* Bethesda, MD: National Institute on Alcohol Abuse and Alcoholism (2007). Surveillance Report no. 80.

Choo, Q.L., G. Kuo, A.J. Weiner, L.R. Overby, D.W. Bradley, and M. Houghton. Isolation of a cDNA Clone Derived from a Blood-Borne Non-A, Non-B Viral Hepatitis Genome. *Science* (1989):244(4902):359–362.

Clark, J.M., F.L. Brancati, and A.M. Diehl. Nonalcoholic Fatty Liver Disease. *Gastroenterology* (2002):122(6):1649–1657.

Clark, J.M., F.L. Brancati, and A.M. Diehl. The Prevalence and Etiology of Elevated Aminotransferase Levels in the United States. *Am J Gastroenterol* (2003):98(5):960–967.

Corrao, G., and S. Arico. Independent and Combined Action of Hepatitis C Virus Infection and Alcohol Consumption on the Risk of Symptomatic Liver Cirrhosis. *Hepatology* (1998):27(4):914–919.

Corrao, G., S. Arico, A. Zambon, et al. Is Alcohol a Risk Factor for Liver Cirrhosis in HBsAg and Anti-HCV Negative Subjects? Collaborative Groups for the Study of Liver Diseases in Italy. *J Hepatol* (1997):27(3):470–476.

D'Amico, G., A. Morabito, L. Pagliaro, and E. Marubini. Survival and Prognostic Indicators in Compensated and Decompensated Cirrhosis. *Dig Dis Sci* (1986):31(5):468–475.

Davis, G.L., J.E. Albright, S.F. Cook., and D.M. Rosenberg. Projecting Future Complications of Chronic Hepatitis C in the United States. *Liver Transpl* (2003):9(4):331–338.

Day, C.P. Who Gets Alcoholic Liver Disease: Nature or Nurture? *J R Coll Physicians Lond* (2000):34(6):557–562.

Debakey, S.F., F.S. Stinson, B.F. Grant, et al. *Liver Cirrhosis Mortality in the United States, 1970–92.* Surveillance Report #37. Bethesda, MD: National Institute on Alcohol Abuse and Alcoholism (1995).

Degos, F. Hepatitis C and Alcohol. *J Hepatol* (1999):31(Suppl 1):113–118.

Dentinger, C.M., W.A. Bower, O.V. Nainan, et al. An Outbreak of Hepatitis A Associated with Green Onions. *J Infect Dis* (2001):183(8):1273–1276.

Diehl, A.M. Alcoholic Liver Disease: Natural History. *Liver Transpl Surg* (1997):3(3):206–211.

Donato, F., A. Tagger, R. Chiesa, et al. Hepatitis B and C Virus Infection, Alcohol Drinking, and Hepatocellular Carcinoma: A Case-Control Study in Italy. Brescia HCC Study. *Hepatology* (1997):26(3):579–584.

Duvnjak, M., I. Lerotic, N. Barsic, V. Tomasic, J.L. Viruvic, and V. Velagic. Pathogenesis and Management Issues for Non-Alcoholic Fatty Liver Disease. *World J Gastroenterol* (2007):13(34):4539–4550.

El-Serag, H.B., and A.C. Mason. Rising Incidence of Hepatocellular Carcinoma in the United States. *N Engl J Med* (1999):340(10):745–750.

Fattovich, G., L. Brollo, G. Giustina, et al. Natural History and Prognostic Factors for Chronic Hepatitis Type B. *Gut* (1991):32(3):294–298.

Finelli, L., J.T. Miller, J.I. Tokars, M.J. Alter, and M.J. Arduino. National Surveillance of Dialysis-Associated Diseases in the United States, 2002. *Semin Dial* (2005):18(1):52–61.

Fiore, A.E., A. Wasley, and B.P. Bell. Prevention of Hepatitis A Through Active or Passive Immunization: Recommendations of the Advisory Committee on Immunization Practices (ACIP). *MMWR Recomm Rep* (2006):55(RR-7):1–23.

Fisher, N.C., J. Hanson, A. Phillips, J.N. Rao, and E.T. Swarbrick. Mortality from Liver Disease in the West Midlands, 1993–2000: Observational Study. *BMJ* (2002):325(7359):312–313.

Freeman, A.J., G.J. Dore, M.G. Law, et al. Estimating Progression to Cirrhosis in Chronic Hepatitis C Virus Infection. *Hepatology* (2001):34(4 Pt 1):809–816.

Frezza, M., C. di Padova, G. Pozzato, M. Terpin, E. Baraona, and C.S. Lieber. High Blood Alcohol Levels in Women. The Role of Decreased Gastric Alcohol Dehydrogenase Activity and First-Pass Metabolism. *N Engl J Med* (1990):322(2):95–99.

Fried, M.W., M.L. Shiffman, K.R. Reddy, et al. Peginterferon Alfa-2a Plus Ribavirin for Chronic Hepatitis C Virus Infection. *N Engl J Med* (2002):347(13):975–982.

Garfein, R.S., D. Vlahov, N. Galai, M.C. Doherty, and K.E. Nelson. Viral Infections in Short-Term Injection Drug Users: The Prevalence of the Hepatitis C, Hepatitis B, Human Immunodeficiency, and Human T-Lymphotropic Viruses. *Am J Public Health* (1996):86(5): 655–661.

Geerlings, W., G. Tufveson, J.H. Ehrich, et al. Report on Management of Renal Failure in Europe, XXIII. *Nephrol Dial Transplant* (1994):9(Suppl 1):6–25.

Gholam, P.M., L. Flancbaum, J.T. Machan, D.A. Charney, and D.P. Kotler. Nonalcoholic Fatty Liver Disease in Severely Obese Subjects. *Am J Gastroenterol* (2007):102(2):399–408.

Hamaguchi, M., T. Kojima, N. Takeda, et al. The Metabolic Syndrome as a Predictor of Nonalcoholic Fatty Liver Disease. *Ann Intern Med* (2005):143(10):722–728.

Hasumura, Y., and J. Takeuchi. Alcoholic Liver Disease in Japanese Patients: A Comparison with Caucasians. *J Gastroenterol Hepatol* (1991):6(5):520–527.

Heron, M. Deaths: Leading Causes for 2004. *Natl Vital Stat Rep* (2007):56(5):1–95.

Holder, H.D., and R.N. Parker. Effect of Alcoholism Treatment on Cirrhosis Mortality: A 20-Year Multivariate Time Series Analysis. *Br J Addict* (1992):87(9):1263–1274.

Hourigan, L.F., G.A. Macdonald, D. Purdie, et al. Fibrosis in Chronic Hepatitis C Correlates Significantly with Body Mass Index and Steatosis. *Hepatology* (1999):29(4):1215–1219.

Hussain, K.B., R.J. Fontana, C.A. Moyer, G.L. Su, N. Sneed-Pee, and A.S. Lok. Comorbid Illness is an Important Determinant of Health-Related Quality of Life in Patients with Chronic Hepatitis C. *Am J Gastroenterol* (2001):96(9):2737–2744.

Ikejima, K., N. Enomoto, Y. Iimuro, et al. Estrogen Increases Sensitivity of Hepatic Kupffer Cells to Endotoxin. *Am J Physiol* (1998):274(4 Pt 1):G669–G676.

Ioannou, G.N., E.J. Boyko, and S.P. Lee. The Prevalence and Predictors of Elevated Serum Aminotransferase Activity in the United States in 1999–2002. *Am J Gastroenterol* (2006):101(1):76–82.

Jacobsen, K.H., and J.S. Koopman. Declining Hepatitis A Seroprevalence: A Global Review and Analysis. *Epidemiol Infect* (2004):132(6):1005–1022.

Jajosky, R.A., P.A. Hall, D.A. Adams, et al. Summary of Notifiable Diseases—United States, 2004. *MMWR Morb Mortal Wkly Rep* (2006):53(53):1–79.

Kerr, W.C., K.M. Fillmore, P. Marvy, et al. Beverage-Specific Alcohol Consumption and Cirrhosis Mortality in a Group of English-Speaking Beer-Drinking Countries. *Addiction* (2000): 95(3):339–346.

Kim, W.R. The Burden of Hepatitis C in the United States. *Hepatology* (2002):36(5 Suppl 1): S30–S34.

Kim, W.R., J.T. Benson, T.M. Therneau, et al. Changing Epidemiology of Hepatitis B in a U.S. Community. *Hepatology* (2004):39(3):811–816.

Kim, W.R., R.S. Brown, Jr., N.A. Terrault, and H. El-Serag. Burden of Liver Disease in the United States: Summary of a Workshop. *Hepatology* (2002):36(1):227–242.

Kim, W.R., J.B. Gross, Jr., J.J. Poterucha, G.R. Locke, 3rd, and E.R. Dickson. Outcome of Hospital Care of Liver Disease Associated with Hepatitis C in the United States. *Hepatology* (2001):33(1):201–206.

Koff, R.S. Clinical Manifestations and Diagnosis of Hepatitis A Virus Infection. *Vaccine* (1992):10(Suppl 1):S15–S17.

Kuo, G., Q.L. Choo, H.J. Alter, et al. An Assay for Circulating Antibodies to a Major Etiologic Virus of Human Non-A, Non-B Hepatitis. *Science* (1989):244(4902):362–364.

Kuper, H., A. Tzonou, E. Kaklamani, et al. Tobacco Smoking, Alcohol Consumption and Their Interaction in the Causation of Hepatocellular Carcinoma. *Int J Cancer* (2000):85(4):498–502.

Lai, C.L., B.C. Wong, E.K. Yeoh, W.L. Lim, W.K. Chang, and H.J. Lin. Five-Year Follow-up of a Prospective Randomized Trial of Hepatitis B Recombinant DNA Yeast Vaccine vs. Plasma-Derived Vaccine in Children: Immunogenicity and Anamnestic Responses. *Hepatology* (1993):18(4):763–767.

Larsson, S.C., and A. Wolk. Coffee Consumption and Risk of Liver Cancer: A Meta-Analysis. *Gastroenterology* (2007):132(5):1740–1745.

Leandro, G., A. Mangia, J. Hui, et al. Relationship between Steatosis, Inflammation, and Fibrosis in Chronic Hepatitis C: A Meta-Analysis of Individual Patient Data. *Gastroenterology* (2006):130(6):1636–1642.

Lelbach, W.K. Cirrhosis in the Alcoholic and its Relation to the Volume of Alcohol Abuse. *Ann N Y Acad Sci* (1975):252:85–105.

Liaw, Y.F., S.L. Tsai, I.S. Sheen, et al. Clinical and Virological Course of Chronic Hepatitis B Virus Infection with Hepatitis C and D Virus Markers. *Am J Gastroenterol* (1998):93(3):354–359.

Loguercio, C., M. Di Pierro, M.P. Di Marino, et al. Drinking Habits of Subjects with Hepatitis C Virus-Related Chronic Liver Disease: Prevalence and Effect on Clinical, Virological and Pathological Aspects. *Alcohol Alcohol* (2000):35(3):296–301.

Mandayam, S., M.M. Jamal, and T.R. Morgan. Epidemiology of Alcoholic Liver Disease. *Semin Liver Dis* (2004):24(3):217–232.

Mann, R.E., R.G. Smart, L. Anglin, and E.M. Adlaf. Reductions in Cirrhosis Deaths in the United States: Associations with Per Capita Consumption and AA Membership. *J Stud Alcohol* (1991):52(4):361–365.

Manns, M.P., J.G. McHutchison, S.C. Gordon, et al. Peginterferon Alfa-2b Plus Ribavirin Compared with Interferon Alfa-2b Plus Ribavirin for Initial Treatment of Chronic Hepatitis C: A Randomised Trial. *Lancet* (2001):358(9286):958–965.

Marchesini, G., E. Bugianesi, G. Forlani, et al. Nonalcoholic Fatty Liver, Steatohepatitis, and the Metabolic Syndrome. *Hepatology* (2003):37(4):917–923.

Mast, E.E., H.S. Margolis, A.E. Fiore, et al. A Comprehensive Immunization Strategy to Eliminate Transmission of Hepatitis B Virus Infection in the United States: Recommendations of the Advisory Committee on Immunization Practices (ACIP) Part 1: Immunization of Infants, Children, and Adolescents. *MMWR Recomm Rep* (2005):54(RR-16):1–31.

Mast, E.E., C.M. Weinbaum, A.E. Fiore, et al. A Comprehensive Immunization Strategy to Eliminate Transmission of Hepatitis B Virus Infection in the United States: Recommendations of the Advisory Committee on Immunization Practices (ACIP) Part II: Immunization of Adults. *MMWR Recomm Rep* (2006):55(RR-16):1–33; quiz CE1–4.

Maynard, J.E. Hepatitis B: Global Importance and Need for Control. *Vaccine* (1990):8(Suppl): S18–S20; discussion S21–S23.

Mbithi, J.N., V.S. Springthorpe, J.R. Boulet, and S.A. Sattar. Survival of Hepatitis A Virus on Human Hands and its Transfer on Contact with Animate and Inanimate Surfaces. *J Clin Microbiol* (1992):30(4):757–763.

Miller, M.E., J.E. Everhart, and J. Hoofnagle. Epidemiologic Research and the Action Plan for Liver Disease Research. *Ann Epidemiol* (2006):16(11):861–865.

Murphy, E.L., S.M. Bryzman, S.A. Glynn, et al. Risk Factors for Hepatitis C Virus Infection in United States Blood Donors. NHLBI Retrovirus Epidemiology Donor Study (REDS). *Hepatology* (2000):31(3):756–762.

Nanji, A.A., and S.W. French. Relationship between Pork Consumption and Cirrhosis. *Lancet* (1985):1(8430):681–683.

Naveau, S., V. Giraud, E. Borotto, E. Aubert, F. Capron, and J.-C. Chaput. Excess Weight Risk Factor for Alcoholic Liver Disease. *Hepatology* (1997):25(1):108–111.

Neuschwander-Tetri, B.A., and S.H. Caldwell. Nonalcoholic Steatohepatitis: Summary of an AASLD Single Topic Conference. *Hepatology* (2003):37(5):1202–1219.

Ni, Y.H., L.M. Huang, M. Chang, et al. Two Decades of Universal Hepatitis B Vaccination in Taiwan: Impact and Implication for Future Strategies. *Gastroenterology* (2007):132(4):1287–1293.

Ogden, C.L., S.Z. Yanovski, M.D. Carroll, and K.M. Flegal. The Epidemiology of Obesity. *Gastroenterology* (2007):132(6):2087–2102.

Ostapowicz, G., K.J. Watson, S.A. Locarnini, and P.V. Desmond. Role of Alcohol in the Progression of Liver Disease Caused by Hepatitis C Virus Infection. *Hepatology* (1998):27(6):1730–1735.

Park, S.C., S.I. Oh, and M.S. Lee. Korean Status of Alcoholics and Alcohol-Related Health Problems. *Alcohol Clin Exp Res* (1998):22(3 Suppl):170S–172S.

Parkin, D.M., F. Bray, J. Ferlay, and P. Pisani. Global Cancer Statistics, 2002. *CA Cancer J Clin* (2005):55(2):74–108.

Parlesak, A. Increased Intestinal Permeability to Macromolecules and Endotoxemia in Patients with Chronic Alcohol Abuse in Different Stages of Alcohol-Induced Liver Disease. *J Hepatol* (2000):32(5):742–747.

Pereira, B.J., E.L. Milford, R.L. Kirkman, and A.S. Levey. Transmission of Hepatitis C Virus by Organ Transplantation. *N Engl J Med* (1991):325(7):454–460.

Pomper, G.J., Y. Wu, and E.L. Snyder. Risks of Transfusion-Transmitted Infections: 2003. *Curr Opin Hematol* (2003):10(6):412–418.

Poynard, T., P. Bedossa, and P. Opolon. Natural History of Liver Fibrosis Progression in Patients with Chronic Hepatitis C. The OBSVIRC, METAVIR, CLINIVIR, and DOSVIRC Groups. *Lancet* (1997):349(9055):825–832.

Ramstedt, M. Per Capita Alcohol Consumption and Liver Cirrhosis Mortality in 14 European Countries. *Addiction* (2001):96(Suppl 1):S19–S33.

Rodger, A.J., D. Jolley, S.C. Thompson, A. Lanigan, and N. Crofts. The Impact of Diagnosis of Hepatitis C Virus on Quality of Life. *Hepatology* (1999):30(5):1299–1301.

Ruhl, C.E., and J.E. Everhart. Determinants of the Association of Overweight with Elevated Serum Alanine Aminotransferase Activity in the United States. *Gastroenterology* (2003):124(1):71–79.

Ruhl, C.E., and J.E. Everhart. Epidemiology of Nonalcoholic Fatty Liver. *Clin Liver Dis* (2004):8(3):501–519, vii.

Ruhl, C.E., and J.E. Everhart. Coffee and Tea Consumption are Associated with a Lower Incidence of Chronic Liver Disease in the United States. *Gastroenterology* (2005):129(6):1928–1936.

Ruiz, J.D., F. Molitor, R.K. Sun, et al. Prevalence and Correlates of Hepatitis C Virus Infection among Inmates Entering the California Correctional System. *West J Med* (1999):170(3):156–160.

Saadatmand, F., F.S. Stinson, B.F. Grant, and M.C. Dufour. *Liver Cirrhosis Mortality in the United States, 1970–1997*. Bethesda, MD: National Institute on Alcohol Abuse and Alcoholism (2000). Surveillance Report no. 54.

Sandler, D.P., R.S. Sandler, and L.F. Horney. Primary Liver Cancer Mortality in the United States. *J Chronic Dis* (1983):36(3):227–236.

Sandler, R.S., J.E. Everhart, M. Donowitz, et al. The Burden of Selected Digestive Diseases in the United States. *Gastroenterology* (2002):122(5):1500–1511.

Sangiovanni, A., E. Del Ninno, P. Fasani, et al. Increased Survival of Cirrhotic Patients with a Hepatocellular Carcinoma Detected During Surveillance. *Gastroenterology* (2004):126(4):1005–1014.

Sato, N., K.O. Lindros, E. Baraona, et al. Sex Difference in Alcohol-Related Organ Injury. *Alcohol Clin Exp Res* (2001):25(5 Suppl ISBRA):40S–45S.

Schiff, E.R., M.F. Sorrell, and W.C. Maddrey. *Schiff's Diseases of the Liver*. Philadelphia, New York: Lippincott-Raven (1999).

Schreiber, G.B., M.P. Busch, S.H. Kleinman, and J.J. Korelitz. The Risk of Transfusion-Transmitted Viral Infections. The Retrovirus Epidemiology Donor Study. *N Engl J Med* (1996):334(26):1685–1690.

Schwimmer, J.B., R. Deutsch, T. Kahen, J.E. Lavine, C. Stanley, and C. Behling. Prevalence of Fatty Liver in Children and Adolescents. *Pediatrics* (2006):118(4):1388–1393.

Shen, L., J.G. Fan, Y. Shao, et al. Prevalence of Nonalcoholic Fatty Liver among Administrative Officers in Shanghai: An Epidemiological Survey. *World J Gastroenterol* (2003):9(5):1106–1110.

Shepard, C.W., L. Finelli, and M.J. Alter. Global Epidemiology of Hepatitis C Virus Infection. *Lancet Infect Dis* (2005):5(9):558–567.

Singh, G.K., and D.L. Hoyert. Social Epidemiology of Chronic Liver Disease and Cirrhosis Mortality in the United States, 1935–1997: Trends and Differentials by Ethnicity, Socioeconomic Status, and Alcohol Consumption. *Hum Biol* (2000):72(5):801–820.

Smart, R.G., and R.E. Mann. Recent Liver Cirrhosis Declines: Estimates of the Impact of Alcohol Abuse Treatment and Alcoholics Anonymous. *Addiction* (1993):88(2):193–198.

Sorensen, T.I., M. Orholm, K.D. Bentsen, G. Hoybye, K. Eghoje, and P. Christoffersen. Prospective Evaluation of Alcohol Abuse and Alcoholic Liver Injury in Men as Predictors of Development of Cirrhosis. *Lancet* (1984):2(8397):241–244.

Steinberg, K.K., M.E. Cogswell, J.C. Chang, et al. Prevalence of *C282Y* and *H63D* Mutations in the Hemochromatosis (HFE) Gene in the United States. *JAMA* (2001):285(17):2216–2222.

Stevens, C.E., R.P. Beasley, J. Tsui, and W.C. Lee. Vertical Transmission of Hepatitis B Antigen in Taiwan. *N Engl J Med* (1975):292(15):771–774.

Stinson, F.S., B.F. Grant, and M.C. Dufour. The Critical Dimension of Ethnicity in Liver Cirrhosis Mortality Statistics. *Alcohol Clin Exp Res* (2001):25(8):1181–1187.

Tang, Y.W., J.X. Wang, Z.Y. Xu, Y.F. Guo, W.H. Qian, and J.X. Xu. A Serologically Confirmed, Case-Control Study, of a Large Outbreak of Hepatitis A in China, Associated with Consumption of Clams. *Epidemiol Infect* (1991):107(3):651–657.

Tassopoulos, N.C., G.J. Papaevangelou, M.H. Sjogren, A. Roumeliotou-Karayannis, J.L. Gerin, and R.H. Purcell. Natural History of Acute Hepatitis B Surface Antigen-Positive Hepatitis in Greek Adults. *Gastroenterology* (1987):92(6):1844–1850.

Terris, M. Epidemiology of Cirrhosis of the Liver: National Mortality Data. *Am J Public Health Nations Health* (1967):57(12):2076–2088.

Thaler, H. Alcohol Consumption and Diseases of the Liver. *Nutr Metab* (1977):21(1–3):196–193.

Tong, M.J., N.S. El-Farra, and M.I. Grew. Clinical Manifestations of Hepatitis A: Recent Experience in a Community Teaching Hospital. *J Infect Dis* (1995):171(Suppl 1):S15–S18.

United Network for Organ Sharing (UNOS). UNOS Data. Available at http://www.unos.org/Data.

Vento, S., T. Garofano, C. Renzini, et al. Fulminant Hepatitis Associated with Hepatitis A Virus Superinfection in Patients with Chronic Hepatitis C. *N Engl J Med* (1998):338(5):286–290.

Wasley, A., A. Fiore, and B.P. Bell. Hepatitis A in the Era of Vaccination. *Epidemiol Rev* (2006):28:101–111.

Wasley, A., J.T. Miller, and L. Finelli. Surveillance for Acute Viral Hepatitis—United States, 2005. *MMWR Surveill Summ* (2007):56(3):1–24.

Weinbaum, C., R. Lyerla, H.S. Margolis, and the Centers for Disease Control and Prevention. Prevention and Control of Infections with Hepatitis Viruses in Correctional Settings. Centers for Disease Control and Prevention. *MMWR Recomm Rep* (2003):52(RR-1):1–36; quiz CE1–4.

Weston, S.R., W. Leyden, R. Murphy, et al. Racial and Ethnic Distribution of Nonalcoholic Fatty Liver in Persons with Newly Diagnosed Chronic Liver Disease. *Hepatology* (2005):41(2):372–379.

Wheeler, C., T.M. Vogt, G.L. Armstrong, et al. An Outbreak of Hepatitis A Associated with Green Onions. *N Engl J Med* (2005):353(9):890–897.

Whitlock, E.P., B.A. Garlitz, E.L. Harris, T.L. Beil, and P.R. Smith. Screening for Hereditary Hemochromatosis: A Systematic Review for the U.S. Preventive Services Task Force. *Ann Intern Med* (2006):145(3):209–223.

Williams, I. Epidemiology of Hepatitis C in the United States. *Am J Med* (1999):107(6B):2S–9S.
World Health Organization. Global and Regional Summary. Available at http://www.who.int/entity/immunization_monitoring/diseases/GS_Hepatitis.pdf.
World Health Organization. WHO Statistical Information System (WHOSIS) Web site. Available at http://www.who.int/whosis/en.
Yang, H.I., S.N. Lu, Y.F. Liaw, et al. Hepatitis B e Antigen and the Risk of Hepatocellular Carcinoma. *N Engl J Med* (2002):347(3):168–174.
Younossi, Z., J. Kallman, and J. Kincaid. The Effects of HCV Infection and Management on Health-Related Quality of Life. *Hepatology* (2007):45(3):806–816.
Zaman, S.N., P.J. Johnson, and R. Williams. Silent Cirrhosis in Patients with Hepatocellular Carcinoma. Implications for Screening in High-Incidence and Low-Incidence Areas. *Cancer* (1990):65(7):1607–1610.
Zarski, J.P., J. Mc Hutchison, J.P. Bronowicki, et al. Rate of Natural Disease Progression in Patients with Chronic Hepatitis C. *J Hepatol* (2003):38(3):307–314.

CHAPTER 20

CHRONIC KIDNEY DISEASE (ICD-10 I12, N18.0)

A. Vishnu Moorthy, M.D. and Jonathan B. Jaffery, M.D., M.S.

Introduction

Chronic kidney disease (CKD) is a common but silent and underdiagnosed health problem contributing to significant morbidity and mortality worldwide, both in the United States and other developed countries and in developing countries (Rettig, Norris, and Nissenson 2008; Barsoum 2006; El Nahas et al. 2005). CKD is typically a progressive disease that can ultimately lead to kidney failure (end-stage renal disease, or ESRD), requiring maintenance dialysis treatments or kidney transplantation for survival. Even more importantly, patients with CKD have a greatly increased risk of death from cardiovascular disease, an outcome more commonly experienced in these patients than kidney failure (Keith et al. 2004).

Pathophysiology

CKD is a term applied to a variety of disorders that cause progressive kidney damage resulting in decreased kidney function. These vary from genetic disorders that may manifest at any age (such as autosomal-dominant polycystic kidney disease), several types of glomerulonephritis that are generally immune in nature, a variety of infections (including HIV/AIDS and hepatitis C), toxicity from medications (including nonsteroidal anti-inflammatory drugs, or NSAIDs) and disorders of organs outside the kidney (e.g., prostate, urinary bladder, uterus) that result in blockage of urine flow.

However, the major causes of ESRD in the United States are diabetes mellitus and hypertension (Figure 20.1). Up to 40% of patients with type 1 and 5% to 10% of patients with type 2 diabetes develop kidney failure from diabetic nephropathy. However, since type 2 diabetes is more prevalent, approximately 50 to 60% of patients receiving renal replacement therapy have type 2 diabetes (USRDS 2006). The kidney damage in patients with diabetes is a consequence of chronic elevations in blood sugar levels that damage the glomeruli in the kidneys. The kidney damage is one component of the widespread microvascular disease seen in patients with diabetes mellitus who develop other complications such as diabetic retinopathy and neuropathy. Urinalysis showing increasing amounts of albumin excretion is the earliest manifestation of diabetic kidney disease. Elevation in blood pressure, which is common in patients with diabetes, compounds the kidney injury and progression of CKD (Cooper 1998).

In addition, hypertension in and of itself continues to be an important cause of CKD. Certain pathologic processes within the kidney can result in hypertension, yet the

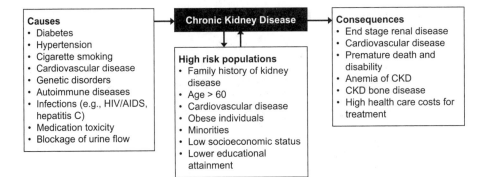

Figure 20.1. CKD causes, consequences, and high-risk populations.

kidney is also very sensitive to the effects of hypertension, and high blood pressure is a key pathogenic factor contributing to deterioration in kidney function. The presence of kidney disease is a common and underappreciated preexisting medical cause of resistant hypertension (Sarafidis and Bakris 2008), and an elevated serum creatinine level is noted in 10% to 20% of patients with hypertension. In 2% to 5% of patients with suboptimally controlled high blood pressure, progression to kidney failure is noted over the subsequent 10 to 15 years (Perry et al. 1995). The risk for kidney disease is greater in African Americans and in the elderly with hypertension, especially in those with systolic blood pressure greater than 160 mmHg (Klag et al. 1996).

The mechanisms for the increase in cardiovascular mortality in patients with CKD are not well-defined, but both traditional and nontraditional cardiovascular risk factors play a role (Kendrick and Chonchol 2008). It is known that younger patients with ESRD on dialysis have an increased cardiovascular mortality (Foley, Parfrey, and Sarnak 1998). Some of the coexisting conditions in patients with CKD that are conducive to development of cardiovascular disease include hypertension, hyperlipidemia, smoking, malnutrition, and diabetes. Impaired kidney function may be a marker for severity of vascular disease as well as being associated with markers of chronic inflammation, itself a risk factor for cardiovascular disease (Shlipak et al. 2005).

Significance

Approximately 13% of the U.S. adult population, or as many as 26 million Americans, may be affected by CKD, and the prevalence has been increasing (CDC 2007; Coresh et al. 2007). As evidence of this, the Medicare ESRD program, which extends Medicare coverage to all Americans with ESRD regardless of age, covered approximately 10,000 patients when it began in 1973. As of December 31, 2005, over 485,000 individuals were covered under this program, and over 100,000 of those were new to the program that year. The majority of people covered were undergoing hemodialysis as a mode of renal replacement therapy, and over 140,000 people are currently living with a functioning kidney transplant (USRDS 2006).

It is noteworthy that recently there has been some slowing in the rate of increase in the number of patients treated for kidney failure (Ruggenenti and Remuzzi 2007).

Although the 1980s saw annual increases in the incident rates of kidney failure of approximately 10% per year, in the mid to late 1990s, these numbers leveled off (Figure 20.2). In fact, the number of patients entering the kidney failure program between 2002 and 2004 has actually decreased by 1%. Regardless, the prevalence of patients with kidney failure remains high. As of 2004, it stood at 339 per million population, far greater than the Healthy People 2010 goal of 217 per million population (USRDS 2006). It is estimated that by 2015, there will be 136,000 incident cases of kidney failure in the United States per year with a prevalence of 712,000 individuals (Gilbertson et al. 2005).

The cost of managing patients with ESRD also remains high. In the United States, the average annual costs for a patient on dialysis is about $60,000, and costs to Medicare for this program exceeded $18 billion in 2005, accounting for approximately 6.5% of the total Medicare budget (USRDS 2006). Despite the enormous expense, both the quality of life and the life expectancy of most patients on dialysis are low. A patient on dialysis spends 14 days per year on average in the hospital, and the annual mortality rate remains approximately 20% (USRDS 2006). Further, the 5-year survival of patients on dialysis is only about 35%, a mortality rate worse than that seen with many cancers (Eknoyan et al. 2001).

Despite the fact that the number of patients with kidney failure in the United States is increasing, most patients with CKD do not survive to reach end-stage and start renal replacement therapy (Kalantar-Zadeh et al. 2007). One reason is that the risk of cardiovascular disease increases dramatically with declining kidney function (Go et al. 2004) (Figure 20.3). Tonelli reviewed 39 studies with a total of 1,371,990 participants. The unadjusted relative risk for mortality in participants with CKD when compared with those without CKD ranged from 0.94 to 5.0 and was significantly more than 1.0 in 93% of cohorts (Tonelli et al. 2006). The absolute risk for death also increased exponentially with decreased kidney function in these studies.

Because patients with CKD do not develop symptoms until they already have significant decline in kidney function, the epidemic of CKD is largely a silent one. In recent

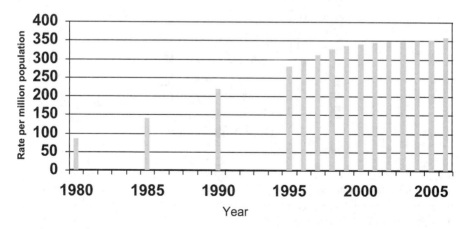

Figure 20.2. Adjusted incidence rates of patients with ESRD by year, 1980–2006. From USRDS (2008).

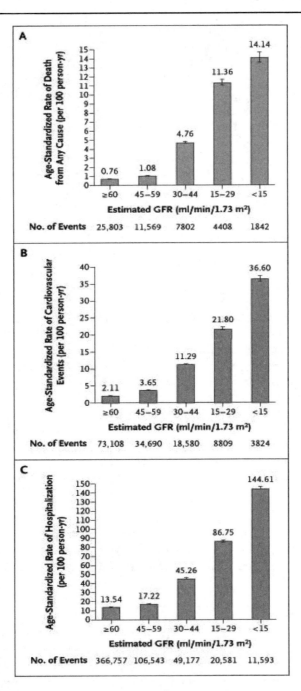

Figure 20.3. Age-Standardized Rates of Death from Any Cause (Panel A), Cardiovascular Events (Panel B), and Hospitalization (Panel C), According to the Estimated GFR among 1,120,295 Ambulatory Adults. A cardiovascular event was defined as hospitalization for coronary heart disease, heart failure, ischemic stroke, and peripheral arterial disease. The association between kidney function (eGFR) and cardiovascular disease is shown in Panel B. Go, A.S., G.M. Chertow, D. Fan, C.E. McCulloch, and C.Y. Shu. Chronic kidney disease and risk of death, cardiovascular events, and hospitalization. *N Engl J Med* (2004):351:1296–1305. Copyright © *[2004] Massachusetts Medical Society. All rights reserved.*

years, the prevalence of CKD has been noted to be increasing. Data from the National Health and Nutritional Examination Survey (NHANES), 1999–2004, revealed that in the U.S. adult population aged greater than 20 years, 16.8% had CKD (CDC 2007). Compared with the NHANES III data from 1988 to 1992, when the prevalence was 14.5%, this represents a relative increase of 15.9%. The number of patients at risk for developing CKD is even greater as conditions such as diabetes and hypertension, the two leading causes of CKD in the United States, are themselves becoming increasingly prevalent (Mokdad et al. 2001).

CKD is also a growing worldwide problem in both developed as well as developing countries (Levey et al. 2007; El Nahas et al. 2005). Moreover, with the aging of the population and the increase in obesity and diabetes, it is expected the problem of CKD will become even greater in the coming years. The prevalence of CKD is also higher in minority populations and the socially disadvantaged (Norris and Nissenson 2008; Bello et al. 2008).

Descriptive Epidemiology

High-Risk Populations

In addition to those with diabetes mellitus and hypertension, the risk of CKD is high in patients with cardiovascular disease, obesity, aged greater than 60 years, and in those with a family history of kidney disease (Figure 20.1). In a recent NHANES report, CKD risk was noted to be greater among persons with diabetes than among those without diabetes by 40.2% versus 15.4%, among persons with cardiovascular disease than among those without cardiovascular disease by 28.2% versus 15.4%, and among persons with hypertension than among those without hypertension by 24.6% versus 12.5% (CDC 2007). CKD was also over twice as prevalent among adults greater than 60 years (39.4%) when compared with the prevalence of 16.8% in the total population studied.

Racial and ethnic features have also been shown to have a great impact on the prevalence of CKD (Figure 20.4). Although African Americans comprise less than 15% of the U.S. population, they account for more than 39% of all patients with ESRD (USRDS 2006). The prevalence of CKD is also greater among non-Hispanic African Americans (19.9%) and Mexican Americans (18.7%) than among non-Hispanic whites (16.1%) (CDC 2007). African Americans have a higher prevalence of hypertension than Caucasians (Davey Smith et al. 1998), and African Americans with diabetes and hypertension who develop CKD have a greater risk of CKD progression and the need for renal replacement therapy compared with Caucasians (Tonelli et al. 2006). Hispanics are more likely to have hypertension and obesity than the general U.S. population (Lorenzo et al. 2002; Raymond and D'Eramo-Melkus 1993). Mexican Americans also have a high risk of developing CKD and may share a common genetic background and "thrifty genotype" with Native American Indians, themselves a group at high risk of developing diabetes and CKD (Benabe and Rios 2004). Mexican Americans with type 2 diabetes are more likely to develop proteinuria and also more likely to progress to kidney failure than non-Hispanic whites (Pugh et al. 1988; Pugh 1996). American Indians are another higher risk group, experiencing a greater burden of CKD than non-Hispanic whites. The prevalence of type 2 diabetes and the metabolic syndrome is higher in American Indians, and in the

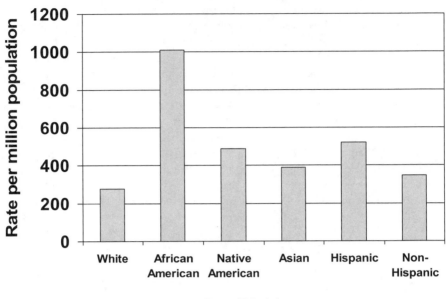

Figure 20.4. Age- and sex-adjusted incident rates of reported ESRD, by race, 2006. From USRDS (2008).

Strong Heart study at 9-year follow-up, the hazard ratio for CKD was 1.3 (Lucove et al. 2008).

Socioeconomic factors also affect the prevalence of CKD, which is seen in greater prevalence among lower income African Americans compared with those at higher income levels (Peralta et al. 2006). CKD is also more prevalent among persons with less than a high school education (22.1%) than persons with at least a high school education (15.7%) (CDC 2007).

Obesity and the metabolic syndrome have been observed in several recent studies as significant independent risk predictors for CKD (Wahba and Mak 2007). In over 7,800 participants who had normal kidney function and who were followed for more than 21 years, Chen et al. found that the multivariate-adjusted OR for CKD was 2.6 for obese individuals when compared with individuals without the metabolic syndrome (Chen et al. 2004). They also found a twofold increase in the risk for microalbuminuria that correlated with the number of traits of the metabolic syndrome (Chen et al. 2004). Wang et al. (2008) in a recently published meta-analysis of 16 previous studies noted that compared with individuals with normal BMI, overweight and obese individuals had a relative risk for kidney disease of 1.40 and 1.83, respectively.

There is also a high prevalence of CKD in individuals who have family members with kidney failure. This is more common among African Americans. A recent study noted a family history of kidney failure in 6.4% of Caucasian participants and 14% of African American participants (Jurkovitz et al. 2002).

Low birth weight—an indicator of an unhealthy fetal environment—has been noted to be a risk factor for chronic diseases in later adulthood (Barker 1995). Low birth weight is also associated with smaller kidney volume and a lower number of nephrons and could predispose to maladaptive changes that initiate and accelerate CKD (Brenner and Mackenzie 1997). In a recent study of records of more than 2 million children born in Norway between 1967 and 2004, births in the lowest decile had an increased risk for kidney failure when compared with other birth weight deciles, with a relative risk of 1.7 (Vikse et al. 2008).

Finally, other risk factors such as elevated levels in serum uric acid and periodontal disease have been noted as risk factors for CKD as well as leading to greater likelihood of progression to ESRD (Obermayr et al. 2008; Shultis et al. 2007).

Geographic Distribution

Since CKD is more common among African Americans and Hispanics than among Caucasians, its geographic distribution tends to be higher in those parts of the country that have a greater proportion of minorities. The prevalence of ESRD is also higher in urban areas than in rural areas and tends to be higher in Southwestern and Midwestern United States (USRDS 2006)

Time Trends

The prevalence of CKD in the United States has grown in recent years. In a recent study, Coresh et al. estimated that 26 million adults in the United States, or 13% of the U.S. population, have CKD, an age-adjusted increase of 3% over previous estimates. This increase is partly explained by the increasing prevalence of diabetes and hypertension (NHANES 1998–1994; NHANES 1999–2004; Coresh et al. 2007). An aging U.S. population and an increase in the proportion of people with obesity are also factors that contribute to the increasing prevalence of CKD.

Causes

Modifiable Risk Factors

As stated previously, diabetes mellitus is the most common cause of CKD (USRDS 2006). Intensive glycemic control can help prevent the development of microalbuminuria, as well as slow the progression of established diabetic nephropathy (UKPDS 1998).

Hypertension is the next most common cause of CKD (USRDS 2006). The presence of inadequately controlled blood pressure in the setting of CKD from any cause has an additive impact on disease progression, and aggressive blood pressure control is recommended for all individuals with CKD, regardless of etiology.

Proteinuria is an independent risk factor for CKD progression. Decreasing proteinuria through the use of drugs that block the renin–angiotensin system (such as angiotensin converting enzyme [ACE] inhibitors and angiotensin receptor blockers [ARBs]) is recommended for all individuals with proteinuric CKD, regardless of blood pressure control. Tobacco use is also associated with the development of proteinuria and more rapid progression of CKD (Orth 2002). Aggressive tobacco cessation programs are recommended to ameliorate this modifiable risk factor.

The utility of dietary changes to slow progression of CKD is unclear. While sodium restriction in hypertensive patients is recommended, the role of protein restriction in those with CKD remains slightly controversial. While animal data suggest a decrease in renal fibrosis with protein restriction, human data have been less clear, and many of these patients already have multiple dietary restrictions to which they must adhere. Despite this, dietary protein restriction (0.6–0.8 g/kg body weight/day) may be advised for the patient with moderately advanced CKD (Fouque and Aparicio 2007).

While animal studies have shown a benefit to lipid lowering on the progression of kidney disease, human studies have not been definitive, as most trials specifically looking at the impact on CKD have been small and inconclusive. However, a recent meta-analysis suggests that lipid-lowering may slow the rate of CKD progression (Fried, Orchard, and Kasiske 2001), and the National Kidney Foundation recommends aggressive lipid control with pharmacologic therapy as needed (KDOQI 2008).

Population-Attributable Risk

The greatest modifiable risk factors for development of CKD are diabetes, hypertension and smoking. In a population based case-control study of white and African American patients with types 1 and 2 diabetes, the overall population-attributable risk for kidney failure was 42% (Perneger et al. 1994). Several large prospective studies (MRFIT and Systolic Hypertension in the Elderly Program) have established that hypertension is an important risk factor for CKD (Pascual et al. 2005; Young et al. 2002). In a prospective study of 23,534 men and women followed for 20 years in Washington County, Maryland, 23% of the CKD cases in this population were attributable to stage 1 hypertension. In addition, this study helped demonstrate the strong link between smoking and CKD, as 31% of cases of CKD in this population were attributed to cigarette smoking (Haroun et al. 2003). Therefore, efforts that successfully target diabetes, high blood pressure and smoking would have the greatest impact on reducing the incidence of CKD in the population.

Prevention and Control

Prevention

Since diabetes mellitus and hypertension together account for greater than 70% of incident ESRD cases in the United States (USRDS 2006), a significant proportion of cases could be prevented through aggressive risk factor modification of these identifiable and controllable diseases. Intensive glycemic control (hemoglobin A1C levels <7%) and blood pressure control (<130/80 mmHg) have been found to slow the development and progression of CKD (KDOQI 2008). Additionally, judicious use of ACE inhibitors or ARB in those with diabetic kidney disease or non-diabetic proteinuric kidney disease can help prevent progression of CKD, even at later stages (Levey et al. 2005).

Other causes of CKD, including genetic (e.g., polycystic kidney disease), immunologic (e.g., lupus nephritis), and urologic (e.g., reflux nephropathy), while modifiable, may be less preventable.

Screening

Who to Screen

While there are no U.S. Preventive Services Task Force recommendations on CKD screening, screening is recommend only for high-risk individuals (Figure 20.1), and not the general population. Mass screening of the general public for CKD is expensive, has a low yield and is not cost-effective. However, targeted screening programs in communities with high-risk populations are effective in detecting previously unidentified persons with CKD. An example of such an approach is the Kidney Early Evaluation Program (KEEP), a free program conducted by the National Kidney Foundation affiliates in the United States. In 135 screening programs conducted in 33 states in over 6,000 persons in 2000–2001, 16% of the participants had CKD. High blood pressure was noted in 47% of the subjects (Brown et al. 2003). In one recent study, the authors concluded limiting screening of CKD to patients with known hypertension, diabetes, aged greater than 55 years or with a family history of CKD would have identified approximately 93% of those with CKD (Hallan et al. 2006). It should be noted that although this study used age 55 years as a cutoff, the generally accepted screening recommendation is that screening should be reserved for individuals aged 60 years and older.

Despite this, in clinical practice the patients at high risk for CKD are not routinely screened. A cross-sectional analysis of laboratory testing in more than 270,000 adult patients in 2003 found that only 19% had serum creatinine measurements (compared with 33% with blood glucose measured, and 71% who had serum lipids assessed). CKD, however, was only identified in 30% of those with serum creatinine measurements (Winkelmayer et al. 2005). This is because the routine determination of estimated glomerular filtration rate (GFR) using the modification of diet in renal disease (MDRD) formula is not in widespread use at the present time in the United States, although this practice is growing.

Physicians are also not routinely aware of the need to consider CKD in patients at increased risk for this condition. In a survey of more than 400 primary care providers, although diabetes and high blood pressure were correctly identified as risk factors for CKD, more than one third did not consider family history of CKD and 22% did not consider African American race to be risk factors (Lea et al. 2006).

While screening for CKD in patients at high risk for this condition is the necessary first step, it is important that adequate subsequent diagnostic procedures and interventions be provided and the patient has access to high quality care (Thomas and Weekes 2007). However, as shown in a recent general practice survey, diabetic patients who have micro-albuminuria are no more likely to receive drugs to block the renin–angiotensin system than those who have urinary albumin excretion in the normal range (Thomas and Weekes 2007). The complex care that must be provided for patients with CKD cannot be over-emphasized (Choudhury and Luna-Salazar 2008). However, the ability of the current U.S. health care system to appropriately manage all of the individuals identified with CKD via effective screening programs remains unclear (McClellan et al. 2003; Thomas et al. 2008).

How to Screen

As CKD is a silent disease, blood and urine tests are necessary for diagnosis. Serum creatinine level alone, a traditionally used blood test, is an inadequate measure of kidney function. Serum creatinine, which is produced from creatine present in the muscle, is normally excreted by the kidney. Therefore, when kidney function declines, serum creatinine levels in the blood increase. As the muscle mass varies in patients differing in age, sex, and ethnicity, a given level of serum creatinine can actually reflect different levels of kidney function in different patients. Timed urine collections to measure creatinine clearance over a 24 hour period have been generally abandoned since they are time consuming, inconvenient and tend to be inaccurate. Formulae to estimate the creatinine clearance such as the Cockcroft–Gault equation are less than adequate in patients with CKD (Shoker et al. 2006; Poggio et al. 2005).

A more sensitive way to assess the kidney function is to estimate the glomerular filtration rate (eGFR) from the serum creatinine level using a formula that takes into consideration the age, sex, and ethnicity of the patient. Currently the four variable modification of diet in renal disease (MDRD) formula for estimating the GFR is used by many clinical laboratories and is reported along with the serum creatinine results (Stevens et al. 2006). CKD is diagnosed in any individual who has an eGFR below 60 mL/min/1.73m^2 for a period of at least three months. Additionally, CKD is diagnosed in patients with any level of eGFR in the presence of structural (e.g., polycystic kidney disease) or functional (e.g., proteinuria or microalbuminuria in a patient with diabetes mellitus) damage that persists for more than 3 months (Stevens et al. 2006).

The MDRD formula performs relatively well in populations that have CKD and mirrors the MDRD cohort from which it was derived. However, there are some limitations of GFR estimates by the MDRD formula that have to be kept in mind. The MDRD formula may be less reliable in persons with normal levels of kidney function, as estimates of GFR by the MDRD method are imprecise at GFR levels greater than 60 mL/min/1.73m^2 and may not represent CKD unless the patient has structural or functional damage to the kidney as noted above (Stevens et al. 2006; Rule et al. 2004). Recently a new equation derived by the CKD Epidemiology Collaboration from a larger and more diverse population (including those with normal kidney function) has been suggested to predict the GFR more accurately, as it reduces the bias at higher levels of kidney function (Levey et al. 2009). Calibration of serum creatinine assays to known standards is crucial to prevent differences in serum creatinine measurements in different laboratories. Isotope dilution mass spectrometry (IDMS) is currently the most appropriate method for serum creatinine assay (Stevens et al. 2007). It must be pointed out that the formula for estimating GFR is unreliable in the hospitalized patient or in the setting of acute kidney injury, when serum creatinine levels can fluctuate daily due to such factors as changes in volume status and disturbances of cardiac function. The measurement of serum cystatin C level holds promise as a possible sensitive measure of kidney function. Its widespread use in clinical practice is, however, limited at the present time due to expense and availability (Shlipak et al. 2006).

In recent years, albumin leakage in the urine (albuminuria) has become a useful tool to detect kidney disease and the increased risk for kidney failure in patients with diabetes mellitus. In a landmark study in 609 Danish patients with diabetes, Mogensen noted that patients with albumin excretion greater than 30 μg/mL in early morning urine specimens had a greater chance of progressive kidney damage with development of overt proteinuria (Mogensen 1984). Healthy persons excrete less than 30 mg of albumin in 24 hours. A 24-hour urine collection is often cumbersome and may actually be inaccurate due to missed collections. Hence, it is recommended that the ratio of albumin to creatinine excreted in a random sample be used to estimate albuminuria (KDOQI 2008). Albuminuria of less than 30 mg/g of creatinine is considered to be in the normal range of albumin excretion and microalbuminuria is defined as albumin excretion of 30 to 300 mg of albumin/g of creatinine. It must be noted, however, that even lower levels of urinary albumin excretion in patients with diabetes may be harmful and may be associated with increased incidence of cardiovascular disease (Danziger 2008). In patients with proteinuria noted by a positive protein test dipstick urinalysis (which usually signifies albuminuria greater than 300 mg/g of creatinine), a protein to creatinine ratio in the random urine sample can be performed to assess the extent of proteinuria (Ginsberg et al. 1983). Combining eGFR and protein-uria may improve prediction of patients with CKD who are likely to progress to kidney failure. In a multivariate analysis of 65,589 adults over a 10.3-year follow-up, Hallan et al. (2009) noted that eGFR and albuminuria were independently and strongly associated with progression to ESRD. Patients with various levels of reduced eGFR and increased albumin excretion in the urine were at increased risk of developing kidney failure with hazard ratios of 6.7 to 65.7.

While the measures to limit progressive kidney damage noted above are important, patients diagnosed with CKD also require regular follow-up and avoidance of exposure to nephrotoxic medications and therapeutic and diagnostic agents, including nonsteroidal anti-inflammatory drugs and iodinated radio-contrast agents used in diagnostic proce-dures (Choudhury and Luna-Salazar 2008). Preventive health measures are underutilized in patients with CKD (Winkelmayer et al. 2002). Preventive goals and treatment strate-gies specific to patients with CKD can differ from those for the general population. Such a move, however, is likely to be useful to decrease the acute morbidity and mortality, in particular the high burden of cardiovascular disease that this population endures (Go et al. 2004).

In summary, the early identification of CKD coupled with an effective intervention and management program to decrease the morbidity and mortality associated with CKD is indeed a worthy goal. However, there are pitfalls in universal screening of all patients for CKD with the laboratory tests available today (Glassock and Winearls 2008; Melamed, Bauer, and Hostetter 2008). At this time it may be prudent to pursue targeted screening of CKD, in subjects at increased risk for this condition (Brown et al. 2003; Grootendorst et al. 2009).

Treatment

Early diagnosis of the patient with CKD is the key to effective management that can pre-vent a progressive decline in kidney function and decrease the patient's cardiovascular mor-bidity and mortality. CKD is further classified into stages depending on the eGFR (Table 20.1). The stages of CKD, referred to as "the roadmap of kidney disease," are useful to improve the management of the patient. In the patient with early stages of CKD a greater emphasis can be placed on diagnosing and managing the conditions causing CKD, while in the patient with advanced stages of CKD, the care shifts to preventing and managing the complications of CKD. An early referral of the patient with advanced CKD to a kidney specialist is recommended to facilitate planning for transition to programs for dialysis and kidney transplantation (Stevens et al. 2006). Despite these guidelines, in the United States, early intervention remains a challenge. A retrospective longitudinal cohort study of over 12,500 older veterans with diabetes found that nearly half the patients had CKD, yet only

Table 20.1. Stages of CKD and Stage-Specific Recommendations for Detection, Evaluation, and Management

Stage of CKD	Description	GFR[a]	Detection, Evaluation, and Management[b]
1	Kidney damage with normal or increased GFR	>90	Diagnosis and treatment Treatment of coexisting conditions Slowing disease progression Cardiovascular disease risk reduction
2	Kidney damage with mild decrease in GFR	60–89	Estimation of progression
3	Moderate decrease in GFR	30–59	Evaluation and treatment of complications
4	Severe decrease in GFR	15–29	Referral to nephrology Consideration for renal replacement therapy
5	Kidney Failure (ESRD)	<15	Renal Replacement therapy

[a]Glomerular Filtration Rate (mL/min/1.73 m^2).
[b]Recommended care at each stage of CKD includes care for less severe stages.

7.2% had a nephrology visit during the 5-year study period. Even among those with stage 4 CKD, only 32% had been seen in the nephrology clinic (Patel et al. 2005).

Numerous studies have shown that effective interventions such as excellent glycemic control in patients with diabetes (UKPDS 1998), aggressive blood pressure control (Ruggenenti et al. 2001), reduction in proteinuria with ACE inhibitors and/or ARBs (Ruggenenti et al. 2001), correction of elevated blood lipids (Fried, Orchard, and Kasiske), and appropriate diet and lifestyle modification (Orth et al. 1998) can prevent kidney disease or delay its progression and decrease its morbidity and mortality rates (Herbert et al. 2001). In a randomized trial of 160 patients with type 2 diabetes and microalbuminuria managed with intensive target-driven treatment (controlling Hemoglobin A1C level to < 6.5%, maintaining normal blood pressure, lowering serum cholesterol to <175 mg%, and using ACE inhibitors and aspirin), Gaede et al. (2008) noted a significant decrease in all-cause mortality and a decrease in cardiovascular events and diabetic nephropathy and retinopathy when compared with the conventional treatment group at 13 years of follow-up.

Hypertension also needs to be closely controlled, as elevated blood pressure is a clear risk for progression of kidney damage in patients with CKD. Clinical guidelines have set target blood pressure values for patients with CKD at less than 130/80 mmHg, with an even lower target of 125/75 mmHg recommended in patients with proteinuria greater than one g/day (Chobanian et al. 2003; KDOQI 2008).

Diurnal variations in blood pressure may play an important role in disease progression in patients with CKD and hypertension. While 24-hour ambulatory blood pressure monitoring can provide a better assessment of the risk for developing kidney failure in these patients (Agarwal and Anderson 2006), clinical use of ambulatory blood pressure monitoring in patients with hypertension is not widespread. Unfortunately, as few as 15% of patients with hypertension in the United States achieve target blood pressure control (Coresh et al. 2001).

Increased urinary albumin or protein excretion is also a risk factor for progression of CKD (Lea et al. 2005). Reduction of proteinuria has been associated with a decreased risk of death and development of ESRD in patients with diabetic as well as nondiabetic CKD (Lea et al. 2005; de Zeeuw et al. 2004). The most common treatments for albuminuria reduction are the use of drugs such as the ACE inhibitors or ARBs. Studies with ARBs in patients with type 2 diabetes have shown that the reduction in albuminuria at 6 months strongly predicted a decrease in adverse renal and cardiovascular outcomes (de Zeeuw et al. 2004). This improvement in outcomes was independent of the blood pressure lowering effects of these medications. African American patients with hypertension, CKD and cardiovascular disease have also been shown to have improved renal and cardiovascular outcomes with a reduction in proteinuria (Ibsen et al. 2005). Reducing albuminuria via treatment with drugs to block the renin–angiotensin system in patients with CKD is recommended even if the blood pressure is at goal (Tuttle 2007).

Experimental studies in animal models of CKD have shown that a decrease in protein intake results in reduced renal fibrosis and a decline in kidney function (Hostetter et al. 1986). Although this beneficial effect in kidney scarring has not been replicated in humans, there is evidence that restriction of dietary protein to 0.6–0.8 g/kg body weight/day in patients with stages 3 and 4 of CKD (eGFR between 60 and 15 ml/min) results in a less rapid decline in the kidney function (Fouque and Aparicio 2007).

There is a lag in the translation of the findings noted in research programs to clinical practice. Hypertension in many persons remains inadequately controlled. Despite treatment, blood pressure control is worse in non-Hispanic blacks and Hispanic persons than in non-Hispanic white persons and among older (ages 70 years and above) versus younger persons (ages 18–40 years) (Ong et al. 2007). In the Kidney Early Evaluation Program screening programs of the patients with hypertension, 64% of patients had inadequate blood pressure control, and only 23% of the patients with a history of diabetes had their blood pressure controlled to JNC 7 recommended level of less than 130/85 mmHg (Brown et al. 2003).

The elevated risk for cardiovascular complications in the patient with CKD is being increasingly recognized (Go et al. 2004). Most patients with CKD do not develop kidney failure requiring dialysis or kidney transplantation, but rather succumb to cardiovascular complications (Berl and Henrich 2006). The importance of including patients with CKD in clinical trials to improve the management of the patient with coexisting cardiovascular disease cannot be minimized.

Examples of Evidence-Based Interventions

Preventive strategies have been shown to preserve kidney function and prevent the development of ESRD and death in affected individuals. However, presently, these preventive programs are not widely used, making CKD a prime example of a chronic health problem that may benefit from a broad based long-term preventive health program. An increase in public awareness of CKD is an essential first step. Only 11.6% of men and 5.6% of women diagnosed with stage 3 CKD reported that they were aware of their decreased kidney function, and even in those with stage 4 CKD, the most advanced stage not yet requiring renal replacement therapy, awareness remained low at only 42% (Coresh et al. 2007). The recent improvement noted in the incidence of patients with ESRD in the USRDS data has been suggested to be due to better secondary prevention of kidney damage with greater glycemic control in patients with diabetes, better blood pressure control and wider use of drugs that block the renin–angiotensin system (Ruggenenti and Remuzzi 2007).

Areas of Future Research

With a high prevalence, an extraordinary cardiovascular disease burden, substantial disparities in affected populations, and extreme associated costs, CKD is a major public health threat (DuBose 2007). The future years are likely to see refinements in the diagnostic tools and in the classification of patients with CKD (Glassock and Winearls 2008). It would be useful to develop tools to better identify those patients with CKD who are at greater risk for developing a progressive decline in kidney function and target them for management programs aimed at preserving kidney function (Tseng et al. 2008). The National Institute of Diabetes and Digestive and Kidney Diseases (NIDDK) has an ongoing study, the Chronic Renal Insufficiency Cohort (CRIC) study. This study has enrolled 4,000 people with reduced kidney function to evaluate traditional and nontraditional risk factors for progression of kidney disease (Feldman et al. 2003). Several genomic studies have been reported that have identified persons at greater risk for developing CKD and also for progression to kidney failure. Recently published reports have shown association between single-nucleotide polymorphism (SNP) in the nonmuscle myosin heavy-chain type II isoform A (*MYH9*) gene on chromosome 22q12 and kidney disease. This association has been suggested to explain much of the increased burden of ESRD in African American individuals (Kao et al 2008; Kopp et al. 2008).

With the growing prevalence of obesity and diabetes in the aging population in the United States, the number of patients with CKD is likely to continue to rise in the future (Felgal et al. 2002). Thus, it is evident that a proactive approach is needed to address the problem of CKD. Diagnosis and management of CKD needs to be a central part of future public health planning in the management of the patient with chronic noncommunicable diseases.

Primary care physicians and other health care providers have an increasingly vital role to play for the patient with CKD, as it is not possible for the number of identified nephrologists to directly manage the ongoing care for the expected increase in the number of patients with CKD. Appropriate guidelines and intervention programs need to be developed and a simplified and streamlined program for management must be devised to include primary care physicians as well as ancillary health care personnel. Pilot clinical programs have shown that such shared care schemes are effective in caring for patients with CKD and effective in preserving kidney function when compared with traditional nephrology-based patient care (Jones et al. 2006). Patient care with multimodal intervention in dedicated remission clinics has been noted to be very effective to prevent progression in CKD patient with proteinuria. In a medial 4-year follow-up of 56 patients with proteinuria of >3 g, Ruggenenti et al. (2008) observed a reduction in monthly GFR of 0.17 mL/min and kidney failure in 3.6% as compared with a monthly decline of 0.56 mL/min and kidney failure in 30.6% in historical control patients.

Public health initiatives with such innovative patient diagnosis and management programs are likely to decrease the suffering, morbidity and mortality in patients with CKD.

Early diagnosis and adequate management of the patient with CKD will also decrease health care expenditures by decreasing the need for dialysis and kidney transplantation. It has been estimated that by decreasing the rate of decline in GFR by 10%, 20% or 30% between 2000 and 2010 the estimated potential cumulative direct health care savings would have been $18.56, $39.02 or $60.61 billion, respectively (Trivedi et al. 2002).

Additional research needs to be done on the detection, management, and, most importantly, prevention of CKD. Interventions directed at the consumer level could include measures to improve the health literacy of the population, empowering patients to be responsible for their own health. Programs in schools focused on healthy living such as avoiding obesity and tobacco use and exposure and ensuring routine health checks for those at high risk for CKD will help people avoid the risk factors for chronic health problems. For the past few years, the International Federation of Kidney Foundations (IFKF) and the International Society of Nephrology (ISN) have worked together to observe the second Thursday of March every year as World Kidney Day. Community activities all over the world have been useful in increasing the awareness of the morbidity of CKD, resulting in efforts to increase its early diagnosis and prevent kidney failure (http://www.worldkidneyday.org). State medical societies, with their experience in preventive programs in infectious diseases, are also beginning to address the problem of CKD (Moorthy and Wegner 2008).

At the provider level, a greater emphasis needs to be placed on prevention of chronic diseases and preservation of health. Many states including New York and Wisconsin have developed programs to improve management of chronic diseases such as diabetes (New York State Department of Health 2009; Wisconsin Department of Health Services 2009). Effective control of diabetes is likely to yield rich dividends in preventing the disabling and often fatal complications of diabetes such as blindness, heart disease and peripheral vascular disease ultimately requiring amputation. Such efforts are also likely to prevent kidney failure in the diabetic patient. Several states such as North Carolina have also set up CKD task forces in an effort to address in a proactive manner the increasing incidence of CKD (North Carolina Institute of Medicine 2009). Such statewide efforts to control chronic noncommunicable diseases are likely to provide long-term benefits to the patient, in addition to decreasing health care expenses.

A greater emphasis also needs to be placed on prevention of chronic diseases in medical school curricula, and by those training allied health personnel. Student clerkships in medical schools should increase the emphasis on continuity of patient care (Hirsh et al. 2007). Public health and preventive medicine programs should include training in development of community-based programs for managing the broad epidemic of chronic disease. On an individual level, the management of the patient with chronic disease requires physicians and other health care workers to have adequate training of how to diagnose chronic diseases early in their course and how to adequately manage protocols that prevent organ damage (Novick and Mays 2001).

Physicians and other health care providers need to stay up to date on new evidence-based measures of integrating chronic disease prevention into their practices. Greater use of web-based resources is likely to be helpful in this endeavor. The increasing utilization of web-based education programs by organizations such as the National Kidney Foundation (http://www.kidney.org/patients/plu/plu_intro/index.cfm) should be useful both to the practicing physician and the patient.

On the health care system level, health maintenance organizations could build in routine screening programs, reminding health care providers to perform routine screenings, and giving them the tools to follow up the results with appropriate care. The growing epidemic of CKD has already resulted in an imbalance between the number of patients with CKD and the number of physicians who are trained specialists in treating kidney disease. One way to relieve the burden of nephrologists would be to ensure adequate training of primary care providers to deliver disease management programs that include additional innovative interventions (e.g., electronic consultation) to manage patients identified with early stages of CKD. In one trial, a primary care–based program was effective in decreasing the referral of patients to kidney specialists by 50% in a 12-month period. The mean decline in the eGFR in 317 patients in various stages of CKD in the 9 months before enrolling in the disease management program was 3.69 mL/min compared with 0.32 mL/min during the 12 months after enrollment (Richards et al. 2008).

Laboratories can greatly contribute to the efficiency of identifying CKD by instituting standard procedures of reporting the eGFR whenever an outpatient serum creatinine is checked, with a simple flag describing the appropriate CKD stage. Urine tests for microalbuminuria should be streamlined and results reported in a standardized manner as mg of albumin/g of creatinine. An improvement in access to health care might be a factor in the management of patients with CKD. While the incidence of CKD is similar in the United States and Norway, a recent report comparing the two countries noted that the progression of the patient to ESRD was three times higher in the United States than in Norway (Hallan et al. 2006). Basic research aimed at understanding the progressive nature of CKD and pathophysiologic processes responsible for tissue damage should be prioritized.

Financial incentives for quality improvement in patient care could be one method to ensure that patients with CKD receive early and appropriate health care. This method has been endorsed by the Institute of Medicine (IOM), which encourages private and public purchasers of heath care to "examine their current payment methods to remove barriers that impede quality improvement and to build stronger incentives for quality enhancement" (IOM 2001). Medical reimbursement systems can be designed to reward quality care for patients with CKD while maintaining appropriate accountability and fairness (Desai, Garber, and Chertow 2007).

Finally, the importance of translational research—applying discoveries generated during research in the laboratory and preclinical studies to studies in human subjects with the disease, and methods aimed at enhancing the adoption of best practices in the community—is now being recognized. Clinical and translational science awards initiated by the National Institutes of Health and development of public–private biomedical research partnerships with the pharmaceutical industry appear to be promising (Zerhouni 2007; Bausell 2006). Clearly, easing the substantial social and economic burden that CKD imposes on both the individual and society will require a multitiered strategy to manage the growing epidemic in the complex population that comprises those with CKD.

Resources

AHRQ National Guideline Clearinghouse, http://www.guideline.gov/summary/summary.aspx?
    doc_id=10828&nbr=5653&ss=6&xl=999.
Kidney Disease: Improving Global Outcomes (KDIGO), http://www.kdigo.org. KDIGO is a
    global non-profit foundation dedicated to improving the care and outcomes of kidney disease
    patients worldwide.

National Diabetes Information Clearinghouse (NDIC), http://diabetes.niddk.nih.gov/dm/pubs/
control.
National Kidney Disease Education Program (NKDEP), http://www.nkdep.nih.gov. The NKDEP
is an initiative of the National Institute of Diabetes and Digestive and Kidney Diseases
(NIDDK), National Institutes of Health (NIH), U.S. Department of Health and Human
Services (DHHS).
National Kidney Foundation, National Kidney Foundation Kidney Disease Outcomes Quality
Initiative (NKF KDOQI), http://www.kidney.org/professionals/KDOQI.
World Kidney Day Website, http://www.worldkidneyday.org.

Suggested Reading

Coresh, J., and J.A. Eustace. Epidemiology of Kidney Disease. In: *Brenner and Rector's The Kidney*
(8th ed.). Philadelphia: Saunders (2008) pp. 615–63.
Menon, V., M.J. Sarnak, and A.S. Levey. Risk Factors and Kidney Disease. In: *Brenner and Rector's
The Kidney* (8th ed.). Philadelphia: Saunders (2008) pp. 633–653.
Hunsicker, L.G. The Consequences and Costs of Chronic Kidney Disease before ESRD. *J Am Soc
Nephrol* (2004):15:1363–1364.
Coresh, J., B.C. Astor, T. Greene, et al. Prevalence of Chronic Kidney Disease and Decreased Kid-
ney Function in the Adult U.S. population. Third National Health and Nutrition Examina-
tion Survey. *Am J Kidney Dis* (2003):41:1–12.
Lei, H.H., T.V. Perneger, M.J. Klag, et al. Familial Aggregation of Renal Disease in a Population-
Based Case-Control Study. *J Am Soc Nephrol* (1998):9:1270–1276.
Freedman, B.I., J.M. Soucie, and W.M. McClellan. Family History of End-Stage Renal Disease
among Incident Dialysis Patients. *J Am Soc Nephrol* (1997):8:1942–1945.

References

Agarwal, R., and M.J. Anderson. Prognostic Importance of Ambulatory Blood Pressure Recordings
in Patients with Chronic Kidney Disease. *Kidney Int* (2006):69:1175–1180.
Barker, D.J. The Fetal and Infant Origins of Disease. *Eur J Clin Invest* (1995):25:457–463.
Barsoum, R.S. Chronic Kidney Disease in the Developing World. *N Engl J Med* (2006):354:997–
999.
Bausell, R.B. Translational Research. *Eval Health Prof* (2006):29:3–6.
Bello, A.K., J. Peters, J. Rigby, A.A. Rahman, and M. El Nahas. Socioeconomic Status and Chronic
Kidney Disese at Presentation to a Renal Service in the United Kingdom. *Clin J Am Soc
Nephrol* (2008):3:1316–1323.
Benabe, J.E., and E.V. Rios. Kidney Disease in the Hispanic Population Facing the Growing Chal-
lenge. *Natl Med Assoc* (2004):96:789–798.
Berl, T., and W. Henrich. Kidney–Heart Interactions: Epidemiology, Pathogenesis and Treatment.
Clin J Am Soc Nephrol (2006):1:8–18.
Brenner, B.M., and H.S. Mackenzie. Nephron Mass as a Risk Factor for Progression of Renal Dis-
ease. *Kidney Int Suppl* (1997):63:S124–S127.
Brown, W.W., R.M. Peters, S.E. Ohmit, et al. Early Detection of Kidney Disease in Commu-
nity Settings: The Kidney Early Evaluation Program (KEEP). *Am J Kidney Dis* (2003):42:
22–35.
Center for Disease Control and Prevention. Prevalence of Chronic Kidney Disease and Associated
Risk Factors—United States, 1999–2004. *MMWR* (2007):56:161–165.
Chen, J., P. Munter, L.L. Hamm, et al. The Metabolic Syndrome and Chronic Kidney Disease in
U.S. Adults. *Ann Intern Med* (2004):140:167–174.

Chobanian, A.V., G.L. Bakris, H.R. Black, et al. Seventh Report of the Joint National Committee on Prevention, Detection, Evaluation and Treatment of High Blood Pressure. *Hypertension* (2003):42:1206–1252.

Choudhury, D., and C. Luna-Salazar. Preventive Health Care in Chronic Kidney Disease and End-Stage Renal Disease. *Nat Clin Prat Nephrol* (2008):4:194–206.

Cooper, M.E. Pathogenesis, Prevention and Treatment of Diabetic Nephropathy. *Lancet* (1998):352:13–19.

Coresh, J., G.L. Wei, G. McQuillan, et al. Prevalence of High Blood Pressure and Elevated Serum Creatinine Level in the United States: Findings Form the Third National Health and Nutritional Examination Survey (1998–1994). *Arch Intern Med* (2001):161:1207–1216.

Coresh, J., E. Selvin, and L.A. Stevens, et al. Prevalence of Chronic Kidney Disease in the United States. *JAMA* (2007):298:2038–2047.

Danziger, J. The Importance of Low-Grade Albuminuria. *Mayo Clin Proc* (2008):83:806–812.

Davey Smith, G., et al. Mortality Differences between Black and White Men in the U.S.A.: Contribution of Income and Other Risk Factors among Men Screened for the MRFIT. MRFIT Research Group. Multiple Risk Factor Intervention Trial. *Lancet* (1998):351:934–939.

Desai, A.A., A.M. Garber, and G.M. Chertow. Rise of Pay for Performance: Implications for Care of People with Chronic Kidney Disease. *Clinc J Am Soc Nephrol* (2007):2:1087–1095.

de Zeeuw, D., G. Remuzzi, H.-H. Parving, et al. Proteinuria a Target for Renoprotection in Patients with Type 2 Diabetic Nephropathy: Lessons from the RENAAL. *Kidney Int* (2004):65:2309–2320.

DuBose, T. D., Jr. Chronic Kidney Disease as a Public Health Threat—New Strategy for a Growing Problem. *J Am Soc Nephrol* (2007):18:1038–1045.

Eknoyan, G., A.S. Levey, N.W. Levin, and W.F. Jeane. The National Epidemic of Chronic Kidney Disease: What We Know and What We Can Do. *Postgrad Med* (2001):110:23–29.

El Nahas, M., R.S. Barsoum, J. Dirks, and G. Remuzzi. *Kidney Disease in the Developing World and Ethnic Minorities.* New York: Informa Healthcare/Taylor and Francis (2005).

Feldman, H.I., L.J. Appel, G.M. Chertow, et al. The Chronic Renal Insufficiency Cohort (CRIC) Study: Design and Methods. *J Am Soc Nephrol* (2003):14(2 Suppl):S148–S153.

Feldman, H.I., L.J. Appel, G.M. Chertow, et al. The Chronic Renal Insufficiency Cohort (CRIC) Study: Design and Methods. *J Am Soc Nephrol* (2003):112:326–328.

Felgal, K.M., M.D. Carrol, C.L. Ogden, and C.L. Johnson. Prevalence and Trends in Obesity among U.S. Adults. *JAMA* (2002):288:1723–1727.

Foley, R.N., P.S. Parfrey, and M.J. Sarnak. Clinical Epidemiology of Cardiovascular Disease in Chronic Renal Disease. *Am J Kidney Dis* (1998):32(3 Suppl):S112–S119.

Fouque, D., and M. Aparicio. Eleven Reasons to Control the Protein Intake in Patients with Chronic Kidney Disease. *Nat Clin Pract Nephrol* (2007):3:383–392.

Fried, L.F., T.J. Orchard, and B.L. Kasiske. For the Lipids and the Renal Disease Progression Meta-Analysis Study Group: Effect of Lipid Reduction on the Progression of Renal Disease: A Meta-Analysis. *Kidney Int* (2001):59(1):260–269.

Gaede, P., H. Lund-Andersen, H.-H. Parving, and O. Pedersen. Effect of a Multifactorial Intervention on Mortality in Type 2 Diabetes. *N Engl J Med* (2008):358:580–589.

Gilbertson, D.T., J. Liu, J.L. Kue, et al. Projecting the Number of Patients with End-Stage Renal Disease in the United States to the Year 2015. *J Am Soc Nephrol* (2005):16:3736–3741.

Ginsberg, J.M., B.S. Chang, R.A. Matarese, and S. Garella. Use of Single Voided Urine Samples to Estimate Quantitative Proteinuria. *N Engl J Med* (1983):309:1543–1546.

Glassock, R.J., and C. Winearls. Screening for CKD with eGFR: Doubts and Dangers. *Clin J Am Soc Nephrol* (2008):3:1563–1568.

Go, A.S., G.M. Chertow, D. Fan, C.E. McCulloch, and C.Y. Shu. Chronic Kidney Disease and Risk of Death, Cardiovascular Events and Hospitalization. *N Engl J Med* (2004):351:1296–1305.

Grootendorst, D.C., K.L. Jager, C. Zocali, and F.W. Dekker. Screening: Why, When and How. *Kidney Interntaional* (2009):76:694–699. doi:10.1038/ki.2009.232.

Hallan, S.I., J. Coresh, B.C. Astor, et al. International Comparison of the Relationship of Chronic Kidney Disease Prevalence and ESRD Risk. *J Am Soc Nephrol* (2006):17:2275–2284.

Hallan, S.I., E. Ritz, S. Lyndersen, S. Romundstad, K. Kvenlid, and S.R. Orth. Combining GFR and Albuminuria to Classify CKD Improves Prediction of ESRD. *J Am Soc Nephrol* (2009):20:1069–1077.

Haroun, M.K., B.G. Jaar, S.C. Hoffman, G.W. Comstock, M.J. Klag, and J. Coresh. Risk Factors for Chronic Kidney Disease: A Prospective Study of 23,534 Men and Women in Washington County, Maryland. *J Am Soc Nephrol* (2003):14:2934–2941.

Herbert, L.A., W.A. Wilmer, M.E. Falkenhain, S.E. Ladson-Wofford, N.S. Nahman, and B.H. Rovin. Renoprotectioon: One or Many Therapies? *Kidney Int* (2001):59:1211–1226.

Hirsh, D., B. Ogur, G.E. Thibault, and M. Cox. "Continuity" as an Organizing Principle for Clinical Education Reform. *N Engl J Med* (2007):356:858–866.

Hostetter, T.H., T.W. Meyer, H.G. Rennke, B.M. Brenner, J.A Noddin, and D.J. Sandstrom. Chronic Effects of Dietary Protein in the Rat with Intact and Reduced Renal Mass. *Kidney Int* (1986):30:509–517.

Ibsen, H., M.H. Olsen, K. Wachtell, et al. Reduction in Albuminuria Translates to Reduction in Cardiovascular Events in Hypertensive Patients: Losartan Intervention for Endpoint Reduction in Hypertension Study. *Hypertension* (2005):45:198–2002.

Institute of Medicine (IOM). Crossing the Quality Chasm: A New Health System for the 21st Century. Washington DC: National Academy Press (2001).

Jones, C., P. Roderick, S. Harris, and M. Rogerson. An Evaluation of a Shared Primary and Secondary Care Nephrology Service for Managing Patients with Moderate to Advanced CKD. *Am J Kidney Dis* (2006):47:103–114.

Jurkovitz, C., H. Franch, D. Shoham, J. Bellenger, and W. McClellan. Family Memebers of Patients Treated with ESRD Have High Rates of Undetected Kidney Disease. *Am J Kidney Dis* (2002):40:1173–1178.

Kalantar-Zadeh, K., C.P. Kovesdy, S.F. Derose, T.B. Horwich, and G.C. Fonarow. Racial and Survival Paradoxes in Chronic Kidney Disease. *Nat Clin Pract Nephrol* (2007):3:493–506.

Kao, W.H., M.J. Klag, L.A. Meono, et al. MYH9 is Associated with Nondiabetic End-Stage Renal Disease in African Americans. *Nat Genet* (2008):40:1185–1192.

Kopp, J.B., M.W. Smith, G.W. Nelson, et al. MYH9 is a Major-Effect Risk Gene for Focal Glomerulosclerosis. *Nat Genet* (2008):40:1175–1184.

Keith, D.S., G.A. Nichols, C.M. Gullion, J.B. Brown, and D.H. Smith. Longitudinal Follow-Up and Outcomes among a Population with Chronic Kidney Disease in a Large Managed Care Organization. *Arch Int Med* (2004):164:659–663.

Kendrick, J., and M.B. Chonchol. Nontraditional Risk Factors for Cardiovascular Disease in Patients with Chronic Kidney Disease. *Nat Clin Pract Nephrol* (2008):4:672–681.

Klag, M.J., P.K. Whelton, B.L. Randall, et al. Blood Pressure and End-Stage Renal Disease in Hypertensive Patients. *N Engl J Med* (1996):334:13–18.

K/DOQI Clinical Practice Guidelines on Hypertension and Antihypertensive Agents in Chronic Kidney Disease. *Am J Kidney Dis* (2004):43(1 Suppl):S1–S290.

Lea, J., T. Greene, L. Herbert, et al. The Relationship between Magnitude of Proteinuria Reduction and End-Stage Renal Disease. *Arch Intern Med* (2005):165:947–953.

Lea, J.P., W.M. McClellan, C. Melcher, E. Gladstone, and T. Hostetter. CKD Risk Factors Reported by Primary Care Physicians: Do Guidelines Make a Difference? *Am J Kidney Dis.* (2006):47:72–77.

Levey, A.S., R. Atkins, J. Coresh, et al. Chronic Kidney Disease as a Global Public Health Problem: Approaches and Initiatives–A Position Statement Form Kidney Disease Improving Global Outcomes. *Kidney Int* (2007):72:247–259.

Levey, A.S., K.U. Eckardt, Y. Tsukamoto, et al. Definition and Classification of Chronic Kidney Disease: A Position Statement from Kidney Disease: Improving Global Outcomes (KDIGO). *Kidney Int* (2005):141:95.

Levey, A.S., L.A. Stevens, C.H. Schmid, et al. A New Equation to Estimate Glomerular Filtration Rate. *Ann Intern Med* (2009):150:604–612.

Lorenzo, C., et al. Prevalence of Hypertension in Hispanic and Non-Hispanic White Populations. *Hypertension* (2002):39:203–208.

Lucove, J., S. Vupputuri, G. Heiss, K. North, and M. Russell. Metabolic Syndrome and the Development of CKD in American Indians: The Strong Heart Study. *Am J Kidney Dis* (2008):51:21–28.

McClellan, W.M., S.P.B. Ramirez, and C. Jurkovitz. Screening for Chronic Kidney Disease: Unresolved Issues. *J Am Soc Nephrol* (2003):14:S81–S87.

McClellan, W., D.G. Warnock, L. McClure, et al. Racial Differences in the Prevalence of Chronic Kidney Disease among Participants in the Prevalence of Chronic Kidney Disease in the Reasons for Geographic and Racial Differences in Stroke (REGARDS) Cohort Study. *J Am Soc Nephrol* (2006):17:1710–1715.

Melamed, M.L., C. Bauer, and T.H. Hostetter. eGFR: Is it Ready for Early Identification of CKD? *Clin J Am Soc Nephrol* (2008):3:1569–1572.

Mogensen, C.E. Microalbuminuria Predicts Clinical Proteinuria in Maturity Onset Diabetes. *N Engl J Med* (1984):310:356–360.

Mokdad, A.H., B.A. Bowman, E.S. Ford, F. Vinicor, J.S. Marks, and J.P. Koplan. The Continuing Epidemics of Obesity and Diabetes in the United States. *JAMA* (2001):286:1195–1200.

Moorthy, A.V., and M.V. Wegner. Chronic Kidney Disease (CKD) in Wisconsin: Time to Address this Public Health Problem. *Wis Med J* (2008):107:16–19.

National Institute of Diabetes and Digestive and Kidney Diseases (NIDDK). US Kidney Failure Stabilizes, Ending a 20-Year Climb. *Troubling Racial Disparities Persist.* Available at http://www.niddk.nih.gov. Accessed June 28, 2009.

New York State Department of Health. *New York State Strategic Plan for the Prevention and Control of Diabetes.* Available at http://www.health.state.ny.us/diseases/conditions/diabetes/strategicplan.htm. Accessed June 30, 2009.

National Health and Nutritional Examination Survey (NHANES). Available at www.nih.gov/news/pr/nov2007/niddk-09.htm. Accessed June 28, 2009.

Norris, K., and A.R. Nissenson. Race, Gender and Socioeconomic Disparities in CKD in the United States. *J Am Soc Nephrol* (2008):19:1261–1270.

North Carolina Institute of Medicine. *Task Force on Chronic Kidney Disease.* Available at http://www.nciom.org/projects/kidney_disease/kidney_disease.html. Accessed June 28, 2009.

Novick, L.F., and G.P. Mays. *Public Health Administration.* Sudbury, MA: Jones and Bartlett (2001).

Obermayr, R.P., C. Temml, G. Gutjahr, M. Knechtelsdorfer, R. Oberbauer, and R. Klauser-Braun. Elevated Uric Acid Increases Risk for Kidney Disease. *J Am Soc Nephrol* (2008):19:2407–2413.

Ong, K.L., B.M.Y. Cheung, Y.B. Man, C.P. Lau, and K.S.L. Lam. Prevalence, Awareness, Treatment and Control of Hypertension among United States Adults 1999–2004. *Hypertension* (2007):49:69–75.

Orth, S.R. Smoking and the Kidney. *J Am Soc Nephrol* (2002):13:1663–1672.

Orth, S., A. Stockmann, C. Condradt, et al. Smoking as a Risk Factor for End-Stage Renal Failure in Men with Primary Renal Disease. *Kidney Int* (1998):54:926–931.

Pascual, J.M., E. Rodilla, C. Gonzales, et al. Long-Term Impact of Systolic Blood Pressure and Glycemia on the Development of Microalbuminuria in Essential Hypertension. *Hypertension* (2005):45:1125–1130.

Patel, U.D., E.W. Young, A.L. Ojo, and R.A. Hayward. CKD Progression and Mortality among Older Persons with Diabetes. *Am J Kidney Dis* (2005):46:406–414.

Peralta, C.A., E. Ziv, R. Katz, et al. African Ancestry, Socioeconomic Status and Kidney Function in Elderly African Americans: A Genetic Admixture Analysis. *J Am Soc Nephrol* (2006):17:3491–3496.

Perkins, B.A., R.G. Nelson, B.E. Ostrander, et al. Detection of Renal Function Decline in Patients with Diabetes and Normal or Elevated GFR by Serial Measurements of Serum Cystatin C Concentration: Results of a 4-Year Follow-Up Study. *J Am Soc Nephrol* (2005):16:1404–1412.

Perneger, T.V., F.L. Brancati, P.K. Whelton, and M.J. Klag. End-Stage Renal Disease Attributable to Diabetes Mellitus. *Ann Intern Med* (1994):121:912–918.

Perry, H.M., Jr., J.P. Miller, J.R. Fornoff, et al. Early Predictors of 15-Year End-Stage Renal Disease in Hypertensive Patients. *Hypertension* (1995):25:587–594.

Poggio, E.D., X. Wang, T. Greene, F. Van Lente, and P.M. Hall. Performance of the Modification of Diet in Renal Disease and the Cockcroft–Gault Equations in the Estimation of GFR in Health and in Chronic Kidney Disease. *J Am Soc Nephrol* (2005):16:459–466.

Pugh, J.A., M.P. Stern, S.M. Haffner, C.W. Eiffer, and M. Zapata. Excess Incidence of Treatment of End-Stage Renal Disease in Mexican Americans. *Am J Epidemiol* (1988):127:135–144.

Pugh, J.A. Diabetic Nephropathy and End-Stage Renal Disease in Mexican Americans. *Blood Purif* (1996):14:286–292.

Raymond, N.R., and G. D'Eramo-Melkus. Non-Insulin Dependent Diabetes and Obesity in the Black and Hispanic Population: Culturally Sensitive Management. *Diabetes Educ* (1993):19:313–317.

Rettig, R.A., K. Norris, and A.R. Nissenson. Chronic Kidney Disease in the United States: A Public Policy Imperative. *Clin J Am Soc Nephrol* (2008):3:1902–1910.

Richards, N., K. Harris, M. Whitfield, et al. Primary Care-Based Disease Management of Chronic Kidney Disease (CKD), Based on Estimated Glomerular Filtration Rate (eGFR) Reporting, Improves Patient Outcomes. *Nephrol Dial Transplant* (2008):23:549–555.

Ruggenenti, P., A. Perna, and G. Remuzzi. ACE Inhibitors to Prevent End-Stage Renal Disease: When to Srart and Why to Never Stop: A Post Hoc Analysis of the REIN Trial Results. *J Am Soc Nephrol* (2001):12:2832–2837.

Ruggenenti, P., E. Perticucci, P. Cravedi, et al. Role of Remission Clinics in the Longitudinal Treatment of CKD. *J Am Soc Nephrol* (2008):19:1213–1224.

Ruggenenti, P., and G. Remuzzi. Kidney Failure Stabilizes After a Two-Decade Increase: Impact on Global (Renal and Cardiovascular) Health. *Clin J Am Soc Nephrol* (2007):146–150.

Rule, A.D., T.S. Larson, E.J. Bergstralh, J.M. Slezak, S.J. Jacobsen, and F.G. Cosio. Using Serum Creatinine to Estimate Glomerular Filtration Rate: Accuracy in Good Health and in Chronic Kidney Disease. *Ann Intern Med* (2004):41(12):929–937.

Sarafidis, P.A., and G.L. Bakris. State of Hypertension Management in the United States: Confluence of Risk Factors and the Prevalence of Resistant Hypertension. *J Clin Hypertens (Greenwich)* (2008):10:130–139.

Shlipak, M.G., L.F. Freid, M. Cushman, et al. Cardiovascular Mortality in Chronic Kidney Disease: Comparison of Traditional and Novel Risk Factors. *JAMA* (2005):293:1737–1745.

Shlipak, M.C., R. Katz, M.J. Sarnac, et al. Cystatin C and Prognosis for Cardiovascular and Kidney Outcomes in the Elderly Persons Without Chronic Kidney Disease. *Ann Intern Med* (2006):145:237–246.

Shoker, A., M.A. Hossain, T. Koru-Sengul, T.L. Raju, and D. Cockcroft. Performance of Creatinine Clearance Equation on the Original Cockcroft–Gault Population. *Clin Nephrol* (2006):66:89–97.

Shultis, W.A., E.J. Weil, H.C. Looker, et al. Effect of Periodontitis on Overt Nephropathy and End-Stage Renal Disease in Type 2 Diabetes. *Diabetes Care* (2007):30:306–311.

Stevens, L.A., J. Coresh, T. Greene, and A.S. Levey. Assessing Kidney Function—Measured and Estimated Glomerular Filtration Rate. *N Engl J Med* (2006):354:2473–2483.

Stevens, L.A., J. Manzi, A.S. Levey, et al. Impact of Creatinine Calibration on Performance of GFR Estimating Equation in a Pooled Individual Patient Database. *Am J Kidney Dis* (2007):50:21–35.

Thomas, M.C., G.C. Veiberti, and P.H. Groop. Screening for Chronic Kidney Disease in Patients with Diabetes: Are We Missing the Point? *Nat Clin Prac Nephrol* (2008):4:2–3.

Thomas, M.C., and A.J. Weekes. *Type 2 Diabetes from the GP's Perspective*. Melbourne Australia: Kidney Health Australia (2007).

Tonelli, M., N. Wiebe, B. Culleton, et al. Chronic Kidney Disease and Mortality Risk: A Systemic Review. *J Am Soc Nephrol* (2006):17:2034–2066.

Trivedi, H.S., M.M. Pang, A. Campbell, and P. Saab. Slowing the Progression of Chronic Renal Failure: Economic Benefits and Patient's Perspectives. *Am J Kidney Dis* (2002):39:721–729.

Tseng, C.L., E.F. Kern, D.R. Miller, et al. Survival Benefits of Nephrologic Care in Patients with Diabetes Mellitus and Chronic Kidney Disease. *Arch Intern Med* (2008):168:55–62.

Tuttle, K.R. Albuminuria Reduction: The Holy Grail for Kidney Protection. *Kidney Int* (2007):72:785–786.

United Kingdom Prospective Diabetes Study (UKPDS) Group. UK Prospective Diabetes Study 33: Intensive Blood Glucose Control with Sulphonylureas or Insulin Compared with Conventional Treatment and Risk of Complications in Patients with Type 2 Diabetes. *Lancet* (1998):352:837–853.

U.S. Renal Data System, USRDS 2006 Annual Data Report: Atlas of End-Stage Renal Disease in the United States, National Institutes of Health, National Institute of Diabetes and Digestive and Kidney Diseases, Bethesda, MD, 2007. *Am J Kidney Dis* (2006):47(1 Suppl).

Vassalotti, J.A., L.A. Stevens, and A.S. Levey. Testing for Chronic Kidney Disease: A Position Statement from the National Kidney Foundation. *Am J Kidney Dis* (2007):50:169–180.

Vikse, B.E., L.M. Irgens, T. Levivestad, S. Hallan, and B.M. Iverson. Low Birth Weight Increases Risk for End-Stage Renal Disease. *J Am Soc Nephrol* (2008):19:151–157.

Wahba, I.M., and R.H. Mak. Obesity and Obesity-Initiated Metabolic Syndrome: Mechanistic Links to Chronic Kidney Disease. *Clin J Am Soc Nephrol* (2007):2:550–562.

Wang, Y., X. Chen, Y. Song, B. Caballero, and L.J. Cheskin. Association between Obesity and Kidney Disease: A Systematic Review and Meta-Analysis. *Kidney Int* (2008):19:1798–1805.

Winkelmayer, W.C., W. Owen, Jr., R.J. Glynn, R. Levin, and J. Avorn. Preventive Health Care Measures Before and After Start of Renal Replacement Therapy. *J Gen Intern Med* (2002): 17:588–595.

Winkelmayer, W.C., S. Schneeweiss, H. Mogun, A.R. Patrick, J. Avorn, and D.H. Solomon. Identification of Individuals with CKD from Medicare Claims Data: A Validation Study. *Am J Kidney Dis* (2005):46:225–232.

Winkelmayer, W.C., S. Schneeweiss, H. Mogun, A.R. Patrick, and D.H. Solomon. Identification of Individuals with CKD from Medicare Claims Data: A Validation Study. *Am J Kidney Dis* (2005):46:225–232.

Wisconsin Department of Health Services. *The Wisconsin Diabetes Prevention and Control Program*. Available at http://dhs.wisconsin.gov/health/diabetes/index.htm. Accessed June 28, 2009.

Young, J.H., H.J. Klag, P. Muntner, et al. Blood Pressure Decline in Kidney Function: Findings from the Systolic Hypertension in the Elderly Program (SHEP). *J Am Soc Nephrol* (2002):13:2776–2782.

Zerhouni, E.A. Translational Research: Moving Discovery to Practice. *Clin Pharmacol Ther* (2007):81:126–128.

INDEX

1% or Less Campaign, 177
5 a Day Power Plus Program (Minnesota), 177–78
5 a Day—Power Play! Campaign (California), 178

A1c, 294
access to healthcare, 12–13
action stage, 65, 214
Active for Life—Increasing Physical Activity Levels in Adults Age 50 and Older, 218
activity dose, 202
administrative data collection systems, 103–4
advertising
food companies, 172, 182
tobacco industry, 130, 133
advertising bans, tobacco industry, 136
Afterschool Snacks, 179
Agency for Healthcare Research and Quality (AHRQ), 526
agriculture policy, and nutrition, 180–81
alcohol dependence, 229, 231–32. *See also* alcohol use
Alcohol Related Disease Impact (ARDI), 250
alcohol use (ICD-10 Z72.1, F10.2), 229, 261
adolescents, 235
as mental disorder, 513, 515
benefits, 230–31
by sex, 236–38, 239
causes, 251–52
cholesterol levels, 368
coronary heart disease (CHD), 393
definitions, lack of, 231–32
descriptive epidemiology, 233–35
genetics, 241–42
geographic distribution, 242–49
homelessness, 240–41
hypertension, 347, 351
intervention examples, 258–59
older Americans, 235–39
oral cancer, 459
pathophysiology, 232–33
personality types, 241
race/ethnicity, 239–40
recommendations, 229
research directions, 259–61
resources, 261–62
screening, 253–55
significance, 229–32
suggested reading, 262
time trends, 249–51
treatment, 255–58
type 2 diabetes and, 302
Alcohol Use Disorders Identification Test (AUDIT), 254
alcohol withdrawal syndrome, 256
alcoholic liver disease (ICD-10 K70–K70.9), 596–99
Alcoholics Anonymous (AA), 256–57
Alzheimer's disease and dementing disorders (ICD-10 G30–G32), 540–42
American Community Survey (ACS), 104
American Legacy Foundation's "truth" media campaign, 135
American Stop Smoking Intervention Study (ASSIST), 441
amyotrophic lateral sclerosis (ALS, ICD-10 G12.2), 546–48
analytic epidemiology, 29, 30, 38–49
ankle-brachial index (ABI), 414
anthrax attacks (2001), 1
antioxidants, 161–62
Apple Project, 278
applied epidemiology, 28
Arizona, tobacco prevention and control program, 140
Arkansas Act 1220, 283
arthritis, costs per employee per year, 73
arthritis and other musculoskeletal diseases (ICD-10 M00-M99), 571–72. *See also* gout; osteoarthritis; osteoporosis; rheumatoid arthritis
ASAM Patient Placement Criteria, 257
asbestosis (ICD-10 J61), 497–98
aspartate aminotransferase (AST), 255
Asperger's syndrome. *See also* autism spectrum disorders
Assertive Community Treatment (ACT), 525
asthma (ICD-10 J45-J46), 473–80
causes, 476–78
costs per employee per year, 73
geographic distribution, 476
high-risk populations, 474–76

asthma (*continued*)
   intervention examples, 479–80
   pathophysiology, 473–74
   prevention, 478–79
   research directions, 480
   screening, 479
   significance, 473
   time trends, 476
   treatment, 479
   See also occupational asthma
atherosclerosis, 385
   and diet, 163
   and tobacco use, 119, 122
   an cholesterol, 363, 364–65, 373–74
   See also cardiovascular disease
Atherosclerosis Risk in Communities (ARIC),
   340, 386, 401
atopy, 473, 476–78
attention-deficit hyperactivity disorder
   (ADHD, ICD-10 F90), 557–58
attributable risk, 47
auras, 532
autism spectrum disorders (ICD-10 F84), 544–46

B readers, 472
back pain. *See* low back pain
behavioral determinants, 60
Behavioral Risk Factor Surveillance System
   (BRFSS), 13, 102, 205, 242
behavioral therapies, and weight loss, 281
Beijing Fangshan cardiovascular prevention
   program (BFCP), 398
Bemidji Cardiovascular Disease Prevention
   Project, 398
benign rolandic epilepsy, 536–37
β-blockers, 353
bias, 44–45
bioethics, 77
biological gradient, 45
BioSense program, 95
bioweapons, concern over, 1
bipolar disorder, 520. *See also* mental disorders
Black Churches Project, 69
black lung disease. *See* coal workers'
   pneumoconiosis
bladder cancer (ICD-10 C67), 458
Bloomberg Initiative to Reduce Tobacco, 17
body mass index (BMI), 269
body weight
   and dairy products, 164
   and fruits and vegetables, 162

breast cancer, 449
   obstructive sleep apnea (OSA), 488
   reduction and diabetes, 280
   reduction and hypertension, 349
   See also obesity and overweight
Bootheel Heart Health Project, 398
Bradford Hill criteria, 45
Brain Attack Surveillance in Corpus Christi
   (BASIC), 401
Breast and Cervical Cancer Mortality Prevention Act (1990), 450
breast cancer (ICD-10 C50)
   and alcohol, 232
   causes, 448–49
   descriptive epidemiology, 447
   estrogen use reduction, 5, 449
   intervention examples, 450
   mortality rates, 37
   pathophysiology, 446–47
   prevention, 449
   research directions, 451
   screening, 449–50
   significance, 446
   treatment, 450
breast-feeding
   and asthma, 477
   and diabetes, 301, 303
   and obesity, 276, 278, 282
brief interventions, 70–71
   on alcoholism, 255
   on tobacco use, 138
built environment
   and low back pain, 560
   and obesity, 61
   and physical inactivity, 209, 212–14
burden of disease, measuring, 32–33
Bush, George H. W., 531
byssinosis (ICD-10 J66.0), 498–99

C-reactive protein (CRP), 391–92, 416
CAGE questionnaire, 253, 254
California, tobacco prevention and control
   program, 139–40
cancer (ICD-10 C00-C97), 429–32
   and alcohol, 232
   and diet, 167
   and dietary fiber, 162
   and red meats, 163–64
   and tobacco use, 123
   causes, 435
   costs per employee per year, 73

pathophysiology, 432–35
prevention, 435–37
resources, 466
suggested reading, 466–67
See also bladder cancer; breast cancer; cervical cancer; colorectal cancer; hepatocellular carcinoma; leukemia; lung cancer;
lymphoma; melanoma of the skin; oral
cancer; prostate cancer
cancer registries, 13, 101–2, 434
Capital Steel and Iron Company cardiovascular
intervention program (CSICIP), 398
carbohydrate-deficient transferrin (CDT), 255
cardiovascular disease (CVD, ICD-10 I20–I25,
I50, I60–I69, I73), 383–84
and diabetes, 292–93, 296, 299–300
and dietary fiber, 162–63
and fruits and vegetables, 161–62
and hypertension, 339
and tobacco use, 119–22
excess weight, 270, 272
pathophysiology, 385
significance, 384–85
See also coronary heart disease; heart failure;
high blood cholesterol; peripheral artery
disease; stroke/cerebrovascular disease
carpal tunnel syndrome (ICD-10 G56.0), 558–59
Cartesian dichotomy, 517
case-control studies, 42
causes of death, 1–2, 3
census data, 104
cerebral palsy (ICD-10 G80–G83), 542–44
cerebrovascular disease (ICD-10 I60-I69). *See*
stroke/cerebrovascular disease
cervical cancer (ICD-10 C53)
causes, 452–53
descriptive epidemiology, 452
intervention examples, 454
pathophysiology, 451–52
prevention, 453
research directions, 454
screening, 453
significance, 451
treatment, 454
cervical intraepithelial neoplasia (CIN), 451–52
channel selection, for media communications,
110–11
chest radiograph, 472, 492
chewing tobacco
time trends, 127
Child and Adult Care Food Programs, 179

Child Nutrition Programs, 173
Children's Food and Beverage Advertising
Initiative, 182
cholesterol. *See* high blood cholesterol
chronic disease
course of, 4–5, 9
definitions, 4–7
Chronic Disease Continuum, 5, 9, 29–31
Chronic Disease Indicators (CDI), 248–49
chronic disease prevention and control
challenges, 13–19
definitions, 8–10
future directions, 21–22
goals, 7–8
integration of programs, 20–21
potential and effectiveness, 10–11
priorities and strategies, 11–12
chronic disease registries, 101–2. *See also*
cancer registries; stroke registries
chronic illnesses, 4
chronic kidney disease (CKD, ICD-10 I12,
N18.0), 623–38
causes, 629–30
geographic distribution, 629
high-risk populations, 627–29
intervention examples, 635–36
pathophysiology, 621–22
prevention, 630
research directions, 636–38
resources, 638
screening, 631–33
significance, 624–27
suggested reading, 636–37
time trends, 629
treatment, 633–35
chronic liver disease (ICD-10 K70-77, E 83,
E 83.1, E 88, B15-19, C22-C22.9), 593–96
causes, 595–96
significance, 593–95
See also hemochromatosis; hepatocellular
carcinoma; nonalcoholic fatty liver
disease; viral liver disease
chronic lung disease, and tobacco use, 123–24
chronic obstructive pulmonary disease (COPD,
ICD-10 J40-J43), 469–70, 480–85
causes, 483
descriptive epidemiology, 481–82
intervention examples, 484–85
pathophysiology, 481
prevention and control, 483–84
significance, 480–81

Chronic Renal Insufficiency Cohort (CRIC)
    study, 636
chronic respiratory diseases (ICD-10 E84,
    G47.3, J40-J47), 469–473
    pathophysiology, 472–73
    resources, 504
    significance, 469–72
    suggested reading, 504–5
    See also asthma; chronic obstructive pulmo-
      nary disease; cystic fibrosis; interstitial
      lung disease; occupational lung diseases;
      sleep apnea
cigar smoking
    significance, 118
    stroke, 404
    time trends, 127
cigarette advertising, 131
cigarette smoking
    and low back pain, 559–60
    and occupational lung diseases, 492
    as an indicator for nationwide surveillance,
      97, 117
    cardiovascular disease, 122
    chronic obstructive pulmonary disease
      (COPD), 483
    significance, 119
    time trends, 127–29
    See also bladder cancer; lung cancer; oral
      cancer
clozapine (Clozaril), 516, 518
clusters, reporting and analysis of, 106–7
coal workers' pneumoconiosis (CWP, ICD-10
    J60-J67), 492–95
colorectal cancer (ICD-10 C18-C21)
    causes, 443–44
    descriptive epidemiology, 443
    intervention examples, 445–46
    pathophysiology, 442
    prevention, 445
    research directions, 446
    screening, 445
    significance, 442
    treatment, 445
Communities Mobilizing for Change on
    Alcohol (CMCA), 259
community-based participatory research
    (CBPR), 75
Community-Based Prevention Marketing
    (CBPM), 84–85
community coalitions, 75–76
confounding, 43

consensus conferences, decision making, 53–54
consequential epidemiology, 28
contemplation stage, 65, 214
Continuing Survey of Food Intakes by
    Individuals (CSFII), 174
contributing causes, 100
control
    and prevention, 9
    meaning of, 30
Coordinated Approach to Child Health
    (CATCH) program, 72
Coors Brewing Company "Lifecheck"
    program, 74
coronary artery disease, 386. See also coronary
    heart disease
coronary heart disease (CHD, ICD-10
    I20–I25)
    and diet, 160, 162, 163
    and Healthy People report, 12
    and physical inactivity, 199–200, 204
    and tobacco use, 117
    calculating incidence rate, 33, 35
    causes, 389–94
    geographic distribution, 387
    high-risk populations, 386–87
    intervention examples, 396–99
    pathophysiology, 386
    prevention, 394–96
    research directions, 399–400
    resources, 418
    screening, 395
    significance, 385–86
    suggested reading, 418
    time trends, 388
    treatment, 395–96
cumulative incidence, 33
cystic fibrosis (CF, ICD-10 E84), 470, 485–87

Da Qing IGT and Diabetes Study, 305
dairy products, 164
Data Resource Center for Child and
    Adolescent Health, 78
DDT residues and breast cancer study, 50
decision making
    assessing a series of studies, 51–52
    expert panels and consensus conferences,
      53–54
    on basis of a single study, 50–51
    risk assessment, 53
    systematic reviews and meta-analysis, 52–53
degenerative diseases, 4

delirium tremens, 256
depression/mental illness
    costs per employee per year, 73
    See also major depressive disorder
descriptive epidemiology, 29, 30, 31–38
detection bias, 46
determinants of chronic disease, 38
    multiplicity of, 60
    See also behavioral determinants;
        environmental determinants; health care
        determinants; social determinants
diabetes (ICD-10 E10–E14), 291–92
    and schizophrenia, 514
    and weight loss, 280
    causes, 301–4
    chronic kidney disease, 623–25, 629
    complications, 303–4
    coronary heart disease (CHD), 392
    descriptive epidemiology, 295–96
    geographic distribution, 298–99
    high-risk groups, 296–97
    intervention examples, 311–16
    nonalcoholic fatty liver disease, 610
    pathophysiology, 293–95
    prevalence, 291–92
    prevention, 304–9
    research directions, 316–19
    resources, 319–20
    screening, 309–10
    significance, 292–93
    stroke, 404
    suggested reading, 320
    time trends, 299–301
    treatment, 310–11
    See also type 2 diabetes
Diabetes Control and Complications Trial
    (DCCT), 310
Diabetes Indicators and Data Sources Internet
    Tool (DIDIT), 313
Diabetes Prevention Program (DPP), 298,
    305–6
Diabetes Prevention Trial (DPT), 305
Diabetes Primary Prevention Initiative (DPPI),
    313
Diabetes Research and Training Centers, 316
DiClemente, Carlo C., 65
diet and nutrition (ICD-10 E40–68), 159–60
    age and life course and, 165
    amyotrophic lateral sclerosis (ALS) and, 548
    breast cancer, 449
    causes of poor nutrition, 168–72

cholesterol, 367–68
chronic kidney disease, 630
    education and, 166
    food price, 169–70, 181
    geographic distribution, 167
    high-risk populations, 165–66
    hypertension and, 351–52
    income and, 166
    industrial development and immigration
        and, 167
    large-scale initiatives, 176–77
    lung cancer, 440
    migraine, 561
    oral cancer, 459
    pathophysiology, 161–65
    policy approaches, 180–82
    primary prevention policy, 172–74
    race and ethnicity and, 165–66
    racial disparity interventions, 180
    research directions, 182–85
    resources, 185–86
    sex and, 165
    significance, 160–61
    site-based interventions, 177–78
    specific population interventions, 178–80
    suggested reading, 185
    surveillance, 174–76
    time trends, 167–68
    type 2 diabetes and, 302
Dietary Approaches to Stop Hypertension
    (DASH), 173–74, 351–52
dietary fat, 163
dietary fiber, 162–63
Dietary Guidelines for Americans, 161, 172–74
dining out, 170–71
diplegia, 543
disability, as consequence of chronic disease,
    17–18
disability-adjusted life-year (DALY), 14
disease latency period, 492
ductal carcinoma in situ (DCIS), 30

emphysema, 470–72, 480–82, 484. *See also*
    chronic obstructive pulmonary disease
employee absence, costs, 73
employee costs to employers, 73–74, 119
environmental determinants, 61
Epidemiologic Catchment Area (ECA) study,
    518
epidemiologic transition, 2
epidemiology, definitions, 27–28

epilepsy (ICD-10 G40–G41), 532–538
  causes, 537
  descriptive epidemiology, 536–37
  prevention and control, 537–38
  significance, 532, 535–36
European Collaborative Trial of Multifactorial
    Prevention of Coronary Heart Disease,
    396
exercise, 201, 202. *See also* physical activity
experimental studies, design, 39–40
expert panels, decision making, 53–54
exposure assessment, 53

failure of success, 5
faith-based organizations
  as venue for intervention, 74
  nutritional interventions, 178
familial adenomatous polyposis (FAP), 442
family-based interventions, 68
"Family Matters" program, 68
farmer's lung, 503
fast-food, 170–71
fast-food establishments, near schools, 171
febrile seizures, 537
fiber. *See* dietary fiber
fibrinogen, 392
Finnish Diabetes Prevention Study, 305–6
"Five As", 138
Florida, tobacco prevention and control
    program, 140
Foege, William, 28
food disappearance data, 174
food frequency questionnaires (FFQs),
    174–75
Food Stamps. *See* Supplemental Nutrition
    Assistance Program
fragile X syndrome, 557–58
Framingham Stroke Profile, 405–6
Fresh Fruit and Vegetable Snack Program, 179
"Friends Can Be Good Medicine" campaign,
    68
Fries model, 5
Fruits & Veggies—More Matters, 176
fruits and vegetables, 161–62
  time trends, 168
Future of Public Health (IOM 1988), 2
Future of the Public's Health in the 21st Century
    (IOM 2003), 3–4, 13

generalized seizures, 532
genomics, 20

gestational diabetes mellitus (GDM)
  high-risk groups, 298
  pathophysiology, 294
  screening, 310
  time trends, 300
Gimme 5 Program (Alabama), 177
Global Alliance for Chronic Diseases, 17
global health, and chronic diseases, 16–22
*Global Strategy on Diet, Physical Activity and
    Health*, 160
gout (ICD-10 M10), 579–80
grain-handlers' disease, 503
Group-Organized YMCA Diabetes Prevention
    Program (GO-YDPP), 308
Guide to Clinical Preventive Services (USDHHS
    1989), 12, 210
Guide to Community Preventive Services
    (CDC), 12, 210
guidelines, for prevention and health
    promotion interventions, 12
Guillain-Barré syndrome (ICD-10 G61.0),
    551–552

haloperidol (Hadol), 517–18
hazard identification, 53
headaches. *See* tension-type headache
Health Belief Model (HBM), 64–65
health care determinants, 60–61
health care systems, as venues for intervention,
    70–71
Health Locus of Control Model, 66–67
health policy, challenges, 15
health promotion, 9–10
health risks, communication of, 15–16. *See also*
    social determinants
health surveys, 102–3
Healthy Eating Index, 176
*Healthy People: The Surgeon General's Report on
    Health Promotion and Disease Prevention*
    (USDHEW 1979), 12
Healthy People 2010, 78, 127, 160, 210–12,
    231, 369
HEALTHY Study, 307
heart disease, costs per employee per year, 73
heart failure (ICD-10 I50.0)
  causes, 411
  descriptive epidemiology, 410
  intervention examples, 414
  pathophysiology, 409–410
  research directions, 414
  significance, 409

Heart to Heart Program, 180
HEDIS® (Healthcare Effectiveness Data and
    Information Set), 103
Helping Patients Who Drink Too Much: A
    Clinician's Guide, 254
hemochromatosis (ICD-10 E83.1), 614–15
hepatitis A (ICD-10 B15), 599–601
hepatitis B (ICD-10 B16, B18.0, B18.1),
    601–5
  causes, 604
  descriptive epidemiology, 602–3
  prevention and control, 604–5
  significance, 602
hepatitis C (ICD-10 B17.1 B18.2),
    605–9
  causes, 608–9
  descriptive epidemiology, 606–8
  prevention and control, 609
  significance, 594, 605–6
hepatocellular carcinoma (ICD-10 C22.0),
    612–14
hereditary nonpolyposis colorectal cancer
    (HNPCC), 442
high blood cholesterol (ICD-10 E78.0–E78.5),
    363
  antioxidants, 373
  causes, 367–68
  children and adolescents, 374–75
  coronary heart disease (CHD), 390–91
  genetic factors, 365
  geographic distribution, 366
  high-risk populations, 366
  hormone replacement therapy (HRT),
    373–74
  intervention examples, 375
  pathophysiology, 363–65
  prevention, 368–69
  research directions, 376
  resources, 376
  screening, 369–70
  significance, 363
  suggested reading, 377
  time trends, 366–67
  treatment, 370–75
high blood pressure (ICD-10 I10-I15), 335–36
  alcohol intake, 347, 351
  causes, 345–48
  chronic kidney disease, 619–20, 626
  coronary heart disease (CHD), 389
  costs per employee per year, 73
  genetic factors, 345

  geographic trends, 344
  high-risk populations, 341–44
  pathophysiology, 336–38
  physical activity, 348, 351
  potassium intake, 347, 350–51
  prevention, 348
    at population level, 355–56
    lifestyle modifications, 349–52
    pharmacological treatment, 352–55
  resources, 356
  salt intake, 346–47, 349–50
  screening, 348–49
  significance, 338–41
  stroke, 403–404
  suggested reading, 356
  time trends, 344–45
high-intensity counseling, 279
high-risk population approaches, 19–20
Hispanic Community Health Study/Study of
    Latinos (HCHS/SOL),
    399–400
Hispanic Health and Nutrition Examination
    Survey, 103
homocysteine, 392
hormone replacement therapy (HRT)
    and Alzheimer's disease, 542
    and high blood cholesterol, 373–74
hospital discharge data, 103
Human Genome Project, 20
Hygeia, 9
hypertension. *See* high blood pressure/
    hypertension

ICD-9-CM 1980 (International Classification
    of Diseases, Ninth Revision, Clinical
    Modification), 103
ICD-10-CM, 103
impaired fasting glucose (IFG)
    high-risk groups, 297–98
    pathophysiology, 294
impaired glucose tolerance (IGT)
    high-risk groups, 297–98
    pathophysiology, 294
inactivity. *See* physical activity
incidence rate, 33
Indian Health Service Diabetes Program,
    315–16
industrialization hypothesis, 519
inequality, and healthcare, 14–15
infant mortality, 1
information bias, 44–45

interpersonal intervention models, 67
 examples, 70
 See also family-based interventions; Social
  Cognitive Theory; social network
  interventions
INTERSALT, 346
interstitial lung disease (ICD-10 J80-J84),
 489–91
intervention, 85
 community-level, 74–77
  planning frameworks, 79–80
   Community-Based Prevention
    Marketing (CBPM), 84–85
   intervention mapping, 82–84
   Mobilizing Action through Planning
    and Partnerships (MAPP), 81–82
   Planned Approach to Community
    Health (PATCH), 76, 81
   PRECEDE-PROCEED framework,
    80–81. *See also* Gimme 5 Program
 interpersonal approaches, 67–70
 intrapersonal approaches, 64–67
 multilevel approaches, 78–79
 organizational-level venues, 70–74
 time required to demonstrate effect, 5
intervention levels, ecological perspective,
 62–64
intervention mapping, 82–84
intervention methods, 59–60
intrapersonal intervention models, 64.
  See also Health Belief Model; Health
  Locus of Control Model; Theory of
  Planned Behavior; Transtheoretical
  Model
ischemic heart disease, 386. *See also* coronary
 heart disease

Joe Camel symbol, 142

Kelloggs. *See* National Cancer Institute/
 Kelloggs Campaign
Keystone Center, 181
Kidney Early Evaluation Program (KEEP),
 631, 635

lay health advisors (LHAs), 69
legal interventions, in health policy, 77–78
leisure-time physical activity, 202
Lennox-Gastaut syndrome, 536
leukemia (ICD-10 C91-C95), 457–58

life expectancy, 1
Lipid Research Clinics Coronary Primary
 Prevention Trial, 396
liver disease, 589. *See also* chronic liver disease
locus of control, 66
Lou Gehrig's disease, 544–46
low back pain (ICD-10 M54.5), 556–57
low-dose aspirin therapy, cost-effectiveness, 11
lung cancer (ICD-10 C33-C34)
 causes, 439–40
 descriptive epidemiology, 438–39
 intervention examples, 441
 mortality rates, 38
 pathophysiology, 438
 prevention, 441
 research directions, 442
 screening, 441
 significance, 438
 treatment, 441
lymphoma (ICD-10 C81-C85), 455–57

mainstream tobacco smoke (MS), 122–23
maintenance stage, 65, 214
major depressive disorder and Parkinson's
 Disease, 536
 descriptive epidemiology, 516–17
 determinants, 518–19
 pathophysiology, 515
 significance, 513–14
 See also mental disorders
mammography, 29
Massachusetts, tobacco prevention and control
 program, 140
mean corpuscular volume (MCV), 255
media advocacy, 76–77
medical care, costs, 3
Medicare
 for preventive services, 61
 patient education billing codes, 61
 spending, 60
 success of, 4
melanoma of the skin (ICD-10 C43), 460–61
mental disorders (ICD-10 F00–F99), 513–26
 alcohol use disorders, 513, 516.
  See also alcohol use
 descriptive epidemiology, 518–19
 determinants, 520–22
 intervention examples, 524–25
 pathophysiology, 517–18
 prevention, 522
 research directions, 525–26

resources, 526–27
screening, 522–23
significance, 513–17
suggested reading, 527
treatment, 523–24
meta-analysis, and decision making, 52–53
metformin, 306, 311
Michigan Alcoholism Screening Test (MAST), 253–54
migraine headaches (ICD-10 G43–G44), 560–61
costs per employee per year, 73
milk, 164
Minnesota Heart Health Program, 375, 396–97
Mobilizing Action through Planning and Partnerships (MAPP), 81–82
modification of diet in renal disease (MDRD) formula, 631–32
Monday morning syndrome. See byssinosis
morbidity compression, 7–8
morbidity data, 13–14
morbidity delay, 7–8
morbidity extension, 7–8
mortality data, collection, 100
motor neuron disease (ICD-10 G12.2), 546–48
MS. See mainstream tobacco smoke; multiple sclerosis
Multiethnic Study of Atherosclerosis (MESA), 399–400
Multilevel Approach to Community Health (MATCH), 398–399
Multiple Risk Factor Intervention Trial (MRFIT), 292, 396
multiple sclerosis (MS, ICD-10 G35), 548–51
musculoskeletal diseases. See arthritis and other musculoskeletal diseases
MyPyramid, 173

National 5 a Day Program, 176–77
National Arthritis Action Plan, 587
National Bone Health Campaign, 587
National Breast and Cervical Cancer Early Detection Program (NBCCEDP), 450
National Cancer Institute/Kelloggs Campaign, 176
National Cancer Institute's Surveillance, Epidemiology, and End Results (SEER) Program, 434
National Coalition for Promoting Physical Activity (NCPPA), 215
National Comorbidity Survey (NCS), 518

National Comorbidity Survey Replication (NCS-R), 518
National Diabetes Prevention and Control Program (NDPCP), 312
National Diabetes Surveillance System (NDSS), 295
National Epidemiologic Survey on Alcohol and Related Conditions (NESARC), 233, 234, 249
National Fruit and Vegetable Program, 176
National Health and Nutrition Examination Survey (NHANES), 102–3, 295
National Health Interview Survey (NHIS), 205
National Health Law Program (NHeLP), 78
National Institute of Diabetes and Digestive and Kidney Diseases (NIDDK), 636
National Longitudinal Alcohol Epidemiologic Survey, 249
National Program of Cancer Registries (NPCR), 101, 434–35
National Registry of Evidence-based Programs, and Practices (NREPP), 526
National Safe Routes to School Task Force, 215
National School Lunch Program (NSLP), 171, 179
National Study of Coal Workers' Pneumoconiosis (NSCWP), 493
National Survey on Drug Use and Health (NSDUH), 233–34
National Tobacco Control Program, 441
National Weight Loss Registry, 282
natural helpers, 69
neurological disorders (ICD-10 F00–F99, G00–G99, M00–M99, S00–T14), 531–32
resources, 561–62
suggested reading, 562
See also Alzheimer's disease and dementing disorders; attention-deficit hyperactivity disorder; autism spectrum disorders; carpal tunnel syndrome; cerebral palsy; epilepsy; Guillain-Barré syndrome; low back pain; migraine headaches; motor neuron disease; multiple sclerosis; Parkinson's disease; spinal cord injuries; tic disorders; traumatic brain injuries
New York Heart Association (NYHA) Functional Classification, 412
New York State Healthy Heart Program, 397
nicotine dependence, and tobacco use, 124
NIH Stroke Scale (NIHSS), 407

nonalcoholic fatty liver disease (ICD-10 K 76.0), 609–12
noncommunicable diseases, 4
normative beliefs, 66
North Carolina Breast Cancer Screening Program, 69
North Karelia Project, 396
Not-On-Tobacco (N-O-T) program, 72
notifiable disease systems, 96–99
nutrition. *See* diet and nutrition
Nutrition and Physical Activity Program to Prevent Obesity and Other Chronic Diseases, 282
Nutrition Fact labels, 181
nutrition safety net, 178–79

obesity and overweight (ICD-10 E66), 1, 8, 19, 269
  and built environment, 61
  asthma, 477
  behavioral determinants, 60
  carpal tunnel syndrome, 558–59
  causes, 275–277
  cholesterol levels, 368
  chronic kidney disease, 627–29
  clinical therapies, 281–82
  coronary heart disease (CHD), 392
  dietary factors, 276
  geographic distribution, 274
  high-risk populations, 273
  hypertension and, 346
  intervention examples, 282–83
  morbidity, 270
  mortality, 271–73
  nonalcoholic fatty liver disease, 609, 611
  of employees, 73
  osteoarthritis, 574–6
  pathophysiology, 272
  prevention, 277–78
  psychosocial outcomes, 269
  research directions, 283–84
  resources, 284–85
  risk factors for chronic disease, 270
  screening, 278–279
  significance, 269–70
  time trends, 274–76
  treatment, 279–280
  weight loss maintenance, 282
  See also body weight
observational studies, design, 40–42
obstructive sleep apnea (OSA), 470–72, 487–89

occupational asthma, 499–502
occupational lung diseases, 491–92. *See also* asbestosis; byssinosis; coal workers' pneumoconiosis; occupational asthma; organic dust-related lung disease; silicosis
omega-3 fatty acids, 163
Online Health Services, 78
oral cancer (ICD-10 C00-C14), 459
oral glucose tolerance test (OGTT), 309, 310
Oregon, tobacco prevention and control program, 140
organic dust-related lung disease (ICD-10 J66), 502–4
orlistat, 281
Oslo Heart Study, 396
osteoarthritis (ICD-10 M15-M19), 573–577
  causes, 574–76
  descriptive epidemiology, 573–74
  pathophysiology, 573
  prevention and control, 576–77
  significance, 573
osteoporosis (ICD-10 M80-M82), 581–588
  causes, 584–85
  geographic distribution, 583–84
  high-risk groups, 582
  intervention examples, 587
  prevention, 586
  research directions, 587–88
  resources, 588
  screening, 586
  significance, 581
  suggested reading, 588
  time trends, 584
  treatment, 587
overweight. *See* obesity and overweight
Oxford Health Alliance, 17

Panacea, 9
Pap test, 452, 453
parental smoking, 132
Parkinson's disease (ICD-10 G20), 538–40
partial seizures, 532
Pawtucket Heart Health Program, 396–97
peripheral artery disease (PAD, ICD-10 I73.9), 383
  causes, 416
  descriptive epidemiology, 415–416
  pathophysiology, 415
  prevention, 417–18
  significance, 414–415

person analyses, 105
pharyngeal cancer (ICD-10 C00-C14), 459
Philip Morris
    "Talk to Your Kids" campaign, 131
    "Think Don't Smoke" campaign, 131
physical activity (ICD-10 Z72.3), 199–218
    breast cancer, 449
    causes, 209–10
    consequences of inactivity, 199–200
    coronary heart disease (CHD), 393
    geographic distribution, 207–8
    high-risk groups, 206–7
    hypertension, 348, 351
    interventions
        environmental and policy factors, 212–14
        examples, 214–16
        prevention, 210–12
    measurement, 216–17
    osteoarthritis, 573
    pathophysiology, 200–204, 582
    recommended activity levels, 199, 206
    research directions, 216–18
    resources, 218–19, 226–27
    stroke, 404–405
    suggested reading, 219–20
    surveillance, 205–6, 216–17
    time trends, 208–9
    type 1 diabetes and, 310
    type 2 diabetes and, 302–3
    weight loss and, 281
physical fitness, 201, 202, 204
pipe smoking
    significance, 119
    stroke, 404
place analyses, 106–7
Planet Health program, 72
Planned Approach to Community Health
    (PATCH), 76, 81
policy, 77
policy analyses, 77–78
population attributable risk, 39, 46–49
population-based approaches, 19–20
PRECEDE-PROCEED framework, 80–81.
    See also Gimme 5 Program
precontemplation stage, 65, 214
preparation stage, 65
President's Council on Physical Fitness and
    Sports (PCPFS), 215–16
President's New Freedom Commission (2001),
    523
prevalence, 33–34

prevention, 252–53
    and control, 7–9
"prevention" media campaigns, 131
primary prevention, 10
primordial prevention. See health promotion
priority populations, as partners for
    interventions, 75
Prochaska, James O., 65
Project Active, 214
Prospective Cardiovascular Munster
    (PROCAM), 393
prostate cancer (ICD-10 C61), 30, 454–55
prostate-specific antigen (PSA) testing, 455
public communications
    health risks, 15–16. See also social
        determinants
    media advocacy, 76–77
    surveillance systems data dissemination,
        108–11
public health
    challenges, 1–4
    mission of, 2

quality-adjusted life-year (QALY), 14
quantitative risk assessment, 53
quasi-experimental studies, 39

Racial and Ethnic Approaches to Community
    Health (REACH) program, 13, 15, 315
racial discrimination, 15
rate difference, 34–35
rates in populations
    calculating, 33–34
    comparing, 34–36
    controlling for differences in age, 36
    small area analyses, 36–38
RCTs (randomized controlled trials), 39
recall bias, 44
recovery from mental disorders, 523–24
red meat, 163–64
regional analyses, 106
registries. See chronic disease registries
relapse stage, 65, 214
relative risk, 34, 42
research dissemination, 14
resilience (mental disorders), 524
respiratory diseases
    and tobacco use, 123–24
    See also chronic respiratory diseases
respiratory disorders, costs per employee per
    year, 73

Reynolds, Thomas, 519
rheumatoid arthritis (ICD-10 M05-06, M08),
    577–79
risk assessment, decision making, 53
risk characterization, 53
risk estimation, 53
risk factors, 4–5, 6
    analyses of, 10–11
risk ratio, 34
R.J. Reynolds Tobacco Company, 142
roadmap of kidney disease, 633
Robert Wood Johnson Foundation, 216

Safe, Accountable, Flexible and Efficient
    Transportation Equity Act (SAFETEA),
    215
SAID principle (Specific Adaptations to
    Imposed Demands), 204
Salud Para Su Corazon community
    intervention, 180
SAMHSA Center for Substance Abuse
    Treatment, 257
saturated fats, 163
"Save Our Sisters" program, 69
schizophrenia
    descriptive epidemiology, 518–19
    determinants, 520–22
    pathophysiology, 517–18
    significance, 513–17
    See also mental disorders
School Breakfast Program, 171, 179
School Foods Report Card, 181
schools
    and physical education, 213
    as venues for intervention, 71–72
    fast-food establishments nearby, 171
    food provision, 171
    nutritional interventions, 177
    screening for excess weight, 279
    tobacco prevention programs, 136
    wellness policies, 181
    See also Afterschool Snacks; National School
        Lunch Program
Screen for Life, National Colorectal Cancer
    Action Campaign, 445–46
SEARCH for Diabetes in Youth Study, 303
SEARCH for Diabetes in Youth Study Group,
    292
secondary prevention, 10
secondhand smoke (SHS), 117
    asthma, 477

cancer, 123
cardiovascular disease, 122
    coronary heart disease (CHD), 389–90
    eliminating exposure to, 136–37
    lung cancer, 439
Selected Metropolitan/Micropolitan Area Risk
    Trends (SMART) project, 205
selection bias, 44
self-efficacy, 67, 214
Senior Farmer's Market Nutrition Program,
    179
Sentinel Event Notification System for
    Occupational Risks, 100
sentinel surveillance, 100–101
Seven Countries Study, 366–67
Shape Up Somerville, 278
silicosis (ICD-10 J62), 495–97
sleep apnea (ICD-10 G47.3), 487–89
    See also obstructive sleep apnea
smokeless tobacco (SLT), 117
    and impact of smoke-free policies, 146
    cancer, 123, 459
    causes
        price, 133
        social norms, 132–33
    geographic distribution, 127
    high-risk groups, 127
    nicotine dependence, 124
    restrictions on tobacco industry marketing,
        142
    significance, 118
    smoke-free policies, 142–43
    See also chewing tobacco; U.S. Smokeless
        Tobacco Company
smoking. See tobacco smoking
Social Cognitive Theory (SCT), 67–68, 214
social determinants, 62
social ecological model of health, 63
social marketing interventions, 183
social network interventions, 68–69
social policy, challenges, 15
societal investment, 8
South Carolina Cardiovascular Disease
    Prevention Project, 398
spasticity, 542–43
Special Diabetes Program for Indians (SDPI),
    316
special populations disparities, 14–15
Special Supplemental Nutrition Program for
    Women, Infants, and Children (WIC),
    173, 178–79

spinal cord injury (ICD-10 S10–S19), 555–56
spirometric testing, 472
Stages of Change Model (Transtheoretical
    Model), 65, 214
Stanford Five City Project, 375, 396–97
Stanford Three Community Study, 180,
    396–97
State Governor's Council on Physical Fitness,
    216
STEPS program, 283
stroke belt, 167, 402
Stroke Belt Elimination Initiative (SBEI), 408
stroke registries, 14
stroke/cerebrovascular disease
    causes, 403–5
    cholesterol and, 364, 366
    descriptive epidemiology, 401–3
    diabetes and, 294–95, 300, 303–4, 309, 317
    diet and, 163, 167
    hormone replacement therapy (HRT) and,
        374
    hypertension and, 335–36, 338–41, 348,
        353–55
    intervention examples, 408
    obesity and, 271
    pathophysiology, 400–401
    physical activity and, 203
    prevention, 405–407
    research directions, 408–409
    screening, 407
    significance, 400
    tobacco use and, 118
    treatment, 407–8
Studies to Treat or Prevent Pediatric Type 2
    Diabetes (STOPP T2D), 307
study design
    evaluating validity of results, 43–45
    evaluating whether associations are causal,
        45–46
    forecasting intervention results, 46–49
    measuring associations between exposures
        and outcomes, 42–43
    types, 39–42
subjective norm, 66
Substance Abuse Treatment Facility Locator,
    257
sudden unexplained death in epilepsy
    (SUDEP), 536–37
sugar-sweetened beverages, 164–65
Supplemental Nutrition Assistance Program
    (SNAP), 173, 179

Supplemental Nutrition Assistance Program
    nutrition education (SNAP-Ed), 179
Surveillance Brief, 110
Surveillance, Epidemiology, and End Results
    program, 101
surveillance systems, 13–14, 95–96, 111–12
    analysis and interpretation, 104–8
    data sources, 96–104
    information dissemination, 108–11
    resources, 112
    See also Behavioral Risk Factor Surveillance
        System; National Diabetes Surveillance
        System; Youth Risk Behavior Surveillance
        System
systematic reviews, and decision making,
    52–53

television, children and diet, 172
tension-type headache (ICD-10 G43–G44),
    560–61. See also migraine headaches
termination stage, 65
tertiary prevention, 10
Theory of Planned Behavior (TPB), 65–66
tic disorders (ICD-10 F95), 552–54
time analyses, 107
tobacco industry advertising, 130, 133
    advertising bans, 136
tobacco smoking, 60
    cancer, 122–23
    cessation counseling, cost-effectiveness, 11
    chronic obstructive pulmonary disease
        (COPD), 482
    diabetes and, 303
    employee costs to employers, 119
    geographic distribution, 127
    high-risk groups, 124–27
    in movies, 131
    major depressive disorder, 521
    nicotine dependence, 124, 133
    obstructive sleep apnea (OSA), 488
    peripheral artery disease, 415
    stroke, 404
    See also cigar smoking; cigarette smoking;
        pipe smoking; secondhand smoke;
        smokeless tobacco
tobacco use (ICD-10 F17), 31, 117
    causes, 129–30
        inadequate understanding, 132, 134
        individual psychosocial factors, 133, 134
        population-attributable risk, 134
        price sensitivity, 134

tobacco use (*continued*)
  ready access to cigarettes, 132
  "safer" products, 132, 133
  smoking in adulthood, 133–34
  smoking in youth, 130–33
  social norms, 132–33
  societal factors, 130, 133
  tobacco industry advertising, 130, 133
  coronary heart disease (CHD), 389
  geographic distribution, 127
  high-risk groups, 124–27
  intervention examples
    comprehensive tobacco prevention and
      control programs, 139–41, 144–45
    countermarketing campaigns and
      restrictions on tobacco industry
      marketing, 141–42
    improving insurance coverage of
      tobacco-use treatment, 143
    minors' access restrictions, 143–44
    smoke-free policies, 142–43
    telephone cessation quitlines, 144
    tobacco excise taxes, 141
  interventions, 134–35
    advertising bans, 136
    countermarketing campaigns, 135–36
    eliminating exposure to SHS, 136–37
    individual cessation interventions, 138–39
    minors' access restrictions, 136, 143–44
    price, 135
    reducing out-of-pocket costs of treatment,
      137–38
    school-based tobacco prevention
      programs, 136
    screening, 137
    telephone cessation quitlines, 138, 144
  pathophysiology, 119–24
  research directions, 145–47
  resources, 147
  significance, 117–19
  suggested reading, 147–48
  time trends, 127–29
  See also tobacco smoking
Tourette syndrome, 552–54
Traffic Light Diet, 280
training issues, 18–19
trans fats, 163, 368
Translating of Research Into Action for
  Diabetes (TRIAD Study), 313
Transportation Equity Act for the 21st
  Century (TEA-21), 215

Transtheoretical Model (Stages of Change
  Model), 65, 214
traumatic brain injuries (ICD-10 S00–S09),
  554–55
Trial to Reduce IDDM in the Genetically at
  Risk (TRIGR), 305
Trials of Hypertension Prevention (TOHP),
  349
type 1 diabetes, 291
  causes, 301
  descriptive epidemiology, 295–96
  geographic distribution, 298–99
  prevention, 304–5
  screening, 309
  smoking and, 303
  time trends, 299
  treatment, 310
type 2 diabetes, 291
  causes, 302–3
  descriptive epidemiology, 295
  dietary fiber and, 162–163
  excess weight and, 270, 273, 291, 302
  pathophysiology, 293–94
  prevention, 305–8
  screening, 309
  smoking and, 303
  treatment, 310–11

underlying cause of death, 100
United Kingdom Prospective Diabetes Study
  Group (UKPDS), 414
U.S. Black Lung compensation program, 493
U.S. health care system
  cost and access, 12–13
  relative performance, 2–3
U.S. Smokeless Tobacco Company
  advertising in youth-oriented magazines,
    131
U.S.–Mexico Border Diabetes Prevention and
  Control Project, 314

vegetables, 161–62
  time trends, 168
viral liver disease, 599. *See also* hepatitis A;
  hepatitis B; hepatitis C
vital statistics, 97–100

Well-Integrated Screening and Evaluation for
  Women Across the Nation
  (WISEWOMAN), 408

What We Eat in America (WWEIA), 174
Who Will Keep the Public Healthy? Educating Public Health Professionals for the 21st Century (IOM 2002), 18–19
WIC Farmers' Market Nutrition Program, 179
Wilson's disease, 614
Wisconsin Collaborative Diabetes Quality Improvement Project, 103–4
Women' Health Initiative, 39, 405
Women's Estrogen for Stroke Trial (WEST), 405
workforce issues, 18–19
Working Well Trial, 171
workplaces
    and Parkinson's Disease, 539
    as venue for intervention, 72–74. *See also*

Capital Steel and Iron Company cardiovascular intervention program (CSICIP)
    carpal tunnel syndrome, 559
    food provision, 171
    lung cancer, 439–40
    nutritional interventions, 177
    physical activity promotion, 215
    See also occupational lung diseases
World Kidney Day, 637

Youth Media Campaign Longitudinal Survey (YMCLS), 206, 207
Youth Risk Behavior Surveillance System, 102
Youth Risk Behavior Survey (YRBS), 205